Management

and Supervisory

Principles for Physical

Therapists

Third Edition

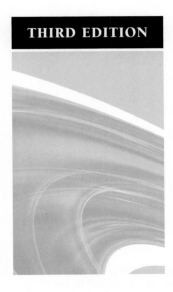

THIRD EDITION

Management and Supervisory Principles for Physical Therapists

Third Edition

Editors and Authors

Larry J. Nosse, MAPT, PhD
President, LJN Therapy, SC
Wauwatosa, WI
Vice Chair
Wisconsin Physical Therapists Affiliated
  Credentialing Board
Former Associate Professor
Department of Physical Therapy
Marquette University
Milwaukee, WI

Deborah G. Friberg, BSPT, MBA
Executive Vice President and Chief
  Operating Officer
WakeMed Health and Hospitals
Raleigh, NC

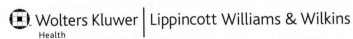

Wolters Kluwer | Lippincott Williams & Wilkins
Health
Philadelphia · Baltimore · New York · London
Buenos Aires · Hong Kong · Sydney · Tokyo

Acquisitions Editor: Emily Lupash
Production Editor: Debra Schiff
Managing Editor: Meredith Brittain
Designer: Stephen Druding
Marketing Manager: Allison Noplock
Compositor: Spearhead Inc.

Third Edition

351 West Camden Street   530 Walnut Street
Baltimore, MD 21201   Philadelphia, PA 19106

Printed in China

9 8 7 6 5 4 3 2 1

Library of Congress Cataloging-in-Publication Data

Nosse, Larry J.
   Management and supervisory principles for physical therapists / Larry J. Nosse, Deborah G. Friberg. — 3rd ed.
     p. ; cm.
   Rev. ed. of: Managerial and supervisory principles for physical therapists / Larry J. Nosse, Deborah G. Friberg, Peter R. Kovacek. 2nd ed. c2005.
   Includes bibliographical references and indexes.
   ISBN 978-0-7817-8132-9
   1. Physical therapy—Practice. 2. Physical therapy—Management. I. Friberg, Deborah G. II. Nosse, Larry J. Managerial and supervisory principles for physical therapists. III. Title.
   [DNLM: 1. Physical Therapy (Specialty)—United States. 2. Practice Management, Medical—economics—United States. 3. Practice Management, Medical—organization & administration—United States. WB 460 N897mb 2010]
   RM713.N674 2010
   615.8′2068—dc22

                                                                            2008051574

DISCLAIMER

Care has been taken to confirm the accuracy of the information present and to describe generally accepted practices. However, the authors, editors, and publisher are not responsible for errors or omissions or for any consequences from application of the information in this book and make no warranty, expressed or implied, with respect to the currency, completeness, or accuracy of the contents of the publication. Application of this information in a particular situation remains the professional responsibility of the practitioner; the clinical treatments described and recommended may not be considered absolute and universal recommendations.

The authors, editors, and publisher have exerted every effort to ensure that drug selection and dosage set forth in this text are in accordance with the current recommendations and practice at the time of publication. However, in view of ongoing research, changes in government regulations, and the constant flow of information relating to drug therapy and drug reactions, the reader is urged to check the package insert for each drug for any change in indications and dosage and for added warnings and precautions. This is particularly important when the recommended agent is a new or infrequently employed drug.

Some drugs and medical devices presented in this publication have Food and Drug Administration (FDA) clearance for limited use in restricted research settings. It is the responsibility of the health care provider to ascertain the FDA status of each drug or device planned for use in their clinical practice.

To purchase additional copies of this book, call our customer service department at **(800) 638-3030** or fax orders to **(301) 223-2320.** International customers should call **(301) 223-2300.**

Visit Lippincott Williams & Wilkins on the Internet: **http://www.lww.com.** Lippincott Williams & Wilkins customer service representatives are available from 8:30 am to 6:00 pm, EST.

PREFACE TO THE THIRD EDITION

What's the Same

Those familiar with the previous edition will find that we have retained its general format. The book is broken into parts, with each part containing related chapters in a logical sequence. The chapter format is also very similar to that used in the prior edition. As before, there is sufficient review of information and cross-referencing of core information in each chapter to allow flexibility in selecting which chapters to read and in which order.

What's New

Contributing Authors

The authors have been very fortunate to have been able to incorporate the thoughts of six very knowledgeable contributors in this third edition. Our collaboration brought about new ideas about how to deepen and organize the content and about which topics to emphasize. In their respective chapters, the contributing authors started with the core material from the second edition and then added their perspectives and expert knowledge. The result is the extensive reorganization of some content from the earlier edition and the incorporation of new material into each chapter.

Organizational Philosophy

Compared to the prior edition, this edition has fewer parts and fewer chapters, but each topic is covered in greater depth and principles are better integrated. The addition of new material led to a redistribution of topics within each part of the book, which resulted in the following topical progression:

- Part I, Broad Perspectives on Providing Health Services, covers essential health service business and legislative background information. This background consists of an overview of international health service systems compared to the U.S. system and an introduction to the U.S. health care industry, with special consideration given to physical therapy as a subsector of this industry.
- Part II, Guiding Behavior: Values, Ethics, Jurisprudence, and Oversight Agencies, introduces management-focused information with emphasis on guiding individual and organizational behaviors. The discussion includes organizational values, ethics, administrative law (licensure), business law principles, governmental and nongovernmental oversight agencies and organizations, and risk management. The information is applied in the context of physical therapy.
- Part III, Business Acumen: Managing, Communicating, Strategizing, Planning, and Decision Making, presents seven practical "how-to" management concepts. The discussion covers principles of leadership, management, communication, strategic planning, organizational design, decision making, and performance improvement. Chapter 16 emphasizes governmental and nongovernmental quality care oversight groups that are of particular interest to physical therapist employees and managers.
- Part IV: Business Acumen: Human Resources, Marketing, and Selling, deals with management knowledge and skills every manager needs. The chapters in this section analyze interactions with job applicants, employees, peers, and customers and offers practical suggestions for meeting common management challenges.

- Part V, Business Acumen: Financial Awareness, deals with money matters. Fundamental economic and accounting principles, physical therapist practice ownership, and personal financial management are the focus of these chapters.

Features

Chapter organization has been retained from the previous edition, as each chapter includes learning objectives, introduction, a summary, and references. The following features have been added or updated for the third edition:

Key Terms

To help the reader develop their business vocabulary, selected key terms appear in bold italics and are defined in the Key Terms section at the beginning of each chapter. The abbreviated forms of some terms are commonly used by managers, so these are included in the Key Terms section and are used throughout. Building a vocabulary takes repetition. Seeing important terms several times, therefore, is a planned learning strategy.

Other important terms are shown in boldface at first instance and are defined by the context in which they are used. There are also terms that are important for integrating concepts covered in other chapters. These important terms are also bolded, but they are defined in the Key Terms section of the chapter where the term is more essential to the discussion. All bolded terms are also defined in the Glossary (on the book's companion website; see "Online Resources").

Additional Resources

At the end of each chapter you will find a list of print and online resources that will add to the understanding of the information presented in the chapter. These resources supplement the cited and referenced sources. Additional resources that are available free of charge are emphasized.

Case Studies

Case studies allow readers to apply the principles emphasized in that particular chapter.

The 42 cases presented help readers to gain skill in dealing with practical physical therapy business and management challenges. The cases can be approached by individuals or groups, in person or online.

Two additional types of case studies are available on this book's companion website (see "Online Resources"). Through the three types of engagement activities (chapter cases, ongoing scenarios [online], and forum role-play [online]), entry level and, transitional Doctor of Physical Therapy students as well as practicing clinicians all have challenging opportunities to apply the principles of leadership, management, and supervision in a physical therapy context. To some extent, the various case studies are scaled in difficulty. The chapter cases are more dependent on the material contained in the related chapter than on practice experience. Solutions to Ongoing Integrated Scenarios and Role Plays (online) are enriched by having at least some time in clinical settings. Manager Forum Scenarios and Role Plays (online) are more suited to experienced physical therapists and first-level physical therapist managers.

Online Resources

Managerial and Supervisory Principles for Physical Therapists, Third Edition, includes additional online resources for both instructors and students that are available on the book's companion website (http://thePoint. lww.com/Nosse3e):

- **Glossary:** An alphabetized glossary of all the terms that are in bold type in the text. Many of the definitions have been expanded in order to provide more complete information than was practical in the chapter discussions. The terms are cross-referenced within the glossary to facilitate integrating related business and management principles. Putting the glossary online allows the reader to quickly access multiple terms using the MS Word Find function. This strategy can also be used by faculty to develop test questions.
- **Ongoing Integrated Scenarios and Role-Play:** These provide a running scenario of the professional and personal challenges, decisions, and accomplishments of a group of physical therapists over time. The man-

agement problems encountered in the situations can be solved as an individual reader or by a collaborating group of readers. These integrated case studies involve application of knowledge and skills gained from more than one chapter of the text.

- **Manager Forum Scenarios and Role-Play:** These features use a manager's forum format with twelve participating managers. The management and personal characteristics of each manager are provided to encourage role-playing, e.g., a group member taking on the character of the manager and playing the part in the scenario. To foster managerial thinking, problem solving, creativity, and so on, role players write some of the script for their character and interact with the group while in character. Assessment forms to score individual and group role-play performances are also included. These integrated case studies involve application of knowledge and skills gained from more than one chapter of the text.
- **Comprehensive Review:** This feature helps to determine the extent of knowledge acquired from this book and how well it can be applied by the reader. The review contains self-assessment questions in various formats. The variety of formats as well as the questions require various levels of cognitive processing. The most superficial cognitive processing (remembering knowledge) is likely to be tested in true-false questions or when an answer is a fact. The deepest level of cognitive processing (creating knowledge [synthesis]) is likely to be invoked when a unique solution or analysis is required in a short essay answer. (A cautionary note is that the online questions reflect the emphasis given in the author's courses. Also, the addition of new information in the textbook necessitated developing many new questions. These new questions have not yet been examined for their reliability, validity, and relative degree of difficulty. Nonetheless, recognizing that a question is not as clear as it might be or, given your experience, that the differences between answer choices are too fine to

confidently make a choice, are both good things. These realizations represent some level of understanding [at least remembering], judgment [application, analysis, or evaluation], and an opportunity to improve the question [creation].)

Instructor Resources

Approved adopting instructors will be given access to the following additional resources:

- PowerPoint presentations
- Image bank

In addition, purchasers of the text can access the searchable full text online by going to the *Managerial and Supervisory Principles for Physical Therapists, Third Edition* website at http://thePoint.lww.com/Nosse3e. See inside the front cover of this book for more details, including the passcode you will need to gain access to the website.

Acknowledgments

To prepare a manuscript of more than a thousand pages requires a great deal of attention to details such as formatting, editing, correcting, and rereading multiple drafts. The authors are indebted to Michael Schilke for his diligence in carrying out these tasks. Michael has 33 years of professional cataloging experience at Marquette University's Raynor Memorial Libraries in Milwaukee, Wisconsin. We thank Michael for his dedication to making our effort a better product for you.

For the second time, the services of Anne Seitz of Hearthside Publishing were invalueable. The organization of the book is an intermingling of her ideas with our own. Her straightforward direction, answers, and wonderfully creative suggestions contributed greatly to what we believe to be our best work to date. It is appropriate that final acknowledgement goes to Molly Morrison of Spearhead. Her timely and diligent efforts contributed to getting this book ready for printing as error free as possible.

CONSULTANT AND CONTRIBUTORS

Subject Matter Consultant

Peter R. Kovacek, BSPT, MSA
President and Chief Executive Officer
Kovacek Management Services, Inc.
Harper Woods, MI

Contributors

Mark Drnach, BSPT, DPT, MBA, PCS
Clinical Assistant Professor
Wheeling Jesuit University
Wheeling, WV
Physical Therapy Pediatric Specialist in OH, PA,
  and WV

Deborah G. Friberg, BSPT, MBA
Executive Vice President and Chief Operating
  Officer
WakeMed Health and Hospitals
Raleigh, NC

Cheryl LaFollette, BSPT, MBA, PhD, GCS
Consultant
Alexandria, MN
Adjunct Faculty
College of St. Scholastica, Duluth, MN;
  University of Phoenix, Phoenix AZ;
  Walden University, Capella University, and
  Globe University, Minneapolis, MN

D. Kathleen Lewis, MAPT, JD
Editorial Board Member: Aon Risk Advisor,
  Physical Therapy magazine, Novicom,
PT Products, and RN Publishing Group
Formerly, Associate Professor
Department of Physical Therapy
Wichita State University
Wichita, KA

John (Jack) R. Nelson, MBA, CFP
District Sales Manager
Harris Investor Services
Mequon, WI

Larry J. Nosse, MAPT, PhD
President, LJN Therapy, SC
Wauwatosa, WI
Vice Chair
Wisconsin Physical Therapists Affiliated
  Credentialing Board
Former Associate Professor
Department of Physical Therapy
Marquette University
Milwaukee, WI

Donald Olsen, MMSc, EdD, OCS
Owner, Homestead Physical Therapy
Cedarburg, WI
North Shore Physical Therapy and Wisconsin
  Orthopedic Rehabilitation Consultants
Milwaukee, WI
Physical Therapy of Sanibel
Sanibel, FL
Founder and Board Member
Midwest Rehabilitation Network, Inc.
Milwaukee, WI

Cheryl Resnik, MSHCM, DPT
Assistant Professor of Clinical Physical Therapy
Director of Community Outreach
Division of Biokinesiology and Physical Therapy
University of Southern California
President, California Chapter of the American
  Physical Therapy Association
Los Angeles, CA

CONTENTS

Social Philosophy and Health Service Systems, Public Policy, Legislation, and Advocacy

LARRY J. NOSSE AND DEBORAH G. FRIBERG

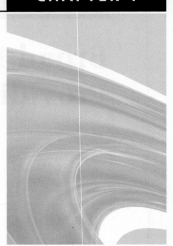

Learning Objectives

1. Begin to develop a professional vocabulary that includes recognition of the names and abbreviations of international and national health service–related government agencies, private organizations, and professional associations relevant to physical therapists and physical therapist assistants.
2. Explain how United States (U.S.) immigration and migration policy relates to health services.
3. In your own words define social philosophy, health service policy, and the core elements of a health service system.
4. Analyze the major elements of social philosophy and public policy related to health services in selected European Union (E.U.) member countries, Canada, and the United States.
5. Use the criteria of control, access, costs, and funding to compare the health service systems of selected European Union member countries, Canada, and the United States.
6. Draw supportable conclusions about the health service systems noted above in terms of benefits and deficits from the point of view of consumers, physical therapists, physical therapist assistants, health service managers, taxpayers, and other interested parties.
7. Evaluate selected examples of U.S. health services legislation in terms of who they affect, e.g., consumers, physical therapists, physical therapist assistants, health service businesses, and so on.

8. Create a personal plan to advocate for health service legislation that is compatible with your beliefs.

Introduction

The purpose of this chapter is to explore the major differences between **health service systems** around the world and the impact those differences have on the delivery of health services to the citizens served. The term **health service** is used broadly as a designation for any activity related, directly or indirectly, to the delivery of health services. This would include planning, financing, delivering, measuring, and analyzing physical and mental health services, and the development and provision of health-related products. A **system** is the integration of a number of interrelated parts, sometimes centrally controlled, that function in concert. A system is something greater than the sum of its individual parts (Shelton, 2000). Some experts even question whether or not the *U.S. health service system* meets the definition of a system due to the lack of a controlling entity to integrate the individual government and private parts (Kronenfeld and Kronenfeld, 2004; Shi and Singh, 2004). System or not, there is general agreement that the U.S. mode of health service delivery is over-due for significant changes. Unfortunately, there is no consensus on what to change or how to change it (Boufford and Lee, 2001; Matcha, 2003; Shi and Singh, 2004;

Key Terms

Note: Key terms are bolded and italicized the first time they appear in a chapter. Other important terms are shown in boldface on first appearance and are defined by the context in which they are used. When either of these types of terms is used several times, its acronym will be identified and subsequently used in the chapter. Both types of terms are listed alphabetically in the online glossary with their definitions and (when applicable) their acronyms.

advocacy/advocating: active support of a cause.

Canada Health Act (CHA): enacted in 1984. It is the governing federal legislation for Canada's Medicare program. The act stipulates the criteria that the provinces and territories must meet in order to qualify for federal funding for publicly insured core health services.

Canadian Medicare: the Canadian single-payer, universal access health service system that covers core services for all citizens of Canada's ten provinces and three territories.

Canadian welfare health service system: the Canadian universal access health service system run by the federal and provincial/territorial government.

comprehensive health service system: a health service system that is publicly funded, universally available to citizens at little or no cost, and offers a complete range of health services. The health care system of the United Kingdom (U.K.).

cost-benefit: measurement of the relationship between costs and benefits.

entrepreneurial health service system: the two-part health service system of the United States, which provides some health services for more than 80% of the population. One part is the large for-profit and not-for-profit private component funded by private insurance, personal resources, philanthropy, and charity and the other part is the smaller government component covering categories of needy citizens and funded through payroll taxes and federal and state general revenues.

European Union (E.U.): a supranational multilevel form of governance with 27 independent and sovereign nation members formed to deal with political, economic, and social matters in a democratic manner to propel E.U. member countries to achieve greater strength and world influence than any single member country could aspire to independently.

gatekeeper: a general practitioner, primary care physician, or family practice physician who has the initial contact with a patient and determines if a referral to a specialist is needed. Physical therapists are among the specialists.

gross domestic product (GDP): the total market value of all services and goods produced in a country in a given month or year. It is the broadest indicator of economic output and growth, therefore it is the most common indicator of a country's economic well-being.

National Health System (NHS): the name of the health service delivery system of the U.K. About 80% of the NHS budget is managed by local primary care trusts to assure community needs are met. Primary care trusts report to local strategic health authorities, which are the administrative centers of the NHS.

Organization for Economic Cooperation and Development (OECD): a unique forum where the governments of 30 market democracies work together to address the economic, social, and governing challenges of globalization as well as to exploit its opportunities.

Pan American Health Organization (PAHO): an international public health agency that is the part of the United Nations working to improve the health and living standards of the people of the Americas.

private health service: service provided by a non-government-owned entity that is for-profit or not-for-profit.

private sector: in reference to health services, the non-government for-profit or not-for-profit business entities or organizations associated with all aspects of health services.

public policies: government policies that express general principles that guide the management of public affairs.

public sector: with regard to health services, this is the portion of society controlled by national, state, and local governments. In the United States, this includes critical services such as the Centers for Disease Control and Prevention, Medicare, Medicaid, and state, county, and city health services.

third-party payers: the payment sources for health services received by but not entirely paid for by consumers.

U.K. health service system: the comprehensive publicly funded and owned health service system of England, Northern Ireland, Scotland, and Wales. See also comprehensive health service system.

U.S. health service system: the government and private system used in the 50 states, District of Columbia, Puerto Rico, and other territories. See also entrepreneurial health service system.

Kronenfeld and Kronenfeld, 2004; Richmond and Fein, 2005; Quadagno, 2005; Gratzer, 2006; Porter and Teisberg, 2006).

Study of the health systems of advanced industrialized free-market countries, particularly those that offer health services for all citizens, is one way to become familiar with the options represented by various health service systems. An increased understanding of how these health service systems operate, opinions of the various systems' users, and the health outcomes they produce can help those who advocate for or against health-related legislative issues at the federal, state, or local level. Proposed legislation can be assessed in light of outcome data from international organizations that study health service systems around the world.

In the United States over half of the money spent on health services comes from government sources. The U.S. legislative process involves the introduction of **bills** (proposed laws), **amendments** (alterations) to bills, and opportunities for public comments for or against a bill. To have a bill introduced, heard, and amended, requires direct or indirect contact with lawmakers. To express one's view of the merits or shortcomings of a bill to legislators and others who have access to lawmakers is to be an **advocate** for or against a bill. The understanding of the impact of a legislative change on health services can be expanded by knowledge of the strengths or weaknesses of other health systems. That knowledge in turn can provide a powerful foundation upon which to base *advocacy* efforts.

To fulfill this chapter's purpose it is necessary to take an international perspective on health service. This perspective includes information on U.S. immigration policies and cultural diversity. Some economic principles and business aspects of health services systems are introduced. The roles of health service personnel will be considered and, where appropriate, related to **physical therapy practice**. Information about health service personnel, particularly physical therapists, who have been educated outside of United States is also presented. The comparable parts of the health service systems of Europe, Canada, and the United States are discussed. The evolution, benefits, and challenges inherent in each health service system are addressed and com-

parisons of social philosophies provide a background for understanding differences between governments and their respective public health policies. *Public policies* are government **policies** that express general principles used to guide the management of public affairs. Public policies have very tangible effects on people. The greater the government involvement in the health service system the greater the need for public health policies. While health policies cover many aspects of a health service system, governments typically have policies that deal with **eligibility**, i.e., who can get health services; **access** and choice, i.e., where and what services and products are available and from whom; **quality-efficiency-effectiveness**, i.e., what service, product, or combination of services and products, provided at what point in time and by whom give the best outcome; and *cost-benefit* or **value-based**, i.e., who pays for services and products, what is the cost, what is the outcome, and whether the outcome is worth the cost. Compared to other major industrialized countries, the U.S. government is less involved in overall health service system **operations**. As a result, its policies have focused on care for selected constituents rather than the totality of the population. This has allowed the health service–related service providers, equipment and supply venders, organizations, for-profit, and not-for-profit businesses in the *private sector* to flourish (see Chapter 2). Differences in the extent of government control of health service systems and the effect of control on health service recipients, providers, manufacturers, and *third-party payers* (those who pay for the health services consumers receive, [see Chapter 2]) are addressed. Attention is drawn to points of particular interest to students and practicing physical therapists (PTs), physical therapy assistants (PTAs), and therapist managers.

Why Learn About Health Service Systems?

Here are seven potential, practical, and positive outcomes that can be reached when PT and PTA clinicians and managers have knowledge about non-U.S. health service systems and act on this knowledge:

1. Fulfill the ethical requirement to practice in a culturally competent manner.
2. Lessen the risk of law suits from immigrants.
3. Increase the likelihood of receiving acceptable customer satisfaction ratings from migrants and immigrants.
4. Enhance intradepartmental and interdepartmental communication with colleagues who were educated outside of the United States.
5. Professional development through increased knowledge of international information resources; education, volunteer, and work opportunities for PTs
6. Become conversant about physical therapy in other countries.
7. Become an informed advocate.

An International Physical Therapy Perspective

Immigration, temporary **migration**, and physical therapy have historical and contemporary connections. For example, Mary McMillan, who is considered the first American PT, trained and worked in England (Pinkston, 1989). Elizabeth Kenny, an Australian military nurse, came to the United States in 1940 and introduced PTs and others to her treatment (heat and exercise) for people with polio (Australian Women, 2007). Stanley Paris is an influential PT who is a citizen of both New Zealand and the United States. He was instrumental in the formation of the Orthopedic Section of the **American Physical Therapy Association** (APTA) and he founded the first professional doctorate program for physical therapy in the United States at the University of St. Augustine in Florida (APTA, 2006).

Immigration and migration move people from one geographical area to another. **Immigrants** are those who seek permanent residence. **Nonimmigrants** come for a limited period and leave. *Refugees* are those who come to the United States to escape persecution. A recent American Community survey estimated that 12.4% of the U.S. population was foreign born. Of this group 42% were naturalized citizens. The majority (53.2%) of immigrants were born in Central America or Mexico, while 26.7% were from Asia and 13.6% were

from Europe (U.S. Census Bureau, 2005). From 2000 to 2005 nearly six million people were admitted as permanent residents. One of the pillars of U.S. immigration policy is to admit applicants with specific skills to fill positions where shortages are believed to exist (Congressional Budget Office, 2007). Of the permanent residents admitted, more than one third were admitted because they had a special occupation that was deemed to be in short supply (Office of Immigration Statistics, 2007). Physical therapy is one of these special occupations (U.S. Citizenship and Immigration Services [USCIS], 2007a). Since 2000, about nine million temporary work visas were issued to workers and their families. Citizens of Canada and Mexico who are PTs are among those eligible for temporary visas under the **North American Free Trade Agreement (NAFTA)** (Office of NAFTA and Inter-American Affairs, 2007) as well as for permanent residence (USCIS, 2007a). In addition, census data suggest that there are as many as 12 million people in the United States without legal documents (Abraham and Hamilton, 2006). Therefore, customers (see Chapters 7 and 18) and coworkers, including physicians, nurses, other health service professionals, and PTs, may comprise immigrants, temporary workers, and undocumented individuals.

In 2007 an estimated 162,000 PTs (Bureau of Labor Statistics, 2009a) and 59,000 PTAs (Bureau of Labor Statistics, 2009b) were working in the U.S. Based on census data, it was estimated about 12% of U.S. PTs and 8% of PTAs and aides were born outside of the U.S. (Abraham and Hamilton, 2006). Bureau of Labor Statistics, (2009a,b) workforce projections for the 2006 to 2016 time period anticipate a need for a 27% increase in the number of PTs (Bureau of Labor Statistics, 2009c) and a 32% increase in the number of PTAs (Bureau of Labor Statistics, 2009d). These figures are based on estimated numbers of graduates, rate of growth in demand for services, replacement needs due to retirements and deaths, and other variables. The growth variables include the first of the baby-boomers (born in 1946) reaching full retirement age before 2016 and the growth of the population overall. If the assumptions underlying the physical therapy workforce needs are accurate, then the projected yearly addition of 6000 plus new PT graduates

(American Physical Therapy Association [APTA], 2007a) and 2500 or so new PTA graduates (APTA, 2007b) are likely to meet the estimated PT workforce needs through 2016, i.e. 6000 new PTs × 10 years + 2500 new PTAs × 10 years. However, these figures are only estimates. Therefore, it is reasonable to suggest that it will be in the nation's best interest to retain the specialized occupation designation status for PTs for immigration and temporary work visa purposes as a hedge against unexpected changes in the variables and assumptions used to estimate workforce need.

Steps for Obtaining a License to Practice Physical Therapy

Licensure is addressed at length in Chapter 8. The aspects of licensure discussed here are limited to licensure of foreign-trained PTs. Legal admission to the United States is an immigration issue dealt with at the federal government level. A license to practice PT and other professions is a state jurisdictional matter. To issue a PT license, all states require evidence of graduation from an educational program recognized by the Commission on Accreditation for Physical Therapy Education (CAPTE) (APTA, 2007c) or from a foreign educational program that is judged to be substantively equivalent (Foreign Credentialing Commission on Physical Therapy [FCCPT], 2007). In recent years CAPTE, the same agency that accredits entry-level U.S. PT educational programs, has accredited some foreign educational institutions. In 2002, 21 non-U.S. programs were accredited (APTA, 2002). In 2007, four non-U.S. institutions, two in Canada, one in Puerto Rico, and one in Scotland, were listed as programs accredited by CAPTE (APTA, 2007d). This decline may be related to the costs associated with CAPTE accreditation and the need to assure a sufficient number of PTs in the home country.

The process for graduates of nonaccredited foreign PT educational institutions to become licensed to practice in the United States is a five-step process: visa, credentialing, language testing, written examination, and other state-specific requirements. Individuals must present evidence that they completed a professional program that was substantially equivalent to a CAPTE-accredited program, that they can communicate in English, that they have proof of licensure and good standing in the country where they were licensed. The education assessment is made by credentialing agencies recognized by the Department of Health and Human Services (HHS) such as the Foreign Credentialing Commission on Physical Therapy (FCCPT) (USCIS, 2007b). English competence is based on the Test of English as a Foreign Language (TOEFL) scores (Educational Testing Service, 2007; USCIS, 2007c). The professional education assessment and English competence information is used by state physical therapy licensing authorities when they decide whether or not to allow a licensure applicant to take the National Physical Therapy Examination (NPTE) (Federated State Boards of Physical Therapy, 2007) and other state-specific examinations. There are two related indications that the educational-equivalency road to licensure may be traveled more frequently in the future by European physiotherapists (physiotherapist and physical therapist are considered equivalent terms) (European Region of the World Confederation for Physical Therapy [ER-WCPT], 2007a; APTA, 2001). The first indicator is the standardization recommendations for the basic educational preparation of physiotherapists. In 2003 the European physiotherapy education community published the European Physiotherapy Benchmark Statement. This document described the desired threshold level criteria for graduates of a physiotherapy preparatory program. The statement described "the nature and standards of programmes of study in physiotherapy that lead to awards made by higher education institutions in Europe and the *European Union (E.U.)* in the subject of physiotherapy" (ER-WCPT, 2007a). Within the target region there are over 500 institutions offering physiotherapy studies (ER-WCPT, 2007a). The benchmark statement laid out the desired knowledge, skill, and attributes expected of physiotherapy graduates. There are unmistakable similarities between the contents of this document, the terminology and concepts in the *Guide to Physical Therapist Practice* (APTA, 2001), and the CAPTE professional practice and client management criteria (APTA, 2007c). In the authors' opinion, the differences in aspirations for future European physiotherapists and U.S. physical therapy graduates in these areas appear very similar. This similarity will make determining educational equivalency for immigration purposes for applicants from the **European Region of the World Confederation for Physical Therapy (ER-WCPT)** countries easier. The second reason for drawing attention to Europe is because of the E.U. The previously quoted educational benchmark identified standards for all members of the ER-WCPT and the E.U. More will be said about the E.U. later in this chapter. For now the key points to understand are: the size of the E.U. and the ER-WCPT membership, and the E.U. general principle of the right of citizens of member countries to migrate to work in any other member country (Europa, 2007a, b). Currently there are 27 E.U. member countries with several more candidate nations under consideration for future E.U. membership (Fig. 1.1) (Europa, 2007c). All of the national physiotherapy associations of E.U. member countries are in the ER-WCPT region. The ER-WCPT (ER-WCPT, 2007b) has formulated a policy for migration of physiotherapists within its geographical area as well as educational recommendations. And the

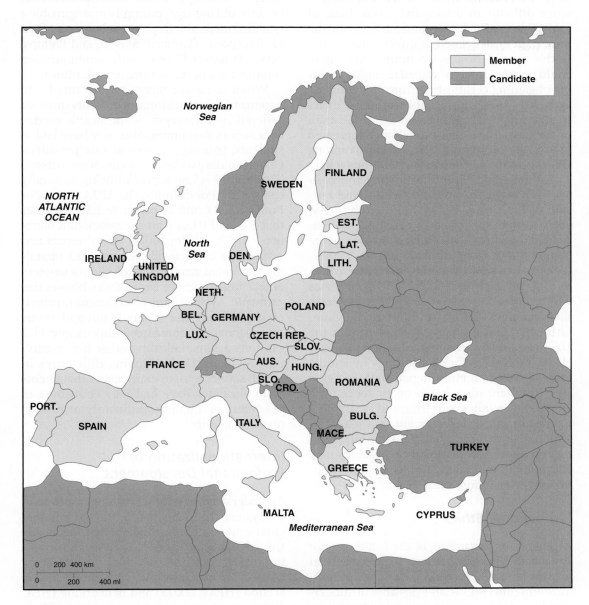

Figure 1.1. The European Union member countries (light gray) and candidate nations (dark gray) as of 2008.

European Commission, which is the E.U. body that protects the overall interests of the union, is making headway on policies for determining how equivalency of professional qualifications of paramedical personnel will be recognized by member nations to facilitate free movement of citizens across borders to work (Europa, 2007b; Chartered Society of Physiotherapy [CSP], 2007a). An outcome of the eventual harmonization of physiotherapist education programs in most of the E.U. member countries may well be that graduates from those programs will have a level of competence difficult to distinguish from those of CAPTE-accredited programs, at least in the important areas related to direct patient care. If this speculation is accurate, then there could be more foreign-trained therapists capable of gaining certification from credentialing agencies. These applicants would be likely to attain higher pass rates on the NPTE than in the past. There will probably be increased interest in joining the U.S. workforce among PTs practicing in foreign jurisdictions where wages are significantly lower than the average U.S. wage. To this end, within and outside of the United States there are business **entities** that specialize in assisting foreign-trained individuals who seek admission to the United States (Jobs Abroad, 2007). A corollary prediction is that the internationalization of physical therapy in the United States will be broadened as qualified therapists from E.U. member countries such as Bulgaria, Lithuania, and Romania attempt to join the U.S. workforce. Internationalization can benefit U.S. physical therapy settings by adding more variety to a multilingual staff, bringing new treatment ideas based on evidence from work done in other countries, and stimulating interest in career development through international study and practice. After all, information about international physical therapy educational, migration, and work opportunities are just a mouse-click away.

Professional Ethics

A general understanding of the health service systems that immigrants have experienced can help to harmonize expectations and to minimize misconceptions and possible misunderstandings. Since immigrants include clients, nonprofessional staff, PTs, physicians, and other health service personnel, there are many possibilities for misunderstandings. Familiarity with the general differences between the health service systems of other nations and the U.S. system, and taking the time to clarify the differences to clients or family members, can contribute to their belief that they have received good care from a knowledgeable, caring professional. People who are treated with respect and understanding are generally more tolerant of imperfect conditions (Scott, 1999) and the risk of a suit is reduced (Chapters 8 and 9). When there is concern about misunderstanding because of language, promptly arranging for a qualified medical interpreter to be present is an ideal response (Lattanzi, Mastin, and Phillips, 2006). (Chapter 12 deals with communication throughout a health service organization.)

When there are recent immigrants in an organization's workforce, cordiality may be fostered by awareness of the health service experiences that immigrants may have had as students, patients, or even as care providers. Understanding a client's or coworker's overall background is one aspect of being culturally competent. For example, the APTA Guide For Professional Conduct principle 1.1A indicates that PTs and PTAs who are association members (APTA, 2007e; 2007f) are to respect and respond to cultural differences. Understanding the broad perspective of client's or coworker's health service experiences honors this principle. With regard to colleagues, principle 11.2 notes that PTs should not undermine professional relationships and principle 11.3 cautions against belittling other health service providers. Understanding differences in health service system experiences that clients and colleagues have had may contribute to practicing in a nondiscriminatory or nonoppressive manner.

Internationalization of Professional Development

An understanding of other nations' health service systems can benefit U.S.-trained PTs that choose to venture beyond the borders of the United States to practice. There is an increasing variety of international volunteering (APTA, 2000; Health Policy and Administration Section [HPA], 2007a) and networking (HPA, 2007b) opportunities for PTs and PTAs. There are employment opportunities outside of the United States (APTA, 2000; HPA, 2007c; CSP, 2007b; International Service, 2007) and country-specific processes for pursuing employment. International service learning programs (Bergman, 1998; Scheuing, 2003; HPA, 2007c) and educational opportunities for student physical therapists also exist (Marquette, 2007; Sawyer and Lopopolo, 2004; University of Colorado, 2007; Williams and Feldman, 2004).

Another component of professional development is reading professional journals and books. The continuing consolidation of the publishing industry has resulted in increased distribution of books written by authors from many English speaking countries. There are also international Web sites with resources for PTs (see Additional Resources at the end of the chapter). Realize that health service information is contextual. The applicability of findings from one country to another can be interpreted more judiciously by the reader who has an understanding of the health service system of the country where the data was generated than a reader who does not. The impression that what works elsewhere, in the U.K. for example, needs to be tempered by the understanding that unlike in the United States, nearly everyone there has had access to free or low-cost health services for decades.

Finally, there are numerous opportunities to mix business and pleasure by attending meetings in different countries. This is a way to learn about different health service systems from those who work in them. There are continuing education courses abroad that are taught in English. International meetings on wound care and other physical-therapy relevant courses |are held in different countries throughout the year. One particularly relevant meeting is the WCPT International Congress, which is held every 4 years in a different country.

Worldwide Concerns About Health Service

Similarities and differences between health service systems are of interest worldwide. Most nations believe that their government is responsible for the well-being of their citizens. However, the breadth and degree of a government's involvement in health services varies from nation to nation. Different countries have different health policies. Unions and other groups that represent workers are concerned about the welfare of their members. They advocate for their members when employer or government policies jeopardize health service and other benefits. The impact of unions on health service policies varies from country to country. Multinational businesses have to be mindful of both the health of their workforce and the costs associated with health-related benefits to maintain a productive workforce. Both are linked to the profitability of the business. Employer health service expenditures also vary by country. And finally, multinational health-related organizations are interested in public health matters worldwide. These interests include comparative analysis and reporting of public health policy matters, health expenditures, health delivery systems, health outcomes, and many other health-related matters.

Multinational Health-Related Organizations and Health Service Policy

A significant amount of data that is cited in the upcoming discussion of health service systems comes from reports produced by multinational health-related organizations. The availability of cross-national data allows government policy makers to compare their health service systems with those of other nations. Four important organizations that collect and disseminate multinational health service data used by government policy makers and others are the **World Health Organization (WHO)**, the *Organization for Economic Cooperation and Development (OECD)*, the **Pan American Health Organization (PAHO)**, and the E.U.

WHO

The purpose of the WHO "... is the attainment by all peoples of the highest possible level of health." Health is defined in WHO's constitution as a state of "complete physical, mental and social well-being and not merely the absence of disease or infirmity" (WHO, 2007a). The focus of WHO is global health and development. This worldwide concern is reflected by the WHO membership, which includes more than 190 countries. All member countries are either members of the United Nations, have been voted in by a majority of WHO members, or have been sponsored by a WHO member country. The United States is a full member of WHO. The widespread representation of this organization places it in the unique position of being able to gather contemporary health information and disseminate it globally. Included among the types of information the WHO gathers are health service developments and outcomes. Table 1.1 contains a sampling of WHO data that deals with spending on health services. Table 1.2 presents sample data on spending per person and selected health outcomes. Both tables show the U.S. health service system to be the most costly. Of the seven countries being compared, people in the U.S. have the highest infant and adult mortality rates and the lowest expected life expectancy.

OECD

The OECD focuses on many issues including democracy, economic development, social issues including health and education, and public governance. Membership is held by 30 nations, all of which have democratic government and a **free market economy** (OECD, 2007b). A free market economy is one in which sellers of services and **goods** (supply) and buyers (demand) make exchanges with limited governmental intervention (see Chapter 20). The OECD is well known for the breadth of its databases, accuracy of its reports, and quality of analysis. For years this organization has collected and disseminated comparative data on access, expenditures, and outcomes, and other

information relevant to health service policy makers. The figures in Table 1.3 come from OECD sources.

The message in this table for government officials in France and Germany is that consumers view their national health service systems relatively favorably. For officials of the other three nations the survey reflects serious consumer concerns about their national systems. (See OECD, 2007c for a complete description of the variables investigated by this organization.) A national survey of Americans that was designed to investigate consumer satisfaction also asked about perceptions of the U.S. health service system. Eighty percent of respondents (N = 1,517) thought the current system had numerous problems and needed improvement (Berk, Gaylin, and Schur, 2006).

PAHO

The PAHO is an international public health agency that works to improve public health and living standards in the the Americas. Its governing body includes the region's WHO representative. There are 35 member countries located in South America, Central America, southern North America (Mexico and the U.S.), and the Caribbean (PAHO, 2007a). Additional data are drawn from 13 other countries and territories in the region (PAHO, 2007b). Economic development varies greatly between countries under the PAHO umbrella. An example would be the economic strength

Member Country	% of GDP Spent on Health	% of Total Gov't Budget for Health	% of All Health Spending Paid for by Gov't	% of All Health Spending Paid for Privately	% of Private Spending Paid for Out-of-Pocket
Canada	9.9	16.7	69.9	30.1	49.6
France	10.1	14.2	76.3	23.7	42.2
Germany	11.1	17.8	78.2	21.8	47.9
New Zealand	8.1	17.2	78.3	21.7	72.1
Sweden	9.4	13.6	85.2	14.8	92.1
U.K.	8.0	15.8	85.7	14.3	76.7
U.S.[a]	15.2	18.5	44.6[b]	55.4	24.3

Table 1.1   Example of Comparable WHO Health-Expenditure Data for Selected Countries, 2003

[a]Data collection preceded U.S.–Iraq conflict. There are numerous discretionary (non legislated) health-related items the government also pays for. See following comment.
[b]Woolhandler and Himmelstein (2002) argue the U.S. government pays for about an additional 15% of all health service costs because it contributes to the payment of government employee health insurance as well as other health-related expenses.
Source: World Health Organization (WHO, 2007b).
Permission to Reproduce from the World Health Report 2006 granted by the World Health Organization (WHO, 2007b,c).

Table 1.2 Example of Comparable WHO Health-Related Outcomes Data for Selected Countries, 2003

Member Country	Per Capita Spent on Health (Dollars)	Life Expectancy at Birth (Years)		Mortality < 5 Years (per 1,000)		Mortality 15–60 Years (per 1,000)	
		M	F	M	F	M	F
Canada	2669	78	83	6	5	91	57
France	2981	76	83	5	4	132	60
Germany	3204	76	82	5	5	112	58
New Zealand	1618	77	82	7	6	95	62
Sweden	3149	78	83	4	3	82	51
U.K.	2428	76	81	6	5	102	63
U.S.	5711	75	80	8	7	137	81

Source: World Health Organization (WHO, 2007b).

of the United States versus that of Haiti. PAHO advocates for universal primary health care for the entire region (PAHO, 2007c). There is recognition that current availability of rehabilitation services in most Latin American countries is inadequate. Only about 2% of Latin Americas' 85 million persons with disabilities have access to appropriate services (PAHO, 2007d). Health service information provided by PAHO includes comparisons of health service systems. Since people from Central America and the 31 states and federal district of Mexico make up the foreign-born majority in the United States, it is informative to note some differences between the Mexican and U.S. health service systems (USCB, 2005). Table 1.4 presents example data from the PAHO for both countries.

The out-patient and hospital bed figures represent all government and *private health service* entities (PAHO, 2007e). While Mexican officials reported nearly four times the number of out-patient facilities as the United States, U.S. officials reported nearly 3.5 times

more U.S. hospital beds. Another difference is that in 2004 out-of-pocket payment for health services in Mexico accounted for a greater percentage of all health care expenditures than in the United States. In fact, Mexicans personally paid for more of their health service costs than the citizens of any other OECD nation (OECD, 2007a). These differences reflect governmental health service policy differences as well as differences in the magnitude of nongovernment entities involved in the health service industry. Health care reform laws were enacted in Mexico in 2004. The results of these changes are preliminary at this point in time (Knaul et al., 2006).

The European Union

The E.U. is a supranational multilevel form of governance. The E.U. currently includes 27 independent countries (Fig. 1.1). The purpose of the E.U. is to deal with political, economic, and social matters in a democratic manor to propel union member countries to achieve

Table 1.3 Example of Comparative OECD Patient Health Service System Satisfaction Data for Selected E.U. Countries, 2002

Questions (Our System . . .)	Responses in %				
	France	Germany	Ireland	Netherlands	U.K.
Runs well	22.0	15.6	3.7	6.5	8.3
Needs minor changes	41.9	31.5	16.7	39.1	22.9
Needs fundamental changes	25.5	34.8	39.3	46.8	49.7
Needs complete rebuilding	7.0	11.1	32.9	6.8	15.8
Uncertain/Do not know	3.6	6.9	7.5	0.8	3.3

Source: Eurobarometer (2007b).

Permission to reproduce from Public's Satisfaction with Health Care System, E.U. countries, 2002, granted by the Office for Official Publications of the European Communities.

Table 1.4   Example of PAHO Data on Health-Related Expenditures, Out-Patient Resources, and Utilization for Mexico and the United States, 2005

Member Country	Tax-Based Health Expenditures as % of GDP[a]	Private Health Expenditures as % of GDP	# Out-Patient Facilities	Out-Patient Visits per 1,000 people	# Hospital Beds per 1,000 people
Mexico	2.8	3.2	18346	2502	1.0
U.S.	6.3	6.0	4807	285	3.3

[a]GDP is a measure of production that includes the total output of all services and goods produced within a country.
Source: Pan-American Health Organization (2007b).
Reproduced with the permission of the Pan American Health Organization (PAHO). This data was originally published in PAHO Regional Core Health Data System Table Generator (PAHO, 2/20/07b)

greater strength and world influence than any single member country could aspire to independently. The E.U. does not have a federal government like the United States. It is a union of member countries that have agreed to allow some of their governmental decisions to be made by shared decision-making institutions—a common elected parliament, a council for individual country representation, and a commission for overall oversight—yet they retain their sovereignty as independent nations (Europa, 2007d). The practical point for citizens of E.U. member countries is that they now have the right to travel, settle, work, study, receive health services, and do business in any member country with a minimum of red tape (Europa, 2007b). Presently, the health services of the 450 million constituents of the E.U. are the responsibility of, and are thus managed by, the governments of their respective home countries. There is an E.U. health insurance card that facilitates payment for services provided to E.U. citizens when they need services outside of their home country (Europa, 2007e). While the general E.U. principle of freedom to work extends to PTs, the directive regarding cross-border physical therapy services is being debated (CSP, 2007a; ER-WCPT, 2007b).

Government Policies and Health Service System Issues

Government health policies are public policies that affect the health of citizens. Boufford and Lee (2001) have identified the key health service policy areas for which the governments of most advanced industrialized nations are responsible:

- Protecting the health of the population
- Building the infrastructure necessary to protect public health
- Managing and regulating health services
- Collecting and disseminating information about the health service system
- Financing all of the above

All advanced industrialized nations struggle to fulfill the noted responsibilities (OECD, 2007d). There are several near universal questions government health policy officials are working hard to answer. These health service questions can be arranged into five general categories:

1. Access (Shi and Singh, 2004)
2. Cost (Kronenfeld and Kronenfeld, 2004)
3. Quantity (Richmond and Fein, 2005)
4. Quality (Brennan and Reisman, 2007)
5. Efficiency (Schoen, et al., 2005)

Access questions refer to whom, where, when, and acceptability: Who should receive health services? Where should they receive them? When should they receive them? And what is the degree of constituent acceptance of the arrangements for health services? Cost is everyone's concern: direct payers, indirect payers (taxpayers), and providers of services. Important cost-related questions include: Who should pay for health services? How much should be paid for services? Are services affordable? What services should be available? And how much service should be provided? The last two questions are evidence-based and **economic value–based** matters. This means that the strength of the evidence for appropriately timed provision or discontinuance of a service or mix of services is weighed against the cost of providing such service(s) for everyone who may need them (Miller, 2007). Quality also has evidence-based and economic value–based components. The quality question refers to what the best mix of services may be for achieving a desirable outcome in most situations. The central efficiency question asks how can performance be improved in all parts of the system. Efficiency addresses concerns about waste, fraud (see Chapters 8 and 9), duplication, errors, right-time services, use of the least costly service appropriate for a condition, and how to minimize or eliminate unproductive activities throughout the system (see Chapter 16).

It is difficult to determine the best answers to the types of questions asked here because the variables are moving targets. Five areas that pose difficulties for health service planners are:

1. Income and budgets. There are the constraints of finite and often unpredictable revenue sources (Wimberly and Thai, 2002).
2. Demographics. Populations are increasing and longevity is increasing. This means there are more people to keep healthy for a longer period of time (OECD, 2007d).
3. Education, service, and product marketing. The availability of medical information on the Internet and in the media contributes to constituents learning about and demanding newer goods and services (Shi and Singh, 2004).
4. Technology and drugs. There are continuous technological improvements and innovations in health service diagnostic, treatment, communication equipment, and new pharmaceutical products (OECD, 2007d).
5. Research. Contemporary practice is dynamic because clinically applicable research is continuously providing additional information to guide practice (Miller, 2007).

In an attempt to fulfill several goals noted in the introduction to this chapter—to provide a comparative overview of health service–related social, political, and economic philosophical principles as well as reflections on differences in health service policy and legislation—the key elements of health service systems under five general socio-political conditions are analyzed. The comparisons that are made will provide background that will help readers to become informed advocates for the health service issues they support. These comparisons allow for more detailed discussions of the U.S. health service system in Chapters 2 through 6.

Beliefs Underlying Health Service Systems

Health service systems differ around the globe because the sponsoring nations differ in their history, social philosophy, available resources (economics), values, beliefs about health care, cultural priorities, and the health status of people (Daniels and Sabin, 2002; Shi and Singh, 2004). Discussions about who should receive health services are philosophical as well as political. In complex systems, e.g., managing the health service of a nation, questions of rights and **justice** are commonplace. These discussions focus on weighing available options. The discussions and final actions taken are subject to political influences (Loewy, 2001). Therefore it is important to recognize that the interests of those in political power and their political ideology do affect major issues, such as what a health service system looks like, how it operates, and whom the system serves. This intermingling of influences that impact public policy merits further discussion. As a reminder, a policy is defined as a broad statement containing goals and objectives that form a framework for organizing specific activities. Public policies are the results of decisions made by an authoritative branch of government that are intended to influence the utilization of resources including political power (Shi and Singh, 2004). Public policy discussions, overtly or otherwise, entail deliberations grounded in ethical principles according to various social philosophies. Taking guidance from a **social philosophy** involves the formal or informal adoption of ethical concepts to form a moral backdrop against which decisions about the allocation of relatively scarce resources are played out. Ethical concepts relevant to fair access to health service generally focus on justice and in particular on issues of social and distributive justice (Austin, 2001) (see Chapters 7 and 8). The ethical concepts that are adopted provide the context for discussions that are part of the process used to develop public health policies.

Social philosophy relates to a wide range of social matters. Assistance programs for the poor, for women and children, for people with disabilities, for people beyond a certain age, and for indigenous peoples are all examples of social welfare programs that benefit various members of society. While there may be a desire to do more for people with real needs for the right reasons, there is the real constraint of limited resources and, of course, varying political philosophies that may impact final decisions. These interacting forces place proposals and programs that meet the needs of a country in competition with one another for funding. Recent examples of competitive health service issues in the United States are the need to increase efforts to bolster homeland security efforts to counter bioterrorism and illegal entry to the country at the partial expense of reductions in biomedical research. Health service is only one of many competing programs on the agenda that government officials and elected legislators must consider when they exert their influence to shape policies and make laws. In democratic countries public policies indirectly reflect voters' wishes. Citizens use their votes to help elect the candidates of their choice. Once elected, constituents have the opportunity to engage their elected officials to express their views on issues that are of importance to them. More will be said about involvement in the legislative process later in this chapter.

The core philosophical issues related to access, allocation, and rationing health services relate to fairness or justice. In its most general sense justice deals with moral issues (see Chapter 7) about access or, stated another way, who "ought" to have access to health services. For health service this can be translated as concerns about who should get what, **distributive justice** (Daniels, 1985) or **social justice** (Shi and Singh, 2004). Health service managers confront distributive justice issues when they allocate funds for one program over another or close a facility and direct resources to services or patients. While there is no consensus on a set of distributive justice principles (Daniels and Sabin, 2002) in public policy discussions, distributive justice versus

social justice is at the core of arguments about access to basic health services and whether they are a right and therefore, a justification for entitlement programs. This boils down to determining how to be fair in meeting health care under the constraint of finite resources (Daniels and Sabin, 2002). Because programs have costs, economic considerations a policy advocates must include a parallel discussion of how the program will be paid for. Given the capitalistic, free market economic philosophy of the United States, the economic cost of health service influences decisions along with consideration of the moral "oughts." In economic terms, health services can be perceived as a commodity, i.e., something to buy and sell in the marketplace (see Chapter 18). In a free market, those who can afford services can buy them. Those who cannot buy standard services find less costly alternatives or do without. This has been called **market justice** (Shi and Singh, 2004). The ethical dialog on health service matters involves reasoned debates about whether or not access to adequate health service is a right of all members of a society. This is a distributive justice debate. Among the advanced industrialized nations of the world, all but the United States have taken a broad social justice perspective that says that constituents have a right to health service and have facilitated access and payment for services. These countries allocate resources systematically to ensure universal or near universal access to adequate health service at little or no out-of-pocket cost to residents.

General Comparison of Health Service Systems

A system is defined as several parts working together such that their interaction produces something greater than could be produced by the individual parts working independently (Shelton, 2000). A useful approach to compare systems is to categorize them based on the relative degree of governmental involvement in the planning, financing, and controlling health service for a nation's residents (Grogan, 1993) and then do a more specific analysis where there are meaningful commonalities (Roemer, 1993). Figure 1.2 and Table 1.5 integrate these thoughts. Figure 1.2 shows

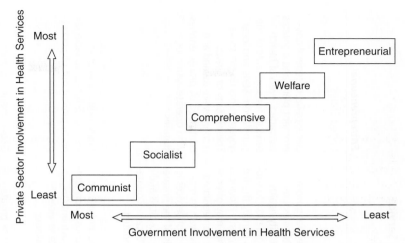

Figure 1.2. Construct names to identify health service systems that result from government policies guided by different social and economic philosophies.

the relative amounts of governmental and private involvement in health services under the different systems. Table 1.5 describes a general progression in degrees of central government control over health service under different social-political-economic philosophies and how the systems differ in terms of financing, payers, patient access, and patient freedom.

Communist Health Service System: The Soviet Union Before 1992

The communism column in Table 1.5 refers to the health service system developed by the Soviets, implemented throughout the former Soviet bloc countries, and ended by the early 1990s. The communism column is first because it represented the system with the most government (public) control over health service and the least availability of alternative health service (private). It represents one extreme in the ways health service can be systematized.

Politically and socially, the Soviet bloc was communist. **Communism** does not recognize the right to private ownership (Loewy, 2001). All resources belong to the central government, which is the caretaker of society (Brinton, Christopher, and Wolff, 1967). In other words, the central government owns the health service system, related resources, and is the employer of all personnel. The central government controls all aspects of health service including planning, education, research, financing, employment, and delivery. Under the Soviet health service system there was very

little privately paid health service available (Roemer, 1993). The central government recognized health service as a right of citizenship. Citizens were entitled to free health service paid for by the government for decades, however, basic medical and acute care for the majority of citizens was not realized until the 1980s (Bourhanskaia, Kubataem, and Paterson, 2002). Care for the general population was provided through regional general and specialty hospitals and ambulatory care centers. The recipients were assigned by home address to local care facilities and had few choices as to where they were treated or by whom. While medical services were free, medications were only conditionally free. Most drugs had to be purchased from government-owned pharmacies. However, drugs considered critical to one's well-being were often provided at no charge (Roemer, 1993). As in most countries, facilities and services were more available in populated areas than in remote areas. In addition to usual medical and nursing staff, patient care was provided by a *feldscher*, a combination nurse practitioner and physician's assistant. Interestingly, physical therapy, along with other services typically provided by nonphysician health professionals, was provided by medical doctors (Bourhanskaia, Kubataev, and Paterson, 2002). Many of the eastern and central European countries that were part of the Soviet bloc are now democracies and members of the E.U. It is also worth mentioning that thousands of people from the old Soviet bloc have immigrated to the United States and elsewhere.

Table 1.5 General Comparison of Important Elements of Health Service Systems Based on Social, Political, and Economic Philosophies

	Communist	Socialist	Comprehensive	Welfare	Entrepreneurial
Example country	Former Soviet Union	Germany	United Kingdom	Canada	United States
Control	Central government owns all resources, employs all providers, plans for and finances all aspects of the health service system, determines where services may be obtained.	Decentralized. Federal and state responsibility for hospital upkeep. State regulates nongovernmental, nonprofit (sickness funds) and private health insurance providers. Access to health services assured. Control through legislation for national insurance tax, mandatory work-related health insurance, availability of private insurance. Actual control can be legislated to local authorities.	Extensive central government control to assure access to quality health services. A single-payer health service system known as the National Health Service (NHS) that plans for comprehensive health services throughout the U.K. to be delivered by local health service authorities. Local authorities in turn arrange for and authorize comprehensive care at the local level. Local accountability is mandated.	Extensive central government control to assure access to quality health services. Legislation to support care in part by the federal government. Provinces and territories may offer and pay for nonlegislated services they wish to provide. Delivery of services is in the hands of the private sector, e.g., hospitals and physicians. Local accountability is mandated.	Decentralized. federal government plans and legislates for varied levels of health services for segments of the population. State and local governments do the same. The majority of health resources are owned and controlled by private entities who operate within legal statutes.
Financing	Federal taxes for specialized care. State payroll taxes and insurance funds to provide care for employed people, territorial taxes for others.	Taxes, and pooled employer and employee premium contributions managed by nonprofit sickness funds. Minimal patient out-of-pocket payments.	Taxes, public and private insurance funds, minimal patient out-of-pocket payments.	Taxes, public and private insurance funds. More out-of-pocket payments as more private services become available.	Taxes, public and private insurance funds, variable levels of patient out-of-pocket payments, charity.
Payer(s)	Government	Government > private	Government > private	Government > private	Government < private
Patient choice	None for most people. Some Communist Party members received care at special hospitals.	Extensive	Assess to hospital and specialists controlled by local general practitioner.	Limitations regarding elective procedures, access to specialists, special diagnostic tests.	None to very restricted. Dependent on health insurance plan and ability to pay out-of-pocket.
Current status	No longer exists.	Undergoing reform. Private insurance growing.	Undergoing reform. Financial shortfalls.	Undergoing reform. Private hospitals and private insurance growing.	Incremental changes being discussed. No current master plan. Number of uninsured going up. Costs up without increase in value to consumers.

Socialist Health Service System: Germany

The socialist column in Table 1.5 shows specifics of the health service system of E.U. member country Germany (Fig. 1.1). Like many E.U. countries, the German government employs elements of socialism in their approach to planning for the health service of its citizens and others in the country. **Socialism** is a term sometimes used interchangeably with the word communism. This is incorrect. Socialism is a political system that recognizes the right to limited private ownership. Communism does not (Loewy, 2001). What the terms have in common is that social conditions are associated with the economic system (Rodwin, 1999). Socialism refers to a system based on the view that there are certain services, products, and institutions that benefit all of society (Brinton, Christopher, and Wolff, 1967). Because these resources represent a good to be used by the greater community of citizens, these assets should be controlled by the central government so they can be put to use to benefit the community (Loewy, 2001). Health service is considered one of these community assets. From a socialist point of view a health service system needs to be under governmental control to ensure equitable distribution of this asset. A related unique feature of socialist-oriented health service systems is the concept of social solidarity. **Solidarity** can be described as a stance taken by a civic community (including those with historically similar ethnic and social backgrounds (Kovner and Jonas, 1999), that socially beneficial programs, e.g., health service, should be "evaluated on more than a materialistic and monetary standard; economic actions are not separated from social morals and actions of society . . ." (Morton, 2001, p. 140). Membership in unions, trade associations, and professional associations is bolstered by the solidarity concept. Such organizations have benefited their members by negotiating very good benefits from employers (sick leave, parental leave, unemployment, social security and pensions, vacations, etc.). The strength of the concept of solidarity is clearly exemplified in Germany where almost all residents, citizens or not, have had mandated health insurance since 1883 (Busse and Riesberg, 2007; Swami, 2002).

In socialist-oriented countries, government assumes the responsibility for centralized health service planning. Planning is done for those areas that are necessary to ensure that universal health service is available free of direct charge for citizens, and in some cases, noncitizens. Socialist-oriented governments finance health service through various combinations of general and special tax revenues, special public and private insurance funds, and small user fees. In Germany's case, the government manages the system in a less centralized fashion than some of its socialist neighbors (Grogan, 1993) but it exerts more control than socialist-oriented Sweden (Kaati, 2002). Germany's health service system is unique because it arranges for near universal health service without taxes, so it neither finances nor pays for health service services. Health service expenditures total about 11% of Germany's *gross domestic product* (*GDP*). For global economic comparisons, the amount spent on health service for each person in a country and the relationship between health service expenditures and the GDP are commonly used. The GDP is the total value of all services and goods produced by labor in a country (Bureau of Economic Analysis, 2007).

Germany uses two types of legislation to pay for and control health service costs. One mandates health insurance and the other controls drug costs. Health insurance legislation mandates that employers, trade associations, and professional associations maintain sickness funds that cover health services for their respective members. Employers and employees share the cost, which is scaled by level of income. For low-income people there is government subsidy. Nearly 500 sickness funds enroll about 90% of the population. Employee contributions are based on income, not health status (Busse and Riesberg, 2007; germanculture.com, 2007; National Coalition on Health Care, 2007). In 2004 over 72% of health funding came from *public sector* sources (OECD, 2007e). There is also private health insurance. Individuals who can afford it, and wish to do so, can opt out of the sickness funds and purchase private health insurance. Payment to providers is a negotiated **fee-for-service** payment. This is per-service payment method with co-payments (see Chapters 2–4). There are co-payments for most services and products (OECD, 2007e). For physical therapy treatment the co-pay is 15% of the total (Busse and Riesberg, 2007). From a management perspective, getting payment is relatively uncomplicated in the German system. There are two payer sources, the sickness fund and private insurance, and the paperwork is standardized for billing. This simplification results in low administrative costs. Another feature of the German health service system is that doctors are limited as to where they treat patients. Doctors who work from their private office cannot see patients in the hospital. Similarly, hospital-based doctors are salaried employees who only see hospitalized patients. Supply and demand forces work to foster competition for patients (see Chapter 20). Admission to German medical schools has been available to all who meet qualifications. Over time this has produced an oversupply of physicians (Swami, 2002).

In terms of outcomes, socialist health service systems, when adequately funded, have met the majority of the basic health service needs of nearly all of their respective constituents (Swami, 2002). While there is no or very minimal out-of-pocket cost to service users, it should be remembered that the cost of health service has been prepaid through contributions to special insurance funds and/or taxes, depending on the country. At present, there is generally a high degree of satisfaction with the socialist health service systems (Eurobarometer, 2007a) but there is also a deep concern about the sustainability of these health service systems (OECD, 2007d). In a survey of patients with health problems, German patients rated ease of access and timeliness as the system's strong points. Poor communication between hospitals and private physicians is a problem that causes significant errors (Schoen et al., 2005).

Comprehensive Health Service System: United Kingdom

The third type of system in the continuum is called comprehensive (Table 1.5). This system is unique to the U.K. The *U.K. health service system* is also a socialist model (Bloor and Maynard, 2002) that is significantly different from the continental European models. It is considered a *comprehensive health service*

system because is provides constituents with the full spectrum of health services (Roemer, 1993). The hallmarks of this system are:

- A great deal of centralized planning and overall management of local government health authorities
- Relatively less governmental control than several continental European socialist systems
- Universally available health service through government-provided services plus privately available health services
- Availability of private insurance to cover elective procedures (Bloor and Maynard, 2002)

Under the U.K. version of a highly centralized, comprehensive health service system, the entire national populations of multiple countries are entitled to complete health service. A recent estimate of how health services and products are paid for found that 86% came from public funds from general taxes, 12% from payroll taxes, and the remainder from users who received dental services and prescription drugs (Bloor and Maynard, 2002; OECD, 2007f). Administratively, the Department of Health is the central government agency overseeing the health service. The coordinating links between the central government and the *National Health System (NHS)* are the **strategic health authorities**. These authorities are charged with helping local NHS staff develop strategies for quality care (NHS, 2007). Local hospital trusts are the actual employers of health service professionals and staff, making everyone a salaried government employee. The government periodically reviews salaries through independent review boards and makes adjustments in the salary schedules. The CSP is the union that represents PTs in salary discussions and other matters. In 2007 the base rate for a full-time new therapist was approximately $20 per hour with the opportunity for location subsidy and other increases (CSP, 2007c). Services are provided at NHS facilities as well as in homes. However, because "Every . . . citizen has the right to be registered with a local GP and visits . . . are free" (NHS, 2002, p. 3), local groups of primary care physicians are the portals of entry into the care system. This places general practitioners in the role of *gatekeeper*. In health services, this is the physician who is responsible for referring a patient to a specialist or for hospital treatment (Bloor and Maynard, 2002) (see Chapters 3 and 4).

The U.K. system is under scrutiny worldwide for several reasons. It is apparently cost effective and has better-than-average outcomes, and has acceptable patient satisfaction ratings. These desirable characteristics of the system are accomplished for about 8.3% of the U.K. GDP. This is less than the mean of all OECD nations (OECD, 2007f). A contributing reason for lower cost is that NHS pay scale is set through periodic negotiation for all NHS health service providers, which includes PTs. This comprehensive system is ranked near the middle of OECD major advanced industrialized member nations based on key desirable health service outcome measures. User satisfaction levels for selected aspects of the system are adequate but varied depending on the specific service they rate. A 2003 survey of 1,000 patients found 59% rated the system satisfactory while 22% rated it unsatisfactory [Department of Health (DOH), 2007a]. A 2003 report of patients who had to wait to see specialists in England after being referred by a general practitioner found 80% of patients waited fewer than 13 weeks (Department of Health, 2007b). The strong point of the U.K. system is that it provides comprehensive care at a relatively reasonable, albeit increasing, cost. The concerns about the NHS system include fewer physicians per 1,000 patients than many other E.U. countries (OECD, 2007f), under-funding evidenced by some health trusts running deficits (CSP, 2007d), and projected increase in demand for services (Pepper, 2006).

Welfare Health Service System: Canada

The fourth column in Table 1.5 is labeled as a welfare health service system with Canada as the unique representative of this system. Its location in the table reflects less central government and more private involvement in health service than the systems discussed thus far. The major commonalities with the other health service systems are that it is primarily a publicly funded health care system (Robertson, 2007) and it affords nearly universal accessibility.

In the *Canadian welfare health service system*, residents have universal access to care (Roemer, 1993). Canadian universal health service insurance is called Medicare (Romanow, 2002). *Canadian Medicare* applies to citizens of all ages and differs from the age and disability limitation requirements of the U.S. Medicare program (see Chapters 2–6, 8, 20). The Canadian welfare health service system is based on a social philosophy that holds health service as a right. This right is reflected in the foundational elements of the *Canada Health Act (CHA)*: Universality, accessibility, comprehensiveness, portability, and public administration (Canadian Physiotherapy Association [CPA], 2007a).

The dual responsibility for health service is clearly stated in the CHA passed by parliament in 1984. In this system health service for citizens is a shared responsibility of the federal, provincial, and territorial ministries of health. This act was formulated to ensure that all Canadian residents would have access to necessary health service on a prepaid basis by establishing criteria and conditions for the provinces and territories to satisfy in order to qualify for their full share of federal funding (Health Canada, 2009). The actual role of the central government in health service is indirect (Kluge, 2001). The CHA made the federal government responsible for setting and administering health service standards as well as assisting with the financing of the health service programs of Canada's provincial and territorial governments. The act mandates that provincial and territorial governments are responsible for actually managing, delivering, and securing additional tax and other revenues to ensure that all residents receive all medically necessary hospital, physician, and allied health services as well as some drugs. Basically, the primary responsibility for the delivery of health services lies with the provincial and territorial governments. They must offer core services, which are medically necessary hospital and physician services. They have the option to offer benefits beyond those mandated by the CHA, and local ministries of health define what services are medically necessary. This means there are regional variations in health services and other benefits. Funding for home care and prescription drugs varies regionally. There is sparse public funding for out-patient prescriptions, long-term, dental, vision, chiropractic, or physical therapy care (Robertson, 2007). In 2004 total spending on Canadian health services was estimated to be 9.9% of GDP (OECD, 2007g). Canadian Medicare paid for about 70% of all health service spending while private insurance covered about an additional 13% and out-of-pocket spending paid for about another 15% [Canadian Institutes for Health Information (CIHI), 2007a]. Because hospital care is a core necessity of Medicare, physical therapists in hospitals tend to be salaried. Out-of-hospital services at private practice clinics are paid primarily through the public provincial health plans, private insurance, or by the patients, with many geographical differences (CPA, 2007b). The increase in private health insurance is an important current and future income source for the approximately 40% of Canadian PTs who own or work in private clinics (WCPT, 2007). The increasing numbers of Canadians purchasing private health insurance and the general repeal of the laws requiring physician referrals to access PTs (CPA, 2007b) have facilitated the expansion of private practice.

In Canada there are 2.1 physicians per 1,000 patients, which is a low ratio compared to other advanced industrialized countries (OECD, 2007g). This contributes to some discontent with the breadth of services available and waiting times in the publicly financed Medicare program. There is a need to meet a broader scope of health service needs than Medicare provides and for access to be more timely as defined by patients. Waiting lists exist for some diagnostic tests and access to specialists and some surgeries and treatments may require a long wait. Across 12 medical specialist areas the average wait was almost 18 weeks (Fraser Institute, 2007). In response to this criticism evidence-based time limits have been set for selected conditions (CIHI, 2007b). To better meet the needs of patients who have private insurance or who can afford to pay out-of-pocket, some Canadians physicians have opened private medical clinics offering an array of services. These clinics do not accept Medicare patients (Maioni, 2007). A legal challenge brought by the Quebec provincial government resulted in the ruling that provincial governments could not prohibit private insurance from paying for services covered under Medicare (Robertson, 2007). Some Canadians purchase private insurance, which may pay for services provided outside of Canada. Alternatively, they pay for out-of-country costs themselves. Emergency care is covered by some provincial health plans (About.com, 2007).

Means of sustaining the Canadian system are currently under investigation. The Commission on the Future of Health Care in Canada is engaged in dialog with a wide range of stakeholders, representatives of other socialist health service nations, and international organizations to determine how the Canadian government can, in the 21st century, sustain a system that will continue to fulfill a core Canadian value associated with providing health service for all residents based on need rather than income (Romanow, 2002; Canadian Health Coalition, 2007).

Entrepreneurial Health Service System: The United States

The last column in Table 1.5 is labeled entrepreneurial. An **entrepreneur** is someone who starts a business knowing that there is the risk of losses if the business fails, but who will be enriched if the business succeeds (Olsen, 1999) (see Chapter 22). The entrepreneurial label was applied by Roemer (1993) in recognition of the importance of private enterprises in the unique, two-part U.S. **health service system** that has a large **private** (nongovernment) component and a slightly smaller public (government) component. The pubic component is funded by payroll taxes and federal and state general revenues, while the income to support the private component comes from individuals paying out-of-pocket, commercial insurance companies, **managed-care organizations** (see Chapters 2–6, 21, 22) that link those seeking services with service providers, and philanthropy (charity and pro bono services). Except for the communist system, all other health service systems have public as well as private health service components, but only in the U.S. system does the private portion predominate. The major related differences between the decentralized entrepreneurial U.S. health service system and the systems of other similarly developed nations include:

1. Extent of government responsibility for health services. The U.S. Constitution is silent on the responsibility of the federal government for health services for citizens. By default, health is the responsibility of the states. The federal government's involvement in health services has been increasing for categories of citizens through its constitutional power to spend (Smith, 2007).

2. Universally available health service. The United States stands out for being the sole advanced industrialized nation where health services are not assured for everyone (Shi and Singh, 2004).

3. Central control. There is no federal government body responsible for health service planning for all U.S. citizens (Boufford and Lee, 2001). The HHS is the federal government department responsible for health-related services that benefit most citizens. However, the role of the HHS in financing and managing health services is limited to government-initiated social and health benefit programs focused on helping the segment of the population least able to help themselves (HHS, 2007a).

4. Expenditures. The per person expenditures for health services in the United States are the highest in the world (OECD, 2007h).

5. Public expenditure for health services. As a result of point number 2, public sources pay for the smallest portion of the total expenditure for health services compared to every other advanced industrialized nation (WHO, 2007a, b).

6. Multiple payer sources. In contrast to similarly developed countries with single-payer systems there are many payers in the U.S. system (see Chapters 2–6, 18, 21, 22). Multiple payers are a source of inefficiencies. This includes increased costs associated with maintaining duplicative management and oversight operations to deal with many different financial arrangements, many different settings to deal with, the need for specialized consultants, and communication breakdowns (Shi and Singh, 2004).

How Did U.S. Health Care Become So Different?

The answer to the question is historical. The United States has a **federalist** form of govern-ment in which there is delineation in the authority of local, state, and federal government and a tendency to favor decentralization of health service (Grogan, 1993). U.S. political ideology is linked to **capitalism**, an economic philosophy that espouses a market orientation, i.e., free-market economy, and competition (Shi and Singh, 2004) plus an orientation that favors individualistic efforts to succeed. Individuals engaged in self-advancing actions are expected to ultimately benefit society (Kronenfeld, 1997). Individual rights are fervently upheld. These economic, political, and orientation factors fostered the development of the U.S. entrepreneurial public-private health service system. The public part of the system caters to those who were most needy, while the part of the system that is privately managed and funded, market-related, and entrepreneurial caters to those who have employer-based insurance or who can afford to pay for services themselves. How health insurance and employment became linked is worth mentioning. The benefit of employer-sponsored health insurance came about after the Second World War as a result of mandated wage controls. The Internal Revenue Service ruled that such programs would not be taxed. Thus, it was a tax-free benefit for employees. Since the benefit remains tax-free, it has become an incentive for employers to attract and retain employees. As health insurance premiums go up, employers offering a health services plan may do so as a trade-off for higher wage increases (Gratzer, 2006). This was an opportunity for the private commercial health insurance industry to flourish. The private component exemplifies many aspects of a market-based economy as well as the U.S. character as described earlier. Examples of these two points in the context of health service providers are: the private system represents the right of individuals to do something to better the human condition, the right to provide charity care, and of course, the right to meet demand for health service as an entrepreneur and make a profit. For consumers, the private system provides an alternative to publicly funded health service, the right to choose where they obtain services, and the right to choose from among competing providers. This freedom of choice however is costly to purchasers (see Chapters 2–6, 14, 21, 22).

Something Good and Something Bad

Questions have been raised about the information that is gathered to determine the public contribution to health services. According to OECD (2007h) data, the public funding in the United States is less than all other developed member nations. This conclusion has been challenged as being underreported and conservative. The crux of the argument is that HHS data does not recognize tax deductions that are allowed for providing health insurance. A deduction from potential tax revenue is actually a loss of tax revenue from the employee (less income and other taxes). Also excluded from the picture are expenditures made from publicly funded budgets of government agencies to pay for private health insurance purchased for several million employees. If these items and some other costs were included as part of the tax-supported contribution to health service the government estimate would be approximately 15% higher than the 45% identified (Woolhandler and Himmelstein, 2002).

Even though the U.S. *entrepreneurial health service system* is the most expensive system in the world, there is no conclusive evidence that health service outcomes are better in the United States than in other advanced industrialized nations (Blumenthal, 2001). For example, among 192 WHO nations, the United States, Costa Rica, Cuba, and Denmark are all ranked 25th in life expectancy (estimated at birth) for each sex (WHO, 2007b).

On the positive side, the general consensus is the U.S. health service system is the most responsive, i.e., lowest wait time, for non-emergency care compared to other wealthy nations employing more governmentally controlled health service systems (Anderson and Hussey, 2002).

All systems exclude some constituents and leave some users unsatisfied with the timeliness of access, outcomes, and costs. Globally, all systems are evolving to better balance resources and needs. A major issue regarding the entrepreneurial bent of the U.S. system, with its foundation based on the ability to pay, is that it contributes to ". . . an ever widening gap between rich and poor" . . . (Institute For The Future, 2000, p. 192). The poor include people who have inadequate health insurance as well as those who have none. Based on census data, approximately 16% of the population was uninsured at the time data were collected (Center on Budget and Policy Priorities, 2007).

Because the U.S. system has no central planner, no single owner, and no single payer, some have questioned whether it should be called a system (Shelton, 2000; Wimberley and Rubens, 2002). Nonetheless, the two-component U.S. entrepreneurial health service system has been superb in developing medical technology, techniques (which increases costs), and new drugs (which also increases costs), has produced a sufficient and well-educated and trained workforce, and has sufficient physical facilities as well as many other wonderful attributes and innovative programs (Pohl, 2002). On the other hand, for all its resources and expenditures, the U.S. system does not serve everyone nor does it produce the best outcomes on some basic health measures compared to other wealthy industrialized nations. In line with entrepreneurial thinking, when it costs more to produce something in the United States costs more to produce, and the local product does not perform better in important measurable outcome than comparable foreign products, innovation has to occur to remain competitive. The point is that there are lessons to be learned from other health service systems. All health service systems continue to evolve as they seek means of balancing the influences of social responsibility and finite resources. Payers, providers, and consumers need to be vigilant when proposed changes are under discussion. Part of this vigilance is to investigate what has occurred in health service systems that have already implemented similar changes. PTs, PTAs, and other health service personnel including rehabilitation service managers need to be knowledgeable about potential effects of proposed health service system legislation so they may take actions as advocates for or against changes that they perceive would benefit or harm their stakeholders or themselves.

Advocacy

The ultimate concern of legislators is how people in their district (constituents) will vote in the next election. For constituents the concern is how their elected officials will vote in the future on issues that are important to them. By voting, constituents help elect the individuals they feel will take actions that are in line with their beliefs and are in their best interests. When issues arise that are contentious, and a legislator must make a decision, it is the responsibility of constituents to express their perspectives to their legislator. Supporting a cause is **advocacy**.

To be clear on what constitutes being an advocate here are some synonyms: associate, adherent, backer, defender, friend, champion, and supporter (Kipfer, 2001; Lewis, 1978). We can add promoter and salesperson to the list. There are a variety of ways to take action: as an individual or as a group member, directly (face-to-face), indirectly (phone, e-mail, text message, fax, letter), and regularly or intermittently. The strength of your belief is what underlies and fuels the extent of your advocacy involvement (see Chapter 7).

How Do Federal and State Policies Affect Me as a Student, Clinician, Educator, or Researcher?

Every year, hundreds of bills are introduced and considered by legislators that can affect you personally. With a stroke of the pen in Washington the lives of PTs as professionals and as citizens can be radically changed. Legislative bills may relate to your work, your pay, your community, insurance, grant money, student aid, and your clients. Since the APTA is the professional advocacy organization for PTs it is not surprising that the association's website (www.apta.org) has an advocacy link to inform you of congressional activities, regulatory issues, state government activities, and other matters it deems important to take action on to fulfill its organizational aspirations. APTA staff meet with federal officials regularly to represent the association's stance, to offer advice, to offer criticism of bills, and to learn about the potential issues. The APTA and its state affiliates also offer practical educational courses on issues that are important to the members and their clients as well as how to advocate.

How to Get Involved

Your involvement in things related to political matters is non-partisan. In other words, you do not represent a political party. You do represent your personal interests, your employer's interests, or your profession's interests. The following discussion of advocating focuses on representing professional interests and uses APTA resources.

There are several ways to express your interests and concerns about bills and pending legislation:

- Contribute financially to political action groups
- Join a political action group
- Join a grassroots network
- Respond to e-mail alerts
- Send e-mails and faxes
- Call or write to legislators
- Volunteer for an elected official or someone running for an office
- Meet with legislators who have or can have influence on a matter of interest

Give Money

You can give financial support to a PT group that will collect funds from many contributors and give to legislators believed to be sympathetic to PT's interests. The APTA, through the **Physical Therapy Political Action Committee (PT-PAC)**, and each state chapter, through its local **political action committee (PAC)**, raises and disperses funds to help finance the election or reelection campaigns of political candidates running for office or those in office, respectively. The PT-PAC focuses on federal legislators in the U.S. Senate, U.S. House of Representatives, the vice president, and the president. The Federal Election Commission (Federal Election Commission, 2007) regulates PACs by requiring them to register, setting maximum contributions allowed and stipulating rules about volunteering. State governments also regulate political action contributions through registration, reporting, and constraints on activities.

Join a PAC and Grassroots Network

You can be actively involved in a PAC at either the national or state level, or at both levels. The PT-PAC and a state PAC consist of volunteer PTs and PTAs who contribute their time and skills to raise money and awareness about issues. The PT-PAC is very active at national meetings and is closely aligned with APTA staff that interact with federal legislators. State level PACs function as a committee which reports to the chapter officers and executive director if there is one. The chapter employs one or more lobbyists as a consultant, advisor, and representative to legislators. The PAC members raise money through creative fundraisers such as legislative days, which bring chapter members and their legislators together, as well as through direct solicitation of donations. They make phone calls, write letters, send e-mails, meet with lobbyists, and so on.

A local **grassroots network** consists of geographically dispersed members who, with little notice, make contact with specific colleagues in their local area. Grassroots committee members educate their contacts about the issue, offer suggestions regarding communicating with their legislator, and encourage making contact with the legislator. A grassroots campaign can result in all legislators hearing their constituents views on a pending legislative item. This can have a broad influence on the outcome of voting on the issue of interest. The support history of your PAC to a candidate can be incorporated into any of the activities that follow.

Respond to E-mail Alerts

Legislative issues are dynamic. Things can change from hour to hour. There are times when a deadline is near and all efforts to advocate for your cause are required. This is when an alert is issued. The timing and volume of communications to legislators are critical variables that can inform and influence their vote. Student and active APTA members may elect to receive alerts from the association. Alerts include a summary of the issue(s) and APTA's view. The position and influence of key legislators are described. With this information in mind you are asked to communicate your perspective on the issue to your legislator. Since e-mail is nearly instantaneous it is often the preferred tool. A sample statement that can be modified is provided in addition to hyperlinks to your legislators' e-mail accounts. The legislators' staff members are likely to be the people who read, tally, and summarize the e-mails for their senator or representative. Federal and state legislators are likely to take the views of residents in their districts seriously.

Send E-mails and Faxes

There are times when a legislator uses his or her constituents as survey participants to sample their perspectives on an issue that remains undecided. Similarly, APTA staff may become aware of legislators whom they believe may be influenced by comments from members. Encouragement to share your perspective with specific legislators may come to you through APTA and chapter communications via e-mail, requests posted on the APTA and chapter advocacy site, requests printed in APTA and chapter publications, and phone call requests from grassroots network members. You would be provided with an issue summary, references, the legislator's position and importance in the decision-making structure, APTA or chapter stance, key points, legislator's address, and information about the timing of the decision-making process. Legislators take note of communications from constituents. Communications can be prepared using topic templates or customized. Paraphrasing and adding personal observations and experiences are often encouraged. The important part is that communications accurately reflect the topic, your position, and key talking points. If you are communicating with regard to a broader coordinated advocacy effort, make sure your group is aware of your contact and any response you may get.

Write Letters or Make Phone Calls

Letters and phone calls are more personal means of contacting a legislator than e-mails and faxes. Letter templates are often available from grassroots network members and other sources. Talking points are also provided for voice communications. Letters and phone calls allow more individualized expressions of good or controversial aspects of a bill or pending legislative item. Both require forethought and planning but a phone call gives the legislator or his or her staff member the opportunity to ask questions. If there is a question you cannot answer, offer to get back to the person later. If the offer is accepted you have the responsibility of responding quickly with accurate information. Inform others who are working for the same purpose of the responses you got and the responses you gave.

Volunteer for a Candidate

As an individual you can help a candidate and their election committee by volunteering your time and skills. You could host a neighborhood meeting, hand out materials, help at events, type, get food, provide transportation, and so on. Participation in these activities is not compensated monetarily. The currencies of value are recognition and potential influence. A supporter known to a legislator is likely to gain attention when issues are discussed. If you have been able to share your views on health service matters, and you have added to the candidate's understanding of the issues, you will have established yourself as a useful source of information. In the future, you may be contacted by your legislator or their staff regarding health service issues. If you initiate communication with your legislator you have a common connection to remind them of as you present your views. You would certainly be a preferred representative of your state chapter if there was a need for a face-to-face meeting with your legislator.

Meet with a Legislator

A face-to-face meeting with a legislator of interest is an effective way to get to know the official and vice versa. Find out from APTA or your state chapter which legislator(s) it would be most helpful for you to meet. Get briefed on the issues and get familiar with the legislator's background, voting history, and current stance on the issue. Formulate your questions and views. If you can address the legislator at a speaking engagement, let them know you will make an appointment to visit them and who you represent.

Since it is more comforting to be with like-minded and experienced people when presenting your point of view to legislative staff members or the senator or representative they work for, schedule the meeting along with at least one other advocate. Ideally, one of you should be a constituent in the district the legislator represents. The discussion is shaped by the stage of the bill, your stance for or against it, the legislator's level of power (chairperson of the committee dealing with the bill, sponsor or cosponsor of the bill, undecided, etc.). Once this information is assimilated, arrange for the meeting. Let the legislators staff know the names of those who will attend with you. A successful meeting encompasses the following:

1. Dress well and arrive on time.
2. Introduce everyone to the legislator or staff member.
3. Be respectful, use the legislator's official title when addressing them.
4. Listen and respond, but don't argue.
5. State your case clearly.
6. Answer the questions that you can.
7. Offer to follow up on unanswered questions.
8. Leave your contact information.
9. Follow up as promised.
10. Send a handwritten thank you note.
11. Reflect on your interaction; accomplishments and areas for improvement.
12. Report on your visit to the APTA if the visit was related to a national issue or to your state chapter officers, lobbyist, and PAC and grassroots committee chairpersons if it was a state issue.

Summary

The U.S. health service system is unique in that there is a duality of driving forces: governmental and private. Currently, a PT can treat publicly funded patients, either by working as a government employee in a government-owned facility or treating patients whose treatment is paid for by the government. Alternatively, a PT can work in privately owned environments and treat patients who have private insurance, government insurance, or pay out of their own pocket. This is why a fundamental understanding of the motivations underlying each component of the U.S. system will be useful as you learn to deal with the idiosyncrasies of each component.

This chapter painted a broad picture of the physical therapy workforce of today and the near future in the United States. Attention was given to immigration and migration rules relevant to PT clinicians and managers. Mobility of E.U. citizens and educational goals of the ER-WCPT were given attention for their potential impact on the U.S. job market. A structure for analyzing cross-national health service systems was used to describe and compare them.

Basic facts on each system were drawn from private international organizations to facilitate making comparisons. Whenever possible, information specific to physical therapy students, clinicians, and managers was included.

Using primarily seven criteria, i.e., socioeconomic philosophy, accessibility, organization, management, financing, satisfaction, and to a lesser extent, health-related outcomes, five general health service systems were defined, compared, and contrasted. Four continue to exist. Of these health service systems three provided nearly universal health service access for their constituents: Germany, the U.K., and Canada. The only advanced industrialized nation without health insurance for all citizens is the United States. Major issues common to all nations involve the availability of timely, appropriate, and affordable health services, how to fund health services, and how to assess that the level of the quality of services. No nation has a perfect system—one that is low-cost, covers everyone, and delivers exceptional quality based on important criteria.

In democratic countries like the United States, legislators are elected. For quality health services to become available to more people it would be in the best interest of PTs and PTAs to become advocates. This includes actively advocating for candidates who indicate willingness to improve health services and advocating to elected officials for social justice.

CASE STUDY 1.1

Immigration

A guest speaker is making a presentation in a class or at a professional meeting on culture and health services. Her opinion is that there should be legislation aimed at increasing the number of immigrants and nonimmigrants with health service education and experience for the next five years. Foreign-trained PTs are included in the speaker's recommendation. Reflect on what she is saying, then formulate three answers:

1. the perspective of a new graduate
2. the perspective of a practicing clinician
3. the perspective of a physical therapy department manager whose department has had staff openings the past several years

Discuss your perspectives with peers. Summarize the discussion.

CASE STUDY 1.2

Employment-Based Health Insurance

In the United States, health insurance has been linked to employment for most workers. Many employers make arrangements for health services for their employees. This linkage however has been weakening because of constant cost increases to the employer. Over the next two years, what are your expectations regarding having health insurance? How much do you expect to contribute to paying for the insurance? Would you opt out of an employer's health insurance plan to increase your take-home pay? If you would, what would you do if you needed health services? Discuss your perspectives with peers. Summarize the discussion.

CASE STUDY 1.3

Social Justice

There are approximately 47 million people with inadequate or no health insurance even though there are federal and state assistance programs for people of certain ages, low income, with certain disabilities, and other categories of need. Discuss your feelings about paying higher federal income taxes to increase revenue for an expansion of the categorical need groups to include uninsured people. Discuss your perspective. Summarize the discussion.

CASE STUDY 1.4

Advocacy

Based on the strength of your personal opinion about immigration or social justice, outline your plan to advocate for your perspective on one of the following topics. You may choose to engage individuals at the state or federal level. Review the advocacy section of this chapter for options to consider.

Building an Advocacy Plan

You need to know how to find out who your legislative representatives are. How will you do this?

It would be informative to know if the APTA or your home state chapter has expressed an opinion on the matter. How will you find out who to ask about this at the APTA office and your home state chapter?

How will you find out if there is a grassroots group to network with and advocate for your perspective?

How will you find out what groups are advocating for your perspective, other than PTs?

Note: Visit thepoint.lww.com/Nosse3e for more cases on topics covered in this chapter.

REFERENCES

Abraham S, Hamilton LH, Co-Chairs. Immigration and America's Future: a New Chapter. New York, NY: Migration Policy Institute. 2006.

About: Canada Online. Nova Scotia's health insurance plan. Available at http://canadaonline. about.com/gi/dynamic/offsite.htm?zi=1/XJ/Ya&sdn=can adaonline&cdn=newsissues&tm=48&gps=384_ 476_994_560&f=00&tt=14&bt=1&bts=0&zu= http%3A//www.gov.ns.ca/health/msi.htm. Accessed 3/03/07.

American Physical Therapy Association. In the best interests of the patient. Physical Therapy. 2006; 86:1541–1553.

American Physical Therapy Association. 2005 fact sheet: Physical therapist education programs. Available at http://www.apta.org/AM/Template.cfm?Section= Home&TEMPLATE=/CM/ContentDisplay.cfm& CONTENTID=23836. Accessed 1/24/07a.

American Physical Therapy Association. 2005 fact sheet: Physical therapist assistant education programs. Available at http://www.apta.org/AM/Template. cfm? Section=Home&TEMPLATE=/CM/Content Display.cfm&CONTENTID=22993. Accessed 1/28/07b.

American Physical Therapy Association. Commission on Accreditation in Physical Therapy Education [CAPTE]. Available at http://www.apta.org/AM/ Template.cfm?Section=CAPTE1&Template=/Tagged Page/TaggedPageDisplay.cfm&TPLID=65&Content ID=20194. Accessed 1/20/07c.

American Physical Therapy Association. Information for: Consumers. Available at http://www.apta.org/AM/ Template.cfm?Section=A_Career_in_Physical_ Therapy&Template=/APTAAPPS/StudentPrograms/ ptprogramselect.cfm. Accessed 1/20/07d.

American Physical Therapy Association. APTA guide for professional conduct Available at http://www.apta. org/AM/Template.cfm?Section=Core_Documents1&

Template=/CM/HTMLDisplay.cfm&ContentID=24781. Accessed 1/20/07e.

American Physical Therapy Association. Guide for conduct of the physical therapist assistant. Available at Http://www.apta.org/AM/Template.cfm?Section=Core_Documents1&Template=/CM/HTMLDisplay.cfm&ContentID=23731. Accessed 1/20/07f.

American Physical Therapy Association. International affairs. Available at http://www.apta.org/advocacy/internationalaffairs. Accessed 8/15/02.

American Physical Therapy Association. International opportunities in Physical Therapy. Alexandria, VA: American Physical Therapy Association. 2000.

American Physical Therapy Association. Guide to Physical Therapist Practice, 2nd ed. Physical Therapy. 2001;81:9–744.

Anderson GF, Hussey PS. Multinational comparisons of health systems data 2000. Available from http://www.cmwf.org/publist/publist2. Accessed 8/22/02.

Austin SE. Medical justice: A guide to fair provision. New York, NY: Peter Lang. 2001.

Bergman R. Theology in the pit of the stomach. Creighton University Window. 1998;15(1):16–21.

Berk ML, Gaylin DS, Schur CL. Exploring the public's views on the health care system: A national survey on the issues and options. Health Affairs. 2006;25:595–606.

Bloor K, Maynard, A. Universal coverage and cost control. The United Kingdom National Health Service. In Thai KV, Wimberley ET, McManus SM, eds. Handbook of international health care systems. New York, NY: Marcel Dekker. 2002:261–286.

Blumenthal D. Controlling health care expenditures. New England Journal of Medicine. 201;344:766–769.

Boufford JI, Lee PR. Health Policies for the 21st Century: Challenges and Recommendations for the U.S. Department of Health and Human Services. New York, NY: Milbank Memorial Fund. 2001.

Bourhanskaia EA, Kubataev A, Paterson MA. Russia's health care system: Caring in a turbulent environment. In Thai KV, Wimberley ET, McManus SM, eds. Handbook of international health care systems. New York, NY: Marcel Dekker. 2002:59–78.

Brennan T, Reisman L. Value-based insurance design and the next generation of consumer-driven health care. Health Affairs. Available at http://content.healthaffairs.org/cgi/content/full/hlthaff.26.2.w204v1/DC1. Accessed2/22/07.

Brinton C, Christopher JB, Wolff RL. A history of civilization 1715 to the present, Volume Two, 3rd ed. Englewood Cliffs, NJ: Prentice-Hall. 1967.

Bureau of Economic Analysis. Glossary GDP. Available at http://www.bea.gov/glossary/glossary.cfm. Accessed 6/22/07.

Bureau of Labor Statistics. Occupational employment and wages, May 2007, physical therapists. Available at http://data.bls.gov/cgi-bin/print.pl.oes291123.hmt. Accessed 1/07/09a.

Bureau of Labor Statistics. Occupational employment and wages, May 2007, physical therapist assistants. Available at http://www.bls.gov/OES/current/oes312021.hmt. Accessed 1/07/09b.

Bureau of Labor Statistics. Occupational Outlook Handbook, 2008-09 Edition, physical therapists. Available at http://bls.gov/oco/ocos080.htm. Accessed 1/07/09c.

Bureau of Labor Statistics. Occupational Outlook Handbook, 2008-09 Edition, physical therapist assistants and aides. Available at http://bls.gov/oco/ocos167.htm. Accessed 1/07/09d.

Busse R, Riesberg A. Health care systems in transition: Germany. Available at http://www.euro.who.int/document/e68952.pdf. Accessed 3/03/07.

Canadian Health Coalition. Romanow commission on the future of health care. Available at http://www.healthcoalition.ca/romanow.html. Accessed 3/03/07.

Canadian Institutes for Health Information. Private insurance represents 13% of health care spending in Canada-twice the OECD average. Available at http://secure.cihi.ca/cihiweb/dispPage.jsp?cw_page=media_26jun2006_e. Accessed 2/20/07a.

Canadian Institutes for Health Information. Informing wait time benchmarks. Available at http://www.irsc.gc.ca/e/31591.html. Accessed 3/03/07b.

Canadian Physiotherapy Association. Improved wait times are only the beginning. Available at http://www.physiotherapy.ca/public.asp?WCE=C=47 K=222578RefreshT=222599RefreshS=LeftNav RefreshD=2225995. Accessed 3/03/07a.

Canadian Physiotherapy Association. Information. Available at http://www.physiotherapy.ca/PublicUploads/222539Direct%20Access.pdf.

Center on Budget and Policy Priorities. Number of uninsured Americans is at an all-time high. Available at http://www.cbpp.org/8-29-06health.htm. Accessed 3/04/07.

Chartered Society of Physiotherapy. Mutual recognition of professional qualifications (2006). Available at http://csp.org.uk/director/newsandevents/physioalerts.cfm?item_ID=75816CE4CBF42C41280828509FED A1BD&module=news&cat=837AA4E9D632ED7770 EC464DD575FDE1. Accessed 1/24/07a.

Chartered Society of Physiotherapy. Job escalator. Available at http://csp.org.uk/director/careersand learning/physiotherapyjobs.cfm. Accessed 1/31/07b.

Chartered Society of Physiotherapy. NHS agenda for change, pay scales, high cost supplements & on-call allowances 1/4/06-31/3/07. Available at http://www.csp.org.uk/uploads/documents/csp_erusfs01_pay scales1.pdf. Accessed 3/03/07c.

Chartered Society of Physiotherapy. NHS reform: Why we need proper debate. Available at http://www.csp.org.uk/director/newsandevents/physioalerts.cfm?item_id=EE765043D7CB9B50779DEB34FCE688F4. Accessed 3/03/07d.

Congressional Budget Office. Immigration policy in the United States. Available at http://www.cbo.gov/ftpdocs/70xx/doc7051/02-28-1mmigration.pdf. Accessed 1/29/07.

Daniels N. Just Health Care. New York, NY: Cambridge University Press. 1985.

Daniels N, Sabin JE. Setting Limits Fairly: Can we Learn to Share Medical Resources? New York, NY: Oxford University Press. 2002.

Department of Health. Public perceptions of the NHS Winter 2003 tracking survey. Available at http://www.ipsos-mori.com/publications/bp/nhs-tracker.pdf. Accessed 3/02/07a.

Department of Health. Health. Outpatient waiting times: Patients seen following GP written referral and time waited from referral to consultation-Quarter ended 30 September 2003 England. Available at http://www.performance.doh.gov.uk/HPSSS/TBL_B19.HTM. Accessed 3/03/07b.

ETS. TOEFL. Available at http://www.ets.org/portal/site/ets/menuitem.fab2360b1645a1de9b3a0779f1751509/?vgnextoid=69c0197a484f4010VgnVCM10000022f95190RCRD. Accessed 1/28/07.

Eurobarometer. European social reality. Available at http://ec.europa.eu/public_opinion/archives/ebs/ebs_273_en.pdf. Accessed 3/02/07a.

Eurobarometer. Public's satisfaction with health care system, E.U. countries, 2002. Available at http://www.ecosante.org/OCDEENG/67.html. Accessed 2/21/07.

Europa. Paramedical (European Union). Available at http://ec.europa.eu/youreurope/nav/en/citizens/education-study/qualificationrecognition/paramedical/index_en.html. Accessed 1/24/07a.

Europa. Living, working, studying - An overview of your E.U. rights (European Union). Available at http://ec.europa.eu/youreurope/nav/en/citizens/services/eu-guide/rights/index_en.html#14134_1. Accessed 2/04/07b.

Europa. 2000 – today a decade of further expansion. Available at http://europa.eu/abc/history/2000_today/index_en.htm. Accessed 2/04/07c.

Europa. E.U. institutions and other bodies. Available at http://europa.eu/institutions/index_en.htm. Accessed 1/30/07d.

Europa. Overviews of the European Union activities: Public health. Available at http://www.Europa.eu/pol/health/print_overview_en.htm. Accessed 1/03/07e.

European Region of the World Confederation for Physical Therapy. European physiotherapy benchmark statement (2003). Available at http://www.physio-europe.org/pdf/Benchmark.pdf. Accessed 1/24/07a.

European Region of the World Confederation for Physical Therapy. Migration policy for physiotherapists in the European region (2002). Available at http://www.physio-europe.org/download.php?document=73&downloadarea=17&PHYSIOEUROPE=c69d0a8395de98fa0b0c41bca58b512b. Accessed 1/25/07b.

Federal Election Commission. Supporting federal candidates: A guide for citizens. Available at http://www.fec.gov/pages/citn0001.htm. Accessed 3/11/07.

Federated State Boards of Physical Therapy. About us. Available at http://www.fccpt.org/aboutus.html. Accessed 1/28/07a.

Federated State Boards of Physical Therapy. Candidate handbook. Available at http://www.fsbpt.org/download/CandidateHandbook2006.pdf. Accessed 1/23/07b.

Foreign Credentialing Commission on Physical Therapy. Available at http://www.fccpt.org/aboutus.html. Accessed 1/28/07.

Fraser Institute. Hospital waiting times continue to increase: Wait to see a specialist pushed back another week. Available at http://www.fraserinstitute.ca/shared/readmore.asp?sNav=nr&id=550. Accessed 3/03/07.

germanculture.com. Health Insurance. Available at http://www.germanculture.com.ua/library/facts/bl_health_insurance.htm. Accessed 3/02/07.

Gratzer D. The Cure: How Capitalism Can Save American Health Care. New York, NY: Encounter. 2006.

Grogan CM. Federalism and health care reform. American Behavioral Scientist. 1993;36:741–759.

Health and Human Services. HHS: What we do. Available at http://hhs.gov/about/whatwedo. html. Accessed 3/03/07a.

Health and Human Services. Department of Health and Human Services organizational chart. Available at http://www.hhs.gov/about/orgchart.html. Accessed 3/03/07b.

Health Canada. Canada Health Act. Available at http://www.hc-sc.gc.ca/hcs-sss/medi-assur/cha-ics/indexed-eng.php. Accessed 1/07/09.

Health Policy and Administration Section (HPA). International physical therapy opportunities: A resource guide. Available at http://www.aptahpa.org/pdfs/2003CCISIGDirectory.pdf. Accessed 1/30/07a.

Health Policy and Administration Section. Cross-cultural and international SIG. Available at http://www.aptahpa.org/sigs/cultural/index.cfm. Accessed 1/30/07b.

Health Policy and Administration Section. Resource guide for international service in physical therapy education programs. Available at http://www.aptahpa.org/sigs/cultural/CCISIG-Resource-Guide.pdf. Accessed 1/30/07c.

Institute For The Future. Health and health care 2010: The forecast, the challenge. San Francisco, CA: Jossey-Bass. 2000.

International Service. Working in development for International Service. Available at http://www.internationalservice.org.uk/. Accessed 2/01/07.

Jobs Abroad. Your search for physical therapy has yielded 7 Jobs Abroad results. Available at http://www.jobsabroad.com/listings.cfm/interntypeID/83. Accessed 2/04/07.

Kaati PG. Sweden's health care system. In Thai KV, Wimberley ET, McManus SM, eds. Handbook of international health care systems. New York, NY: Marcel Dekker. 2002;287–331.

Kipfer BA. The Original Roget's International Thesaurus, 6th ed. New York, NY: Harper-Collins. 2001.

Kluge EHW. Health care as a right. A brief look at the Canadian health care system. In Loewy E, Loewy RS. Changing health care systems from ethical, economic, and cross-cultural perspectives. New York, NY: Kluwer Academic. 2001;29–48.

Knaul FM, Arreola-Omelas H, Méndez-Camiado O, et al. Health system reform in Mexico 4: Evidence is good for your health system: Policy reform to remedy catastrophic and impoverishing health spending in Mexico. The Lancet. 2006;9549:367–368.

Kovner AR, Jonas S, eds. Jonas and Kovner's Health Care Delivery in the United States, 6th ed. New York, NY: Springer. 1999.

Kronenfeld JJ, Kronenfeld MR. Healthcare Reform in America. Santa Barbara, CA: ABC-CLIO. 2004.

Kronenfeld JJ. The changing federal role in U.S. health care policy. Westport, CN: Kraeger. 1997.

Lattanzi JB, Mastin H, Phillips A. Translation and interpretation services for the physical therapist. HPA Resource. 2006;6:1, 3–5.

Lewis N. The New Roget's Thesaurus in Dictionary Form, Revised ed. New York, NY: G P Putnam's Sons. 1978.

Loewy E. Health care systems and ethics. In Loewy E, Loewy RS. Changing health care systems from ethical, economic, and cross cultural perspectives. New York, NY: Kluwer Academic. 2001:1–14.

Maioni A. A hybrid health-care system. For-profit medicare forays in Quebec raise concerns for public system. Toronto Star. February 2, 2007. Available at http://www.healthcoalition.ca/quebec2tier2.pdf. Accessed 3/03/07.

Marquette University. International opportunities for MUPT students. Available at http://www.marquette.edu/chs/pt/activities/international_opportunities.shtm. Accessed 6/22/07.

Matcha DA. Health Care Systems of the Developed World. How the United States' System Remains an Outlier. Westport, CN: Praeger. 2003.

Miller W. Value-based policy in the United States and the United Kingdom: Different paths to a common goal. National Health Policy Forum. Available at http://www.nhpf.org/pdfs_bp/BP_VBCoveragePolicy_11-29-06.pdf. Accessed 2/22/07.

Morton LW. Health care restructuring: Market theory vs. civil society. Westport CN: Auburn House. 2001.

National Coalition on Health Care. Health care in Germany. Available at http://www.nchc.org/facts/Germany.pdf. Accessed 3/03/07.

National Foundation for Australian Women. Australian Women. Available at http://www.womenaustralia.info/biogs/AWE0056b.htm. Accessed 2/25/07.

National Health Service. NHS in England. Available at http://www.nhs.uk/England/AuthoritiesTrusts/Sha/Default.aspx. Accessed 4/09/07

National Health Service. The NHS explained. Available from http:// www.nhs.uk. Accessed 8/15/02.

Office of Immigration Statistics. 2005 Yearbook of immigration statistics. Available at http://www.dhs.gov/xlibrary/assets/statistics/yearbook/2005/OIS_2005_Yearbook.pdf. Accessed 1/21/07.

Office of NAFTA and Inter-American Affairs. Temporary entry for business purposes. Available at http://www.mac.doc.gov/nafta/chapter16.html. Accessed 2/05/07.

Olsen D. Entrepreneurship: Ownership and private practice physical therapy. In Nosse LJ, Friberg DG, Kovacek PR. Managerial and supervisory principles for physical therapists. Baltimore, MD: Lippincott Williams and Wilkins. 1999:278–298.

Organization for Economic Co-operation and Development. OECD health data 2006. How does Mexico compare. Available at http://www.oecd.org/dataoecd/30/36/36959446.pdf. Accessed 3/01/07a.

Organization for Economic Co-operation and Development. Overview of the OECD: What is it? History? Who does what? Structure of the organisation? Available at http://www.oecd.org/document/18/0,2340,en_2649_201185_2068050_1_1_1_1,00.html#what. Accessed 1/30/07b.

Organization for Economic Co-operation and Development. A system of health accounts. Available at http://www.oecd.org/dataoecd/41/4/1841456.pdf. Accessed 2/21/07c.

Organization for Economic Co-operation and Development. Health at a glance 203-OECD countries struggle with raising demand for health spending. Available at http://oecd.org/Documentprint/0,2744,en_2649_201185_16560422_1_1_1_1_,00.html. Accessed 2/12/07d.

Organization for Economic Co-operation and Development. OECD health data 2006. How does Germany compare. Available at http://www.oecd.org/dataoecd/31/5/36957221.pdf. Accessed 3/02/07e.

Organization for Economic Co-operation and Development. OECD health data 2006. How does the United Kingdom compare. Available at http://www.oecd.org/dataoecd/29/53/36959993.pdf. Accessed 3/02/07f.

Organization for Economic Co-operation and Development. OECD health data 2006. How does Canada compare. Available at http://www.oecd.org/dataoecd/19/13/36956887.pdf. Accessed 3/03/07g.

Organization for Economic Co-operation and Development. OECD health data 2006. How does United States compare. Available at http://www.oecd.org/dataoecd/29/52/36960035.pdf. Accessed 3/03/07h.

Pan American Health Organization. About PAHO. Available at http://www.paho.org/English/PAHO/about_paho.htm. Accessed 1/30/07a.

Pan American Health Organization. Regional core health data initiative. Table generator system. Available at http://www.paho.org/English/SHA/coredata/tabulator/newTabulatorFirst.htm. Accessed 2/20/07b.

Pan American Health Organization. Draft declaration of the Americas on the renewal of primary health care. Available at http://www.paho.org/english/ad/ths/os/phc-regionaldeclaration-sep05.pdf. Accessed 2/01/07c.

Pan American Health Organization. Disabilities: What everyone should know. Available at http://www.paho.org/English/DD/PIN/ptoday17_aug06.htm. Accessed 2/20/07d.

Pan American Health Organization. Indicators glossary. Available at http://www.paho.org/English/SHA/coredata/tabulator/glossary.htm. Accessed 2/20/07e.

Pepper D. U.K. doctors' anger over NHS cash crisis. Lancet. 2006;367:2047–2048.

Pinkston D. Evolution of the practice of physical therapy in the United States. In: Scully RM and Barnes MR, eds. Physical Therapy. Philadelphia, PA: JB Lippincott. 1989.

Pohl CM. The United States health care system. In Thai KV, Wimberley ET, McManus SM, eds. Handbook of international health care systems. New York, NY: Marcel Dekker. 2002;99–133.

Porter ME, Teisberg O. Redefining Health Care. Creating Value-Based Competition on Results. Boston, Mass: Harvard Business School. 2006.

Quadagno J. One Nation Uninsured. Why the U.S. Has No National Health Insurance. NY, NY: Oxford University Press. 2005.

Richmond JB, Fein R. The Health Care Mess. How We Got into it and What it Will Take to Get Out. Cambridge, Mass: Harvard University Press. 2005.

Robertson EC. Major trends in health legislation in Canada 2001–2005. Available at http://www.paho.org/english/DPM/SHD/HP/health-legislat-trends-CAN05.pdf. Accessed 3/03/07.

Rodwin VG. Comparative analysis of health systems: An international perspective. In Kovner AR, Jonas S, eds. Jonas and Kovner's health care delivery in the United States, 6th ed. New York, NY: Springer. 1999:116–151.

Roemer MI. National health systems throughout the world. American Behavioral Scientist. 1993;36:694–708.

Romanow RJ. Interim report 2002. Shape the future of health care. Available from http://www.healthcarecommission.ca. Accessed 8/18/02.

Sawyer KL, Lopopolo R. Perceived impact on physical therapist students of an international pro bono experience in a developing country. Journal of Physical Therapy Education. 2004 (Fall). Available at http://www.findarticles.com/p/articles/mi_qa3969/is_200410/ai_n9463175. Accessed 2/04/07.

Scheuing KM. International service learning program connects communities abroad and on campus. Marquette, the Magazine of Marquette University. 2003;21(3):20–25.

Schoen C, Osborn R, Huynh PT, Doty M, et al. Taking the pulse of health care systems: Experiences of patients with health problems in six countries. Health Affairs. Available at http://content.Healthaffairs.org/cig/cpmtemt/full/hlthaff.w.5.509/DC1. Accessed 11/04/05.

Scott RW. Health Care Malpractice: A Primer on Legal Issues for Professionals, 2nd ed. New York, NY: McGraw-Hill. 1999.

Shelton MW. Talk of power, power of talk: The 1994 health care reform debate and beyond. Westport, CN: Praeger. 2000.

Shi L, Singh DA. Delivering health care in America: A systems approach, 3rd ed. Boston, Mass: Jones and Bartlett. 2004.

Smith JA. Health legislation trends in the United States of America 2001–2005. Available at http://www.paho.org/english/DPM/SHD/HP/health-legislat-trends-USA05.pdf. Accessed 3/03/07.

Swami B. The German health care system. In Thai KV, Wimberley ET, McManus SM, eds. Handbook of international health care systems. New York, NY: Marcel Dekker. 2002:333–358.

University of Colorado. International Health Opportunities. Available at http://www.uch.edu/cancercenter/content/IHOP/default.asp?index=IHOP&title=About%20SGH. Accessed 2/07/07.

U.S. Census Bureau. American community survey. 2005. Available at http://factfinder.census.gov. Accessed 1/21/07.

U.S. Citizenship and Immigration Services. Additional authorization to issue certificates for foreign health care workers [64 FR 23174] [FR 20-99] \ What is the purpose of this interim rule? Available at http://www.uscis.gov/propub/ProPubVAP.jsp?dockey=912b7bc41b422395599ae21229160e56. Accessed 1/28/07a.

U.S. Citizenship and Immigration Services. How do I apply for health care worker certification? Available at http://www.uscis.gov/portal/site/uscis/menuitem.5af9bb95919f35e66f614176543f6d1a/?vgnextoid=c55878a814f0e010VgnVCM1000000ecd190aRCRD&vgnextchannel=48819c7755cb9010VgnVCM10000045f3d6a1RCRD. Accessed 1/23/07b.

U.S. Citizenship and Immigration Services. Certificates for certain health care workers [67 FR 63313] [FR 56-02]. http://www.uscis.gov/propub/ProPubVAP.jsp?dockey=03eb28054c644e6333a870fd1a1ddd1d. Accessed 1/23/07c.

U.S. Citizenship and Immigration Service. INA: ACT 212 - General classes of aliens ineligible to receive visas and ineligible for admission; waivers of inadmissibility. Available at http://www.uscis.gov/propub/DocView/slbid/1/2/31?hilite=. Accessed 1/08/09.

Williams M, Feldman R. Physical therapy education: The feasibility of international collaborative assignments using e-mail. Journal of Physical Therapy Education. 2004 (spring). Available at http://www.findarticles.com/p/articles/mi_qa3969/is_200404/ai_n9399081/pg1. Accessed 2/04/07.

Wimberley ET, Rubens AJ. Like plugging the holes in a colander. Health policy and provision in the United States circa the millennium. In Thai KV, Wimberley ET, McManus SM, eds. Handbook of international health care systems. New York, NY: Marcel Dekker. 2002:135–206.

Wimberley ET, Thai KV. Introduction to international health care systems. Themes and variations on themes. In Thai KV, Wimberley ET, McManus SM, eds. Handbook of international health care systems. New York, NY: Marcel Dekker. 2002:1–28.

Woolhandler S, Himmelstein DU. Paying for national health insurance—And not getting it. Health Affairs. 2002;21:88–98. Retrieved from ABI-INFORM database 8/20/02.

World Confederation for Physical Therapy. WCPT news. Congress focus. Available at http://www.wcpt.org/common/docs/WCPTNews/WCPTNewsJan07.pdf. Accessed 3/03/07.

World Health Organization. About WHO. Available from http://www.who.int/about/en/. Accessed 1/30/07a.

World Health Organization. World health report 2006 Annex table 2: Selected indicators of health expenditure rations, 1999–2003. Available at http://www.who.int/whr/2006/annex/06_annex2_en.pdf. Accessed 2/11/07b.

World Health Organization. World health report 2006 Annex table 3: Selected national health accounts indicators: measured levels of per capita expenditure on health, 1999–2003. Available at http://www. who.int/whr/2006/annex/06_annex1_en.pdf. Accessed 2/03/07c.

ADDITIONAL RESOURCES

A book that specifically addresses physical therapists and cultural competence is Lattanzi JB, Purnell LD. Developing Cultural Competence in Physical Therapy Practice. Philadelphia: FA Davis. 2006.

A free continuing education offering on cross-cultural issues in physical therapy authored by Ronnie Leavitt and titled Developing Cultural Competence in a Multicultural World, Parts 1 & 2 is available at http://www.apta.org/Content/ContentGroups/Education/ContinuingEducation/OnlineCoursesText/CEU_25_Cultural.pdf.

The National Center for Cultural Competence offers numerous free products. One product of interest is an extensive measurement instrument titled Self-assessment of Cultural and Linguistic Competence. Available at http://www11.georgetown.edu/research/gucchd/nccc.

For an in-depth discussion of the status of the U.S. health service system and recommendations for the future there are several books that address the issues with solutions. See references for complete information on books by: Gratzer, 2006; Porter and Teisberg, 2006; Quadagno, 2005; Richmond and Fein, 2005.

For an in-depth international perspective on health service systems read Matcha DA. The journal Health Affairs publishes articles on many topics relevant to PTs and PTAs. Access through a university library subscription or institutional subscription is needed for access to complete articles.

To keep up on U.S. legislation on health services check the Federal Register: access at http://www.gpoaccess.gov/. For examples of international education opportunities (U.K.) access http://www.csp.org.uk. For examples of international work opportunities for experienced PTs access http://www.umn.org.np, http://www.international service.org.uk; http://www.aptahpa.org/sigs/cultural/index.cfm; and http://www.physioihd.com.

CHAPTER 2

OVERVIEW OF THE BUSINESS OF HEALTH CARE DELIVERY

DEBORAH G. FRIBERG AND LARRY J. NOSSE

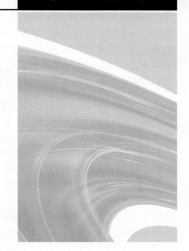

Learning Objectives

1. Define common business terms applicable to the U.S. health care industry.
2. Examine the characteristics that differentiate the U.S. health care market from other consumer markets.
3. Explain the market forces driving the growth of the U.S. health care market.
4. Describe the size and scope of the U.S. health care industry in relation to the U.S. national economy.
5. Explain how the U.S. health care industry operates in terms of who provides services, spending patterns, payment sources, and financial contributors.
6. Explain the economic impact of the U.S. health care industry on our national and local economies as well as on individual households.
7. Discuss what the U.S. health care industry needs to improve performance by addressing specifically the role of the health care leadership and what leaders need to consider in order to improve.
8. Explain current payer initiatives to encourage quality improvement.

Introduction

Chapter 1 provided an overview of the entrepreneurial free market U.S. **health service system** model in relation to other health service system models. The characteristics of different models were discussed in relation to their success at meeting the **health service** needs of the people. In conclusion, all current models pose financial risks but they also have strengths, weaknesses, and opportunities for improvement. There is as yet no perfect delivery model.

In Chapter 2 we turn our attention to the U.S. **health care system**, but this time the focus is on business and economic impact. This statement makes two points:

1. The perspective provided in this chapter is that the provision of health care is a business.
2. The **health care industry** is very important to the U.S. **economy** because of its large workforce as well as the amount of money earned, invested, and spent.

The general characteristics of economic systems, e.g., scarcity, growth, distribution of **services** and **goods**, production, and consumption are used to depict the health care industry. For the current discussion, when we speak of an economy we are referring to the amount of services and goods that are produced and available, how services and goods are distributed, and how many and which types of services and goods are consumed (Gale, 2006). These introductory concepts are built upon in Chapter 20, which deals specifically with economic principles.

This chapter explores the true nature of the U.S. health care **market** and how it differs

Key terms, which are defined below, are bolded and italicized the first time they appear in the chapter. Other important terms are shown in boldface on first appearance and are defined by the context in which they are used. When either of these types of terms is used several times, its acronym will be identified and subsequently used in the chapter. Both types of terms are listed alphabetically in the online glossary with their definitions and (when applicable) their acronyms.

Baldrige criteria: the (Malcolm) Baldrige National Quality Program criteria for health care performance excellence are leadership, strategic planning, focus on patients, other customers, and markets, measurement, analysis, and knowledge management, workforce focus, process management, and results.

Centers for Medicare and Medicaid Service (CMS): a federal agency under the Department of Health and Human Services formerly known as the Health Care Financing Administration (HCFA). This agency is responsible for the Medicare (Title XVIII), Medicaid (Title XIX), SCHIP (Title XXI), and other programs.

coinsurance: after the deductible has been met a proportion of the cost is paid by the individual (coinsurance) with the remainder paid by their health insurance plan. The proportion paid by the individual varies by plan.

co-payment/copay: the amount the individual or a third party, if covered by a supplemental insurance plan, must pay each time services or drugs or both are accessed. Co-payments vary by insurer and by insurance contract.

deductible: the annual amount the individual must pay before their health care plan begins to pay according to the plan's coinsurance stipulations.

evidence-based practice (EBP): the decision of health service professionals to use the most appropriate information available coupled with their clinical expertise to make clinical decisions regarding the care of individual patients.

for-profit (FP): a business entity owned by someone or a group organized for the purpose of making more money than it spends. After expenses and taxes are paid, the owner(s) may use the remaining money as they choose.

free market competition: competition between service and product vendors in the same markets that tends to lead to moderating prices while quality tends to increase.

health care industry/sector: A government and financial industry term for the economic sector related to health care services and products. The economic sector that includes anything and anyone related directly or indirectly to health promotion, injury or disease prevention, and diagnosis or treatment of mental or physical pathologies, impairments and functional limitations, or the production, distribution, or sales of health service goods.

managed care models: health care delivery systems that (1) strive to control the cost of services, (2) utilization of services, (3) regulate access to the services a particular health care plan offers and, (4) maintain or improve their quality.

market economy: an economy characterized by the voluntary exchange between buyers and sellers that is not planned or controlled by any central authority. Also see free-market economy.

Medicaid: also known as Title XIX, Title 19, or T 19. A jointly funded federal and state program that helps with medical costs for some people with low incomes and limited resources. Benefits and eligibility varies state to state.

Medicare: also known as Title Title XVIII, Title 18, or T 18. This is a fee-for-service health insurance plan that lets beneficiaries (those over 65 and some under 65) go to any doctor, hospital, or other health service supplier who accepts Medicare payment as the full payment and is accepting new Medicare patients. There are five parts designated by letters A–D.

not-for-profit/non-profit (NFP/NP): a business or organization whose primary purpose is some form of community service that has been granted tax-exempt status by the Internal Revenue Service. Organizational funds may not provide financial benefit to any private individual. Excess funds must be reinvested to support its community services.

private health care insurance: a health care plan offered by a nongovernment insurer.

self-insured/self-funded: an organization that assumes the risk of covering medical costs for its employees itself rather than purchasing a plan from an insurer. Self-funded plans are allowed by the Employee Retirement Income Security Act (ERISA). Such plans are exempt from state insurance plan laws and regulations.

self-pay/out-of-pocket: paying with personal funds.

(continued)

spending patterns: in health care this includes all money spent for hospital care, physician and clinical services, medical laboratory services, nursing home care, prescription and nonprescription drugs, nondurable medical products, medical, dental, and other professional health care provider services, home health care, and nonpersonal spending like administration expense.

third-party payment/payer system: in the U.S.health service system, most payments are made through health insurance. Services are a three party transaction. The consumer (service recipient who pays the coinsurance, copay, etc.) is the first party in the transaction. The service provider (seller) is the second party, and the health insurance plan (payer) is the third party in the transaction.

from other U.S. **consumer markets**. The U.S. market for health care is like no other U.S. consumer market for services and/or products. In a traditional consumer market, the relationship between **supply and demand** works effectively to control price and limit market growth. The U.S. health care system does not function this way. The majority of U.S. health care consumers have employer- or government-sponsored insurance that pays for their health services. This *third-party payment system* has caused a "disconnect" between price and consumer demand. Another difference is the relationships between **value** (quality/cost), price, and payment. In a typical market, the better the quality, the more the consumer values it and is likely to pay more for it. If quality is less than expected, the consumer may pay less than full price or return the product. *In the health care market, poor quality can and will result in higher prices and payments for services.* These market differences have resulted in runaway growth in the demand for and cost of medical and health services (Porter and Teisberg, 2006). Attempts to control the growth of the medical and health services market have taken the form of *free market competition* as well as regulatory control of competition, **market entry**, investment, and/or price. To date no approach has proven to be effective at controlling the growth and related **expenditures** for medical and health care services (Gaynor and Vogt, 1999). As a result, the medical and health care services industry has grown to become the largest industry in the United States (Bureau of Labor Statistics [BLS], 2007a). Due to its size, this industry is now driving the growth of the U.S. economy and employis more people than any other industry. Many experts believe that our nation's level of investment in health services and products cannot be sustained without grave long-term

economic consequences (Favro, 2006; Heffler et al., 2004).

As this chapter explores the impact U.S. health care businesses have on national and local economies, it also looks at forces driving U.S. **health care providers** to improve their **productivity**. Hence, the reader will appreciate the importance of having health care business managers who are knowledgeable and innovative leaders. The reader also gains an understanding about the businesses and occupations that contribute to the delivery of our nation's health care services and products, where health care dollars are spent, and who spends them. It will become clear that health care industry leaders will need knowledge and skills to lead their businesses through a **transformation**. Health care businesses will need to do more than grow. They will need to adapt to a **pay for performance (P4P)** market where both quality and price will drive consumer choice and only well-managed businesses will be strong enough to survive. Over the next several years, the health care industry can expect intense scrutiny of cost and quality as well as more government policy geared toward slowing growth in the cost of health care. Those who pay for health care will find ways to shift their financial burden to the health care consumer, and provider payments will be linked more closely to quality of services received (The Advisory Board, 2006). It will be up to our industry leaders to address these challenges in innovative ways.

U.S. Economic Market for Health Care

A *market economy* is characterized by the voluntary exchange between buyers and sellers that is not planned or controlled by any central authority. The typical market is a forum for transactions where the buyer, influenced by income and the price of services and goods, will make purchases. The seller, influenced by costs and buyer demand, will determine the supply of services and goods they will offer. The amount of services or goods that a buyer is willing to purchase will typically rise with increases in income and fall with increases in price. The price the purchaser is willing to pay is influenced by their perception of value. By value we mean the relationship between quality and price. The higher the value, the more they are willing to pay. The sensitivity of demand to changes in price is referred to as **price elasticity** (Moffatt, 2007) (Chapter 21).

The market for health care services is atypical in several ways.

- The relationship between the buyer and seller of medical and health services is indirect. The party requesting the health service (e.g., physician, therapist, parent) may be different than the party consuming the health service (e.g., patient) who is often different from the party paying for the health service (e.g., private or public health care insurer), and the payer may be different than the party who funds the bill payer (e.g., employer, government, philanthropist). Often, the health care service customer does not even know the price of the services they are purchasing. *Under these circumstances price becomes meaningless and has no influence on consumer demand* (Porter and Teisberg, 2006).
- The majority of medical and health services provided to consumers are paid for by employer- or government-sponsored health care insurance plans. For those without insurance, access to emergency medical services is guaranteed regardless of the patient's ability to pay under the **Emergency Medical Treatment and Active Labor Act (EMTALA)** and other government-sponsored programs (Chapter 9). Other nonemergency services may be provided through charity care programs. *Under this system income becomes less meaningful and has limited influence on consumer demand.*
- Depending on the circumstances, the purchase of health care may not be considered to be a discretionary purchase regardless of the price or income.

- It is hard for the consumer to judge the technical quality of the medical and health care services they receive. The quantity of services received, interpersonal interactions, speed of service, easy access, personal convenience, consumer amenities, the latest technology, and the physical appearance of the health care service facilities are often used as surrogate measures of quality and overall value (Chapter 6).
- Health service providers are driven by this unlimited demand to provide more services with higher consumer amenities. Supply often exceeds consumer demand. The health care provider can cover the cost of providing extra **market capacity** by charging higher prices. *This works because the price of medical and health services does not impact consumer demand* (Porter and Teisberg, 2006).
- Payment for medical and health services is not tied to value (quality/cost) being delivered. In fact, it can be just the opposite. For example, a patient who acquires an infection while in the hospital will pay more for their hospital stay than a patient who experiences an uncomplicated stay. *The current payment system actually rewards health service providers for providing inefficient or ineffective care* (Porter and Teisberg, 2006).

As a result of these market characteristics, the consumer demand for health care has no market-driven barriers and the demand for medical and health services is essentially unlimited. Unlimited demand creates a pressure on the medical and health services industry to continually increase supply. No wonder the U.S. medical and health services market has continued to grow unchecked.

Scope and Size of the U.S. Health Care Industry

As physical therapists, the authors are particularly interested in the management and provision of **direct care** to consumers. Because of this bias, we have often used direct-care-related terms such as *medical and health services, health services,* and *health care services,* as well as nonspecific term *health care.* When government and private investment companies report on the economy they divide the economy into contributing parts called industries. An **industry** is defined as a distinct group of productive or profit-making enterprises (Merriam-Webster, 2001). Government and commercial financial businesses refer to health care services and products as the *health care industry*. The U.S. health care industry is big business. But how big is big? The U.S. health care industry is comprised of several categories, or **sectors**, including direct health care service delivery, pharmaceuticals, health care products, and health insurance. For investment purposes sectors are often divided further into **subsectors**. For example, health care can be divided into a specialized services category that includes rehabilitation, which includes physical therapy businesses (BusinessWeekOnline, 2007). In the broadest sense, the health care industry includes anything and anyone related directly or indirectly to the care of consumers. This includes health promotion, injury or disease prevention, and diagnosis or treatment of mental or physical pathologies, impairments and functional limitations, or the production, distribution, sales, and application of health service goods. In addition to the direct care professionals and technicians, this broad definition includes faculty who educate health care–related personnel and provide for their clinical training, health care facility architects and construction companies, manufacturers and vendors of health care equipment and supplies, as well as support personnel such as security, sales clerks, cooks, and volunteers. The industry also includes an array of consultants, which includes accountants, attorneys, insurance and risk management representatives, and technical experts (Chapters 1, 9, 13, and 22).

U.S. gross domestic product (GDP) is a measure of the output of services and goods produced by labor and property in the United States as calculated by the U.S. Bureau of Economic Analysis (2007). This agency produces the GDP-by-industry accounts, a set of accounts that present the contribution of each private industry and government to the nation's GDP. An industry's contribution is a measure of its size relative to other U.S. industries and the government. According to data released in 2006 by the *Centers for Medicare and Medicaid Services (CMS)*, in fiscal year (FY) 2005 U.S. expenditures for all sectors of the health care industry rose 7.2% to $2.0 trillion dollars or $6,697 per person. That represented 16.0% of the total U.S. GDP (CMS, 2007a). As a point of reference, during the same period, total **federal revenues**, which equal federal receipts minus contributions of government social insurance, represented 16.3% of total U.S. GDP (California Health Care Foundation [CHCF], 2007).

Given the amount of money the United States spends on health care it should be no wonder that the business of health care is of significant national concern. Business activity of the U.S. health care industry can be better understood by examining:

- Who provides health care services (health care providers)
- Where the money is spent (*spending patterns*)
- Who pays health care bills (payment source)
- Who finances the bill payers (financial contributors)

Health Care Providers

Health care providers include places where care is given, such as a hospital and the people who provide the care, e.g., physical therapists. According to the BLS (2007a) the health care industry comprises more than 545,000 business establishments that vary greatly in size and structure. Health care is our nation's largest industry, providing more than 13.1 million jobs. In addition, there is a multiplier effect. In 2004, hospitals represented 2% of all establishments, but employed 40% of all health care workers. The **American Hospital Association (AHA)** projects that every hospital job supports another 1.6 additional jobs due to the related and unrelated business activity generated by the hospital and the people it employs (AHA, 2006). The remaining health care provider business establishments include nursing and residential care facilities, physician and dental offices, home health providers, offices of other health practioners, outpatient centers, ambulatory health care services, and medical/diagnostic laboratories. These businesses range greatly in size from single employee businesses to health systems that employ thousands of people in diverse positions. It would not be unusual for a large health system to employ individuals in over 700 different job titles and nonclinical roles ranging from architects to industrial engineers. The pharmaceutical and medical manufacturing sector is one of the fastest growing of the manufacturing industries. The pharmaceutical sector provides an additional 291,000 jobs (BLS, 2007b).

Health Care Enterprise Ownership

A legal definition of an **owner** is a person who has ownership, control, or proprietorship (Nolan and Nolan-Haley, 1990). Ownership of health care businesses can be classified in several ways (Fig. 2.1). Health care provider **enterprises** owned by the government are known variously as governmental, public, or tax-supported facilities.

Privately owned health care businesses likewise have several designations, however, there are major differences between private **entities**. The first distinction is based on the Internal Revenue Service (IRS) requirements for being classified as a *for-profit* or a *not-for-profit* entity (Chapters 1 and 14). A for-profit entity

is formed to make a profit. The owner(s) of a for-profit organization may take the profit for their own use. Shares of stock in some for-profit corporations may be offered for sale to the public through stock exchanges. Such corporations are known as publicly traded corporations. Owners of shares are **stockholders**. Stockholders buy shares with the expectation that they will earn dividends while they own the shares and a profit when they sell their shares. Taxes are paid by corporations as well as by the individuals who gain from the operation of for-profit businesses. There are also some private businesses that provide health care services directly to their employees and their employees' dependents (e.g., SAS, Raleigh, North Carolina).

The IRS may also designate health service businesses as not-for-profit. Not-for-profit businesses have the same business need to make more than they spend in order to grow and improve their offerings to their constituents. The difference between for-profit and not-for-profit status lies in the rules governing the distribution of business profits

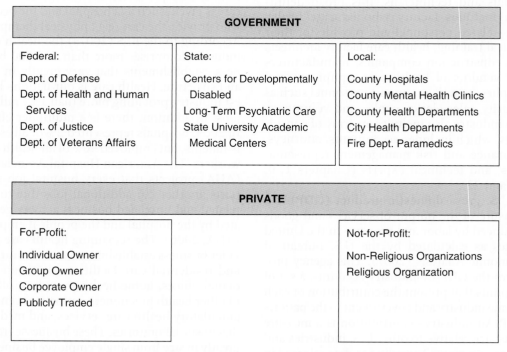

Figure 2.1. Centers for Medicare and Medicaid Services (2007h): Health care spending by payment sources.

or losses. Other than the receipt of market competitive compensation for services provided, no individual or group of individuals are allowed to benefit from a not-for-profit business. A not-for-profit entity is required to invest profits back into the not-for-profit business rather than provide income to its stockholders. Not-for-profit businesses are tax exempt (Chapter 4). Charities (e.g., Shriners), religious groups (e.g., Catholics), and businesses formed to help the community at large are often not-for-profit. Not-for-profit associations or corporations are formed for reasons other than for making a profit (IRS, 2007). These reasons usually are associated with meeting the needs of a particular community or constituency (Nolan and Nolan-Haley, 1990).

Health Care Provider Occupations

The U.S. Department of Labor (2007) categorizes the numerous health occupations as follows:

1. **Management**, business, and financial occupations includes executives, business owners, marketing and sales managers, and health services mangers.
2. Professional and related occupations—includes professionals such as nurses, pharmacists, social workers, dental hygienists, industrial engineers, biochemists, microbiologists, chemists, and computer systems analysts. Therapists accounted for 2.7% of jobs in this category.
3. Sales and related occupations—includes sales representatives.
4. Production occupations—include occupations such as assemblers, chemical plant operators, testers, packing and filling machine operators, and inspectors.
5. Service occupations—includes occupations such as home health aides, nursing aides, food preparation, and service occupations.
6. Office and administrative support occupations—includes occupations such as billing clerks, medical secretaries, bookkeepers, shipping and receiving clerks, secretaries, and receptionists.
7. Transportation and material moving occupations—includes laborers and material movers.

Health Service Spending Patterns

Figure 2.2 shows 2005 U.S. health care spending by category. Based on 2005 data, spending on personal health accounts for greater than 79% of all health service expenditures. The major spending categories as defined by the North American Industrial Classification System and the Standard Industrial Classification System (CMS, 2007b) include:

1. Hospital care. Includes all services provided by public and private hospitals to patients. The value of hospital services is measured by **net revenue**. Net revenue is equal to gross patient charges less **contractual adjustments**, **bad debt**, and charity care. It includes **nonoperating** and nonpatient **revenues (Chapter 21)**.
2. Physician and clinical services. Covers services provided in establishments operated by Doctors of Medicine (M.D.) and Doctors of Osteopathy (D.O.), outpatient care centers, and portions of medical laboratories services that are billed independently by the laboratories.
3. Nursing home care. Covers services provided in private and public freestanding nursing home facilities.
4. Prescription drugs and nondurable medical products. Covers the retail sales of prescription drugs, nonprescription drugs and medical sundries.
5. Dental and other professionals. Covers services provided by a Doctor of Dental Medicine (D.M.D.) or Doctor of Dental Surgery (D.D.S.) or a Doctor of Dental Science (D.D.Sc.).
6. Home health care. Covers medical services provided by private and public non-facility-based home health care agencies (HHAs).
7. Nonpersonal spending. Includes **administration expense**, investment, and government public health activities.

Health Care Payment Sources

Figure 2.3 shows health care paid for by direct payment source for the same period. *Private health insurance* paid the greatest portion followed closely by tax supported *Medicare, Medicaid,* and the **State Children's Health**

Spending Category	Percent
Hospital Care	30
Physician and Clinical Services	21
Nursing Home	6
Prescription Drugs	10
Dental and Other Professional	10
Home Health	2
Program Administration and Net Cost	7
Other Spending	14

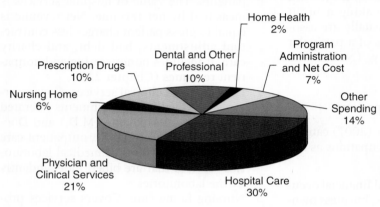

2005 Health Care Spending by Category

Home Health 2%

Program Administration and Net Cost 7%

Dental and Other Professional 10%

Prescription Drugs 10%

Nursing Home 6%

Other Spending 14%

Physician and Clinical Services 21%

Hospital Care 30%

Figure 2.2. Centers for Medicare and Medicaid Services (2007h) estimates of health care spending by category.

2005 Health Care Spending by Payment Source	Percent
Medicaid and SCHIP	16
Medicare	17
Out-of-Pocket	13
Private Insurance	35
Other Private	7
Other Public	13

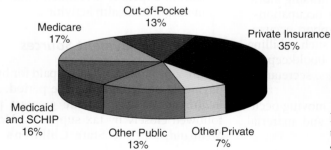

2005 Health Care Spending by Payment Source

Out-of-Pocket 13%

Medicare 17%

Private Insurance 35%

Medicaid and SCHIP 16%

Other Public 13%

Other Private 7%

Figure 2.3. U.S. health care system categorized by ownership with selected examples.

Insurance Program (SCHIP). Health service consumers pay for 13% of the service directly. Payments received directly from the consumer are referred to as *out-of-pocket* or *self-pay* **payments** (CMS, 2007b).

Private health insurance payment for health service is calculated by subtracting the insurer's cost of doing business, including the cost of paying health care bills for covered conditions and administrative costs, from the **premiums** earned. Private health insurance pays for 35% of health care bills (CMS, 2007a).

According to the Department of Health and Human Services (HHS; HHS, 2007) the original Medicare program, also known as Title 18 of the Social Security Act, (T 18 for short) is a **fee-for-service** health plan that allows **beneficiaries** visit any doctor, hospital, or other health service supplier who accepts Medicare and is accepting new Medicare patients. The beneficiary must pay the *deductible*. Medicare pays its share of the Medicare-approved amount, and the beneficiary pays their share (*coinsurance*). In some cases the beneficiary may be charged more than the Medicare-approved amount. This is discussed in detail in Chapters 20–22. The original Medicare Plan has two parts: **Part A** (hospital insurance) and **Part B** (medical insurance) (HHS, 2007). The Medicare program has expanded since its inception and now offers coverage through private insurers, in both fee-for-service and *managed-care models*. Under a fee-for-service model, Medicare pays for their beneficiary health services based on a preset fee schedule that the health care provider agrees to accept. The beneficiary may use any participating provider. Under the managed-care model, the beneficiary selects a managed-care plan and agrees to use only those providers included in the managed-care plan's **provider panel**. Medicare pays the managed-care plan a set fee per beneficiary. The managed-care plan pays the health provider based on the terms of the provider's contract with the managed-care plan. For more information on insurance see Additional Resources section at the end of this chapter.

Medicaid is a joint federal and state program that helps with medical costs for some people with low incomes and limited resources. *Medicaid programs vary from state to state,* but most

health care costs are covered if you qualify for both Medicare and Medicaid (CMS, 2007c).

SCHIP is a CMS-administered program that was established by **Title XXI** of the Social Security Act and is jointly financed by the federal and state governments and administered by the states. Within broad federal guidelines, each state determines the design of its program, eligibility groups, benefit packages, payment levels for coverage, and administrative and operating procedures. SCHIP provides a capped amount of funds to states on a matching basis for federal fiscal years 1998–2007 and extended to March 2009 (National Conference of State Legislatures, 2008). Federal payments under Title XXI to states are based on state expenditures under approved plans effective on or after October 1, 1997 (CMS, 2007d).

Out-of-pocket (self-pay) payments represent direct cost to the health care consumer. These include payments made for all health care services and goods including insurance-related payments paid by consumers from their own resources. Common out-of-pocket charges are:

- *The deductible*: the annual amount the individual must pay before the health care plan begins to pay according to the **health insurance plan**'s coinsurance stipulations
- *Coinsurance*: after the deductible has been met a proportion of the cost is paid by the individual with the remainder paid by their health insurance plan. For example, after a $300 deductible is paid, 25% of the additional costs are paid by the individual and 75% are paid by the insurance plan. Plans may have a maximum after which they will pay 100% of additional costs incurred by the insured patient.
- *Copayment*: the amount the individual must pay each time services or drugs or both are accessed.

Other public spending covers programs such as **workers' compensation**, public health spending, Department of Defense, Veterans Affairs, Indian Health Services, state and local subsidies, and school health programs. Other private spending includes industrial in-plant, privately funded construction, and nonpatient revenues including philanthropy (CMS, 2007a).

Health Care Financial Contributors

The financial burden for the $2 trillion dollars per year spent on health care service falls on businesses, households, and the government. Ultimately, it is up to these contributors to health care spending to determine what health care insurance coverage is offered, who is eligible, the terms of eligibility, and how much the individual consumer will have to pay out of pocket for the coverage offered and services they use. As the cost of health care rises the financial burden grows. Health care expenditures have been growing as a percentage of GDP each year, from 13.8% of GDP in 2000 to 16.0% in 2005. Growth in health care spending is projected to continue (CHCF, 2007; CMS, 2007a). As health care costs rise, the choices these financial contributors make and the public policy that shapes them can be expected to change as well.

Employers

For many people less than 65 years of age, health insurance is a work-related benefit that is fully or partially paid for by employers (Chapter 1). Employers may purchase insurance from a health insurance plan, directly from health care providers, or pay for health care costs for employees from company funds set aside for this purpose. This latter method is called being *self-insured* or *self-funded*. When self-insured, the employer assumes the risk for covering medical and other costs rather than purchasing health insurance (Kongstvedt, 2002). Employers also bear the cost for the Workers' Compensation program. There is a separate set of workers' compensation laws in each state to cover nonfederal employees. These laws are designed to:

- Deal with payment of wages lost because of incapacitation
- Deal with payment for medical treatment
- Ensure that employees who are injured or disabled from job-related events are awarded a fixed amount in lieu of suing
- Ensure that there are death benefits for dependents of workers who die from work-related illnesses or accidents

"Each state develops its own workers' compensation laws, which produces state-to-state variations in the dollar amount of awards and other program areas" (Department of Labor, 2007). No state law covers all workers. Employers can buy insurance through contributions to a state fund, purchase insurance from commercial sources, or self-insure. Depending on the state, employers may have all three options. See Additional Resources at the end of this chapter for more detailed information on workers' compensation statutes for each state.

The business portion of total health care spending has been relatively stable at 26% but has increased in real dollars as total expenditures have grown. The majority of expense is related to the purchase of private health insurance plans for employees. Employers have been actively working to control the cost of health care benefits by promoting managed care plans as an alternative to fee-for-service insurance plans. Employers have also focused on insurance plan redesigns that shift an increasing amount of the financial burden onto employees through higher coinsurance and deductible payments (CMS, 2007e).

Government

The federal government's financial burden has grown faster than that of other contributors because of the growth in the tax-funded Medicare and Medicaid programs. Health care expenditures, as a percent of federal revenues, grew from 17.3% in 2000 to 30.0% in 2005. As this financial burden has grown the health care industry has seen substantial changes in Medicare and Medicaid payment methodology and payment levels. For example, changes that resulted from the adoption of the Balanced Budget Act of 1997 were projected to result in a $116.4 billion dollar federal spending reduction (Congressional Budget Office, 1997). In this regard, the government is the proverbial 800-pound gorilla. Because consumers with government health insurance represent the largest portion of the health care market few providers can afford to forego the patient volume that they represent. However, the rules governing provider participation in government-sponsored health plans carry the force of law. This means that the government can pay providers whatever they want for the health care provided to the Medicare and Medicaid beneficiaries. *For most providers the amount the government pays for health care is less than the cost of providing the care they purchase.* The payment deficit created by government is shifted to other purchasers of health care including employers and households. As an employer, the federal government has been less successful at controlling the growth in cost of providing health care insurance to its employees (CMS, 2007e).

Individual state and local governments are engaged in a variety of health care activities. All 50 states have public health authorities. The focus of local public health agencies is on the health of the population. Interventions typically include disease prevention and education programs, plans for dealing with epidemics, and other emergencies. There are also state-run health care institutions for individuals with developmental disabilities, psychiatric problems, those who are in prison. At the local level there are tax-supported community health centers, clinics, and city and county hospitals for the care of eligible residents (CMS, 2007e).

Household

Households have seen a decline in percentage of total expenditures; but the true financial burden of out-of-pocket health care expenditures is on the rise. Over the same 2000–2005 period, the share of household health spending to personal income has grown from 5.3% to 6.0%. Households are spending more of their income on health services and have less money to cover other costs (CMS, 2007c). The increase in household spending can be directly attributed to a decline in the number of employers offering health service coverage and employer efforts to transfer some of their financial burden to the employee through increased deductibles, coinsurance, and copayments. Indirectly, these trends can be attributed to the rising cost of health services (Clemans-Cope, 2006).

Economic Impact of the Health Care Industry

In Chapter 1 the reader learned that the United States spends more money on health care than any other country. The relationship between health care spending growth and the U.S. economy is inherently complex and multidimensional. Depending on the point of view, growth of health care spending can be described as having a negative impact on the U.S. economy or as a driver of local and regional economic prosperity (Office of the Assistant Secretary of Planning and Evaluation [ASPE], 2007). In fact, the economic impact of the medical and health services industry on the U.S. economy are mixed. To understand how that might happen, let's look at some of the impacts. Since 1998, health care spending has increased at a faster growth rate than the GDP, the rate of inflation, and overall population (Pauly, 2003). Efforts to control health care spending have been numerous but have been largely unsuccessful. Changes in health care utilization, population demographics, price inflation, and advances in medical technology are all factors that contribute to spending growth (The Lewin Group, 2002; Newhouse, 1993). Some economists suggest that rising health care spending has the effect of lowering the rate of growth in GDP and employment, while increasing inflation (Monaco and Phelps, 1995). The economic arguments are:

- Businesses unable to absorb the growing cost of health care benefits may opt to reduce wages, increase work hours, reduce the workforce, not replace employees who quit, and/or increase the number of part-time and temporary workers. Practical experience has shown that health care cost increases are in fact offset by direct wage reductions, cost shifting to employees, or, where wages are fixed, increases in the number of working hours (Goldman et al., 2003).
- Businesses may need to cover increased costs by charging higher prices. In 2007, General Motors estimated that providing health insurance for its workers and retirees added $1,500 to the price of cars built in the United States (Froetschel, 2009).
- Business leaders responding to a 2004 survey identified employee health care costs as their foremost cost concern (Business Roundtable, 2007). The 2006 Kaiser/Hewitt survey on retiree health benefits found that the employer cost of providing health benefits to retirees increased an average of 12.7%

from 2003 to 2004 (Kaiser Family Foundation, 2007).

- The burden of government health care spending is reflected in higher taxes and/or increases in the government's long-term borrowing. As government borrowing increases, it negatively impacts the availability of resources for other activities and drives up interest rates (the cost of borrowing) for businesses and households. As the cost of borrowing increases, business and personal investments are deferred (ASPE, 2007).

- Federal, state, and municipal governments facing health care costs that are increasing more rapidly than revenues will scrutinize all discretionary spending more closely. Employers, to counter the rising health care expenditures, may cut other **expenses**, reduce wage increases, reduce health insurance benefits, or require employees to pay a greater share of the costs. As more costs are shifted to consumers, they will weigh the value of health care services more closely against other purchases (ASPE, 2007).

- Consumers with employer-sponsored health insurance may experience reductions in real wages or growth in wages. Household finances will be affected as fewer resources are available for purchasing consumer goods, savings, education, or retirement. For less affluent households, this could result in forcing tradeoffs between health care and other normal necessities of living. A 2003 survey found that 63% of families reported problems with paying medical bills as well as paying for other household necessities, such as food, clothing, and rent (May and Cunningham, 2004).

- Households may also benefit from increased health spending through improved health status, increased access to care, wage and employment growth in the health care sector, and improved local economic activity. Improvements in health status may have a positive economic impact on households through increased productivity, reduced absenteeism, and enhanced independence.

- "One American's rising medical spending is another American's rising income" (Pauly, 2003, pp. W3–16). The health sector is a significant source of employment for American workers, employing 13.1 million workers (BLS, 2007a).

- At a local level, health care spending growth is more likely to be viewed as beneficial. It creates health care jobs, increases wages for health care workers, expands local tax revenues, and increases demand for related services and goods (Business Roundtable, 2007).

The experts believe that the impact of health care on the U.S. economy is double-sided. On one side there are those who see the growth in health care spending as an economic driver, powering the majority of growth in our national economy. On the other hand, there are those that see the negative impact of this same growth in spending on the viability of other industries and the overall economy. On balance there does seem to be agreement that U.S. health care businesses need to reduce their cost of **operations**, be more productive with the resources they have, be more accountable for delivering quality care, and do so at a reasonable price (Favro, 2006). Health care industry experts estimate that the costs of delivering medical and health services will have to decrease by as much as 30% while demand for services continues to escalate (The Advisory Board, 2006). Payers will continue their efforts to tie payment to performance as defined by measurable patient outcomes (see Chapter 16). Cost related to poor care will no longer be covered (CMS, 2007f). However, there does not seem to be any consensus on how that will be achieved.

Improving the Performance of the U.S. Health Care Industry

Efforts to counter the negative impact of rising health care costs have been unsuccessful to date. Industry leaders will be challenged to reduce costs, improve quality, and improve access, while they find the capital resources and workforce to meet the ever-increasing demand for health care services. Now more than ever medical and health service businesses are being pushed to do more with fewer resources.

There are resources that leaders can turn to for help in meeting this challenge. The

Baldrige National Quality Program, Criteria for Performance Excellence is one of those resources. The Malcolm Baldrige National Quality Improvement Act of 1987, Public Law 100–107, established this program. There are three versions of performance criteria that offer a framework for businesses to use in pursuit of improved overall performance. One version is specifically written for health care businesses. The *Baldrige criteria* cover seven categories including:

Leadership: how leaders guide their organizations and fulfill their citizenship responsibilities.

Strategic planning: how to set strategic directions and action plans.

Customer and market focus: how to determine needs and expectations of customers, how to meet customer expectations and keep them coming back.

Measurement, analysis, and **knowledge management**: how to effectively manage, analyze, use, and improve data and information.

Human resource management: how the workforce is enabled to develop its full potential and their efforts aligned with strategic initiatives.

Process management: how key processes are designed, managed, and improved.

Business results: how the business performs.

These criteria, available through the National Institute of Standards and Technology (NIST), provide leaders with a guide for performance improvement (NIST, 2007). Regardless of the tools used, to be successful, a medical and health service business should have:

- Strong leaders
- Strategic plans
- Good information
- Quality service/product
- Financial resources

Health Care Leadership

Leadership is the key to the future success of the U.S. health care industry. Health care is a business that has a tremendous impact on the nation's health but also on the health of our nation's economy. There should be no doubt that strong leaders are needed to bring about the type of improvement in the health care delivery system that will provide the highest quality of care at an affordable price. While health care businesses are diverse in size and function the roles of their leaders share common characteristics. Leaders are vested with the formal authority to plan, organize, control, and direct an organization in the pursuit of its **mission**, the reason it exists.

According to Mintzberg (1975), leaders fulfill several roles. Their interpersonal role requires them to act as an organization's figurehead, acting as a leader within the organization and a liaison with customers and other parties outside of the organization. In their informational role, leaders monitor internal and external forces impacting organizational performance and, acting as the spokesperson, they disseminate that information to key **stakeholders**. Finally, leaders are decision makers. In this role, leaders act as **entrepreneurs**, they handle disruptions affecting organizational performance, allocate resources, and negotiate on behalf of the organization. In Chapters 11, 16, and 22 more will be said about the concepts of leading and managing the performance of organizations and entrepreneurs, respectively.

According to the BLS (2007c), the outlook for medical and health service managers is a good one. Job opportunities for health care services managers will grow at a faster than average rate through 2014. In 2004, there were about 248,000 individuals employed as medical and health service managers. Private hospitals employed about 30% of these mangers while another 26% worked for private physician offices and nursing care facilities. The remainder were employed by HHAs, federal government health care facilities, ambulatory facilities run by state and local government, outpatient care centers, insurance carriers, and community care centers for the elderly.

Health care managers can be generalists or specialists. **Management generalists** have responsibilities for an entire facility or health system. They often have job titles such as administrator, president, vice president, executive director, or director. Depending on the size of the health care facility or system, a general manger may have more or less direct responsibility for daily operations. In large businesses it is usual to have several assistant general managers (e.g., senior vice presidents, vice presidents, executive directors, etc.) to support the senior general manager (e.g., a president and chief executive officer [CEO]). In a smaller business the senior general manger may have less support and more responsibility for daily running of the business or the business operations.

Management specialists have focused responsibilities for a segment of a business such as a clinical department or health information. Management specialists will usually have specialized training and/or experience in a clinical or business area. Their job will require them to perform more specific duties that relate to those areas of expertise. For example, a manager of rehabilitation services would require expertise and experience in one of the physical rehabilitation fields of physical therapy, occupational therapy, speech therapy, or psychology. A highly specialized or **start-up** health care service business such as a physical therapy private practice may require a leader with the skills of both the generalist and specialist manager to be successful. Chapter 14 deals specifically with organizational design and levels of management, and Chapter 22 provides a more thorough discussion about private practice.

The work life of the health care manager is not an easy one. When compared to other industries, earnings are high but so is the workload (BLS, 2007a). Many medical and health services facilities operate 24 hours a day, 7 days a week 365 days per year. That generally means that managers at all levels have to be "on call" and prepared to respond to everything from a customer concern to a facility flood at all times. In larger facilities with multiple management levels, managers may share being on call with others. In smaller health care businesses a single manager may bear that burden alone. Physical working conditions are usually good but may involve a lot of walking to or driving for managers with multilocation or multisite responsibilities. The need for cost control is also having an impact on the working conditions of health service managers (Chapters 20–22). Health service businesses often constrain the growth (and cost) of management resources while other parts of the business grow. When this happens, man-

agers experience an increased workload often with no change in compensation or resources to get the job done. This cascades down to the individual service-providing departments, such as physical therapy where productivity expectations increase while pay does not.

The U.S. Department of Labor projects that the demand for qualified managers exists in all areas but will be greatest for hospitals and health systems, private practice offices, HHAs, and outpatient care centers. For up-to-date information on the job outlook and earning potential for medical and health services managers refer to the BLS, Occupational Outlook Handbook noted in Additional Resources (BLS, 2007d).

Strategic Plan

The importance of planning in a business is introduced here and planning as a process will continue to be addressed in several upcoming chapters. Basically, a **strategy** is a plan to meet organizational goals. Leaders have several tools that they can use to help them meet their diverse obligations. One of the most important tools is a **strategic plan**. The foundation of the strategic plan is a **mission statement** that clearly defines why the business exists. The strategic plan states in writing the mission of the organization and its **vision** for the future. It defines the business **goals**, **objectives**, and **action plans** that will allow it to meet its mission and achieve its vision of a future state (see Chapter 7). Strategic planning should be a dynamic process continually supported by new information and adjusting the business' actions accordingly. An effective strategic plan is based on good information about the **strengths and weaknesses** of the business and external **opportunities and threats** it is facing in its **external environment**. This is known as a **SWOT analysis** (McConkey, 1976). Information is used to develop measurable goals. Goals are supported by a plan of action that will, if undertaken successfully, allow the business to achieve its goals. One of the most important elements of a strategic plan is the assignment of responsibility. Assignment of responsibility sets clear expectations for management performance and serves to align the efforts of all segments of a business toward achievement of common goals. SWOT analysis and strategic planning are addressed in more detail in Chapters 3–6.

Good Information

To be successful, leaders need good information upon which to base their decisions and plan for the future. Good information is current, accurate, complete, and available when needed. In an ideal world, health business leaders would have access to information about all aspects of their business including, but not limited to, their market, customers, workforce, business processes, business performance outcomes, and financial performance. In addition, information is available about the performance of similar businesses against which leaders can compare their own performance. Terms frequently used to describe the use of such comparative information include **benchmarking,** *evidence-based practice,* and **best practice benchmarking**. Unfortunately, good information is often lacking in even the largest of health care businesses. The use of **business intelligence systems** that can link and integrate data from a variety of sources is on the rise, but is not yet available to the majority of health care businesses.

Quality Health Care Services

As a way to control their rising health care costs, health care payers, led by both employer groups and the federal government, focus on **quality outcomes** (Chapters 6 and 16). The belief is that elimination of waste through increased **efficiency** and reduction in medical errors will reduce the cost of health care services while improving patient outcomes. To motivate health service providers to participate in quality improvement initiatives two complementary initiatives are being pursued. The first initiative is public reporting of common quality indicators. The second is payment based on clinical outcomes. The latter is commonly referred to as **pay-for-performance** (CMS, 2007f).

Public reporting of clinical outcomes is on the rise. Information, typically Internet-based, covers a variety of clinical performance measures presented in a way that allows comparison between health care providers. Depending on the source, type, and age of the information, the use of the provided information is variable. CMS provides information on a hospital's performance in providing prescribed bundles of care for specific patient populations. The bundles of care are thought to represent best practices but do change from time to time. See Additional Resources for more information. Hospitals are required to audit their own performance and submit performance measures to CMS on a monthly basis. The information submitted is validated by CMS and used to provide the comparative information found at the website mentioned earlier.

P4P programs are also expected to motivate health care providers to give more attention to quality through adoption of evidence-based practices as well as reduction of unnecessary complications and medical errors. The concept is simple. P4P recognizes the powerful motivation of enhanced reimbursement. It uses that motivation by offering financial rewards to health care providers who can demonstrate consistent use of evidence-based care practices and/or improved patient outcomes. However, there are some P4P programs that are gearing up to withhold payment for preventable medical complications like infections. CMS has been mandated to change the methodology to eliminate the extra payment. Hospital-acquired infections are a likely target for this initiative (CMS, 2007g). P4P initiatives are coming from both government and private payers. They are targeting the performance of physicians, hospitals, and integrated delivery systems. At present, P4P initiatives are tied to process conformity more than to the outcomes of services (Porter and Teisberg, 2006).

Financial Resources

Health care businesses are under a lot of pressure to expand services, improve quality, and, in competitive markets, provide their customers with personal services that extend well beyond the delivery of health care services. All of those activities will, at least in the short run, add cost to their operations. These pressures to increase costs come at a time when they are facing significant external pressures to reduce costs, charge less for their services, and provide for an increasing number of patients who are uninsured or underinsured. No matter what their mission, health care businesses need to have the financial resources to recruit and retain the best workforce, support growth, replace aging equipment and facilities, and offer new technology. While some health care providers receive some support through grants, government subsidies, philanthropic contributions, and investments, most still need to make additional money from the services they provide (revenues) over what they spend to survive (expenses). It is up to health care managers to balance these competing pressures so that their business can make a profit. Financial planning and resource management are critical skills for the health care leader. These topics are addressed in detail in Chapters 20, 21, and 22 and include an overview of economic principles, accounting and finance practices, and entrepreneurship (private practice ownership), respectively. This is knowledge that can be used to manage any health care business.

Summary

The first step in understanding the U.S. health care industry is to learn the terms and acronyms used, its characteristics, and operation. Common business terms applicable to the U.S. health care industry have been used and defined throughout the chapter. The U.S. health care market is different from other consumer markets in several ways. Transactions between the health care consumer and providers are disconnected from price, income, and quality due to the third party payment system. In reality, health care is not considered a discretionary purchase but rather a human necessity to be obtained at any cost. The consumer often uses amenities and convenience as surrogate measures of quality and overall value. Payment for medical and health services is not tied to value (quality/cost) being delivered. In fact, it can be just the opposite; the current payment system actually rewards health service providers for providing inefficient or ineffective care. Driven by unlimited demand, the health service market continues unrestrained growth. The U.S. health services industry is the country's largest industry accounting for 16% of the

U.S. GDP and employing more than 13 million people. According to the BLS (2007a), the health care industry comprised over 545,000 business establishments that vary greatly in size and structure. Health service occupations include management, business and financial occupations, professional and related occupations, sales and related occupations, production, service occupations, office and administrative support occupations, and transportation and material moving occupations. Therapists accounted for 2.7% of the health service jobs. Health services spending categories include hospital care, physician and clinical services, nursing home care, prescription drugs and nondurable medical products, dental and other professional services, home health care, and nonpersonal spending which includes administration expense, investment and government public health activities. Private health insurance, Medicare, Medicaid, and SCHIP pay for these services. Health service consumers pay out-of-pocket for 13% of the service directly. Ultimately the burden of all health care spending falls to businesses, households, and the government. Naturally, there is an economic impact on the national and local economies as well as on individual households. On one side, businesses, government and private households struggle to meet the growing health care cost burden. As a result, businesses, government, and even private individuals are searching for ways to control the growth in health care expenditures and hold health care providers more accountable for providing higher value. On the other hand, the health care industry is the fuel behind the nation's economic development, contributing more new jobs and financial investment than any other industry. There should be no doubt that strong leaders are needed to bring about the type of improvement in the health care delivery system that will provide the highest quality of care at an affordable price. It will be the responsibility of health care leaders to devise initiatives to control cost, while at the same time addressing the opportunities to improve patient outcomes and ensure patient safety. To do this, leaders will need an exceptional grasp of management best practices.

CASE STUDY 2.1

What Next?

You are the owner/manager of a small private practice physical therapy clinic, Therapy A. Your business employs two other physical therapists and a small support staff. Business has been good primarily because of your location. You are across the street from a large retirement community. In addition, you are located in an industrial area and your location is attractive to workers who need to receive services in close proximity to their job site. There are no local competitors. The one issue that is constraining your growth is parking. Even now your patients are sometimes late because they could not find a place to park. For years your patients have complained of walking long distances or spending extra time waiting for a parking space to open up. Your business makes about $100,000 a year after salaries and all other routine expenses.

You have recently learned that a new competitor has moved in a few blocks away. The new competitor, Therapy B, offers the same services in a comparable facility at a comparable price. Therapy B also offers free valet parking service. Your business volumes are dropping off. At current levels your business will only clear a $60,000 profit this year. To the best of your knowledge you are losing business to Therapy B and suspect it is related to the parking situation. It will cost you $45,000 to rent additional parking spaces or $55,000 to add a comparable valet parking service. Considerations:

- You cannot increase your prices to offset the additional cost.
- The only way you can cover the cost is through increased patient volume.
- If you do nothing, you risk further erosion of your business.
- If you add parking or a valet service, at this point there is no guarantee that it will reverse the trend.
- If the trend continues, you are at risk of losing money this year. More if you add the cost of parking or a valet.
- You fear that if you match Therapy B's service strategy they will just add other amenities at more additional cost.

The Questions:

What are your incentives?

What are your customers' incentives?

What other information might help you make your decision about the parking situation?

If you can't get the additional information you desire, what is your decision right now?

What will you do in the near future to deal with this matter?

CASE STUDY 2.2

It Happens All the Time

The Situation

You are the manager of the rehabilitation department of a small home care agency. Your agency is the home health safety net for your community, a mission that you and your fellow employees embrace. All of the other area home care providers are for-profit and do not provide charity care. Historically, your agency has been able to pay the bills and set a little money aside with help from philanthropy and the local health department. You have just learned at a management meeting that Medicare payment has been cut 5%. What you know:

(Continued)

CASE STUDY 2.2

It Happens All the Time (continued)

- Your agency is now facing an annual budget deficit equal to 5% of your operating costs.
- Your patient payer mix is 60% Medicare, 20% private health plans, and 20% charity care.
- Your agency has no financial reserves because you convinced your agency director to spend existing reserves on a new mobile computer system.
- At current spending levels your agency will need to close within 24 months.
- You need to reduce total spending by 7% to finish the year with a small financial reserve.

You believe that agency staff work at full productivity (on average they see five patients a day).

The Questions

What is the payer's incentive?
What is the organization's incentive?
What is your incentive?
What else do you need to know to develop a survival strategy?
What are the information sources you will pursue immediately?
Write six test questions based on the stated objectives.
Write suggested answers to the questions.

REFERENCES

Advisory Board (Health care advisory board). Hospital of the future: Briefing for the board and medical executives. Washington, DC: Author. October 22, 2006.

American Hospital Association. Beyond health care: The economic contribution of hospitals. 2006. Available at www.aha.org/aha/content/2006/pdf/ECONRPT#.pdf. Accessed 3/04/07.

Bianco A. BusinessWeek Online.com. Healthcare's busiest empire builder. Available at http://www.businessweek.com/archives/1991/b323764.arc.htm. Accessed 1/09/09.

Bureau of Economic Analysis. Glossary. Available at http://www.bea.gov/glossary/GDP. Accessed 2/05/07.

Bureau of Labor Statistics. Health care. Available at http://www.bls.gov/oco/cg/cgs035.htm. Accessed 3/04/07a.

Bureau of Labor Statistics. Pharmaceutical and medicine manufacturing. Available at http://www.bls.gov/oco/cg/cgs009.htm. Accessed 3/04/07b.

Bureau of Labor Statistics. Medical and Health Services Managers. Available at http://www.bls.gov/oco/pdf/ocos014.pdf. Accessed 3/04/2007c.

Bureau of Labor Statistics. Occupational outlook handbook, 2006-07 edition, Medical and Health Services Managers. Available at http://www.bls.gov/oco/ocos014.htm. Accessed 3/04/07d.

Business Roundtable. CEO economic outlook survey. Available at http://www.businessroundtable.org/newsroom/Document.aspx?qs=5866BF807822B0F1AD7468422FB51711FCF50C8. Accessed 3/04/07.

California Health Care Foundation. U.S. health care spending, quick reference guide. Available at http://www.chcf.org/documents/insurance/QuickReferenceGuide06.pdf. Accessed 2/04/07.

Centers for Medicare and Medicaid Services. National health expenditure projections 2006 2016. Available at http://www.cms.hhs.gov/NationalHealthExpenddata/downloads/proj2006.pdf. Accessed 3/04/07a.

Centers for Medicare and Medicaid Services. Category definitions, national health expenditures. Available at http://www.cms.hhs.gov/NationalHealthExpendData/downloads/quickerf.pdf. Accessed 3/04/07b.

Centers for Medicare and Medicaid Services. Medicaid program general information. Available at http://www.cms.hhs.gov/MedicaidGenInfo/. Accessed 4/15/07c.

Centers for Medicare and Medicaid Services. State children's health insurance program (SCHIP). Available at www.cms.hhs.gov/LowCostHealthInsFamChild. Accessed 3/06/07d.

Centers for Medicare and Medicaid Services. Sponsors of health care costs, national health expenditures. Available at http://www.cms.hhs.gov/NationalHealthExpendData/Downloads/bhg07.pdf. Accessed 3/04/07e.

Centers for Medicare and Medicaid Services. Medicare "pay for performance (P4P)" initiatives. Available at http://www.cms.hhsgov/apps/media/press/release.asp?Counter=1343. Accessed 3/24/07f.

Centers for Medicare and Medicaid Services. Medicare Program. Proposed changes to the hospital inpatient prospective payment systems and fiscal year 2007 rates. Available at http://www.cms.hhs.gov/AcuteInpatientPPS/downloads/cms1488p.pdf:363. Accessed 3/24/07g.

Centers for Medicare and Medicaid Services. The nations health care dollar, calendar year 2005: Where It Went. Available from http://www.cms.hhs.gov/NationalHealthExpendData/downloads/PieChartSourcesExpenditures2005.pdf. Accessed 3/24/07h.

Clemans-Cope L. Changes in employer-sponsored health insurance sponsorship, eligibility, and participation: 2001 to 2005. Washington, DC: The Kaiser Family Foundation. December, 2006.

Congressional Budget Office. Congressional Budget Office Memorandum. Budgetary implications of the balanced budget act of 1997. Washington, DC: Author. December 1997:18.

Department of Labor. State workers' compensation officials. Available at http://www.dol.gov/esa/regs/compliance/owcp/wc.htm. Accessed 5/04/07.

Favro T. Nothing short of a complete overhaul will cure America's health care system. City Mayor Health Report. August 24, 2006.

Froetschel S. Globalization forces a health-check of US auto industry. Available at http://yaleglobal.yale.edu/display.article?id=8785. Accessed 1/09/09.

Gayle. Encyclopedia of business information sources. Detroit, MI: Author. 2006.

Gaynor M, Vogt William B. Antitrust and competition in health care markets. Cambridge, Mass: National Bureau of Economic Research. May 1999.

Goldman DP, Sood N, Leibowitz A. The reallocation of compensation in response to health insurance premium increases. NBER working paper no. 9540. Cambridge, MA: National Bureau of Economic Research. March 2003.

Health and Human Services. Medicare. Available at http://www.medicare.gov/Glossary/search.asp?SelectAlphabet=S&Language=English. Accessed 3/09/07.

Heffler S, Smith S, Keehan S, Clemmens MK, Zezza M, Truffer C. Health spending projections through 2013. Health Affairs. 2004;23(1):1-10.

Internal Revenue Service. Tax-exempt status for your organization. Available at http://www.irs.gov/pub/irs-pdf/p557.pdf. Accessed 3/10/07.

Kaiser Family Foundation. The 2006 Kaiser/Hewitt retiree health benefits survey. Available at http://www.kff.org/medicare/retiree.cfm. Accessed 3/19/07.

Kongstvedt PR. Managed Care. What it is and How it Works, 2nd ed. Gaithersburg, MD: Aspen. 2002.

Lewin Group. Drivers of healthcare costs associated with physician services. Falls Church, VA. Author. October 16, 2002.

May JH, Cunningham PF. Issue Brief 85. Tough trade-offs: Medical bills, family finances and access to care. Washington, DC: Center for Studying Health System Change. June, 2004.

McConkey DD. How to manage by results, 3rd ed. New York, NY: AMACOM. 1976.

Merriam-Webster's Collegiate Dictionary, 10th ed. Springfield, MA: Author. 2001:595.

Mintzberg H. The manager's job: Folklore and fact. Harvard Business Review. 1975;53(July-August):49-61.

Moffatt M. Your guide to economics: Price elasticity of demand. Available at http://economics.about.com/cs/micfrohelp/a/priceelasticity.htm. Accessed 3/19/07.

Monaco RM, Phelps JH. Health care prices, the federal budget, and economic growth. Health Affairs. Summer 1995;14(2):248-259.

National Conference of State Legislatures. SCHIP reauthorization resources. Available at http://www.ncsl. org/programs/health/chiphome.htm. Accessed 10/06/08.

National Institute of Standards and Technology. Baldrige National Quality Program. Available at http://www.quality.nist.gov/PDF_files/Improvement_Act.pdf. Accessed 3/20/07.

Newhouse JP. Medical care costs: How much welfare loss? Journal of Economic Perspectives. 1993;6(3):3-21.

Nolan JR, Nolan-Haley JM. Black's Law Dictionary. St. Paul, MN: West. 1990.

Office of the Assistant Secretary for Planning and Evaluation. Effects of health care spending on the U.S. economy. Available at http://www.aspe.hhs.gov/health/costgrowth. Accessed 3/04/07.

Pauly MV. Should we be worried about high real medical spending growth in the United States? Health Affairs Web Exclusive. January 8, 2003;W-3:15–27. Available at http://content.healthaffairs.org/cgi/reprint/hlthaff. w3.15v1?maxtoshow=&HITS=10&hits=10&RESULTFORMAT=&author1=pauly&andorexactfulltext=and&searchid=1&FIRSTINDEX=0&resourcetype=HWCIT. Accessed 3/26/07.

Porter ME. Teisberg O. Redefining health care: Creating Value-based competition on results. Boston, MA: Harvard Business School. 2006.

ADDITIONAL RESOURCES

The Federal government occupational outlook handbook on line is available at http://www.bls.gov/oco/. To find out more about workers' compensation log on to http://www.law.cornell.edu/wex/index.php/Workers_compensation. For information on your own state's program use a general search engine such as Ask.com or Google.com. Patients do look up information about Medicare on the Internet. Up to date Medicare information for patients is available at http://www.medicare.gov/publications/pubs/pdf/10050.pdf. For Medicare provider information the site is http://www.cms.hhs.gov/. The address for Medicaid program information is http://www.cms.hhs.gov/home/medicaid.asp. Access to a particular state's Medicaid and SCHIP programs is available at this address also. More on the Baldrige criteria is available at http://www.baldrige.com. For a look at the information available to consumers about hospital performance from the Centers for Medicare and Medicaid Services see http://www.hospitalcompare.hhs.gov. A recent report on the development and testing of a model for P4P for physical and occupational therapists treating Medicare B patients is available at http://www.cms.hhs.gov/TherapyServices/downloads/P4PFinalReport06-01-06.pdf.

CHAPTER 3

STRATEGIC MANAGEMENT AND EXTERNAL FORCES INFLUENCING HEALTH SERVICE PROVIDERS

DEBORAH G. FRIBERG AND LARRY J. NOSSE

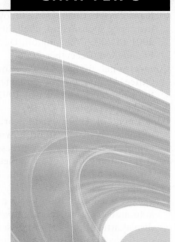

Learning Objectives

1. Explain the relationship between strategic planning and business success.
2. Describe the characteristics and elements of a strategic plan.
3. Become familiar with a variety of strategic planning models and the business characteristics that influence an organization's approach to strategic planning.
4. Follow a basic strategic planning process.
5. Be able to identify internal and external resources available to support the strategic planning process.
6. Describe the components of the strengths, weaknesses, opportunities, threats (SWOT) analysis and relate them to environmental scanning.
7. Explain the key elements of an external environmental scan using the politics, economy, social, technology (PEST) analysis to assess externally driven opportunities and threats.
8. Discuss the major external influences that impact the strategic decision-making process for medical and health service businesses.
9. Analyze the differences between a strategic plan and a business plan.

Introduction

Ideas and actions that focus on securing a desired future for an organization are often called *strategies* (Macmillan and Tampoe,

2000). Thinking in terms of strategies is a hallmark of a management philosophy known as *strategic management* (Swayne et al., 2006). *Strategic thinking* addresses the questions of *what* one should be doing and *why* one should be doing it. Strategic thinking starts with the organization's *mission statement*, which defines the purpose of its existence Chapters 4–7, and 14). *Strategic planning* considers the questions of *how* and *when* a business should take action, but without a lot of detail. Operational or tactical planning answers the questions of *how* and *when* in detail (Kane, 2007). The operational plan also addresses the question of responsibility and defines *who* will get the job done. The *strategic plan* documents the planning process and its results. Why do organizations develop strategic plans?

> "Would you tell me please, which way I ought to go from here?"
> "That depends a great deal on where you want to get to," said the Cat.
> "I don't much care where-" said Alice.
> "Then it doesn't matter which way you go," said the Cat.
> "-so long as I get somewhere," Alice added as an explanation.
> "Oh, you're sure to do that," said the Cat, "if you only walk long enough."
> *(Carroll, 1866).*

Unlike Alice, business leaders generally want to get somewhere specific. The hard part is, of course, defining where that "somewhere"

Key Terms

Key terms, which are defined below, are bolded and italicized the first time they appear in the chapter. Other important terms are shown in boldface on first appearance and are defined by the context in which they are used. When either of these types of terms is used several times, its acronym is identified and subsequently used in the chapter. Both types of terms are listed alphabetically in the online glossary with their definitions and (when applicable) their acronyms.

benchmarking: a structured approach for identifying the outstanding performers in a field, learning and understanding what they do that makes them outstanding, and adapting what they do to improve your own performance.

chief executive officer (CEO): a member of the top level of management of an organization chosen by the board of directors or trustees. A primary person responsible for formulating the strategic direction of an organization.

complexity: the degree of external environment variation among customers, services offered, regulations, and competitors. In such environments, managers must have in-depth knowledge and expertise to plan the organization's future.

external factors/variables: anything outside of a person, group, or business entity that can impact positively or negatively on their/its efforts to succeed in fulfilling their goals. Factors that may be opportunities or threats.

mission statement: or mission is a written document identifying why an organization exists. It tells the reader what the business does (services and products), who the customers are, the geographical location(s), its specialty, and it may contain goals and values. One of the fundamental guiding documents of an organization.

outcome measure(s): means of quantifying outcomes like HEDIS for managed care plans and PORI for a variety of providers treating Medicare beneficiaries.

political, economic, social, and technological (PEST/STEP) analysis: basic components of an external environmental scan.

sector environment: the variables that affect the success of all members of a specific industry such as health care.

strategic goal(s): the ultimate quest of organizational efforts as described in the vision, values, and mission statements.

strategic management: a management philosophy based on thinking in terms of strategy formation.

strategic objective(s): written statements related to critical success factors that provide sufficient detail so that when enacted, the organization will move closer toward fulfillment of its strategic goals.

strategic plan: the result of an organizational decision-making and planning process intended to fulfill the organization's values and mission and move the organization toward the realization of its vision.

strategic planning: a strategic management decision-making process based on analyses of intrinsic and extrinsic variables to develop step-by-step action plans (strategies) to fulfill the organization's mission and vision.

strategic thinking: upper management engaging in disciplined mental processing to select and synthesize large amounts of data relevant to the organization gathered through the strategic planning process to answer the questions what should we be doing and why should we be doing it.

strategy(ies): integrated plan(s) for achieving SMART(ER) goals informed by analysis of information internal and external to the organization.

SWOT analysis: a mnemonic for a method of analyzing the results of external and internal environmental analyses: (S)trengths, (W)eaknesses, (O)pportunities, (T)hreats. S and W information is obtained from examination of the organization's internal environment. O and T information is obtained from examination of the organization's external environment.

tactical action plan(s): also called an operational plan. Operationally specific assignments that have set timelines for achievement (implementation schedule), assign responsibility, and are tracked by defined measurable outcomes. Developed as part of a strategic planning process.

values statement/philosophical statement: a narrative presentation or a list of core values expressing the principles that are deemed most important by the organization in all human interactions. One of the fundamental documents of an organization.

vision statement: a simple, brief, written document intended to advance a futuristic view of an organization, to inspire internal stakeholders, to strive for progress toward the desired state, and to share this future view with external stakeholders.

is with enough specificity to figure out how to get there. In addition, for those who want to get to their destination quicker than trial and error will allow, a road map is advisable. In business, the strategic plan is the road map. Strategic planning is the process one goes through to define the destination and draw the road map to that desired destination. A good strategic planning process will be dynamic enough to adjust for detours and unexpected road hazards along the way.

This chapter covers the major components of strategic management. It describes the elements of an effective strategic planning process that is applicable to any business endeavor. The value of the strategic plan in communicating to internal and external audiences, aligning efforts at all levels of the business, and motivating employees to contribute to the success of a business are discussed. Through the planning process, an organization's desired outcomes are identified and guidelines developed for making decisions about actions intended to better the organization's future (Swayne et al., 2006). A successful strategic planning process starts with a clear statement of mission and finds its foundation in the gathering and analyzing of information about the business itself and all external factors that affect its viability. The process of gathering and the use of information internal and external to the organization are explored, followed by a more complete discussion of the essential elements of strategic management, a strategic planning process, and the use of external information to support management decisions. The concepts presented in this chapter are used extensively in Chapters 4–6.

Why Plan?

Strategic planning is a management tool used by all types and sizes of businesses. Whether a business is large or small, for-profit or not-for-profit, private or public makes no difference. The approach to planning may differ but the value to the business is the same. The strategic planning process is used by business managers to answer three basic questions: Where are we now? Where are we going? And, how will we get there? (Mystrategicplan, 2007). Strategic planning serves to improve business performance in several ways. Table 3.1 summarizes six benefits of strategic planning.

Table 3.1 Expected Benefits of Strategic Planning	
Focuses thinking	The strategic planning process serves to focus the thinking of an organization away from "what is happening today" and onto "what might or could happen tomorrow." This happens as business leaders develop and/or revise their organization's mission, vision, and values statements (Chapters 5 and 7).
Prioritizes efforts	The strategic planning process can help a business prioritize efforts. Businesses are often faced with a multitude of opportunities to improve what they are doing today and expand into new areas tomorrow. Most businesses lack the resources to "do it all." The strategic planning process allows business leaders to explore a wide range of possibilities and identify opportunities that have the greatest potential to contribute to long-term success.
Aligns efforts and goals	Strategic planning helps a business align the efforts of all its members toward the achievement of common goals. As the strategic plan is communicated, everyone in the organization is looking at the same road map. They see how their efforts contribute to reaching the desired destination. Alignment can be enhanced when all employees are included in the planning process. Those who help select the destination are more motivated to support the journey (Bourgeois and Brodwin, 1984).
Scans external environment	Because the strategic planning process includes a continuous environmental scan (Chapters 4–6), and a review of the external environment, a business is better positioned to recognize and respond to unexpected external changes such as new technology, changes in governmental regulations, or a new competitor.

(Continued)

Table 3.1 continued	
Can share plan with external audiences	The strategic plan is a communication tool for external audiences. It might be used to communicate the direction of the organization for the purposes of obtaining external funding from philanthropic sources or financial lending institutions. It may also be used to engage the community in cooperative dialog.
To implement the plan needs action plans	The strategic plan is a management tool. Strategy formulation is only half the story. Implementation is the essential other half. A strategic plan is only beneficial if management can use it as a tool to understand and communicate the strategic goals and objectives. Employees at all levels must be able to use the strategic plan as a guide for the implementation of detailed tactical action plans.

Characteristics of the Strategic Plan

Up to this point, we have been talking about the strategic planning process in the context of whole organizations. It is important to note that strategic plans may vary in scope. They can be written for an entire organization. However, some businesses are so large or diverse that to make the plan usable, strategic plans are also written to address the needs of a specific segment of the business. For example, a large national health care provider may undertake strategic planning on a geographical basis. Each region may develop a geographically specific plan that better reflects local markets (Chapter 18). Alternatively, if the same health services provider operates hospitals, home health care agencies, long-term care facilities, and ambulatory care centers, they may opt for strategic planning by business division (Chapter 14). In fact, strategic planning may be segmented by both **market** (customer characteristics) and **service line** (deliverables) (see Chapter 18). The goal is to develop strategic plans that are meaningful and actionable.

Strategic plans may also cover variable time periods. The time frame chosen is influenced by the organizational size, complexity of service mix, market, and environmental volatility. Given the speed and degree of change in the health care industry, it is hard to believe that any prediction for more than 5 years into the future is reliable. This is a key reason for adopting a cyclical strategic planning process that calls for the review and update of plans on an annual basis (Swayne et al., 2006).

Elements of a Strategic Plan

An effective strategic plan should include at a minimum:

- A mission statement
- A vision statement
- Strategic goals
- Strategic objectives
- Tactical action plans or operational plans
- Implementation planning schedule
- Outcome measures

Other elements that can add clarity and facilitate efficient enactment of a strategic plan include a **value statement**, list of **critical issues**, and a **planning schedule**.

The **mission statement** states the purpose of the business. The *vision* defines its ideal future state. *Strategic goals* are areas of focus that, when addressed, will close the gap between the current and ideal state. *Strategic objectives* are statements that, when enacted, will move the business toward its goals. Objectives are achieved through action plans. *Tactical action plans* are specific, have set timelines for achievement (implementation schedule), assign responsibility, and can produce measurable outcomes. An implementation planning schedule defines the annual planning cycle that is followed (Center for Strategic Planning, 2007).*Outcome measures* are the specific indicators of success for each implemented strategy (Chapter 16). **Value statements** describe the forces that motivate a business and the behaviors it promotes in its employees. **Critical issues** describe internal weaknesses or external threats that must be addressed. An

implementation planning schedule defines the annual planning cycle that will be followed (Center for Strategic Planning, 2007).

About Mission Statements

Strategic thinking starts with the mission statement of the business. This statement defines the purpose for which the business exists. As businesses grow and develop, their mission statements need to evolve with them. Mission statements should be short, to the point, and written in a way that will energize a business' internal and external audiences. Jones (2007) suggests that a good mission statement will answer three questions:

1. Who are we?
2. Who are our customers?
3. What sets us apart from the competition?

The last question gets to the heart of what a business does to retain customers (Jones, 2007). Let us take Google as an example. Google is possibly the world's largest search engine. According to their website, Google has two business lines, highly targeted advertising and online search services. Customers use their product to find information on almost any topic. Google's stated mission is to "organize the world's information and make it universally accessible and useful" (Google, 2007).

Balanced Score Card

Another approach to focus on the implementation of strategies is the use of a **Balanced score card** (Swayne et al., 2006). A balanced score card (Table 3.2) is a management tool that can be used to share and report outcome measures important to achieving an organization's goals. The importance of this approach to evaluate the results of specific efforts can be for the business as a whole or for a specific business unit or department. Balanced score cards are typically segregated into goal or topic areas. Topic areas for health service organizations might include financial performance, key process performance such as clinical outcomes, customer service measures such as patient satisfaction, and workforce related measures such as turnover. Selected performance areas and related outcome measures stated in terms of targeted and actual performance represent each topic area (Kaplan and Norton, 1992). Table 3.2 provides a template for a balanced

Table 3.2 Balanced Score Card				
		Performance		
Goal	**Performance Outcome Measures**	**Target**	**Actual**	**Status**
Clinical Excellence	Percent patients who achieved goals	95%	90%	–5%
Service Excellence	Percent patients who would return	90%	93%	3%
Financial Viability	Cost per outpatient visit	$45	$47	$2

score card that can be used to track and communicate targeted performance outcomes. Such performance outcomes are used to evaluate and revise the strategic objectives and tactical action plans on an annual basis. This template shows the alignment between the business' strategic goals and outcome measures. It provides a clear performance target and compares the actual and desired target performance. The arrows are used as a quick reference to show the direction for improved performance.

Strategic Planning Models

The literature approaches the question of strategic planning models from two different perspectives. The first approach addresses the question of models from the perspective of leadership and inclusion. Bourgeois and Brodwin (1984) describe five strategic planning models that find their basis in the style of the business's *chief executive officer* (CEO). These five models are defined by the role the CEO plays and/or the extent of involvement of others within the strategic planning process.

1. Commander model: thinking is done at the top without input from lower level management or those doing the work. This model is characterized by CEOs who are powerful and able to command performance.
2. Change model: based in behavioral science methods and engages other managers in the process to increase the chance of success.
3. Collaborative model: employs a group process and techniques such as brainstorming to get broader input and inclusion of differing management opinions. As each of these models limits input from frontline workers, they often encounter limited success and are difficult to implement.
4. Cultural model: expands on the collaborative model and includes input from all levels of the organization.
5. Crescive model: *crescive* is derived from the Latin term meaning "to grow." This model takes participation even further by inviting strategy to flow from the **operating core** (direct service/clinical providers) of the organization. This model encourages a higher level of innovation and places the

CEO in the reactive role of selecting from the strategic proposals that come from others. Both the cultural and crescive models require more planning effort but are more effective during implementation.

The second approach to strategic planning models is based on the perspectives of scope and *complexity*. McNamara (2007) also describes five models for strategic planning:

1. Basic model: a top-down model that is best suited to **small businesses** with little strategic planning experience. It has five chronological steps, (1) development of a mission statement, (2) setting goals, (3) developing operational strategies, (4) setting tactical or action plans, and (5) monitoring success and updating the plan.
2. Issue-based model: expands on the basic model to include (1) design or update of mission, vision for the future, and values; (2) an assessment of internal and external factors that have the potential to impact success; (3) identification of major issues and goals; (4) design of major strategies; (5) develop tactical or action plans; (6) document planning in the form of a strategic plan; (7) develop yearly operating plan; (8) develop an annual financial plan (budget); (9) monitor annual performance; and (10) update plan on an annual basis based on performance measures.
3. Alignment model: this model is focused on alignment of resources and efforts to achieve the stated mission. It is suited to organizations that need to refine strategies that are not achieving the desired outcomes or address significant internal inefficiencies. The steps in this model include (1) creating an outline of current mission, programs/services, current resources, and areas in need of support; (2) identification of areas in need of improvement; (3) determination of how improvements should be achieved; and (4) add these as refinements to the strategic plan.
4. Scenario model: this model incorporates the results of environmental scans into the development of "what if" scenarios. Scenarios for the best, worst, and most reasonable cases are used to develop possible response or contingency strategies. The organization is then asked to determine the most likely

scenarios and implement protective strategies.

5. Organic model: this model contrasts with the more traditional cause and effect approach to planning. It calls on the organization to (1) focus on its mission and values, (2) engage in frequent dialog around these values, and (3) share its reflections about the organization's current processes. These discussions identify the changes needed in the process that will bring the organization closer to its shared vision for the future. This method requires considerable time and is more of a learning endeavor than a planning method.

Ultimately, the model is less important than the outcomes following their application. The keys to a functional strategy are that it has to be realistic, customer oriented, understandable, easy to communicate, and flexible (Padgaonkar, 2007).

The choice of a strategic planning model is dependent on the perspective of an organization's leaders, the upper level managers.

The importance of these perspectives and the expected employee responses to different leadership and management approaches require a more complete discussion. This discussion is provided in Chapters 11 and 15.

The Strategic Planning Process

The process of strategic planning is a continuous cycle of questioning and decision making. In this process, the business takes into consideration what and who they are today (mission and values), what they might become (vision) (Chapter 7) and all of the internal and external factors that might impact their journey to realize their aspirations. Figure 3.1 depicts the elements and cyclic nature of a basic strategic planning process. Input is translated into a few high-level strategic goals. The strategic goals are further defined by strategic objectives. Strategic objectives are put into action through the implementation of detailed tactical action plans. The effectiveness of the action

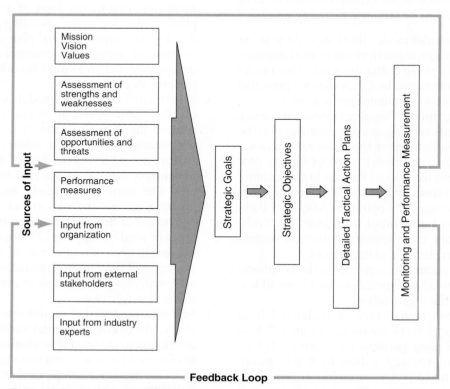

Figure 3.1. Continuous planning cycle.

Strategic Planning Example: Mission Through Measurement

Mission: Provide home-based pediatric physical therapy services.

Vision: Remain a sole practioner's private practice with a nine month per year operating schedule that generates a reliable, above-average income.

Strategic Goal #1: Reliable Financial Performance

Strategic Objective #1A: Cultivate a minimum of 30 elementary school-aged clients whose parents are interested in September thru May treatment schedules.

Tactical Action #1A1: Develop a referral relationship with the five largest pediatric practices in the market area.
Tactical Action #1A2: Obtain provider contracts with a majority of managed-care plans.
Tactical Action #1A3: Produce a service brochure with parent testimonials.
Tactical Action #1A4: Become a Medicaid provider and accept future state-funded clients.

Outcome Measure #1A1: Receive one successful referral per month from each of the targeted pediatric practice groups.
Outcome Measure #1A2: Have contracts with 75% of managed-care plans within one year.
Outcome Measure #1A3: Produce service brochure with a minimum of 3 testimonials.
Outcome Measure #1A4: By August 1, have a Medicaid provider number.
Global Measure: Number of elementary school-aged clients whose parents are interested in September thru May treatment schedules.

Figure 3.2. Strategic planning example: Mission through measurement.

Table 3.3   Annual Strategic Planning Cycle and Schedule[a]

Activity	Start Date	Finish Date
Implement annual plan	January 1	December 31
Monitor/measure outcomes	January 1	December 31
Update balance score card	April 1	April 15
October 1	October 15	
Jan 1	Jan 15	
Evaluate current initiatives	May 1	June 30
Review/update strategic plan	July 1	July 31
Prioritize initiatives	August 1	August 30
Develop annual budget	September 1	November 15
Plan and budget approval	November 15	December 15
Start over	January 1	

[a]Based on a January 1–December 31 fiscal year.

plans is monitored and measured. The performance results are used to modify strategy and action plans and the process starts again. This process depicted in Figure 3.2 is an example of content and flow for a simple strategic plan that is used by a small private physical therapy practice. Notice the complementary mission and vision, the specific goal, strategies to achieve the goals, tactical action plans, measurable outcome measures for each action plan as well as an overall outcome measure. The next process example is the strategic planning schedule. Table 3.3 demonstrates an annual strategic planning cycle of activities, and the linkage of strategic planning activities to the annual financial planning. Such an example of a planning schedule is used for businesses that follow a January to December fiscal calendar otherwise referred to as a **fiscal year**.

Organizational Structures That Support the Strategic Planning Process

Organizational structures refer to the legal designation assumed by a business (Chapter 14). Each organizational structure has a hierarchy of management. Each level of the managerial hierarchy has a different degree of planning responsibility. The responsibility for overall organizational planning is held by the upper level managers. Progressively narrower, focused and more specific planning responsibility is carried out by managers lower in the hierarchy. In general, there are more levels of managers in a larger organization. Businesses, depending on size, may have several organizational structures that have authority over the strategic planning process. Most large, middle, and some **small businesses** are legal corporations. **Corporations** are businesses whose operations have been legally separated from its owners (see Chapters 11 and 14). All corporations have an elected **board of directors** (BOD). The BOD, as a group, controls the corporation and appoints the corporate officers to manage operations (Clarkson et al., 1995). The BOD is ultimately responsible for the success of the business and, in that capacity, have direct responsibility for strategic planning. Many corporations have a **board committee** that is charged with the responsibility to oversee the development and implementa-

tion of the strategic plan. The board appointed CEO is responsible for supporting the board in meeting this responsibility. As discussed in the previous section, strategic planning models can be more or less inclusive. The choice of planning model is often driven by the style of the CEO with guidance from the board and **senior leadership**. Senior leadership is usually charged with managing and facilitating the strategic planning process. Depending on the size of the organization, there may be a senior leadership level position that has designated responsibility for this function such as a Vice President of Planning. Operational managers like directors of physical therapy, support managers like directors of human resources, and staff may have more or less of a role as determined by the planning model employed. Current best practice in management suggests that the more inclusive model is more likely to engage employees at all levels, take ownership of the completed strategic plan and be motivated to support a successful implementation (Baldrige National Quality Program, 2007).

Planning Support

Support for strategic planning can come from a variety of internal and external sources. The availability of internal resources is dependent on the size and capability of the business. Businesses that lack internal resources may obtain planning support by the use of external consultants, academic-based programs, or government sponsored business services. Types of support services that may prove to be of value include:

Process facilitation. The use of facilitators to guide the planning process can be of great value. An effective facilitator can make the planning process more organized and efficient. They can pull in a variety of opinions while balancing any personal agendas or passionate positions of participants. Facilitators should be objective and neutral. Facilitators who are also content experts may have a tendency to discourage input and drive the process in a single direction. External facilitators may have a tendency to "know what is best" and should not be allowed to exclude input from within the organization.

Performance data gathering and analysis. The reader has learned that effective strategic planning is dependent on timely, complete, and accurate information about internal and external factors that have the potential to impact performance. Accurate information about the current performance of the business is essential. This information may come from internal sources such as financial planning, clinical performance analysis, customer and staff surveys, or outcome measurement systems. Information may also be acquired from external rating and evaluation services such as industry performance *benchmarking* services (Chapters 6 and 16).

Market data gathering and analysis. Input from customers is essential. Market information may come from a variety of internal and external services. Types of information that may be of value include market trends, competitor analysis, performance benchmarks, customer feedback reports, and best practice benchmarks.

Implementation support. **Operational managers** of clinical departments have patient care skills that are generally stronger than their business skills. These managers may need support from nonclinical managers for implementation of tactical action plans.

External Sources for Planning Support

Businesses can turn to external consultants, academic-based programs, or government-sponsored business services to obtain support for their strategic planning efforts. For more information about the use of consultants, see Chapters 22 and 23. The **U.S. Small Business Administration** (SBA) also provides information and educational programs on most business management topics (SBA, 2007a). Information on SBA offerings can be found in the SBA Small Business Directory by state. A free copy of the SBA directory can be obtained from any SBA office. The SBA also sponsors services through **Service Corps of Retired Executives** (SCORE), an organization of over 13,000 volunteers business executives who provide free support to small businesses (SCORE, 2007). Moreover, **Small Business Development Centers** (SBDC) offer services in partnership with local and state governments (SBA, 2007b), and **Small Business Institutes** (SBI) on more than 500 college campuses nationwide provide counseling by students and faculty to small businesses (Policastro, 2007).

Getting Started

The first step in the strategic planning process is to affirm the mission. Then the task is to reach an agreement on the vision for the future. The next step is to carry out an assessment to define the gap between the current and desired state. This is known as gap analysis. This assessment needs to take into consideration factors that are external and internal to the organization. *External factors* are considered to be out of the direct control of the organization and are often referred to in terms of **opportunities** or **threats** (see Chapters 4, 15, and 22). Out of direct control does not mean that external factors cannot be influenced by the business. Political advocacy with the intent of promoting legislative activity that is favorable to a business as discussed in Chapter 1 is a good example of how a business might influence external factors. **Internal factors** are considered to be under the control of the organization. Internal factors are often referred to in terms of **strengths** and **weaknesses** (see Chapters 5, 6, and 22). A total assessment of both external (opportunities and threats) and internal (strengths and weaknesses) factors that have the potential to impact an organization's success is called a *SWOT analysis* (Learned et al., 1969; McConkey, 1976) (see Fig. 3.3). The information gained through the completion of a SWOT analysis is used to guide the development of strategic goals, objectives, and action plans. External and internal information subjected to SWOT analyses can assist strategy development by raising key questions including:

How can we take advantage of opportunities to achieve our goals?

How can we protect the business against potential threats?

How can our strengths be leveraged to achieve our goals?

How can our weaknesses be eliminated or, better yet, turned into future strengths?

The focus is on the assessment of external factors that represent opportunities or threats to a business. The examination of the external environment starts with the SWOT process

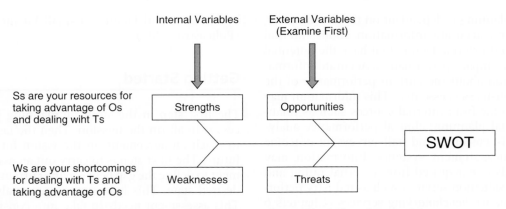

Figure 3.3. Strengths, weaknesses, opportunities, threats (SWOT) analysis model.

because it is the variables outside of the organization that are to be dealt with using internal resources. Chapters 5 and 6 will explore the internal influences on health service businesses and physical therapy, respectively, to complete the discussion of the SWOT analysis and its application in strategic planning.

Assessing External Influences

The external analysis can be divided into general factors that have the potential to influence any organization in a community and business specific factors. In this case, the business and its market define the term community. Depending on the business, its community could be local, regional, national, or international. An example of a general environmental factor would be the national, state, or local tax laws that apply to all businesses in a community. Tax laws can be favorable or unfavorable to business growth and development. They can encourage or discourage capital investment (Chapters 20 and 21) and business growth.

Business-specific factors are those that could reasonably be expected to impact businesses in a particular industry. Hannagan (2002) refers to the business specific factors as the *sector environment*. Some examples of health sector specific factors include availability of a trained workforce, changes in reimbursement or service coverage by third party payers, advances in health services technologies, and laws that regulate health service business and professional practices. This last example is of

particular importance in the countries where the medical and health care service industries are highly regulated.

There are several models available that businesses can use to guide the analysis of external factors. Among the most basic models is the *Political, Economic, Social, and Technological (PEST) analysis* (Internet Center of Management and Business Administration, 2007). An alternative to is rearrange the word order to Social, Technological, Economic, and Political or a **STEP** analysis (Hannagan, 2002; Quick-MBA, 2007). Both mnemonics make intuitive sense since pests can pose dangers and steps can be taken toward resolutions. Elements in a PEST/STEP analysis are:

Political analysis includes factors related to the type, stability, and regulatory activity of national, regional, or local governing bodies.

Economic conditions include factors that might have an effect on customer spending patterns, business operating costs, or access to investment capital.

Social conditions includes information about the population including their characteristics, living conditions, interests, attitudes, and preferences.

Technological developments include information about the business impacts of technology, both current and potential.

Table 3.4 provides a list of some of the possible **macroenvironmental** and sector-specific **microenvironmental** factors that might be included in a PEST analysis.

Table 3.4   Elements of a PEST Analysis

Element	Macroenvironment (any business)	Micro-environment (health services)
Political	Political climate and stability Tax rates and incentives Pricing regulations Trade regulations Wage legislation Mandatory employee benefits Industrial safety regulations Environmental regulations Business operation regulations Budget deficit or surplus Labor laws Payroll taxes	Political climate related to health services and health spending Political issues that may divert funding away from health care Reimbursement regulations Health business regulations Health safety regulations Zoning and building regulations Licensure/professional practice regulation
Economic	Type of economic system State of the economy Free versus regulated market Economic growth rate Unemployment rate Inflation rates Interest rates Infrastructure quality Consumer confidence Workforce skill and availability Discretionary income Future economic trends	Household income levels Wage rates Regulation of not-for-profit status Reimbursement rates and trends Labor cost and trends Malpractice insurance rates Insurance coverage rates Supply/equipment costs trends Competitor trends
Social	Market demographics Population size Population distribution Age and gender Education levels Ethnic origin Cultural preferences Religious affiliations Education levels Consumer attitudes Consumerism Environmentalism Work attitudes Role of church and religion Leisure interests	Health-specific demographics Health care utilization trends Cultural makeup of target market Language Health preferences Health-specific consumer trends Diet and nutrition Health conscious Health education Housing and general living conditions
Technological	Efficiency of infrastructure Industry productivity Recent technology developments Impact of technologies on cost Rate of technology diffusion	Impact of emerging technologies on current market demand and business processes Competitor deployment of new technology Cost of new technologies

The actual content of the macro- and micro-environmental items is chosen by upper-level management based on multiple factors including experience, the type of business, the scope of the business, and other factors.

Accessing Information for Strategic Analysis

Management's decisions about strategic goals, objectives, and tactical action plans should reflect the organization's mission and vision and be guided by the adopted values (Chapter 7). These decisions should be based on management's experience, and information about the internal and external factors that may influence the organization's success. Strategy decisions should be informed decisions that are based on the analysis of real time, accurate, and well-analyzed data transformed into usable information. Managers use this information and interpret its significance by filtering it through their screen of judgment supported by intuition, insight, gut feelings (Helms, 2000), and personal values (Mintzberg et al., 1995). However, getting the information that is needed might require significant investment in time and financial resources. A guide to determining the scope of an environmental assessment needed is to start with known or anticipated factors that can be expected to have an effect on the organization's ability to carry out its strategic objectives (Dunn, 1998).

Information needed for a complete environmental scan can be obtained from a variety of sources. Information about the external environment, particularly related to competitors or competitive services, may be difficult to obtain because they come from sources outside the organization. Most businesses try to limit access to sensitive information such as costs, litigation, competitive strategies, first to market technologies, and other future plans. Some information is available because it is publicly circulated. Examples of source documents for publicly available information include annual reports, announcements in trade journals, presentations by top-level managers to customers or community stakeholders, and government reports. Other sources of external information include:

- Consultant reports
- Customer feedback
- Financial annual reports
- Financial consultants/brokers
- Government agency reports and publicly shared databases
- Human resources reports
- Information technology reports
- Investor groups
- Market research
- Marketing and consumer trend reports
- Professional associations
- Professional publications
- Professional seminars
- Publicly reported clinical outcome reports
- Trade associations
- Treatment outcome reports
- Vendor feedback

Determining the quantity of information needed is a management responsibility. The degree of risk associated with making a poor decision must be balanced against the cost and effort associated with obtaining more information. That is a decision the leadership of individual businesses must make for themselves. The number of influential and relevant variables to consider in an external environment can be difficult for inexperienced managers to identify. To help guide new managers in their external environment scanning efforts, general PEST categories are expanded into more specific groupings in Chapter 4.

Strategic Versus Business Planning

The strategic plan defines a business's road map for success in qualitative terms with minimal quantitative support. It addresses in broad terms why the business should focus its attention on specific markets, products, services, technologies, processes, or other opportunities. In contrast, a **business plan** builds on the strategic plan. A business plan is more specific and contains highly detailed information about a specific element of the operational plan (Rubenstien, 2007). Key elements of the business plan include:

- Market plan
- Operations plan
- Financial plan

The basic elements of these plans are introduced here and expanded in Chapters 14, 18, and 22. A market plan starts with a clear definition of the opportunity under consideration. The market plan includes analysis of such things as market size, market characteristics, growth trends and projections, customer preferences, service locations, partnering opportunities, the competitive environment, and so on. It also includes strategies to product/service positioning within the market, communication, and promotional strategies (see Chapter 18).

An operations plan addresses issues related to governance, business structure, relationship of new services/products to other components of the business, human resource requirements, business capacity, technology requirements, infrastructure requirements, building and equipment requirements, the proposed implementation strategy, and post implementation methodology for tracking performance and measuring success (Chapters 11, 13, 14, 16, 17, and 22).

A financial plan includes a detailed analysis of capital expenses, operating budgets inclusive of revenues, expenses, profit/loss projections, and return on investment (see Chapters 20–22). The financial plan should also address the **opportunity cost** of the project under consideration. Opportunity costs are those opportunities that must be bypassed in order to pursue one strategy rather than another. For example, a business may not have the resources or capacity to pursue two attractive expansion opportunities. One opportunity must be chosen. The other opportunity must be delayed or not pursued at all. The benefits of the forgone project represent what are called opportunity costs.

Summary

Strategic planning offers business leaders a tool to improve the performance of their organizations in several ways. A good strategic plan can be used to focus leaders on the future, prioritize their efforts, align the effort at all levels of the organization, incorporate environmental factors into their plans, communicate to internal and external audiences, and support the implementation of tactical action plans. In short, strategic planning can improve the odds in favor of a business's success. Strategic plans must be individualized to the needs of the business. There are several models that can be used as guides. Effective strategic plans share some common elements. These include, at a minimum, a mission statement, vision statement, strategic goals, strategic objectives, operational or tactical action plans, an implementation schedule, and outcome measures. Other elements that can add value include a values statement, list of critical issues, and a planning schedule. The planning schedule lays out the steps of the strategic planning process to keep the organization on track and insure continuity over time. There is a variety of internal and external resources available to support the strategic planning process. Many of these can be accessed by small businesses at minimum expense. Of great importance is management's recognition of the internal and external factors that can impact their success. Tools that can be used to assess external factors include the PEST analysis and SWOT analysis. The PEST analysis helps in the recognition and evaluation of externally driven opportunities and threats, the O and T of SWOT. External influences that impact the strategic decision-making process for health service businesses may be general, affecting all businesses, or specific to the health service sector businesses. Finally, the differences between a strategic plan and a business plan are discussed. The tools to complete a comprehensive business plan found in later chapters. For a comprehensive situational analysis, the information from the external environment analysis must be coupled with an examination of the internal resources and limitations of an organization. The internal environment is the focus of Chapters 5 and 6.

CASE STUDY 3.1

The External Environment for a Private Practice

Task

Conduct a PEST analysis for the following scenario. You get to choose the state where this scenario takes place. This may be your state of residence or where you might have an internship, where you would like to practice or where you have practiced. Specific comments for you to consider are italicized.

The Organization

This is a private physical therapy practice owned by four physical therapists. It is a for-profit limited liability corporation (Chapters 9 and 14) with 25 locations in the state of [*you choose the state*]. The organization's vision is to become the largest privately owned outpatient provider in the state. The mission is to provide same day, quality physical therapy services to adult clients with orthopedic conditions in all major cities in the state. The values (Chapters 5–7) espoused by the organization are respect, honesty, and professionalism. All sites are linked to a central server. There are computer templates for all usual paper work duties. Each clinic has video conferencing capabilities, online mentoring, consultation, continuing education, and other professional development activities. All therapists have attended at least two manual therapy continuing education courses in the past 2 years.

External Environment: PEST

P: The organization that pays Medicare B claims in the state is in the middle of making changes in their computer system to accommodate new provider code regulations. It is necessary to add new servers and link them to the old servers. Computer hardware and software problems have occurred. The payer organization has let it be known that processing of claims for services may be irregular or delayed over the next few months. The state has had a budget shortfall the past . . . years (*check on your state's financial status*). Most states provide advice and assistance to business owners (*check on your state's offerings*). The state licensure act allows physical therapists to . . . (*check your state's referral statutes–do clients have direct access to physical therapists or not. If not, who can prescribe*). Physical therapist assistants are allowed to . . . (*determine if they licensed or not and if so, what can they do?*)

E: Overall, unemployment in the state is low. Interest rates are X (*check current rates*) as they are today. The outlook for establishing new practices in several of the large cities shows mixed potential. City A will experience a workforce cutback at a large automotive plant as sections of the plant will be modeled to accommodate more robots. When this work is completed, many employees will not be called back to work. The union has worked out a deal with another automobile company to offer employment for some people if they are willing to relocate. In city B management failed to get a federal grant to explore making ethanol from wood pulp. The company will continue to operate but without external research funds it will not be able to expand. Unemployment has been above state average for a decade. There is no union at the mill but the mill is self-insured–it pays for health services out of a special fund it maintains. City C has more office employees than the other cities. The city provides tax incentives for new businesses of all types and sizes who establish offices within the next 12 months. Currently there are numerous small financial, banking, accounting, and job placement businesses. This city has affordable housing and a stable and relatively well-paid workforce. Its residential and school taxes are high. It is considering a city income tax.

(Continued)

CASE STUDY 3.1

The External Environment for a Private Practice (continued)

S: Comparative populations are: City A 100,000 with slow growth, median age 45, 38% college graduates, obesity, chronic diseases common; City B 25,000 and unchanged for several years, median age 52, 20% college graduates, typical workers are hardy but wood products industry employees are subject to accidents; City C population 55,000 and growing rapidly, median age 34, 60% college graduates, generally high out-of-pocket cost health insurance plans.

T: Health care in City A is provided by two large not-for-profit community hospitals that are in a technological war. When one gets new equipment the other obtains the newer model. This holds for the physical therapy departments also. Equipment wise there are 10 well-equipped hospital outpatient physical therapy clinics. There are four small physical-therapist owned clinics with varying degrees of technological and equipment sophistication. A therapist-owned clinic is the only paper free clinic. In City B, there is one medium size for-profit and two small not-for-profit general hospitals. The latter two are affiliated with larger hospital organizations in other cities.

They are the best equipped, most technologically advanced, and have the benefit of the resources of their parent corporations. All hospitals offer inpatient and outpatient physical therapy in their main buildings. The medium-size hospital also has an outpatient clinic 2 miles from the mill. A private practice physical therapist is across the street from the mill, another is 10 minutes away to the north of the mill and a third clinic is 15 minutes away to the south of the mill. The private clinics treat everyone from pediatric to hospice clients. All practices are paper and pen oriented. City C has two for-profit specialty hospitals. One is for orthopedics. The other is a heart hospital. There are several ambulatory care/emergency clinics around town. There are five private physical therapy practices. One concentrates on home care clients, three list themselves as orthopedic-sports clinics, and one is a geriatric and pediatric physical therapy clinic that also contracts with the school system. Attempts to gather information about these practices were unrewarding for various reasons. *Formulate a list of reasons you feel might account for this difficulty.*

CASE STUDY 3.2

SWOT Analysis

Task

Use the PEST analysis scenario plus the information you gathered about your state and conduct a SWOT analysis for the practice that wishes to expand. Do a cursory strengths and weaknesses analysis of the organization and an in-depth opportunities and threats analysis for EACH of the cities (do three SWOTs). Based on your SWOTs, choose one of the following options:

- Move forward in one of the cities
- Move forward in two cities
- Move forward in all three cities
- Delay a decision until the payer's computer troubles are resolved
- Expand the search to (*your choice of how many*) other cities
- Another option you wish to pursue not listed

CASE STUDY 3.3

Strategic Plan

Task

Take the choice you made in the preceding scenario and develop a strategic plan. Use Table 3.1 as your guide. You already have

the external environment scanned. If you need more information to complete this task use your creativity and experience to fill in the voids.

REFERENCES

Baldrige National Quality Program. Health care criteria of performance excellence. Gaithersburg, MD: Baldridge National Quality Program National Institute of Standards and Technology, Technology Administration, U.S. Department of Commerce. 2007.

Bourgeois LJ, Brodwin DR. Strategic implementation: Five approaches to an elusive phenomenon. Strategic Management Journal. 1984;5:241–264.

Carroll L. Alice's adventures in wonderland. New York, NY: D. Appleton and Company. 1866.

Center for Strategic Planning. Outcome-based strategic planning approach for schools. Defining elements of actionable strategic plans. Available at http://www.planonline.org/planning/strategic/planningmodel.htm. Accessed 4/02/07.

Clarkson KW, Miller RL, Jentz GA, Cross FB. West's business law: Text cases, legal, ethical, regulatory, and international environment, 6th ed. Minneapolis/St. Paul, MN: West. 1995.

Dunn RT. Haimann's supervisory management for health-care organizations, 6th ed. Boston, MA: McGraw-Hill. 1998.

Google. Company overview. Available at http://www.google.com/intl/en/corporate/index.html. Accessed 4/02/07.

Hannagan T. Mastering strategic management. New York, NY: Palgrave. 2002.

Helms MM, ed. Encyclopedia of Management, 4th ed. Detroit, MI: Gale Group. 2000.

Internet Center of Management and Business Administration. PEST analysis. Available at http://www.netmba.com/strategy/pest/. Accessed 4/10/07.

Jones J. The CEO Refresher. When is it time to rewrite your mission statement? Available at http://www.refresher.com/!jjmission.html. Accessed 4/13/07.

Kane M. The CEO refresher: The world of strategic thinking, it's not about time. Available at http://www.refresher.com/!mjkstrategic.html. Accessed 4/2/07.

Kaplan RS, Norton DP. The balanced scorecard-measures that drive performance. Harvard Business Review. 1992;72(1):71–79.

Learned EP, Christensen CR, Andrews KR, Guth WD. Business policy text and cases, Revised ed. Homewood, IL: Richard D. Irwin. 1969.

Macmillan H, Tampoe M. Strategic management. New York, NY: Oxford University Press. 2000.

McConkey DD. How to Manage by Results. New York, NY: AMACOM. 1976.

McNamara C. Basic overview of various strategic planning models. Adapted from the Field Guide to Nonprofit Strategic Planning and Facilitation. Minneapolis, MN: Authenticity Consulting, LLC. 1997–2007.

Mintzberg H, Quinn JB, Voyer J. The strategy process, Collegiate ed. Englewood Cliffs, NJ: Prentice Hall. 1995.

Mystrategicplan. How to create a strategic plan. Available at http://mystrategicplan.com/strategic-planning-tools/how-to-create-a-strategic-plan.shtml. Accessed 4/2/07.

Padgaonkar A. The CEO refresher. Invent your future with strategic planning. Available at http://www.refresher.com/aabpinvent.html. Accessed 4/1/07.

Policastro ML. U.S. Small Business Administration (SBA) Introduction to strategic planning. Management and Planning Series 21. Available at http://www.sba.gov/idc/groups/public/documents/sba_homepage/pub_mp21.pdf. Accessed 4/1/07.

QuickMBA. Strategic Management. PEST Analysis, 1999–2007. Available at http://www.quickmba.com/strategy/pest/. Accessed 4/9/07.

Rubenstien H. The CEO Refresher. Business planning and strategic planning revisited. Available at http://www.refresher.com/!hrrrevisited.htm. Accessed 4/1/07.

Senior Corps of Retired Executives (SCORE). About SCORE. Available at http://www.score.org/explore_score.html. Accessed 4/18/07.

Small Business Administration. Manage your business from start to finish. Available at http://www.sba.gov/smallbusinessplanner/plan/writeabusinessplan/SERV_STRATPLAN.html. Accessed 4/18/07a.

Small Business Administration. Entrepreneurial development. Available at http://www.sba.gov/aboutsba/sbaprograms/sbdc/index.html. Accessed 4/19/07b.

Swayne LE, Duncan WJ, Ginter PM. Strategic management of health care organizations, 5th ed. Malden, MA: Blackwell. 2006.

ADDITIONAL RESOURCES

For readers who would like to read some original papers on strategic management or strategic planning here are a few informative sources:

Eisenhardt JM. Strategy as strategic decision-making. Sloan Management Review. Spring 1999;40:65–72.

Hogan B. Stuck in the mud. Executive Excellence. 2003;20(8):15.

Middleton J. The Ultimate Strategy Library: The 50 most influential strategic ideas of all time. Chichester, West Sussex, United Kingdom, Capstone Publishing Ltd. 2000.

Mintzberg H. Patterns in strategy formation. Management Science. 1978;24(9):934.

Mintzberg H, Lampel J. Reflecting on the strategy process. Sloan Management Review. 1999;Spring:21–30.

Porter ME. What is strategy? Harvard Business Review. 1996;74:61–78.

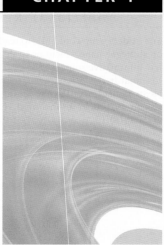

CHAPTER 4

EXTERNAL INFLUENCES: PHYSICAL THERAPY

LARRY J. NOSSE AND DEBORAH G. FRIBERG

Learning Objectives

1. Relate environmental scanning and analysis principles to the examination of the external environment of selected areas of the field of physical therapy.
2. Identify the components of an expanded adaptation of the PEST analysis called DEPT SPACES to examine external environmental factors.
3. Identify common sources of external environment information.
4. Given a case study, use the DEPT SPACES mnemonic and a related template as a guide to conduct an external scan of selected areas of the field of physical therapy.
5. Given a case study and a related template, begin a SWOT analysis by identifying opportunities and threats.
6. Given a case study, a related template, and data, practice estimating the degree of importance of identified opportunities and threats for specific organizations and concurrently estimate the probability of each opportunity and threat.
7. Interpret the results of item 6.

Introduction

This chapter will use many of the terms and concepts presented in Chapter 3 related to examining, assessing, and planning responses to external influences that can impact on the success of health service businesses. The two chapters differ in the *scope* of the **external environment**. The focus shifts from the general external forces on businesses, the **macro-environment** (Porter et al., 2006), to the macro- and micro-environments of physical therapy. Figure 4.1 represents this macro- and micro-environmental perspective. The circles embedded within circles reflect the multiple layers of extrinsic variables that could be examined. Analogous to a microscope, an examination of the microenvironment allows for a detailed examination of specific segments of physical therapy. In Figure 4.1 physical therapy is listed twice, first as a generic term, and then as an individual business. Within the "your setting" circle another smaller circle could have been added to represent individual physical therapists (PTs) or physical therapists assistants (PTAs) who are **sole proprietors** (Chapter 14).

Remember that *environmental scanning* is a continuous process used by large and small organizations as well as individual business owners for the same purpose, to guide planning the steps that will lead to achieving desired **goals**. The difference between large and small businesses is often the breadth of the surrounding external environment. Some organizations offering physical therapy services have the need, personnel, and expertise to perform broad-scope external scanning that looks at the macro-environment from the international through local levels of the industry. An example is Extendicare (2007) which has long-term care and outpatient health care

Key Terms

Key terms, which are defined below, are bolded and italicized the first time they appear in the chapter. Other important terms are shown in boldface on first appearance and are defined by the context in which they are used. When either of these types of terms is used several times, its acronym will be identified and subsequently used in the chapter. Both types of terms are listed alphabetically in the online glossary with their definitions and (when applicable) their acronyms.

accountability: responsible for one's actions.

competition: two or more parties concurrently striving to achieve the same end through the same object(s) of interest.

competitor analysis: a more discrete part of the environmental analysis process that focuses on gathering and assessing data on service area competitors for strategic decision making.

competitor(s): a rival for an object of common interest. Competitors are those who provide, intend to provide, and might provide similar services and products to the same target market(s), in the same service area(s).

demographic(s): characteristic(s) of the population of interest that influence their consumption of services and products. Examples of common demographic variables are: age, family size, health, income, level of education, marital status, occupation, location of residence, race, and gender.

DEPT SPACES: a mnemonic for categorizing important external environment elements. The letters stand for (D)emographics, (E)conomics, (P)olitics, (T)echnology, (S)takeholders, (P)erceptions, (A)ccountability,(C)ompetition, (E)cology, (S)ocial.

environmental scanning: gathering data from external environments that impact on the viability of an organization and then examining internal organizational assets that can be used to take advantage of discovered opportunities and minimize threats to the organization.

external stakeholders: individuals, groups, or organizations external to an organization who may wish to influence management decisions that will or may affect them.

fundamental documents: the core guiding documents of an organization. These are the vision, values, and mission statements; also called fundamental guiding statements/documents.

interface stakeholders: members of the organization that have a legal identity outside of the organization. For example, a physical therapist who treats clients in their homes in their free time.

internal stakeholders: individuals, groups, or organizations within an organization who may wish to influence management decisions that will or may affect them.

opportunities: the O in a SWOT analysis. Factors/variables identified through external environmental scanning and analyses processes that may be options for an organization to advance toward its goals.

physician-owned physical therapy services (POPTS): financial arrangements based on a physician's referral for physical therapist services when the referral is of financial benefit to the referring physician.

politics: processes for determining how decisions are made, how power is used, the rules for behavior, and procedures for dispute resolution.

reliable: the consistency of the results of measurements.

scope: the breadth, reach, or range of interest. Scope can be broad or wide, or narrow. For an organization or part of the organization there can be differences in terms of geographic markets, number of markets, and diversity of services or products.

stakeholders: individuals, groups, or organizations within and external to an organization who may wish to influence management decisions that will or may affect them.

threats: the T in a SWOT analysis. Factors or variables identified in the external environment that are likely to have a negative effect on the success of an organization.

valid: the meaningfulness of measurements made for specific purposes. Measurements that measure what they were intended to measure.

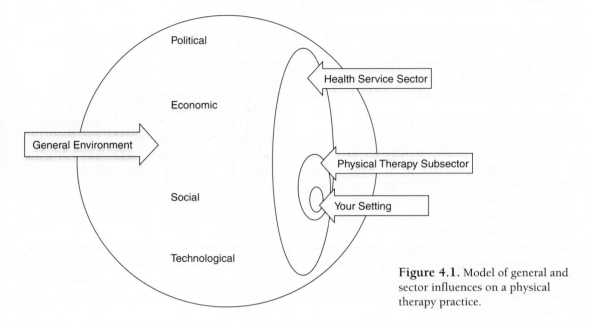

Figure 4.1. Model of general and sector influences on a physical therapy practice.

businesses in Canada and the United States. Compared to an international organization, the external surrounding of a national corporation is not as broad. Concentra (2007), which operates in 40 states and specializes in workers' compensation and occupational medicine, would be U.S.-focused. A less broad external environment would be relevant to a large regional rehabilitation business such as Novacare Rehabilitation (2007). This division of a corporation operates outpatient rehabilitation services in 19 states and the District of Columbia. It also offers on-site industrial rehabilitation. The relevant external interests would be in the overall health service industry and selected states, particularly those where Concentra also operates. MJ Care (2007) is a smaller regional rehabilitation business with contracts primarily in Wisconsin, Illinois, and Virginia. MJ Care provides rehabilitation services in multiple settings including hospitals, Veterans Administration centers, skilled nursing facilities, and schools. The variety of services and consumer types makes for a broad spectrum of external influences that could impact on this organization. A single state not-for-profit hospital system is WakeMed (2007). This organization is a network of medical and ambulatory care centers and outpatient facilities in North Carolina. The **operations** are geographically limited so interest in

external variables is relatively local. However, WakeMed uses national quality comparison data to gauge its performance. The most constrained external environment is that of a small physical therapy practice. A practice with one or two owners who **manage** the practice(s) and treat patients have little time to scan more than their local environment. Northshore and Homestead Physical Therapy located in two Wisconsin cities is an example practice. Besides time limitations, a small practice may not generate enough expendable income to purchase consultant services or reports from data resource centers to help with *environmental scanning*. Under these constraints the objective of a scan is likely to be to gain an understanding of the few most important external variables relevant to the practice(s). The most important matters are often those related to garnering enough clients to stay in business (Chapter 22).

Another reminder from Chapter 3 is that an external environmental scan provides half of the **strategic planning** information. External influences are usually determined first to identify *opportunities* and *threats*. The second half of the information comes from examining the organization's **internal environment** (Chapters 5 and 6). This scan identifies the organization's **strengths** and **weaknesses**, allowing it to move forward take advantage of potential opportunities or to buffer threats (Helms, 2006). In other words, health service managers need to learn what's out there that may help or hurt their business before they can determine the availability and adequacy of their resources to do something about their findings (Chapters 5 and 6).

Environmental scanning is ongoing. It is not something that starts and stops. The information gathered has to be kept up-to-date when strategic planning takes place. Ideally, most of the information gathered will be relevant and interpretable. For our external scanning and analysis examples we use a variety of physical therapy situations. By looking at the external environment from these different physical therapy perspectives the reader will have the opportunity to experience the mental challenges involved in selecting external variables relevant to a specific organization, department, or practice. Guided by the *DEPT SPACES* mnemonic, most external variable categories that are relevant to these physical therapy subsectors can be identified, thoughtfully discussed, and analyzed.

PEST to DEPT SPACES

Table 3.4 in Chapter 3 was built on a (P)olitical, (E)conomic, (S)ocial, (T)echnolgical (**PEST**) analysis to introduce the general components of an environmental scan. This table provided lists of examples of the kinds of external variables that generally impact on businesses including health service businesses. Managers and staff with little prior scanning experience may find it easier to carry out a scan with a more precise list of environmental components. To this end the PEST categories were incorporated into a more explicit memory aiding mnemonic, DEPT SPACES. The mnemonic's letters represent ten external environments:

1. **D**emographic
2. **E**conomic
3. **P**olitical
4. **T**echnology
5. **S**takeholder
6. **P**erceptions
7. **A**ccountability
8. **C**ompetition
9. **E**cology
10. **S**ocial

The expansion of external influence categories offers three potential benefits. First, it may produce a more exact analysis of the external environment by identifying more variables to consider. Second, because variables can have an influence in more than one category, listing them in more than one category may make it easier to see each variable's breadth of influence. Third, identifying variables with cross-category influences can help selecting and prioritizing the variables to focus in the relevant portion of the SWOT analysis. The mnemonic letters were chosen to form PT-relevant words. They do not suggest a fixed order of environments to scan. However, demographic information is a reasonable place to begin because of the variety of economic, social, income, and employment-related information typically included in demographic databases. The mnemonic is a guide. Which specific variables actually chosen to investigate is a management decision fueled by a combination of personal values, experience, informed judgment based on subjective and objective evidence, intuition, and current circumstances (Helms, 2006; Swayne et al., 2006) (Chapters 7, 11, and 15).

D: Demographic Environment

The statistical characteristics of a group of people are called their *demographics* (Random House, 1999). In business, demographic characteristics of interest are those that correlate with a specific segment of the population's consumption of particular services and products. Examples of demographic information that is helpful for developing health service strategic plans for marketing and advertising plans (Chapters 18 and 19), services to offer, business expansion or retraction (Longest et al., 2000), and other purposes are listed in Table 4.1. A great deal of demographic information is collected by various governmental agencies. Relevant information is publicly available from agencies such as:

• Bureau of Labor Statistics (2007a,b): National occupational growth projections and average salaries

- Census Bureau (2007a,b): Population estimates by age and gender and economic information on 886 metro and micropolitan areas.
- Economic Development Board (County of Sonoma, 2007): Local economic and demographic information including health care providers
- Federal Bureau of Investigation (2007): Crime rates for cities with populations >100,000
- Health and Human Services (2007): Poverty rates by geographical area
- National Center for Health Statistics (2007): Age and health, injuries, trends, future projections, selected disease information, and expenditure information

A practical use for demographic information for students is examining the cost of off-campus housing in areas around the universities they might be interested in attending. In addition to cost, information about neighborhood, social, cultural, and safety considerations may also be sought. PTs looking for a new position could compare the average salary in the **metropolitan statistical areas** (MSA) they would consider moving to. A private practice owner looking for a clinic space to rent would do well to consider the insurance and income information of the population within a few miles of each potential location as well as the locations of like providers. Rehabilitation managers considering new service lines would find the incidence of major diseases by age group for their service delivery area powerful supportive information. An organization wishing to explore new service lines would certainly examine the demographic data of their service area, income, insurance, and other utilization and payment-related information.

E: Economic Environment

In personal life and in business, economic considerations are included in strategic plans. Essentially, **economics** is the study of consumption and production (Porter et al., 2006). To be able to consume and provide services or products requires money. Economic data therefore includes how consumers, providers of services, producers of goods, and government

Table 4.1 Examples of Demographic Items of Interest to Health Service Businesses

Item	Sample Correlations of Interest
Age group	Number of people Gender distribution What media they use to inform themselves? What are the chronologically related health service needs? Level of disability
Educational level	Average educational attainment Preferred media used for health information
Employment	Major employers Occupational title Common injury/disease risks Location Benefits Unemployment
Health	Functional level Average number of physician visits/ physical therapist visits Medical history Number of major diagnoses Usual providers of medical and physical therapy services Who pays for the services? Use what complimentary health services/products
Housing	Home Zip code Total monthly payment for housing Own home House value Rental housing
Income	Salary/hourly rate/annual income Average debt Discretionary funds
Social/cultural	Religion Base language Other languages spoken Country of birth Immigration status Marital status Dependents Life style
Transportation	Total monthly payment for transportation Usual mode Who usually drives? Number of cars Own/lease/borrow Frequency of public transport use

choose to use their limited financial resources (Chapter 20). Economists use historical and current data on production, income, spending, price, **supply and demand**, employment and unemployment, and other areas to predict future economic trends. The **inflation rate** (price increases) and **interest rate** (borrowing cost) are two important trends.

Macroenvironmental information is essential for physical therapy providers that operate in multiple states, deal with payer sources that cover large areas of the country, and provide services to large national corporations. For example, national corporate **management** needs to know current regional salary ranges, pending payment rule changes, employment outlook, and health benefit trends in their economic sector(s). While widespread economic factors can have similar impact on comparable physical therapy corporations, each will develop unique strategies to deal with them based on their internal resources and limitations (Chapters 5 and 6). Management of regional physical therapy businesses who have a vision of growth beyond the current service area(s) likewise need to look at the broader economic trends. Smaller localized practices are critically affected by the local economic variables. An example of local external influence is the sale of a nearby company to new owners who have announced the need to reduce the number of employees and increase employee contribution to health insurance.

National, regional, and local economic information is often included in demographic studies and can be found at the governmental sources noted earlier. Specific economic information and analysis of many regions of the country are available through the following agencies:

- Bureau of Economic Analysis (2007): Produces BEARFACTS which consists of narratives for states, counties, MSAs, and BEA economic areas. These narratives describe an area's personal income using current estimates, growth rates, and a breakdown of the sources of personal income down to the city level.
- Census Bureau (2007b,c): Economic information available includes personal income, wealth, and health service utilization

- Economic Development Administration (2007a,b): Narrative reports on selected areas of the United States noting economic related strengths, weaknesses, opportunities, and threats. Rural communities have been of interest for the past several years
- FedStats (2007): Website links to 100 government agencies with descriptions of the available statistics

P: Political Environment

Politics is the art and science of influencing decisions. The main elements of politics include rules for the use of power, behavioral expectations, procedures for dispute resolution, and strategies to influence decisions. External environment scanning is most often associated with the activities of government (Beech and Chadwick, 2005; Random House, 1999). We recognize that politics is part of most group interactions between friends, family members, students and teachers, colleagues, and grass roots political groups (Chapter 1). Here we will emphasize external politics using physical therapy examples.

The APTA advocacy site is an excellent place to begin looking for "legislative hot topics" specific to physical therapy (see Additional Resources). There are links to the association's governmental affairs office and their communications about congressional issues, federal regulatory issues, and state government issues. The top five congressional issues for APTA members in 2007 were

1. Support for payment for appropriate services, less burdensome payment process, consideration of additional payment methods, and **pay for performance**.
2. **Medicare therapy cap**: support for alternatives to a yearly maximum on payment for physical therapy services to **Medicare B** beneficiaries served by PTs in private practice.
3. Referral for profit/ *Physician-owned physical therapy services (POPTS)*: support enactment and enforcement of federal laws that would prohibit financial arrangements where referral sources refer patients to physical therapy services in which they have ownership and thus profit from the referral.

4. Direct access under Medicare: support federal legislation that allows Medicare beneficiaries to be able to access PTs without a referral where state jurisdictions allow direct access.
5. Clinical coverage and compliance: support legislation and regulations to ensure that the spectrum of medically necessary services provided by PTs are covered (paid for).

Tip O'Neill (1994), former speaker of the U.S. House of Representatives, said all politics is local. For licensed PTs and PTAs the local regulating body is the state. The health service political issues at the state level related to physical therapy affects the practice of every PT, and where licensed, every PTA licensee (Chapter 8). States define the terms physical therapy, PT, and, where licensed, PTAs. They also set requirements for initial licensure, relicensure, referral/direct access, and other issues critical to the regulation of physical therapy practice. Sources of information on local matters are available from each state's APTA affiliate (see http://www.apta.org and click on communities). All state governments have a department that deals with regulated professions. Their websites often have information about changes in licensure laws, relevant Q & A site, and a link to a regulatory digest that provide minutes of meetings, summaries of new legislation, and other useful information like a link to information from the state's physical therapy examining board. All **jurisdictions** are members of the **Federated State Boards of Physical Therapy** (**FSBPT**). The FSBPT's website provides information about the **National Physical Therapy Examination** (**NPTE**), a recommended definition of physical therapy for state licensure bodies, and links to state licensing authorities (http://fsbpt.org/licensing/index.asp).

T: Technology Environment

Technology includes ideas, equipment, methods, and anything else that helps expand human capabilities (Massachusetts Department of Education, 2007). As technology evolves it produces a continuous flow of new methods for developing, producing, and delivering services and products. Computer hardware and software programs are familiar technologies that change regularly. These changes bring about change in other technologies. For example, there are computer-based products and services for: communicating, accumulating, accessing, examining (**mining**), interpreting, and sharing information (data), making decisions (**decision support system**), leading and managing people, fostering creativity, increasing profitability, productivity, efficiency and effectiveness, and so on. All these technologies have potential application across the spectrum of physical therapy environments from the individual clinician level through the professional organizational level. Individual therapists and assistants may find that inexpensive voice recognition software can meet their documentation needs while reducing time spent writing or keyboarding and transcription cost. Some department managers have the authority to purchase major pieces of equipment. Distance-learning training in sales techniques can enhance a PT manager's confidence when negotiating with equipment vendor representatives. Some department managers provide valued input on major equipment purchases. The ability to use spreadsheet software to present reasonable estimates of **costs** (initial costs, training costs, maintenance and extended warranty costs) and **revenue** over time would be helpful when making the request. Skill with basic architectural drawing and flow chart programs can help managers make their point. Training in sales techniques can enhance the likelihood of gaining favorable responses to data supported recommendations (Chapter 19). A health service organization with a sense that its clinical services are falling short of meeting the mission to provide services that meet or exceed its patients' expectations may contract with an outside consultant group. Trained consultants can lead **focus groups** to get a variety of community members' perspectives on issues such as waiting times, courtesy, billing accuracy, and respect for dignity. The information can be coded by the consultants directly from the interview or later from video recordings. The coded information can be scanned and analyzed by statistical programs. Another available technology is consultant groups. Consultant groups are able to conduct surveys or interview statistically desirable numbers from the target community using *valid* and *reliable* proprietary instruments to gather data to formulate their recommendations (Chapter 6). Recommendations often include changes in work methods and service processes (Helms, 2006). The APTA used a consultant research group to scan the environment relative to workforce needs (Vector Research, 1997). This association also sought expertise in software development. It partnered with a medical software corporation to develop a user-friendly physical therapy computerized patient record system that will feed into a national outcomes data base for system subscribers (APTA, 2007a).

Technology is a strategic resource. If new technology is to expand PT and PTA capabilities it needs to be adopted at the appropriate time. An early adoption in the evolution process will likely mean costly upgrades and additional training time to maximize the usefulness of the technology. If it is adopted late, others will have had more experience with it, which may give them a competitive advantage (Swayne et al., 2006). Early, on-time, or late, technology adaptation changes how things are done. Since technological change seems to be one of the few constants in the external environment, how well other organizations have responded to change should not be overlooked in an external environmental scan. Sources of technology relevant to PTs include:

- APTA publications including those of sections and state chapters
- APTA conferences and meetings including exhibitors, posters, and platform presentations
- Buyers guides, e.g., Fitter First Professional Products; Patterson Medical Sammons Preston Professional Catalog
- Professional Rehab Catalog, PT Magazine Buyers Guide, and Invacare Wheelchairs
- Consultants, e.g., APTA consulting services; Images and Associates; Kovacek Management, Services; Rehabilitation Consulting and Resource Institute; Service Corps of Retired Executives (SCORE)
- Educational programs, e.g., individual faculty members from various departments including bioengineering, business, computer science, exercise science, and physical therapy

- Manufacturer websites, e.g., Chattanooga Group (electrotherapy), Cybex (fitness and testing equipment), Hoggan Health Industries (ergonomic measurement equipment), Neurocom International (balance measurement system), Tekscan (gait analysis system)
- Meetings of other professional organizations, e.g., National Prevention and Health Promotion Summit, Annual Federal Occupational Health Conference, Annual Meeting of the American Academy of Orthopaedic Surgeons, and Symposia of the American Medical Informatics Association
- Research centers, e.g., Trace Center at the University of Wisconsin-Madison, Robotics Laboratory, Sensory Motor Performance Center at the Rehabilitation Institute of Chicago, Civitan International Research Center, the University of Alabama at Birmingham (see Additional Resources)
- Trade association meetings, e.g., National Consumer Driven Summit, Annual National Forum on Quality Improvement in Health Care, Augmentative-Alternative Communication and Assistive Technology Conference
- Trade publications, e.g., Advance for Physical Therapists and PT Assistants, Newsline for Physical Therapists and PT Assistants, Physical Therapy Products, PT/OT Insider, and Rehab Management

S: Stakeholder Environment

Whenever an organization's management makes decisions there are individuals, groups, and other organizations who want to influence them because they may have something to gain or lose depending on the decision (Nosse et al., 2005). The individuals, groups, and organizations that have a stake in the success of an organization are known as its *stakeholders* (Swayne et al., 2006). Longest et al. (2000) categorizes stakeholders according to their relationship to the organization of interest. *Internal stakeholders* (Chapters 5 and 6) are members of the organization, such as rehabilitation department managers and staff PTs. *Interface stakeholders* are also part of the organization but they have a legal identity outside of the organization. Contract PTs, consultants, and stockholders of for-profit businesses are examples of interface stakeholders.

Stakeholders outside of the organization make up the last group, *external stakeholders*. Examples of external stakeholders likely to have interest in rehabilitation service businesses are listed in Table 4.2.

Keeping the three categories in mind (internal, interface, and external) can help ensure that all relevant stakeholders have been identified and their views examined in the decision-making process. This is difficult to do. Organizational leaders have to deal with the competing interests and demands of multiple stakeholders as each exerts their own degree of influence. Internal stakeholders (Chapters 5 and 6) tend to be interested in issues related to formulating and implementing strategies. External stakeholders tend to be interested in outcomes (Porter et al., 2006). Interface stakeholders may be interested in strategies and outcomes. Ultimately, it is the organization's governing body that is responsible for achieving balance between advancing the organization's vision and mission, social responsibility and ethics, and stakeholders' belief that their views have been heard and considered (Swayne et al., 2006). Whether or not the balance is achieved often remains a difference in perception.

P: Perceptions Environment

The term *perceptions* is used here to mean the understanding that stakeholders, potential stakeholders, and others have about an organization whose success they have a stake in. There are also people who may have an interest in the organization succeeding in the future—potential stakeholders (Swayne et al., 2006). Perceptions are the points of view these interested and potentially interested individuals, groups, and organizations have about what the organization is, what it does, and what it should do. In an external environmental scan the perceptions of interface and external stakeholders are of greatest interest. These stakeholders have intermittent or indirect contact with the organization, respectively. They form their perceptions on limited actual experience as part of the organization or from information the organization allows to circulate. Nonetheless, analysis of stakeholder perceptions can provide opportunities for the organization to:

Table 4.2   Categories of Physical Therapy–Related External Stakeholders

Categories	Examples
Accreditation agencies	Commission on Accreditation of Physical Therapy Education (CAPTE) Commission on Accreditation of Rehabilitation Agencies (CARF)
Competitors	Athletic trainers Physical therapy businesses in your service area with similar offerings aimed at your targeted consumers Holistic complementary health services
Consumers	Legal referral sources (state statute dependent) Internal (staff, other department members [actual and potential users and verbal referral sources]) Patients, their family and friends (actual and potential users)
Labor groups	Employer groups formed to lower health service costs Federal Employees Health Benefits Program Labor unions
Local community	City finance/assessor's office Fire, police, emergency, and recreation departments Lenders Major employers
Regulatory bodies	Centers for Medicare and Medicaid Services (CMS) Internal Revenue Service State Departments of Health, Regulation and Licensing
Special interest groups	American Physical Therapy Association State chiropractic associations Paralyzed Veterans Association
Suppliers	Durable medical goods providers Temporary staffing agencies Private transport companies
Third-party payers	Medicare intermediaries (Part A) and carriers (Part B) United Health Care Blue Cross Blue Shield Self-insured companies

- Alter the relative degree of influence among stakeholders by fostering or rebutting the ideas they put forward. This can elevate or reduce the relative status of a stakeholder.
- Enact a strategy to manage stakeholder perceptions. The more that is known about stakeholder perceptions the more precise a strategy can be crafted.
- Incorporate new insights offered by stakeholders into strategic plans. This can lead to further good will, more cooperation, and more give and take.
- Provide more information and arrange for individual meeting opportunities with stakeholders to counter their misperceptions. This can be promoted as a sincere effort to increase organizational transparency and foster cooperation.

Finding out what stakeholder perceptions are can be assessed either directly or indirectly. A direct approach entails gaining information directly from the stakeholder through attending gatherings where stakeholders express their views, e-mail or fax communications, interviews, letters and memos, and phone conversations. An indirect approach might include anonymous and unidentified third-party comments, general publications, news reports, organizational documents, sponsored focus groups, and surveys (Chapter 3).

The following is a physical therapy–related example of directly acquiring knowledge of stakeholder perceptions.

Background: Management of a regional rehabilitation center is currently ordering and buying its own equipment and supplies as well as directing patients to the five local medical equipment vendors. It has been documented that the time spent by the rehabilitation services manager, PTs and PTAs, occupational therapists and assistants, social workers, accounting office staff, secretaries, clerks, and nursing staff in dealing with five vendors averages 1.5 hours per patient. It is proposed that purchasing might be consolidated with a single national vendor approved to participate in Medicare's competitive bidding program (see Additional Resources) who can meet the organization's and patients' needs through online ordering. Management believes that one vendor, one extensive catalog, one order-ing template, one phone call, and one shipper will increase efficiency.

Vendor stakeholders: The local vendors learned of the consolidation discussion by seeing it listed as an agenda item published in the center's monthly newsletter. Based on this item their perception was that the center, which had a very favorable reputation in the business and resident communities, was about to do something that would detract from its good standing. Basically, going to a national vendor was not in keeping with the center's commitment to the community. The vendor's spokesperson noted that the community had always seen the center as a supporter of local businesses as well as a significant contributor to the well-being of injured and disabled people. In the vendor group's opinion, the proposed consolidation would be detrimental to patients and businesses. Patients would no longer receive the individual attention they currently received from local vendors. With less business, the vendors would have to downsize their workforce, increase employee contributions for health insurance, and reduce inventory. The largest local vendor added that it was doubtful that a national vendor's prices would be significantly lower on all items when transportation costs were added. To support this statement he provided a list of 100 items he "shopped" for from national vendor catalogs. The overall price differential between the national vendors and his prices was less than 1%. When the director of rehabilitation services reviewed the list she noted that about half of the chosen items were seldom ordered from any of the local vendors and several of the brands were lesser known brands. Another vendor suggested that the vendors might jointly order from the same sources to obtain better prices on the commonly ordered items and then be able to lower their prices accordingly. The group was invited to continue the discussion over lunch in the center's cafeteria.

Dealing with vendor perspectives: During lunch it was clarified that the purpose for consolidating was more a matter of improving service efficiency and value than it was the price of equipment and supplies. Consolidation would automate some aspects of service and would enhance an aspect of organizational integration. The key points presented were

- Dealing with five independent vendor businesses is expensive for the center.
- It would be a benefit to patients and their caregivers to have a single vendor with an extensive online catalog that included video clips showing the equipment in use.
- The total cost and the ability to order online 24 hours per day, 7 days a week, would facilitate timely discharge planning.
- A reduction in labor costs, a potential increase in therapist billable time, and more timely discharges would increase many facets of organizational efficiency.

Stakeholder influence: In recognition of the center's obligation to be a good corporate citizen, the chief financial officer told the group that a final decision would not be made for 90 days. He told the local vendors that the center would welcome a plan from them that realized the desired benefits and efficiencies that had been outlined. To assist them, the rehabilitation services director would be available to consult with the group as needed. The interaction with interface and external stakeholders reminded the center's management that they are answerable to a variety of stakeholders regarding their actions.

A: Accountability Environment

The essence of *accountability* is to be answerable to someone else (who), in some way (how), for something that was said, done, or omitted (what) (Swisher and Krueger-Brophy, 1998), at some point in time (when). In an external environment context accountability begins with identifying the primary individuals, groups, and organizations that make up the "who." The categories listed in Table 4.2 can serve to guide identification of who the organization is accountable to. The similarity of categories underscores the connection between an organization's stakeholders and organizational accountability (Chapters 7–11, 16, 17, and 21).

Accountability for individual PTs has also been defined by the APTA. The description is more behaviorally specific than the preceding description. The act of being accountable includes (1) acknowledging and accepting consequences for one's actions, (2) acting in accord with the association's **code of ethics**, policies, and procedures, (3) actively seeking and responding to feedback, (4) communicating accurately, and (5) responding to consumer needs (APTA, 2007b). These behaviors can be extrapolated to a business that offers physical therapy service and is engaged in environmental scanning. To help identify the accountabilities of the organizations the following questions may be helpful:

- To whom does the organization have legal responsibilities (e.g., consumers, contractors, payers)?
- What do the mission and values statements say about whom we serve and how we will interact with them (e.g., customer satisfaction records, risk management reports, patients bill of rights)?
- With whom has there been proactive follow-up on unfinished business that the organization agreed to complete (e.g., check minutes, correspondence, phone logs)?
- Have public and private communications been candid, clear, and truthful (e.g., news releases, e-mail, annual reports)?
- Have the needs of those in our service area been met (e.g., marketing data, consultant reports, competitor challenges)?

Some competitors may challenge the accuracy or completeness of information available about any part of their organization's operations. The challenged organization has the responsibility to respond within the guidelines of accountability. The broader issues of identifying and examining competitors' intentions are addressed next.

C: Competition Environment

In Chapter 3, we noted that the forces in the general external environment act on all businesses in the same **sector** of the economy. The important regulations pertaining to business *competition* are deferred until Chapter 9, which will discuss all types of regulations. The discussion in this section deals mostly with the competitive **microenvironment** of selected subsectors of physical therapy. This level of data gathering and assessment is often called a *competitor analysis* (Swayne et al., 2006).

So, what is **competition**? When two or more individuals or groups seek the same thing, a rivalry or competition to acquire the item of common interest exists. To successfully complete the quest for the object of mutual interest, information about competitors is needed in order to formulate appropriate strategies (Chapters 3 and 13). Who are business *competitors*? Competitors are those who provide, intend to provide, and might provide similar services and products to the same **target market**(s), in the same service area(s) (Chapter 18). The continued success of a business is dependent in part on identifying, examining, and formulating appropriate strategies to deal with its actual and perceived competitors (Longest et al., 2000) (Chapters 13, 14, 16, and 18).

Example sources for identifying competitors are noted in Table 4.3. Competitor information can come from multiple sources (also see Table 3.4) but it should be precise and timely. A good place to get familiar with a competitor is through their **fundamental documents** (vision, values, and mission statements) (Nosse et al., 2005). These statements say what the organization aspires to become, what it considers most important in its dealing, what it does well and for whom, respectively (Chapter 7). These documents are often available online, in organizational publications, on display at the competitor's facilities, and shared with consumers. These documents are also often in the organization's annual reports along with general financial information. Annual reports may be included in the reading material in reception or waiting areas, at an information desk in their facility, or available if requested. Annual report summaries contain how each part of the business or each location has done financially, patient demographics and volume, and other useful information. If the organization has a foundation, foundation reports provide additional future direction, accomplishment, and financial information. Organization and foundation websites may have more current data than published reports. Local media may also report on some aspects of your competitor organizations. If the service area is geographically large, media scanning service can be purchased to track information about competitors. Consultant groups may be hired to gather competitor data rather than taking employees away from their normal tasks.

Table 4.3   Potential Sources for Identifying Competitors
Advertisements
Attorneys
Board members
Billing services
Brochures
Building permits
Computer installers
Construction workers
Direct competitor contact
Employment agencies
Informational mailings
Interviewees
Internal and external networks
Letter carriers/post office
Organizational publications
Other competitors
Patients and their caregivers
Real estate agents
Real estate sales information
Referral sources
Search engines/websites
Suppliers/vendors
Trade publications/directories
Unplanned discovery/luck

The type of information to look for is whatever will help identify competitor areas of excellence and advertising, expansion, and other strategies and their "soft spots." A competitor's areas of excellence and strategies may pose threats to your organization's success and their soft spots may become opportunities that your organization can take advantage of to advance toward goals. Table 4.3 provides examples of information sources that offer this kind of information (see also Chapter 3). Notice the similarities between the stakeholder examples in Table 4.2 and the information source examples in Table 4.3. This suggests that a cordial relationship with stakeholders can be an asset when scanning the competitive environment.

The scope and intensity of competitor efforts and the **tactics** they have and are likely to use is important information. The key questions to answer are, *how have our competitors competed in the past, how are they competing now, and how are they likely to compete in the future?* The answers come from the scanned sources (e.g., Tables 4.2 and 4.3). At one end of the philosophical spectrum of health services completion is to compete by offering consumers more value for their dollar and consistently high quality outcomes. In this vein competition could be based on continuity of care from admission through discharge. It could be based on safety indicated by low unintended injury rate. Superior functional outcomes for patients with strokes would certainly be of interest to consumers (Chapter 16). Such desirable and distinguishable characteristics are achieved by health service organizations that are innovative. Innovations that improve quality and reduce costs add value for the consumer (Porter and Teisberg, 2006). Innovations that attract more consumers are likely to be adopted by competitors. This customer-value driven competition is constructive, as it can bring more value to more customers. It is a win-win type of competition.

The other end of the spectrum is probably a more familiar description of competition. In this version, there is a winner and a loser. In this type of competition a win is someone else's loss because the object of interest gained by one competitor is a loss to one or more another competitors. Consider for example the Milwaukee, Wisconsin MSA, which has about 1.5 million residents. There have been four major health service systems competing for insured and **self-pay** consumers. To gain more targeted consumers from a fixed number of such consumers means the gain of one system is a loss for one or more of the others. One system lauds itself on providing state of the art diagnostic, surgical, and rehabilitation services. It uses technology coupled with specialized services in its strategy to increase market share rather than competing on price. The other health service systems feel compelled to purchase the same equipment out of concern for losing consumers. This means costs and spending go up for all systems. There are concerns about underutilization of the expensive equipment. Also, initially, the first

system with the equipment and training has the most experience which it claims lead to superior outcomes. This technology warfare depicts investment inefficiencies and potential patient safety concerns at three of the four systems. Competition for staff also occurs. All of the systems have unfilled physical therapy management and staff positions. A common win–lose scenario is that one system begins offering higher salaries and bonuses to "win-over" some local PTs. Rather than risk losing valued personnel the other systems match these incentives. Cost goes up but value for most physical therapy consumers does not. Consumers may receive appropriate care in the better staffed "winning" system's facilities but consumers of the "losing" system(s) may be wait listed or scheduled less often than is optimal for their condition. In this scenario the sum total of consumer value gained minus the consumer value lost is zero. In the four systems, physical therapy services were not improved by win–loss competition. Competition that does not improve value for consumers perpetuates the known problems in the U.S. health services sector: inefficiencies, high cost, a relatively poor safety record, and less than optimal outcomes (Porter and Teisberg, 2006). Keeping track of competitor strategies and trends can be aided by entering information into a matrix such as that found in Table 4.4. The information can then be digested before it is analyzed further.

E: Ecology Environment

This topic could have been included in the competition environment but it was felt that doing so would have minimized the potential importance of including this area in the internal scan. There are two aspects of an ecological environment scan: (1) public health and (2) the natural and man-made surroundings. The more common of these is how health service organizations, particularly hospitals and medical offices, deal with human tissue, and infectious and radioactive wastes. In the microenvironment of physical therapy, the relatively few biohazards, such as contaminated bandages, disposable gowns, soiled absorbent pads, used gloves, and similar items, must be disposed of. The handling and disposal of potentially hazardous and contaminated

Table 4.4   Sample Competitor Matrix

Selected Variables	Competitors				
	New to Area	East Side	West Side	North Side	South Side
Background Date(s), Source(s)					
Leadership Date(s), Source(s)					
Org. Goals Date(s), Source(s)					
Location(s) Date(s), Source(s)					
Target Market(s) Date(s), Source(s)					
Volume Date(s), Source(s)					
Reputation Date(s), Source(s)					
Personnel Date(s), Source(s)					
Financial Info. Date(s), Source(s)					
Strategies Date(s), Source(s)					
Others					

materials is a public safety and ecology matter. How much waste is produced? Where does it go? What is the risk of harm to others? These are questions that an external scan may include when looking at competitors when there is a community concern about air pollution (burning waste) or land fill contamination of water. A related health concern is the risk posed by a competitor's physical facilities and grounds. It is often more efficient for a business to rent space than to build or buy. It is common to rent space for outpatient clinics. Older facilities near business and residential areas that are being upgraded may be reasonably priced. However, there are potential health risks if extensive renovation including removal of hazardous materials has not been done yet. Older buildings may have been recently painted but without removal of underlying lead-based paint. Very old buildings may have some functioning lead water pipes. False ceilings may cover old ceiling tiles with asbestos in them. Asbestos was also used as insulation around heating and hot water pipes. Mold is common where basements are damp. Poor ventilation can lead to high accumulated levels of pollutants. Inadequately grounded outlets and the absence of ground-fault interrupters in outlets near water is another hazard. Finally, the ground around an older (or new) building may be contaminated from prior businesses that operated at the site. Information about the extent of a building's renovation and hazard removal is available at the city or county building permit department. When authorized work has been adequately completed an occupancy permit is issued by the city. Some building owners skirt these permits by doing the work themselves or having unlicensed contractors do the work without a permit. This leaves the question of facility safety unanswered.

The second view of ecology deals with harmony. Looking at the way a business interacts with its natural and man-made surroundings can be a benefit or liability in a SWOT analysis. A facility that is congruent with the organization's mission (services, location, and target market) is a threat to a competitor with a less ideal facility. This is because at some level of consciousness consumers have expectations about what a hospital physical therapy department or an outpatient physical therapy clinic should look like, how it should be maintained, and how it fits in with its neighbors and natural surroundings. Basically, a facility and its location should match the expectations of the targeted consumers (Chapters 18 and 22). An opportunity could exist if a competing sports and orthopedic practice operated in or near a skilled nursing facility. A sports and orthopedic practice that operated within or near a health club would be a threat to a competitor who was not in this type of location.

Construction of a new facility can have negative ecological effects as well as be a threat to competitors. New facilities can improve an organization's income but they can also alter a neighborhood's appearance, the natural topography, and strain local resources. These issues can be raised during the planning phase of the project and may lessen the immediate threat of a competitor's expansion by delaying approval or terminating the construction. Any of the sources in Table 4.3 can be the source of competitor's plans. An opportune time to raise ecological questions is at city planning committee meetings. These are open meetings with pre-announced agendas that are often attended by local reporters. Consider the following scenario: A **not-for-profit** physical therapy organization wishes to build a three-storey satellite facility for a state-of-the-art children's rehabilitation center. The intent would be to lease office space on the upper floors to medical and other health service providers. The plan includes 300 outdoor parking spaces. The building site is surrounded by single-story ranch style office buildings each surrounded by trees and flower gardens. These buildings blend well with the natural surroundings. A concern that could be raised is that the building and parking area would change the neighborhood architecture and the natural vista.

The size of the proposed facility would likely bring increased traffic (noise, pollution, and safety concerns), increased utilization of gas, water, and electricity, and a potential increased burden on the resources of the local infrastructure, e.g., traffic lights and road signage, road changes, and fire and police services. It could be pointed out that no direct tax dollars would be generated to cover governmental expenses because the facility would be tax-exempt. This in itself might delay the facility. This delay would allow time to explore opportunities for competing organizations to: expand services for children, investigate the need for more medical office space and options for providing space, and develop grassroots networks to contact legislators to advocate for termination of the building project.

S: Social Environment

Many social variables are found in demographic data provided by sources such as those noted earlier in the demographic section. These variables are less income related than those discussed so far. Social environment includes age, base language, country of birth, immigration status, lifestyle, marital status, number of dependents, religion, organizational memberships, and more. These external variables can impact on staff selection, facility location, adjunct services provided, community groups to support, marketing, and other business decisions.

SWOTing and Evaluating Likelihoods

Once collected, the external environment data musst be organized, sifted, and prioritized. The initial step in the analysis process is to list the opportunities (O) and threats (T) for a SWOT analysis. Opportunities compatible with the organization's **mission** and **values statements** are listed. Figure 4.2 is a template for organizing information for SWOT analysis. The external environment O and T findings are entered in the two lower boxes. These lists are then examined to estimate their impact on the organization and their probability of occurring.

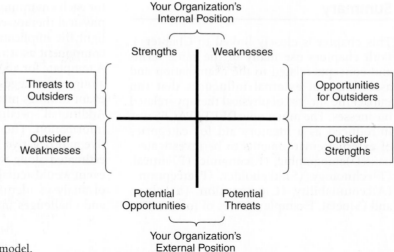

Figure 4.2. Annotated SWOT model.

This step results in estimates of the degree of strength or benefit and severity or challenge to each O and T, respectively, along with the likelihood of the events actually happening (Helms, 2006). Figure 4.3 is a matrix template for entering O and T strength/severity and probability estimates. The completion of the upper boxes of the SWOT template requires examination of the organization's capabilities to leverage O and deal with T. These internal environment scanning topics will be addressed in Chapters 5 and 6.

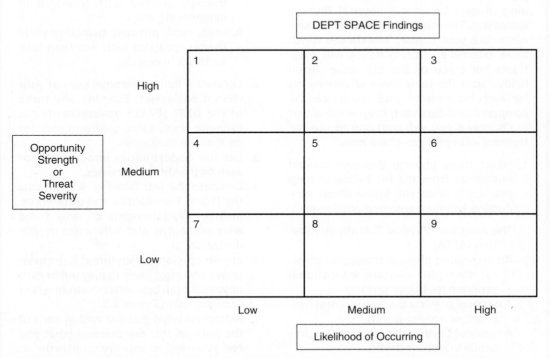

Figure 4.3. Matrix template for qualifying external environment findings according to their anticipated impact on the organization and their likelihood of occurring.

Summary

This chapter is closely linked to Chapter 3. Both chapters use many of the same terms and concepts related to the examination and assessment of external influences that can impact the success of physical therapy–related businesses. The mnemonic DEPT SPACES was introduced as a memory aid for categories of external environments to be investigated, i.e., (D)emographic, (E)conomic, (P)olitical, (T)echnology, (S)takeholder, (P)erceptions, (A)ccountability, (C)ompetition, (E)cology, and (S)ocial. Example sources of information for each environment were identified. Various physical therapy examples were used to highlight the implications of each environmental component as it related to a SWOT analysis. A template for a SWOT analysis was provided along with suggestions about organizing relevant findings into opportunities and threats. Additional specificity was then added to this information. The anticipated degree of positive and negative impact of each finding was estimated along with the probability that the event would actually happen. This progression of analyses identified the potential benefits and challenges in the external environment,

CASE STUDY 4.1

Conduct a Portion of the External Environment Scanning and Analysis Process of Selected Physical Therapy Businesses

Instructions and Options

This case gives you the opportunity to apply part of the external environmental scanning process to several physical therapy businesses. The environments and the businesses are your choice. You choose which three external environments you will investigate for three of the businesses listed below. Scan the same three environments for each business so your results can be compared and discussed. *Keep in mind that in Chapter 6 you will continue to use the business examples you chose now.*

1. Select three physical therapy—related businesses from the list below to help you apply what you know about conducting a limited environmental scan.

   The American Physical Therapy Association (APTA)

   An accredited physical therapy or physical therapist assistant educational program (public or private)

   A national physical therapy business (for-profit or not-for-profit)

   A regional physical therapy business (for-profit or not-for-profit)

   A multiple location single state physical therapy business (not-for-profit hospital system)

   A large local privately owned physical therapy practice with locations in neighboring cities

   A small, local, privately owned physical therapy practice with less than four locations in one city

2. Conduct a limited external scan of your chosen businesses. Examine any three of the DEPT SPACES environments but examine these same environments for each of the businesses.

3. List the opportunities and threats for each of the three businesses.

4. Compare the lists (see Fig. 4.2). Discuss the O and T similarities and differences. Include your thoughts on why there were similarities and differences in your discussion.

5. In your opinion, which threat is the most severe and most likely to play out in each of your chosen businesses environments? Consider using Figure 4.3.

6. Reflect on what you did well in each of the parts of this exercise and what you feel you need to improve on in order to complete an external scan.

it prioritized them, and it identified those that were most probable. This three-step process will be used again in the next two chapters, which deal with internal environmental scanning. The internal position of a business provides the resources for dealing with the opportunities and threats discovered in the external environment.

REFERENCES

American Physical Therapy Association. Get connected with APTA connect. Available at http://www.apta.org/AM/Template.cfm?Section=Info_for_Clinicians&TEMPLATE=/CM/ContentDisplay.cfm&CONTENTID=36088. Accessed 5/11/07a.

American Physical Therapy Association. Professionalism in physical therapy: core values. Available at http://www.apta.org/AM/Template.cfm?Section=Policies_and_Bylaws&TEMPLATE=/CM/ContentDisplay.cfm&CONTENTID=36073. Accessed 5/14/07b.

Beech J, Chadwick S, eds. The Business of Tourism Management. New York, NY: Financial Times/Prentice Hall. 2005.

Bureau of Economic Analysis. Available at http://www.bea.gov/bea/regional/bearfacts/. Accessed 5/05/07a.

Bureau of Labor Statistics. Nonfarm Employment by Industry from the current employment. Charleston, W.Va. Available at ftp://ftp.bls.gov/pub/special.requests/philadelphia/fax_9460.txt. Accessed 5/03/07a.

Bureau of Labor Statistics. Local area Bearfacts. Available at http://www.bea.gov/bea/regional/bearfacts/countybf.cfm?areatype=MSA&sublist=next. Accessed 5/05/07b.

Census Bureau. Service annual survey: data for NAICS 62 health care and social assistance. Available at http://www.census.gov/svsd/www/services/sas/sas_data/sas62.htm. Accessed 3/24/07a.

Census Bureau. 2002 economic census: Geographic area series schedule. Available at http://www.census.gov/econ/census02/guide/geosumm.htm. Accessed 5/03/07b.

Census Bureau. The 2007 statistical abstract. Available at http://www.census.gov/compendiastatab/health_nutrition/health_care_utilization/. Accessed 5/05/07c.

Concentra. About Concentra. Available at http://www.concentra.com/About/. Accessed 5/05/07.

County of Sonoma. Sonoma county 2006 economic and development report. Available at http://www.sonoma-county.org/edb/pdf/2006/2006_sonoma_profile.pdf. Accessed 5/04/07.

Economic Development Administration. Research. Available at http://www.eda.gov/Research/Research.xml. Accessed 5/05/07a.

Economic Development Administration. Cluster based economic development. Available at http://www.eda.gov/Research/ClusterBased.xml. Accessed 5/05/07b.

Extendicare. About us. Available at http://www.extendicare.com/aboutus/aboutus.html. Accessed 5/05/07.

Federal Bureau of Investigation. Crime in the United States 2006. Available at http://www.fbi.gov/ucr/prelim06/table4index.htm. Accessed 5/16/07.

FedStats. International, state, county & local area statistics. Available at http://www.fedstats.gov/regional.html. Accessed 5/05/07.

Health and Human Services. Frequently asked questions related to the poverty guidelines and poverty. Available at http://aspe.hhs.gov/poverty/faq.shtml many. Accessed 5/03/07.

Helms MM. Encyclopedia of Management, 5th ed. Detroit, MI: Thompson Gayle. 2006.

Longest BB, Rakich JS, Darr K. Managing Health Services Organizations and Systems, 4th ed. Baltimore, MD: Health Professions Press. 2000.

Massachusetts Department of Education. Science and technology/engineering curriculum framework. Available at http://www.doe.mass.edu/frameworks/scitech/2001/resources/glossary.html. Accessed 6/17/07.

MJ Care. Programs and services. Available at http://www.mjcare.com/mj1/. Accessed 5/05/07.

National Center for Health Statistics. Health, United States, 2006. Available at http://www.cdc.gov/nchs/hus.htm. Accessed 5/03/07.

Nosse LJ, Friberg DG, Kovacek PR. Managerial and supervisory principles for physical therapists, 2nd ed. Baltimore, MD: Lippincott Williams & Wilkins. 2005.

Northshore Physical Therapy. About us. Available at http://www.worc.net/. Accessed 5/05/07.

Novacare. Company information. Available at http://www.novacare.com/flash_frameset.html. Accessed 5/05/07.

O'Neil T, Hymel G. All Politics Is Local: And Other Rules of the Game. New York, NY: Times Books. 1994.

Porter K, Smith P, Fagg R. Leadership and Management for HR Professionals, 3rd ed. Burlington, MA: Butterworth-Heinemann. 2006.

Porter ME, Teisberg EO. Redefining health care: Creating value-based competition on results. Boston, MA: Harvard Business School. 2006.

Random House. Webster's Unabridged Dictionary, 2nd ed. New York, NY: Random House. 1999.

Swayne LE, Duncan WJ, Ginter PM. Strategic management of health care organizations, 5th ed. Malden, MA: Blackwell. 2006.

Swisher LL, Krueger-Brophy CK. Legal and ethical issues in physical therapy. Boston, MA: Butterworth-Heinemann. 1998.

Vector Research, Inc. Physical therapy workforce study: Executive summary. Ann Arbor, MI: Author, 1997.

WakeMed. About us. Available at http://www.wakemed.org/. Accessed 5/05/07.

ADDITIONAL RESOURCES

An example of a general home use version of voice recognition software is Dragon Naturally Speaking (http://www.nuance.com/naturallyspeaking). There are also professional versions for business and medical fields. For information on paid and volunteer internship opportunities in the APTA Government Affairs department contact davemason@apta.org. APTA also provides current information on legislative issues relevant to PTs at http://www.apta.org/advocacy. The Department of Health and Human Services commissioned a study on health information technology. The report summary is available at http://www.hhs.gov/news/ press/2005pres/20050511.html. Thomson Gale has produced a guide to research centers and services. General information is available at http://www.gale.com/world. The Centers for Medicare and Medicaid Services have solicited bids from vendors of durable medical equipment, prosthetics, orthotics and supplies (DMEPOS) to compete for business from its beneficiaries. As of May 2007, approval to submit a bid was required. For more information see http://www.cms.hhs.gov/CompetitiveAcqforDMEPOS.

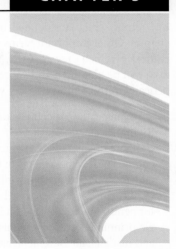

CHAPTER 5

INTERNAL ENVIRONMENT OF
HEALTH SERVICE PROVIDERS

DEBORAH G. FRIBERG

Learning Objectives

1. Explain the relationship between strategic planning, business success, and the internal business environment.
2. Compare the purposes of external and internal environmental scanning and analyses.
3. Identify major internal influences that impact the strategic decision-making process for a health services business.
4. Describe how the major internal influences of the internal environment can impact the success of a health services business.
5. Become familiar with the impact of resource allocation for decision making on the internal environmental assessment.
6. Become familiar with the impact of internal elements on the workforce.
7. Utilize the use of strengths, weaknesses, opportunities, and threats (SWOT) analysis in evaluating the internal environment of a health services business.

Introduction

Chapter 3 explored the application of **strategic thinking** to address the questions of what a business should be doing to fulfill its **mission** and achieve its **vision** of success. Strategic thinking starts with the organization's **mission statement**, which defines the purpose for which it exists (Chapters 7 and 14).

Its **vision statement** defines its desired future state. **Value statements** describe the forces that motivate a business and the behaviors it promotes in its employees (Chapter 7). *Critical issues* describe internal weaknesses or external threats that must be addressed. Business leaders utilize **strategic planning** as a tool to help them consider the questions of how and when a business should take action. Strategic planning is used to develop **strategic goals**, **strategic objectives** and, finally, specific **operational or tactical plans** that answer the questions of how and when in detail (Kane, 2007). The operational plan also addresses the question of responsibility and defines who will get the job done. The **strategic plan** documents not only the planning process but also its results. In business, the strategic plan is the road map. Strategic planning is the process we go through to choose the destination and draw the map to that desired destination. In preparing for the strategic journey, we must do our best to plan and prepare for detours and unexpected road hazards along the way. In Chapter 3, we explored the **external environmental** factors that can impact success. In this chapter we turn our attention inward to the *internal factors* that determine whether our business is prepared to take us to our destination. The internal environment scan and analysis focuses on the organization itself, to (1) understand its resources and capabilities and (2) to identify its *core competencies*, which can be developed into a **competitive advantage** (Porter et al., 2006; Swayne et al., 2006).

Key terms, which are defined below, are bolded and italicized the first time they appear in the chapter. Other important terms are shown in boldface on first appearance and are defined by the context in which they are used. When either of these types of terms is used several times, its acronym will be identified and subsequently used in the chapter. Both types of terms are listed alphabetically in the online glossary with their definitions and (when applicable) their acronyms.

Baldrige criteria: the Malcolm Baldrige National Quality Improvement Act of 1987 was established to promote quality awareness, to recognize quality and business achievements of U.S. organizations, and to publicize these organizations' successful performance strategies. For health care, criteria for performance excellence are leadership, strategic planning, focus on patients, other customers, and markets, measurement, analysis, and knowledge management, workforce focus, process management, and results.

best practice(s): best generally denotes recognition by peer organizations. In business, this means organization processes, practices, and systems that are performed exceptionally well and are recognized as improving an organization's performance and efficiency in specific areas. In health care, this refers to approaches to care or organizational management that are innovative, effective based on evidence, and are good models. In medicine, this is a treatment that experts agree is appropriate, accepted, and widely used. Also called standard therapy or standard of care. See also comparative benchmarking, evidence-based practice, and standards.

competitive advantages: services or products that are difficult for competitors to duplicate, imitate, or develop substitutes for that can be quickly and continuously improved and are perceived by consumers to be an excellent value. It is what an organization can do that others cannot.

core competencies: in business these are the sum total of the knowledge, skill, and special expertise (strengths) the members of the business have that make or can make their services or products distinguishable from those of competitors for long periods of time.

critical issues: in business these are internal weaknesses or threats identified in an internal environmental scan that must be addressed.

fiduciary/fiduciary duty(ies): the legal and ethical responsibility of a board of directors (BODs) or trustees to act primarily for stockholders' or stakeholders' benefit, respectively.

governance: the process whereby societies or organizations make important decisions, determine whom they involve, and the outcomes of the process.

internal environment/factors/variables: the information a business has about itself, including resources and performance relative to the industry as a whole.

key processes: according to Baldrige criteria these are means that provide for the direct delivery of health services, support the delivery of health services, and processes that help the business

key requirements: according to Baldrige criteria these are design elements that are critical to success. They may include but are not limited to desired health outcomes, efficiency targets, cycle times, ease of access, continuity, timeliness, environmental impact, level of patient involvement, facility characteristics, capacity, and/or regulatory requirements.

mutual accommodation: ongoing interaction between individuals to facilitate continuous adjustment between themselves in order to achieve their shared work-related goals.

organizational chart: graphic depiction of an organization's management, coordination, and communication structure.

organization structures and designs: strategically designed organizational management hierarchies and functional relationships that are organized to facilitate mission-driven activities.

policy: a broad statement that contains goals and objectives that form a framework for achieving an organization's mission and shaping human behaviors. Health policy deals with all factors that affect the health of the public. A policy may also mean an insurance contract.

procedure(s): describes how a policy is enacted. It is a detailed statement of when, where, and how an activity should be accomplished.

(Continued)

productivity/productivity rate: in accounting, this is the relationship between the cost of resources used to the value of the outcome produced. In the clinical setting productivity is commonly determined by calculating the relationship between the amount of time a staff member spends providing billable services in an eight-hour day divided by the number of units billed.

standardized work plans: treatment plans. A way to standardize work processes to reduce variation and minimize errors.

strengths: organizational variables identified through internal environmental scanning and analysis as assets for reaching organizational goals. The S in a SWOT analysis.

supervision: the provision of direction, instruction, constructive feedback, and other means intended to have a positive influence on work-related knowledge, skills, and behaviors. A part of a manager's responsibility toward his or her subordinates.

weaknesses: organizational variables identified through internal environment scanning and analysis to be shortcomings that impede reaching goals. The W in a SWOT analysis.

work standardization: formalizing work-related processes, tasks, output, and worker skills to minimize variation in performance and output. This is commonly accomplished by policies, procedures, protocols, special training, treatment plans, written guidelines, educational and experience requirements, licensure, and other means.

A successful strategic planning process finds its foundation in the gathering and analyzing of information about the business itself. Every business needs to be positioned to leverage its strengths and be protected against weaknesses. To be successful, health services managers need to understand the relationship between strategic planning, business success, and the internal business environment. They need to be able to identify the major internal influences that impact their business's ability to follow its strategic plan and achieve its strategic vision. In this regard, each business is unique and must rely on close self-examination to determine which internal factors are important as well as how much of what kind of information is needed to position the business for success. The concepts presented in this chapter are used extensively in Chapter 6 to look at the internal environment of selected physical therapy subsectors.

Internal Analysis as Part of the Strategic Planning Process

Strategic planning is a continuous cycle of questioning and decision making. In this process the business takes into consideration what and who they are today (mission and values), what they might become (vision), and all the external and internal factors that might impact their journey to realize their aspirations. Figure 5.1 depicts the elements and cyclic nature of a basic strategic planning process. Input is gathered from both external and internal sources.

The internal sources reviewed include:

1. Mission, vision, and values statements
2. Assessment of strengths and weaknesses
3. Performance outcome measures
4. Input from across the organization

Input from the organization is translated into a few high-level strategic goals. The strategic goals are further defined by strategic objectives. Strategic objectives are put into action through the implementation of detailed tactical action plans. The effectiveness of the action plans is monitored and measured. Outcome measures are the specific indicators of success for each implemented strategy (Chapter 16). The performance results are used to modify strategies and action plans. Then the process starts again. The effectiveness of the strategic planning process lies in the quality of the information available upon which business leaders make their strategic decisions.

Characteristics of an Internal Environmental Analysis

Scope

Just as strategic plans may vary in **scope**, so might the analysis of internal environmental factors. The scope of the analysis should be

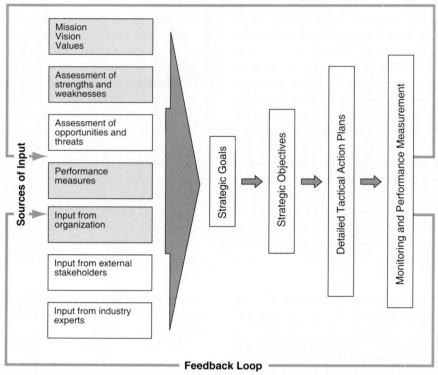

Figure 5.1. Continuous strategic planning cycle.

driven by the scope of the strategic plan. The scope can cover an entire organization or be written to address just the needs of a segment of the business. Take once again the example of a large national health care provider that operates hospitals, home health care agencies, long-term care facilities, and ambulatory care centers. **Management** may undertake an internal environmental analysis on a geographical basis to better reflect local markets (Chapter 18) or **service line** (deliverables) basis to optimize planning by business division (Chapter 14). In fact, the internal environmental assessment may be segmented by both **market** (customer characteristics) and service line (see Chapter 18). The goal is to obtain information that is meaningful, reflects the current state of the business, and is actionable.

Time Frame

The internal environmental assessment represents the characteristics of the business at a specific point or period in time. Given the speed and degree of change in the external

environment impacting the health care industry, the internal environment of a health services business may change rapidly in a short period. Some high-impact internal changes can substantially affect the internal environment of a business. Some examples of internal changes that may lead to a rapid, temporary, or permanent change in the internal environment of a business are listed in Table 5.1.

Strategic planning needs to take into consideration the potential for rapid internal change. This is a key reason for adopting a cyclical strategic planning process as presented in Figure 5.1 that calls for the review and update of plans on an annual basis (Swayne et al., 2006).

Assessing the Internal Health Services Business Environment

Internal factors are considered to be under the control of the organization. Internal factors are often referred to in terms of *strengths* and *weaknesses* (Chapters 6 and 22). A

	Table 5.1 Examples of Internal Changes That Affect the Internal Environment	

Changes	Impact
Business performance	Significant changes in performance can impact leadership style, resource availability, employee recruitment and retention, vision, strategic initiatives, and more.
Business structure	Changes such as transitioning from for-profit to not-for-profit, single to multisite, centralized to decentralized operations
Labor availability	Changes in the availability of people with the needed skills and expertise to perform the work. Labor availability can change swiftly due to such things as union actions, employee illness, economic changes, or natural disasters. Slower changes occur due to regulatory changes or other factors that influence the total demand or availability of professional or skilled workers.
Leadership	Changes in senior leadership, especially the CEO can have dramatic influences. At a minimum, it may slow down the implementation of the strategic action plan while the organization adjusts to new leadership.
Market position	A change in market position in either direction may bring about considerable changes such as rapid expansions or retractions in workforce, market locations, and so on.
Ownership	Changes in ownership through either an acquisition or merger can affect every aspect of a business including its mission, vision, and goals. Mergers can result in cultural clashes if two very different businesses are brought together.
Regulatory requirements	A change in regulation may bring about a revamping of business processes, change in market position, and/or change in business performance.

total assessment of both external (opportunities and threats) and internal (strengths and weaknesses) factors that have the potential to impact an organization's success is called a **SWOT** analysis (Learned et al., 1969; McConkey, 1976). The information gained through the completion of a SWOT analysis is used to guide the development of strategic goals, objectives, and action plans. Internal information subjected to SWOT analyses can assist strategy development by raising key questions including:

- How can our strengths be leveraged to achieve our goals?
- What is the competitive advantage we have or can have?
- How can our weaknesses be eliminated or, better yet, turned into future strengths?

These questions serve to focus attention on the factors internal to the business that can influence success.

Elements of an Internal Organizational Assessment

There are many aspects of the organization that management needs to consider during an internal organizational assessment. How much attention needs to be paid to any individual element will vary by organization. Management must weigh the cost of investing resources in the gathering of information against the benefit that additional information will add to the strategic decision-making process. **Management style**, available **discretionary resources**, and management's perception of the risk of making poor decisions will influence this decision. Discretionary resources refer to resources such as time or money that the management has to expend without impacting the operations of the business. One of the most important and difficult aspects of the internal review process can be **best practice comparative benchmarking**. Comparative benchmarking involves the use of information from other comparable businesses, identified as having the best performance in the industry. The information is used to assess the performance of the business under review against the reference entity. This approach will help a business identify opportunities for process and outcome improvement (Government Accountability Office, 2007). Internal assessment is effective when divided into topic areas including:

1. Mission, vision, and values (Chapters 6 and 7)
2. Regulatory compliance (Chapters 6, 7, 8, and 9)
3. Governance and management model (Chapters 6, 11, 12, 13, and 15)
4. Organizational structure (Chapters 6 and 14)
5. Operational processes (Chapters 15 and 16)
6. Human resources (Chapters 6 and 17)
7. Customer satisfaction (Chapters 6, 18, and 19)
8. Financial operations and resource availability (Chapters 6, 20, 21, and 22)

Mission, Vision, and Values

The internal assessment should start with the **mission**, **vision**, and **values statements**. These statements provide guidance when judging behavior and choosing options. These statements should be reviewed annually and updated as needed. This should be the first step in the strategic planning process and involve input from all levels of the organization and key **stakeholders** (Darr, 2005). An annual assessment should determine if these statements

- Reflect current reality
- Send a clear and actionable message to the employees
- Represent the needs of the customers

The mission statement defines the purpose for the business to exist. As businesses grow and develop, their mission and vision statements need to evolve with them. Mission statements should energize a business' internal and external audiences. A good mission statement will answer the questions of who we are, who are our customers, and what sets us apart from our **competitors**. The last question serves to differentiate a business from its competitors and gets to the heart of what a business does to keep customers coming back (Jones, 2002). The vision defines its ideal future state. A clear vision for the future will serve to focus and align the efforts of the business toward a common goal. Value statements describe the forces that motivate a business and the behaviors it promotes in its employees. Value

statements can also change over time. Value statements are updated periodically to synchronize with business changes and current employees. They also change considerably at times of significant and rapid changes in the internal business environment as described above. Mission, vision, and value statements are addressed in greater detail in Chapter 3 and discussed further in Chapter 7.

Regulatory Compliance

Health services businesses are highly regulated. **Compliance** with applicable regulatory requirements is essential and must be included in any assessment of the business' internal environment. Health services providers face several types of regulatory risk areas in addition to the regulation associated with the health services delivery. Health services providers face regulation related to almost every aspect of their operation including but not limited to:

- Employment
- Environmental impact
- Financial management and taxation
- Health services delivery (licensure, registration, service regulations, etc.)
- Heath services coverage and reimbursement
- Occupational health and safety
- Securities and Exchange

For health services providers, the risk is raised because of sponsored health care programs of the federal and state governments. For government-sponsored programs almost any level of noncompliance with coverage and reimbursement guidelines represents substantial risk to the health care provider. Sanctions can range from having to return improper payments to imprisonment for health care businesses that engage in fraudulent practices (Chapters 8–10, and 17). In addition to criminal and civil monetary penalties, health care providers that are found to have defrauded the federal health care programs are excluded from participation in these programs (OIG, 2007).

We are in a current social environment that is focused on corporate responsibility. This responsibility for regulatory compliance rests with the **board of directors** (BOD) and the senior leadership. All employees must be knowledgeable of compliance requirements, risks, and how to avoid compliance violations. Health care businesses, to protect themselves, must take an organized approach to regulatory compliance. This often takes the form of a **corporate compliance program** designed to help mitigate risks of intentional or unintentional regulatory noncompliance. The Office of Inspector General (OIG) of the U.S. Department of Health and Human Services (2007) recommends that health services businesses have in place a corporate compliance program that includes the elements presented in Table 5.2.

These OIG (2007) recommendations can be used to assess a business's ability to protect against regulatory compliance violations. The actions listed under the Measures to Prevent Violations heading are the assessment tools to ensure that the compliance program is working and violations are avoided where possible; recognized and corrected when they occur.

Regulatory compliance is addressed in more detail in Chapters 7–9.

Governance and Management Model

Governance refers to the act or process of governing (American Heritage Dictionary, 2003). For corporations, governance is the responsibility of the **BOD** (see Fig. 5.2).

Governing a corporation includes setting the vision, monitoring upper-level management's performance, quality services or products, financial performance, and self-assessment. The BOD, as a group, controls the corporation and appoints the corporate officers to manage **operations** (Longest et al., 2000). The BOD is legally charged with the governance of the corporation (Clarkson et al., 1995). In a **for-profit** company, the BOD is responsible to the **stockholders**. In a **not-for-profit** company the BOD is responsible to the **stakeholders**, usually the community served (McNamara, 2007). According to United Way of Canada (2007) while the BOD may perform

Table 5.2 Elements of a Corporate Compliance Program Based on OIG Recommendations	
Elements	**Meaning**
Code of conduct	A code of conduct documents the principles, values, and actions related to compliance within the organization that articulates the business's commitment to ethical behavior.
Compliance infrastructure	The corporate compliance program is typically led by a designated **compliance officer** with the authority and accountability to manage all aspects of the organization's compliance program. The compliance officer should be (1) supported by adequate organizational resources and (2) report on a regular basis to the senior leadership and the BOD.
Compliance-related policies and procedures	Documents to guide the organization's day-to-day management of high-risk activities.
Measures to prevent violations	Measures include (1) organization-wide training on compliance standards, policies, and procedures, (2) ongoing efforts to recognize and respond to regulatory developments, (3) mechanisms to measure the effectiveness of the compliance program and adherence to related policies and procedures, and (4) mechanisms to respond to identified compliance program weaknesses.
Measures to respond to violations	Measures to guide the organization in (1) monitoring the organization to identify compliance violations, (2) responding to suspected compliance violations, (3) reporting suspected compliance violations, (4) protecting employees who report compliance violations (**whistleblowers**) to the organization and/or outside regulators, (5) forming policies to govern the reporting to the government of probable compliance violations, and (6) retaining relevant documents and information in the event of a violation.

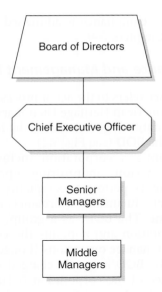

Figure 5.2. General upper-level governance schema of a health service corporation.

a wide range of tasks, their role falls into two categories. The first is the mandated role that includes all of the duties that a BOD must perform to meet the minimum legal requirements for all board members. The BOD has legal obligations to the

- Corporation, **stockholders**, and its members (referred to as *fiduciary duties*)
- Government
- People or organizations with whom the corporation interacts

The second is the chosen role that the BOD elects to perform. This depends on the following:

- The decisions the BOD will make versus the decisions it will delegate
- The BOD's involvement in operations
- The relationship between the BOD and staff

Based on the answers to these questions, the model the BOD adopts may one of the following:

Policy board: This model is characterized by a collaborative relationship between the BOD and the board-appointed chief executive officer (CEO). Board committees, supported by the CEO and senior manage-

ment, carry out the work of the BOD. The BOD assumes responsibility for defining the mission, strategic planning, and the corporation's image in the community.

Policy governance board: This model is characterized by a structure that sets limits on the CEO. The BOD assumes responsibility for determining the relationship between the BOD and the CEO, the board process, strategic goal, objectives, and tactical action plans.

Working board: In addition to providing policy and planning, the members of a working board assume some responsibilities for operations including human resources, general operations, and community relations.

Collective board: This is a group of people working toward a common goal that assume responsibility for planning, finance, human resources, operations, and community relations.

The size, complexity, mission, and vision of the business should drive the chosen board model. The wrong model will negatively impact the business.

Management models are founded on assumptions about human attitudes, aptitudes, and behaviors. There are literally hundreds of management models that profess to help leaders impact employee performance, satisfaction, and motivation on the job. Tannenbaum and Schmidt (1973) suggest that management style is influenced by three **contextual elements**:

1. The employee(s)
2. The manager(s)
3. The situation(s)

Table 5.3 lists some of the contextual forces that may influence management style.

Business leaders want to adopt a management style that best meets the needs of the business and its employees. Management's success can be evaluated by assessing such factors as employee satisfaction, employee turnover, absentee rates, workers' compensation claims, and employee *productivity* rates. Governance and management models are addressed in greater detail in Chapters 11, 12, 13, and 15. For this discussion, in a corporate

Table 5.3   Contextual Factors Influencing Management Model

Manager Characteristics and Competencies	Employee/Work Group Characteristics and Competencies	Internal and External Business Environment
Decision-making style	Acceptance of responsibility	**Organizational:**
Experience	Autonomy	Available resources
Knowledge of business	Availability	Board model
Knowledge of employees	Competencies	Culture
Leadership style	Education	History
Management skills	Experience	Mission
Perception of risk	Initiative	Ownership
Performance history	Level of satisfaction	Practices
Sense of security	Level of interest in job	Strategies
Situational comfort	Manager's expectations	Values
Values	Reliability	Vision
	Seniority	**Job Characteristics:**
	Skills	Importance
	Values	Scope
		Urgency

health service business it is the BOD that is the highest level of governance and the CEO answers to the BOD.

Organizational Structure

To organize is to arrange elements into a whole of interdependent parts. Businesses, to be effective, must organize their employees into a cohesive structure by defining the role of each employee in relation to every other employee. Mintzberg (1979) suggests that *work standardization, supervision,* and *mutual accommodation* are the three methods used to coordinate work between individuals.

Work standardization can be accomplished through standardization of work processes, outputs, and worker skills (Mintzberg, 1979). Work processes can be standardized through the use of *policies, procedures,* work (treatment) **protocols,** or *standardized work (treatment) plans.* Output (outcome) standardization is on the rise in the health care industry. An example would be the use of mobility status as the criteria for discharge from treatment. Skill standard-

ization uses criteria such as education, training, demonstrated competencies, and licensure as tools to standardize the work of health services employees.

Supervision refers to the control and direction of the work of one or more employees by another employee (Chapter 11). Supervision can be used to coordinate the work of the organization. The *organizational structure* defines the supervisory relationships between individuals at all organizational levels (see below).

Mutual accommodation is the simplest method of work coordination because it is the result of ongoing interaction between individuals. This interaction results in continuous adjustment between individuals toward the achievement of their shared goals.

Organizational structure is a term that describes how management constructs the organization to fulfill its mission. The organizational structure defines the relationships between individuals and/or groups of individuals and the hierarchy of management's decision-making authority (Chapters 6 and 14). A graphic depiction of an organization's structure is called an *organizational chart*. The organizational structure must define the way work is divided and the method for coordination of those divided efforts. In a small business with few employees this may require a relatively simple structure. Consider a physical therapist in private practice that employs a receptionist and physical therapy aide. This is a business that can rely on verbal sharing of information with little documentation of roles and responsibilities. The owner educates the employees about their roles, responsibilities, and how their roles are related to the business's other roles. Their work is coordinated by consistency of their duties and direct supervision by the owner. When their efforts need coordination, they talk to each other. In larger, more complex organizations, the act of organizing demands a more formal approach. Supervision becomes more important. Supervisors must be supported by:

- Documented organizational structure
- Job **competency** requirements
- Outcome measures
- Policies and procedures
- Tools to support interpersonal and interdepartmental communications.
- Written role descriptions

The topics of leadership and supervision and organizational structure are addressed in more detail in Chapters 11 and 14.

Operational Processes

Baldrige National Quality Program's Health Care Criteria for Performance Excellence (*Baldrige criteria*) encourages health services business to start the assessment of operational processes by identifying their *key processes and requirements* for those processes (Baldrige National Quality Program, 2007). Key processes are those that (1) provide for the direct delivery of health services, (2) support the delivery of health services, and (3) help the business achieve success. Support includes processes for such things as medical records, environmental services, building management, grounds, public relations, and administration. Other nonpatient care processes include research, teaching, **supply chain** management, legal services, sales, government relations, and fund raising.

The Institute of Healthcare Improvement (IHI, 2007) suggests several areas of focus for assessing process effectiveness. These key process focus areas and related questions are presented in Table 5.4.

Key requirements are design elements that are critical to success. Sometimes these are referred to as critical success factors. They include, but are not limited to, desired health outcomes, efficiency targets, cycle times, ease of access, continuity, timeliness, environmental impact, level of patient involvement, facility characteristics, capacity, and/or regulatory requirements. The topics of operations management and performance improvement are addressed in more detail in Chapters 15 and 16.

Human Resources

The most important resource that any business has is its people. This is especially true in health services businesses where employee-related labor costs represent more than 50% of all **expenditures** (Haugh et al., 2007). It is management's responsibility to recruit and retain the employees needed to perform the work of the business. Therefore, a workforce assessment is a critical component of any internal environmental assessment. Some questions that guide this assessment include:

- Do we have the right employees?
- Do we have the right number of employees?
- Do they have the right skills?
- Are they available at the right times?
- Are they doing what they are supposed to do?
- Are they doing only what they are supposed to do?

Ideally, every business can answer "yes" to each of these questions. Research and an honest assessment are often needed to answer these questions with a definitive "yes." When the answer is "no" then further investigation is often needed to determine why the answer is not yes and how the "no" can become a "yes"! The internal assessment should show how

Table 5.4 Helpful Questions for Assessing the Performance of Key Processes	
Key Items	*Example Questions*
Customer interface	Will the customer recognize and appreciate the improvements?
Error	Can processes be improved to reduce the likelihood of employee error?
Information systems	Are we able to communicate throughout the organization? Are there improvement opportunities related to the use of improved information technologies? Can we use **simulation technology** to improve health care service provider education and performance during the health delivery process (Issenberg et al., 1999)?
Inventory	Does the inventory of resources needed to support the process match the demand? Is it available throughout to facilitate process flow?
Process variation	Are there opportunities to reduce process variation to improve the predictability and quality of process outcomes?
Service improvement	Can our services/products be improved?
Time management	Can the business gain a **competitive advantage** by reducing the time needed for new service or product development, customer wait times, supply delivery times, and/or other key process cycle times?
Waste	Does the activity add value to an external customer? Is there excess inventory or waste in any area?
Work environment	Will a change in the work environment make a process more effective?
Work flow	Does the flow of work within the process improve the quality of the services and goods produced by those processes?

the business has performed in areas related to employees including:

- Career development and promotion
- Compensation and benefits
- Discipline and grievance procedures
- Diversity management
- Productivity (cost–benefit analysis)
- Performance assessment and feedback
- Performance recognition and reward
- Recruitment (availability) and retention
- Role descriptions and performance goal setting
- Training and development

The topic of human resources management is addressed in more detail in Chapter 17.

Customer Satisfaction

A business is nothing without its customers. For the purposes of the internal assessment, it is reasonable to define the customer as any person, group of people, or business that either directly or indirectly purchases a service or product. Some of the questions to be answered in relation to customer satisfaction include:

- Who are our customers? (mission)
- What services or products do they purchase?
- How do our customers rate our services and products and why these ratings?
- How do they rate other providers of the same services and products?
- Do they say they would return?
- Do they say they would recommend us to someone else?
- What other options do they have to meet their service or product needs?
- How do we compare to those options?
- If there were currently no options, what would our customers do if an option became available?
- Do our customers have needs that we are not meeting?

Understanding the customers, their level of satisfaction, and what drives that satisfaction will reinforce the things that the customer likes and allow the business to change the things the customer dislikes. Customer feedback can also be used to identify market opportunities or risks. A valuable, but sometimes difficult to access, element of the customer satisfaction assessment is access to comparative data from similar businesses that are not competitors (Chapter 6). Knowledge about how other providers of the same services or products are rated by their customers can help the business set reasonable performance targets for their own services. The topics of customer satisfaction, marketing, and sales management are addressed in more detail in Chapters 18 and 19.

Financial Operations and Resource Availability

Effective financial operations are important for any business. Financial management can be defined as "the process of managing the financial resources, including accounting and financial reporting, budgeting, collecting accounts receivable, risk management, and insurance for a business" (Small Business Notes, 2007). The effectiveness of these functions has a great impact on the success of the business. Many of these functions are evaluated as part of a financial audit of statements and records. An audit is an examination by an independent third party of the financial statements of a company that results in the publication of an independent opinion on whether or not those financial statements are relevant, accurate, complete, and fairly presented. The audit process will also look at the financial management policies, procedures, and practices of the business to assess whether the business is following generally accepted accounting principles (GAAP). Beyond the audit process, financial performance can be evaluated using comparative performance outcome benchmarks. The faster a business collects its accounts receivable, money owed to the business by creditors, the more financial resources will be available to pay its bills, for investment, or to meet other business needs. The topics of financial planning, accounting, financial management, and practice ownership are addressed in more detail in Chapters 20–23.

Support for an Internal Environmental Analysis

A guide to determining the scope of an internal environmental assessment is needed in the initial stages. It is best to begin with known or anticipated factors that can be expected to have an effect on the organization's ability to carry out its strategic objectives (Dunn, 1998). Support for internal environmental analysis can come from a variety of internal and external sources. The availability of internal resources is dependent on the size and capability of the business.

Upper levels of management hold the responsibility for overall organizational planning. Managers, lower in the hierarchy, carry more specific planning responsibility. Businesses, depending on size, have several organizational structures that have authority over the strategic planning process, including the internal environmental assessment. Owners or, for corporations, the BOD, are ultimately responsible for the success of the business and, in that capacity, have direct responsibility for strategic planning. While it may vary based on the structure of a business, **senior leadership** typically manages and facilitates the strategic planning process (see Fig. 5.2). In large businesses, there may be a senior leadership level position that has designated responsibility for this function such as a vice president of planning. Operational managers (e.g., director of physical therapy) and support managers (e.g., director of human resources) as well as staff may have more or less significant roles as determined by the planning model employed. Current *best practice* for management suggests that the more inclusive the model the more likely employees at all levels will be engaged, take ownership of the completed strategic plan, and be motivated to support a successful implementation (Baldrige National Quality Program, 2007). Managers at all levels are likely to have a role in the assessment of the internal environment.

Businesses that lack internal resources may obtain planning support from external consultants, academic-based programs, or government-sponsored business services. Types of consultant support services that may prove to be of value include:

- Implementation support
- Market data gathering and analysis
- Process facilitation
- Performance data gathering and analysis

For more information about the use of consultants, see Chapters 22 and 23. The **U.S. Small Business Administration (SBA)** sponsors several programs on business management topics (SBA, 2007a). In addition the SBA sponsors services through **Senior Corps of Retired Executives (SCORE)** (SCORE, 2007), an organization of over 13,000 volunteer business executives who provide free support to small businesses (SCORE, 2007), **Small Business Development Centers (SBDCs)** that offer services in partnership with local and state governments (SBA, 2007b), and **Small Business Institutes (SBIs)** on more than 500 college campuses nationwide provide counseling by students and faculty to small businesses (Policastro, 2007). The SBA *Small Business Directory*, organized by state, is a good resource.

Information needed for a complete internal environmental scan can be obtained from a variety of sources including:

- Consultant reports
- Customer feedback
- Financial annual reports
- Financial consultants/brokers
- Government agency reports and publicly shared databases
- Human resources reports
- Information technology reports
- Publicly reported clinical outcome reports
- Trade associations reports
- Treatment outcomes reports
- Vendor feedback

Once again, determining how much of any type of information is needed is a management responsibility. The degree of risk associated with a poor decision must be balanced against the cost and effort associated with obtaining more information. It is a decision the leadership of individual businesses must make for themselves. The number of influential and relevant variables to consider in an internal or external or internal environment can be difficult for inexperienced managers to identify, but there are ways to lessen the difficulty as noted in Chapters 4–6 and 15.

Summary

Effective health service managers understand the relationships between strategic planning, assessment of the internal business environment, and a successful business. In this chapter, the value and application of external and internal environmental scans as a foundation for strategic planning were explored. The major internal influences that impact the strategic decision-making process for a health services business were discussed along with their potential impact on the success of a health services business. Recognizing that there is a cost in terms of both human and financial resources to performing an internal environmental assessment, the scope of an assessment is directly impacted by management's decisions about resources allocated to support the decision-making process. Because significant changes in the internal environment can happen quickly, it is important for management to become familiar with the internal environmental factors that can have a significant impact on a business' workforce. To provide the health services manager with an appropriate framework the use of a SWOT analysis that examines the internal strengths, weaknesses, as well as externally driven opportunities, and threats of a business is discussed. The discussion of internal environment analysis will continue in the next chapter and focus on physical therapy businesses.

CASE STUDY 5.1

The Inside Story

Background

Good Care Corp (GCC) is a for-profit, multi-city, multi-facility hospital and long-term care organization in a central state. Internal environmental scanning is a year-round activity in this organization.

The Issue

An external event of interest occurred this week. A not-for-profit competitor began using the previous two years of it's customer satisfaction ratings to attract patients to its facilities. Based on their internally developed survey they found that their cardiac and stroke rehabilitation services had the highest satisfaction ratings of all their services. They proclaim themselves as the number one provider of cardiac and stroke care in the state. The quandary for GCC is that patient satisfaction information for all their locations is known to be sparse and generally inadequate based on Baldrige (2007) criteria for customer relationships and satisfaction. This matter has been on agendas twice before, but it was tabled each time because it was felt that there were more pressing internal issues to work on. The possibility of losing market share to a competitor is real. This places a high priority on developing a strategic plan to gather, assess, and disseminate customer satisfaction information particularly for customers who had cardiac and stroke diagnoses. A strategic plan is urgently needed for the measurement of overall customer satisfaction.

Patience Wearing, director of marketing, noted that the current GCC marketing strategy was based on a high degree of patient satisfaction. This criterion was in line with the mission statement that proclaims, "we meet our stakeholders' needs and expectations, especially those of patient stakeholders." She reminded everyone that there is not adequate information available to determine whether patients believe that GCC does the things they say they do as well as they say they do them.

Starting a Strategic Plan: Resources

Link Systems, of the information technology department, suggested that his department could provide older computer terminals at selected locations to get consumer feedback before they leave the facilities. Terminals could be placed at information desks, in main waiting areas, and at the transporter/security locations. All computers would be linked to a single server. For protection Link noted that he would use an old server to keep the satisfaction information separated from the regular institutional servers. Jorge Duboyou, vice president of GCC, asked Patience if she would take on this customer satisfaction endeavor and he asked Link if he would estimate the cost for the hardware setup, questionnaire software development, personnel training, and data analysis. Patience said yes and was given leeway in putting together a team. Link said he could have a budget laid out within the week. Hi Tower, GCC CEO, asked Patience to be sure to look into the options for getting a large sample of the patients who have been discharged in the past two years. He offered to make available past Baldrige Health Care Criteria for Performance Excellence information on customer satisfaction and funds from his discretionary monies. A motion was made for Patience and Link to go forward with these initial tasks and report to VP Duboyou within seven working days.

Working Days 1–3

Patience asked the director of rehab services, Manny Talents, PT, to look into the physical and occupational therapy literature on patient satisfaction to generate optional survey questions. Next, he went to Emma Climber, RN, director of mursing, and asked her to investigate the criteria for patient satisfaction from a nursing perspective. Finally, Patience spoke to the medical staff president (physicians) to secure his views on patient satisfaction. Her impression was

(Continued)

CASE STUDY 5.1

The Inside Story (continued)

that each physician had his or her specialty benchmarks. To try to put all of these quality indicators into one instrument would make it so long that few people would fill it out.

Working Day 4

Patience reviewed the Baldrige information provided by the CEO. Manny reported that he found a 2000 general PT satisfaction instrument (Goldstein et al., 2000) and a 2002 PT outpatient satisfaction instrument (Beattie et al., 2002) but nothing on inpatient physical therapy. Emma suggested that the group look at the past GCC Press Ganey (2007) survey results to get a better picture of inpatient perspectives. She mentioned that a new instrument from the Agency for Healthcare Research and Quality (2007) produced for the Centers for Medicare and Medicaid Services would be available shortly. Her inclination was to go with a reliable and valid instrument administered by a consultant group because they were the trained instrument development professionals. This would be a superior approach than was taken by the competition. It would also rate GCC on a wider scale because its satisfaction data would be compared to benchmarks of similar successful hospitals and long-term care facilities on a national scale. Emma's strongest points were that there was inadequate expertise at GCC and insufficient time to develop a survey, administer it, and analyze it. Manny added that the competition only measured consumer satisfaction at its hospitals; it did not include it's rehabilitation or long-term care facilities. He believed that GCC was doing an excellent job when the whole continuum of care was considered. This raised the issue of there being a possible need for multiple surveys.

Working Day 5

Link Systems announced that he had 50 operational computers and keyboards and the server ready. The cost estimate could not be completed until it was known how long the questionnaire was, how many questionnaires were expected to be completed, and what types of analyses were required. His best guess was to allocate $15,000 for IT maintenance and other services.

Your Tasks

1. Review the chapter section on consumer satisfaction. What additional questions do you think would be of interest in dealing with the issues presented in this scenario?
2. Access Press Ganey to get an idea of hospital criteria for patient satisfaction.
3. Access the Baldrige criteria. What do they say about customer complaints? How do complaints fit into this scenario?
4. Consider mission, leadership, labor availability, market position, financial resources, and so on, and determine GCC's strengths and weaknesses.
5. Based on the limited information in this scenario, what, if any, is/are the potential competitive advantage(s) of GCC?
6. Identify the parts of the strategic planning process that have been completed thus far.
7. If you were Patience Wearing, what would you do on Day 6 in preparation for your progress report and recommendations for the V.P., Jorge Duboyou?

Agency for Healthcare Research and Quality. CAHPS Surveys and tools to advance patient-centered care. Available at https://www.cahps.ahrq.gov/content/NCBD/PDF/HCAHPS_Chartbook_2007.pdf. Accessed 6/04/07. Baldrige National Quality Program. Health care criteria for performance excellence. Gaithersburg, MD: Baldrige National Quality Program National Institute of Standards and Technology, Technology Administration, U.S. Department of Commerce. 2007. Beattie PF, Pinto MB, Nelson MK, Nelson R. Patient satisfaction with outpatient physical therapy: Instrument validation. Physical Therapy. 2002;82:557–565. Goldstein MS, Elliott SD, Guccione AA. The development of an instrument to measure satisfaction with physical therapy. Physical Therapy. 2000;80:853–863. Press Ganey. Hospital press report 2007. Available at http://www.pressganey.com/hospital-report.pdf. Accessed 6/04/07.

REFERENCES

American Heritage Dictionary of the English Language, 4th ed. Boston, Mass: Houghton Mifflin. 2000, Updated 2003.

Baldrige National Quality Program. Health care criteria for performance excellence. Gaithersburg, MD: Baldridge National Quality Program National Institute of Standards and Technology, Technology Administration, U.S. Department of Commerce. 2007.

Clarkson KW, Miller RL, Jentz GA, Cross FB. West's business law: Text cases, legal, ethical, regulatory, and international environment, 6th ed. Minneapolis/ St. Paul, MN: West. 1995.

Darr K. Ethics in health services management, 4th ed. Baltimore, MD: Health Professions Press. 2005.

Dunn RT. Haimann's supervisory management for health-care organizations, 6th ed. Boston, MA: McGraw-Hill. 1998.

Government Accountability Office. Business process re-engineering (BPR) team: Glossary of terms 1998. Available at http://www.gao.gov/special.pubs/bprag/ bprgloss.htm. Accessed 4/15/07.

Haugh R, Larkin H, Serb C, Towne J. Special report: Cost drivers. Hospitals & Health Networks, Health Forum, Chicago, IL. June 16, 2004. Available at http:// www.hhnmag.com/ hhnmag_app/hospitalconnect/ search/article.jsp?dcrpath=AHA/PubsNewsArticle/ data/0406HHNCover_Story&domain=HHNMAG. Accessed 5/31/07.

Institute of Healthcare Improvement. Improvement Methods at http://www.ihi.org/IHI/Topics/Improvement/ImprovementMethods/. Accessed 5/19/07.

Issenberg SB, McGaghie WC, Hart IR, et al. Simulation technology for health care professional skills training and assessment. JAMA. 1999;282(9):861–866.

Jones J. The CEO Refresher. When is it time to rewrite your mission statement? 2002. Available at http://www. refresher.com/!jjmission.html. Accessed 4/13/07.

Kane M. The CEO Refresher. The world of strategic thinking, it's not about time. Available at http:// www.refresher.com/!mjkstrategic.html. Accessed 4/2/07.

Learned EP, Christensen CR, Andrews KR, Guth WD. Business policy text and cases, Revised ed. Homewood, IL: Richard D. Irwin. 1969.

Longest BB, Rakich JS, Darr K. Managing health services organizations and systems, 4th ed. Baltimore, MD: Health Professions Press. 2000.

McConkey DD. How to manage by results. New York, NY: AMACOM. 1976.

McNamara C. Basic overview of various strategic planning models. Adapted from the Field Guide to Nonprofit Strategic Planning and Facilitation. Minneapolis, MN: Authenticity Consulting, LLC. 1997–2007.

Mintzberg H. The structuring of organizations. Englewood Cliffs, NJ: Prentice Hall. 1979.

Office of Inspector General. Corporate responsibility and corporate compliance: A resource for health care boards of directors. Available at http://oig.hhs.gov/fraud/docs/ complianceguidance/040203CorpRespRsceGuide. pdf. Accessed 4/15/07.

Policastro ML. Introduction to strategic planning. Management and Planning Series 21. Available at http://www. sba.gov/library/pubs/mp-21.txt. Accessed 4/1/07.

Porter K, Smith P, Fagg R. Leadership and Management for HR Professionals. Boston, MA: Butterworth-Heinemann. 2006.

Senior Corps of Retired Executives (SCORE). About SCORE. Available at http://www.score.org/explore_ score.html. Accessed 4/18/07.

Small Business Administration. Manage your business from start to finish. Available at http://www.sba. gov/smallbusinessplanner/plan/writeabusinessplan/ SERVSTRATPLAN.html. Accessed 4/18/07a.

Small Business Administration. Office of Small Business Centers. Entrepreneurial development. Available at http://www.sba.gov/aboutsba/sbaprograms/sbdc/ index.html. Accessed 4/19/07b.

Small Business Notes. Definition of financial management. Available at http://www.smallbusinessnotes. com/glossary/deffinancialmanagement.html. Accessed 5/19/07.

Swayne LE, Duncan WJ, Ginter PM. Strategic management of health care organizations, 5th ed. Malden, MA: Blackwell. 2006.

Tannenbaum R, Schmidt WH. How to choose a leadership pattern. Harvard Business Review. May-June 1973;51:162–180.

United Way of Canada – Centraide Canada. Board basics kit manual. Available at http://www.board-development.org. Accessed 5/14/07.

ADDITIONAL RESOURCES

The following is a list of informative sources with original papers on strategic management or strategic planning:

For a list of hundreds of change concepts, as well as examples of how they were applied in process improvement, both inside and outside of health care see Langley GJ, Nolan KM, Nolan TW, Norman CL, Provost LP. The Improvement Guide. San Francisco, CA: Jossey-Bass. 1996. An article that relates to board decision-making, internal scanning, benchmarking, strategic planning, and other topics is Hollis SR. Strategic and economic factors in the hospital conversion process. Health Affairs. 1997;16:131–143.

In this chapter we used the term leverage in reference to organizational strengths discovered in the internal examination. An article in this vein is Hamel G, Prahalad CK. Strategy as stretch and leverage. Harvard Business Review. 1994;71:75–84.

A witty discussion of competency can be found in Federation Forum. 2006;22(1):1, 18–21.

CHAPTER 6

INTERNAL ENVIRONMENT: PHYSICAL THERAPY

LARRY J. NOSSE

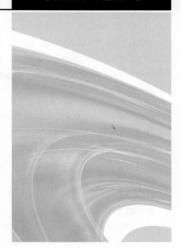

Learning Objectives

1. Relate environmental scanning and analysis principles to the examination of the internal environment of the field of physical therapy.
2. Identify common information categories of an internal environmental scan represented by the mnemonic CORE STATUS.
3. Identify common sources of internal environment information in physical therapy businesses.
4. Use the CORE STATUS mnemonic and a related template as a guide to conduct an internal scan for the self-selected physical therapy businesses you examined in the Chapter 4 case study.
5. For the businesses you choose, combine your Chapter 4 case study external scan (O and T) information with the new internal scan (S and W) information from this chapter and complete SWOT analyses.
6. Prioritize the strengths and weaknesses of your self-selected physical therapy business.
7. Develop an initial strategic plan for one of your self-selected businesses to take advantage of what you determine to be the greatest strength or a plan to improve in the area you consider the greatest weakness.
8. Discuss how the plan in # 7 relates to the concept of developing a competitive advantage for your self-chosen physical therapy business.

Introduction

This chapter uses the principles of **external** and *internal environmental scanning* presented in Chapters 3–5 and applies them to the physical therapy field. The products of this integration are the ability to complete **SWOT analyses** and the opportunity to develop more complete strategic plans than were requested in earlier chapters. To accomplish these tasks it is beneficial to review some core information.

In Chapters 3 and 4, we learned that the factors outside of an organization that can help or hurt it in its quest for success are identified by scanning the **external environment**. A key point made in Chapter 5 was that an organization's responses to external events are dependent on factors within the organization itself. Such factors are identified by scanning the internal environment. Internal scanning has also been appropriately called an *internal capability analysis* (Longest et al., 2000). An organization's internal environment is defined by its **fundamental documents**: its **mission**, **vision**, and **values statements**. The internal environment of a business consists of everything the business has available to advance toward achieving its mission as well as what it lacks to adequately respond to external **opportunities** and **threats**.

The internal environment includes the organization's human and other resources. Human resources include owner(s) if the business is **for-profit**, the **corporate govern-**

Key terms, which are defined below, are bolded and italicized the first time they appear in the chapter. Other important terms are shown in boldface on first appearance and are defined by the context in which they are used. When either of these types of terms is used several times, its acronym will be identified and subsequently used in the chapter. Both types of terms are listed alphabetically in the online glossary with their definitions and (when applicable) their acronyms.

compensation: bonuses, continuing education allowance, expense allowance, on-call pay, relocation allowance, shift premium, tuition repayment, wages, and other forms of payment made in exchange for work.

CORE STATUS: a mnemonic for categorizing organizational variables to organize an internal environmental scan: The letters stand for (C)ulture/(C)haracter, (O)bjectives, (R)esources, (E)xcellence, (S)tructure, (T)echnology, (A)uthority, (T)alent, (U)niqueness, and (S)atisfaction.

employee/employment benefits: in addition to compensation employees may be offered some of the following: group discounts, insurance (dental, disability, health, and life), paid health club fees, paid parking, paid time off (bereavement, family care, holidays, illness, and vacation), subsidized child care, tax-deferred savings plans, with or without employer contributions, retirement plan, travel subsidy, and other options.

First-level manager(ment): those responsible for the work of nonmanagers. May have the title supervisor, senior therapist, team-leader, or other title. Also called lower level manager(ment).

goodwill: an intangible asset of a business that includes the positive reputation consumers have of a business, its past earnings performance, and location.

internal capability/assessment analysis: examination of internal environmental scan data to determine what the organization is able to do given its current resources and shortcomings.

internal environmental scan(ing): examination of an organization's capabilities (strengths) and limitations (weaknesses) for dealing with external opportunities and threats.

job description/written role description: a written description of the organizational relationships of the position, list of general duties, decision-making authority, work standards, minimum job requirements for the job, responsibility for the work of others, and methods of coordinating with others.

labor: the workforce.

objectives: statements, when enacted, will move the business toward achievement of its goals. Mini-goals.

operational manager(s): those with responsibility for the day-to-day activities of an organization. Managers of clinical services like physical therapy are engaged in operations and are considered operational managers.

operation(s)/business operations: all of the day-to-day activities of an organization. Each activity that can be associated with money spent, money earned, or both.

organizational culture: the learned implicit and explicit assumptions, behavioral expectations, and values shared by management and staff that underlie how work is accomplished in an organization. The formally (written) and informally (coworker networks) communicated ways by which members are told and shown what is important, how to behave, how to treat one another, how work gets done, who to go to for what, salient history of the organization, and other information so they fit in socially and organizationally. Entities have unique cultures.

physical plant: a business' buildings, equipment, and fixtures.

report(ing) relationships: the solid lines connecting job titles, individuals or groups that signify direct oversight and upward communication responsibilities on an organizational chart.

return on equity (ROE): an evaluation of the relationship between income available to common stockholders and the stockholders' equity.

satisfaction: a subjective, emotional, and cognitive evaluation of the degree to which personally salient aspects of an object or event matches what the object or event was expected to be like.

variance(s): in accounting this is the positive or negative difference(s) between expected and actual results.

ing board/board of directors (BOD)/board of trustees, **managers**, and **professional** and **nonprofessional** staff (Longest et al., 2000). Nonhuman aspects of the internal environment are diverse. For example, ambiance, equipment, financial resources, **operational** systems, **organizational structure**, patents, *physical plant* [building(s) and land:, services and products offered, and more. The many components of the internal environment can be grouped to minimize the likelihood of missing any of the important ones. To facilitate conducting an internal environmental scan we have developed a mnemonic aid. We rearranged and expanded the internal categories presented in Chapter 5 to produce the mnemonic *CORE STATUS*. The letters represent: culture or character, objectives, resources, excellence, structure, technology, authority, talent, uniqueness, and satisfaction. Each of these categories is discussed in the next section in the context of physical therapy businesses. The internal environmental scanning process is consistent in the physical therapy businesses used as examples, but there are variations in the importance given to each internal category. These variations are due to different external forces, unique mission and vision statements, and differences in capabilities and challenges. The process and variations are clearer as we add content to the letters of the mnemonic.

CORE STATUS as a Guide for Studying Internal Position of a Business

The mnemonic letters stand for individual categories of an organization's framework and operations. This may give an unintended impression that it is the individual components of the organization that are the focus of the internal assessment rather than the organization in total. Internal assessment is an integrative process through which components of the organization are scrutinized individually for determining the contribution of each to fulfilling the mission. When examining a portion of the organization, it is important to remember that one part relates to the other parts as well as to the ultimate organizational **goal**. In Table 6.1 the CORE STATUS categories are identified along with some of the internal organization components that are included in each category.

Culture/Character

It is appropriate to start with an examination of an *organization's culture* because culture is linked to **values** (Darr, 2005) and values are indicators of motives (Nosse and Sagiv, 2005). An organization's culture reflects what is

Table 6.1 CORE STATUS Guide for Internal Environmental Scanning

Internal Categories	Example Components to Examine
Culture/character	Workplace culture, core values, transmission of values and culture
Objectives	Mission statement, vision statement, strategic objectives, strategic goals
Resources	Financial operations, available capital, labor supply, physical plant, goodwill, reputation
Excellence	Accreditation, licenses, certifications, benchmarking, awards, compliance, risk management
Structure	Organizational configuration, organizational chart, tax status, liability
Technology	Purposes, acquisition issues, upkeep, use, replacement
Authority	Policies, procedures, job descriptions, written communications, meetings, reports
Talent	Adequacy of human resources (number), competencies, knowledge, recruitment, retention, and development
Uniqueness	Actual and potential customer distinguished strengths competitors lack, competitive advantages
Satisfaction	Customer perspective as part of overall outcomes measurement system, physical therapy measurement instruments, relationship of satisfaction to clinical outcomes

expected and valued throughout an organization. The culture is a reflection of upper management's value hierarchy (Sherman, 1999) (Chapter 7). An organization's culture is the management's means of transmitting expectations, shaping attitudes, shaping behaviors, and motivating everyone to do their part to make the organization successful. The proper culture for a business facilitates employee performance while an improper culture hinders their performance (Joyce et al., 2003).

It has been suggested that there are six essential elements of business culture. Paraphrasing and building on the ideas of Deal and Kennedy (2000) the elements of business culture include:

- An informal *workplace network that transmits and reinforces* behaviors congruent with the organization's stated values and expectations
- Meaningful *events and ceremonies that exemplify* what the organization stands for and where it is going
- Members who understand the business environment and the importance of *fitting into* it
- Organizational *values* are stated, shared, understood, and accepted
- The presence of *exemplars* whose work is clearly guided by and representative of the culture's values
- Unique ways through which the organization tangibly *demonstrates* to employees what the behavioral expectations are

An organization that has these mechanisms in place is likely to have a cohesive work environment in which there is a widespread common understanding of "what it's like to work here, how we do things, what is right and what is wrong, and what the organization stands for." Organizational cultures differ because the core values differ. Note the variations in values espoused in the values statements of five physical therapy related organizations presented in Table 6.2.

Organizations that have a culture that promotes high- level performance and ethical behavior are more successful than those that do not (Joyce et al., 2003). A culture of high expectations and appropriate treatment of others is an internal strength. However, since management and staff personnel change over time it is important to check regularly the match between what is currently desired and what is actually practiced. Checking entails reviewing the formal values statement to see if it needs revision, and seeking evidence of management and staff compliant and noncompliant behaviors. Internal sources of behavior information include customer *satisfaction* surveys, complaints, the human resource department, department heads, and accreditation reports. If there is a change in the organization's core values, or there are sufficient incidences of noncompliant behavior, then strategies to communicate the changes and to review the core values are needed.

If issues related to cultural expectations are a concern, then there is a related weakness in the next category of internal items. The related weakness is an incomplete understanding of what the organization stands for and where it is going. The organizational documents that most clearly express this are the mission and vision statements. These documents are discussed in the next internal category, called *objectives*.

Objectives

Objectives are action statements which, when enacted, will help move an organization toward achievement of its goals. An organization's mission statement sets parameters for objectives and goals because it defines the organization's existence. An organization's vision statement is the ultimate goal.

Mission

A physical therapy organization's mission statement identifies at least:

Who we are (e.g., a private physical and occupational therapist company)

Whom we serve (e.g., adults with upper-limb movement and musculoskeletal problems in Orem, UT)

What we do best (e.g., integrate motor-learning and specialized manual therapy techniques)

What is unique about us (e.g., all professional staff members are certified hand therapists, all PTs are doctors of physical therapy)

Table 6.2 Sample Value Statements of Organizations Providing Physical Therapy Services	
Private Practice We believe in: "Uncompromising commitment to excellence . . . Ethical business practices and value integrity Respect for people Employer/employee work-life balance Listening to our customers and patients for oppor tunities to add value Innovation and creativity Responsive communication Fact based management Purposeful action" (PRORehab, 2007) *Specialty Rehabilitation Hospital* The Shepherd Center's (2007) code of ethical conduct applies to all professional and business interactions with customer groups. Staff behavior is guided by the following ideals: "Competence Integrity Professional responsibility Respect for people's rights and dignity Maintaining expertise Accountability (documentation) Non-discrimination (admissions) Fairness (fees) Honesty (refusal to offer inducements) Confidentiality Promote ethical decision making" (Shepherd Center, 2007)[a] *Urban Not-For-Profit Rehabilitation Hospital System* We value: "Innovation: New ideas, creative approaches; continu- ous improvement. Integrity: Behavior reflecting the highest ethical standards. Accountability: Personal responsibility for achieving goals. Service: Provide superior compassionate service and care. Teamwork: Respect others; work together.	Excellence: Demonstrate pride as you add quality and value to all we do" (Brooks Rehabilitation, 2007). *Sectarian Not-For-Profit Hospital* "The core values of the Providence Health System: Compassion: Caring for each person as part of our family. Justice: Working for a fair and equitable society. Respect: Affirming the God-given dignity and worth of each person. Excellence: Continually improving all that we do. Stewardship: Wisely caring for and sharing human, environmental and financial resources held in trust" (Providence Health and Services Alaska, 2007).[b] *Mult-State For-Profit Hospital System* "Successful partnerships require that the parties share certain beliefs; that they hold philosophies, expectations and standards in common. These are our tenets: Meet the needs of each and every patient whose care is our primary purpose and mission Maintain and enhance cooperative relationships with affiliated physicians to better serve the health care needs of our communities Forge strong partnerships with those who share our values Achieve standards of excellence which become the benchmark of industry practices Use innovation and creativity to identify and solve problems Apply quality management and leadership princi- ples to foster continued employee development Treat each other, our patients, and our partners with respect and dignity Hold integrity and honesty as our most important principles and perform at all times at the highest ethical standards Achieve competitive return for our investors Strive for improvement day in and day out in everything we do" (Tenet, 2007a)[c]

[a-c]Permission to reprint granted.

There are additional items that can be included in a mission statement. These are listed in Table 6.3. This template can be used to draft, assess, or revise a mission statement.

Vision

The vision statement is included as a component of objectives because it is the ultimate goal statement for **stakeholders**. It is the least tangible of an organization's guiding documents because it is something to strive to achieve rather than something that has eas-

ily measurable properties. Leadership uses the vision to inspire members to work to their capacity through good and bad times to move the organization toward a worthy and desirable future position. When management communicates what the organization can become they also imply that what is good for the organization is good for its individual members. Vision statements should be communicated effectively, so that stakeholders have a clear and vivid mental image of what the organization will look like when its mission has been accomplished (Swayne

Table 6.3   Template for Formulating, Analyzing, and Editing a Mission Statement

Element	Current Key Term(s)	Possible Change(s)
Core services offered		
Core values honored		
Geographical area(s) served		
Our philosophy		
Targeted consumers		
Our unique feature(s)		

et al., 2006). Examples of vision statements from six different practice settings are presented in Table 6.4. These examples were chosen because they represent small to large physical therapy–related businesses, the information was available on line, and each vision statement presented a different view of the future.

Ideally, the mission and vision statements are distributed, displayed, and reiterated continuously so their meaning and intent are understood by all members of the organization who, in turn, perform in accord with these **fundamental documents**. This is a strength. However, in health services organizations this often is not the case (Darr, 2005;

Table 6.4   Sample Vision Statements of Organizations Providing Physical Therapy Services

Two-Site Private Practice
"Valley Physical Therapy will be recognized as a leader in physical therapy practice in Santa Cruz County, providing cutting edge, state of the art, evidence based physical therapy" (2007).

Multi-Site Private Practice
"Saco Bay Orthopaedic & Sports Physical Therapy will be a leader in the provision of autonomous physical therapy services. We will demonstrate leadership and develop alliances within the Northern New England consumer and medical communities through innovative practice, education and research, quality of care, professionalism, socio-economic adaptability and financial responsibility. These criteria will be pursued indefinitely by our dedicated staff" (2007).[a]

Large Metropolitan Area Rehabilitation Hospital
"The Rehabilitation Institute of Chicago (RIC) will set the standards in patient care, . . . research, professional and public education, and focused advocacy and will disseminate knowledge and expertise throughout the world. RIC will create a culture of knowledge and excellence by rewarding innovation and by investing in its core assets, its staff" (2007).

Local Not-For-Profit Hospital System
"Middlesex Health System through best practices and innovation, will measurably improve the health of individuals in the communities we serve. In partnership with our physicians, employees, volunteers and patients, and in collaboration with other institutions and agencies that share our goals, we will commit our resources to programs that are ethically, socially and financially responsible. We will be a center of excellence in healthcare and wellness services" (2007).[b]

Multi-State For-Profit Hospital System
"Tenet will distinguish itself as a leader in redefining health care delivery and will be recognized for the passion of its people and partners in providing quality, innovative care to the patients it serves in each community" (2007).[c]

National Workers' Compensation Treatment Provider
"Concentra brings together talented, compassionate people to solve the highly complex issues of healthcare delivery, accessibility, and affordability. Every day, we make a difference in the lives of thousands of people through our ability to improve healthcare efficiency and outcomes" (2007).

[a-c]Permission to reprint granted.

Swayne et al., 2006). If members are not clear about the meaning or intent of the words in the mission or vision, or if the mission and vision are not synchronized, or if members are not in agreement with these statements, the strategic efforts to fulfill the organizational mission are diminished.

As noted in the introduction to strategic planning in Chapter 3, **strategic thinking** begins with the mission and vision statements as the foundation for the development of **strategic goals** and **strategic objectives**. It is appropriate therefore to review these goals and objectives with the intent of assuring currency and cohesiveness relative to the guiding documents. This is done to assure that resources are utilized to serve the same ultimate purpose. Areas of discrepancy between the basic directions set by the mission and vision and the strategic goals and objectives require realignment. The following physical therapy scenario describes an example of vision–mission–strategic goal discord.

The owner of a private practice has emphasized sports and orthopedic physical therapy in the fundamental documents of his organization. Over the years, he has recruited and hired appropriate professional staff to provide services to these target groups. His clinic locations and buildings are spacious, attractive, and house fitness and rehabilitation equipment in separate areas. His current concern is that the reimbursement amount per visit and per service has continued to decrease during the past three years. If this trend continues, he doubts that he will be able to make much of a profit next year. His accountant verified this conclusion.

By chance, the owner was approached by a local **home health** agency with a request to provide services to patients who are homebound. Soon after this inquiry, he met with his employees to summarize what was being discussed with the home health agency and the reason he was willing to continue talking with them. He let the staff know that most home health agency patients have multiple diagnoses, are elderly, and payment is through **Medicare Part A**. He clearly stated that staff members would have to do some traveling to treat these patients and that evaluation and reimbursement regulations for home health agencies were quite different from the outpatient

regulations they were familiar with [American Physical Therapy Association (APTA), 2007a]. The reaction of the employees in response to this information was a unanimous disapproval of this possible change in business direction. They reminded the owner that they had been hired because they were highly qualified and experienced in treating sports and orthopedic cases. It was obvious that the group's collective passion for care giving was derived from this segment of the market and not from treating geriatric patients or working as traveling therapists. The central issue for the owner is inadequate financial resources to continue in business.

Resources

Anything an organization has (a strength) or lacks (a weakness) could be a resource. However, loading one category would counter the intention to present a precise and easy-to-remember guide for conducting an internal scan. We chose to limit the discussion of component parts of resources to those related to financial matters, real estate, and *goodwill* and to deal with the additional important resources in other categories.

Financial

Circulation of financial information about an organization is guarded (Chapters 5 and 21). Owners, the **BOD, senior management**, and financial officers have access to all current and projected financial information. *Operational managers*, such as the manager of physical therapy, may only get information related to their department. Dated information is available to other stakeholders and interested parties in published annual reports. See Additional Resources for an example. Important areas to consider in the assessment of the financial status of a health service organization include **accounts receivable, cash flow, expenses, financing mix, gains, income/revenues, losses,** *return on equity*/**investment,** and **working capital** (Cleverley and Cameron, 2002). These accounting terms, their general calculation, and where they are found in reports are covered in Chapter 21. At this time, it is sufficient to know that any organization has to have sufficient money coming in to pay the bills (**cash flows**) to be able to carry out its mission. In general terms the **income** from *operations* and **nonoperating** sources has to be sufficient to pay current and estimated expenses and also provide some extra to invest for future growth, maintenance, and special projects. For-profit businesses also have to pay taxes and **dividends** to stockholders. Varying amounts of money are irregularly available as payments for services provided. There is potential income on investments made from past gains. Donations and grants are other sources of income. Expenses include the cost of maintaining buildings and grounds, contractual obligations, interest payments, *labor* (*compensation* and *employee benefits*), new equipment and supplies, and more (Chapter 21). Information available to operational department managers usually includes daily, weekly, monthly, quarterly, and year-to-date reports comparing what was budgeted for various expense and income- related categories to what was actually spent, collected, or produced. A critical comparison for physical therapy managers is the labor cost compared to the revenue generated by department professionals. *Variances*, the positive or negative differences between expected and actual performance, require further examination to determine their causes (Chapter 21). Financial systems for accounting, billing, collecting, recording, retrieving, and disseminating can be an organizational strength when these systems are integrated to produce accurate, timely, pertinent, and lucid information according to organizational needs.

Physical Plant

The physical plant refers to the business's buildings, fixtures, grounds, large equipment, and their condition. A building or department that is attractive both inside and outside and easy for people with limitations to access can be a comparative strength. Buildings and grounds that enhance the neighborhood help set consumer expectations that services provided inside will also be top-notch. The functionality of the physical plant such as sufficient number of elevators, signage, proximity of related departments, and sound control are additional potential strengths.

Goodwill

Goodwill is an intangible that can be a competitive advantage because it is something very difficult for competitors to duplicate (Swayne et al., 2006). The past earnings record, a positive reputation, and impressions communicated by customers to potential customers about an organization make up goodwill. Goodwill is a potential asset that can increase the value of a business when it is sold. It is also a consideration in valuation of the business when another owner joins the ownership group. In a physical therapy business, two likely situations where goodwill is a factor are when a private practice is for sale or an employee is interested in becoming a partner-owner. The latter situation is more complicated because the extent of goodwill is probably known by the aspiring partner. The question that may come up is how much of the goodwill is associated with the prior efforts of the aspiring partner. It may take an independent practice valuation to fix a fair price.

Excellence

To be considered excellent requires a comparison to the standard. The primary markers of internal excellence come from external bodies. These markers are accreditations, licenses and certifications the health service organization has earned, its relative position compared to industry benchmarks, awards, and adherence to professional standards. The frequency of legal actions (Chapters 8–10) the organization has been involved in is a more subtle indicator of excellence.

Accreditation

Seeking accreditation is voluntary on the part of an organization's leaders but accreditation is often necessary to have access to patients who are members of most health insurance plans. Potential consumers also may consider accreditation status when deciding on the hospital, rehabilitation center, long- term care facility, home health agency, or other types of facilities. The major institutional accreditation agencies include the **Commission on Accreditation of Rehabilitation Facilities** (CARF; 2007) and the **Joint Commission on Accredi-**

tation of **Healthcare Organizations** (JACHO; 2007) (Chapter 16). CARF's mission is to promote quality, value, and optimal **outcomes** of health services to clients. This commission emphasizes integrated interdisciplinary care. Physical therapy is examined as part of the overall criteria for medical rehabilitation accreditation in rehabilitation centers and on other criteria in assisted living communities and nursing homes. JACHO offers accreditation and specialty certifications. Physical therapy is examined as part of the criteria for JACHO accreditation for home care agencies, hospitals, and long- term care facilities. Physical therapy is not one of the specialty certification programs.

Licenses and Certifications

State governments issue licenses to operate a health service facility and certification to participate in the **Medicare** and **Medicaid** programs (Chapter 10). For Medicare and Medicaid certification, outpatient or rehabilitation services are optional programs that a facility may offer. An organization's strength lies in how well it monitors and meets licensure and certification regulations. Continuous timely responses are reflected in satisfactory ratings by state inspectors and ignorance can result in closure, public notice of deficiencies, loss of customers, and loss of employment.

Benchmarking

Benchmarking involves gaining insights from the performance of health service organizations considered to be the best in the industry (Chapter 5). Besides the application of general health service organization quality measures like the **Baldrige criteria** (2007) and the federal government, an organization may subscribe to a benchmarking service like Thompson Reuters (2009). For physical therapy specific benchmarking data, contracting with a group like Focus on Therapeutic Outcomes (FOTO; 2007), Care Connections (2007) or APTA Connect (2007b) can be informative. There is a limited amount of publicly available comparative information. An example is a Texas physical therapy benchmarking study involving mostly small physical therapy clinics (Davis, 2007). There are also research articles

on outcomes for specific conditions treated by PTs (Friesner et al., 2005) and a book on rehabilitation outcomes for PTs (Finch et al., 2002).

Awards

Awards for individual PTs can come from the APTA, its state affiliates, or its sections. Recognition from civic, commercial, and government groups for excellence in service, participation in research, or consideration for research funding, respectively, are plausible awards. A financial award for meeting specific quality criteria is available through federal government programs (see Additional Resources). PTs may participate in the Centers for Medicare and Medicaid Services (CMS) and Physician Quality Reporting Initiative (PQRI) program (CMS, 2007). Independent and employed PTs who screen their Medicare patients for future fall risk may receive up to a 1.5% reimbursement bonus. Organizations often give financial and other types of awards to departments and individual employees. Physical therapy departments and individual therapists are eligible for financial and recognition awards from their own health service organizations. Recognition for having achieved excellence in areas that are considered to be important to the organization also recognizes a contribution to the good of the organization.

Professional Standards

Another internal excellence marker is professional staff members subscribing to the standards of their profession. There are ethical and moral matters that cannot be dealt with by regulatory or accreditation requirements. It is the adherence to the standard of a profession that serves as an additional set of guidelines to help deliver quality care (Chapter 7). For PTs the professional standards are those of APTA and contained in the *Guide to Professional Conduct and the Code of Ethics* (APTA, 2007c).

Risk Avoidance

From a health services organization perspective **risk** is the mathematical probability that something bad will happen because of the actions or inactions of an employee, faulty equipment, inadequately designed facility for its customers, visitors and employees, unlawfulness, and other activities (Chapters 3, 8–10). A good risk management program is one that is supported by senior management, involves a committee with organization wide representation that regularly identifies and analyzes risks and reduction options, has authority to make changes, and monitors progress. Risk management in physical therapy can enhance the patient's experience in many ways by improving safety through infection control, short response time to emergencies, and adequate number of professional staff members. Employee, customer, and visitor falls are reduced if there is quick cleanup of wet areas, if exterior surfaces are level, and wheelchairs are readily available. Physical therapy is a department with many risks for patients and staff—falls, equipment failure, and burns are a few of the risks. Examples of risk management practices in physical therapy are disinfecting treatment surfaces and equipment after each patient, annual calibration of electrical equipment and temperature gauges, policies on the used of a gait belt, supervision, reporting unusual occurrences, emergency procedures, enforcing the policies, and training to ensure competence in these areas. An internal strength is having low levels of **civil** actions due to accidents with injuries and low numbers of **workers' compensation** claims compared to industry norms, meeting accreditation criteria, and compliance with regulations. All these reflect a strong risk management profile. As discussed in Chapter 3 regulatory compliance covers most aspects of health service business operations from ownership to financial practices to hiring and firing. This important topic is revisited in Chapters 9 and 17. The part of compliance that are of interest here are the regulatory requirements for hiring, promoting, disciplining, and discharging employees. For risk management purposes, it is a judicious practice for PTs and other organizational members who participate in interviews, assessments, and evaluations to have training by qualified individuals such as human resource professionals on the legal constraints associated with personnel matters (McConnell, 2006). In physical therapy especially, understanding regulations that deal with job applicants and employees with disabilities,

those who are older, and labor union members is a good risk management practice.

Looking for internal strengths and weaknesses as presented here involves assessing accreditations, certifications, licenses, regulatory compliance, benchmarked status, awards, adherence to professional standards, and risk management procedures. There certainly are other important areas, such as human resources, that could have been included in the discussion of excellence. Such components are highlighted in other categories in this mnemonic approach to internal scanning.

Structure

Organizational structure has two parts. The first part is the way organizational segments and employees relate to each other in the performance of their work to fulfill the mission. This is what the organization looks like on an **organizational chart**. This part of the structure is a management tool for communicating working relationships, defining levels of decision making, scope of responsibility and control, and showing how the work of the organization is distributed (Longest et al., 2000). These activities together are an organization's operational **configuration**. Figures 6.1 through 6.3 depict three common physical therapy organizational operational configurations.

Figure 6.1 represents a typical single-owner practice where the owner manages the business and treats patients. Some key internal questions for this practice include:

Is the owner-manager able to keep up his or her clinical and business knowledge and skills?

Has the flow of patients been acceptable given the organization's mission?

Is there quality control supervision and follow-up?

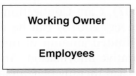

Figure 6.1. Small-size physical therapy organization.

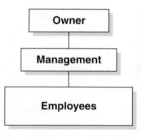

Figure 6.2. Intermediate-size physical therapy organization.

Are employees being mentored?

Are bills being sent and payment received in a reasonable amount of time?

Does documentation meet contemporary standards?

If the answer to these sample questions is yes, the structure is likely to be appropriate. The structure allows decisions to be made quickly because the owner has intimate knowledge and control over all aspects of the organization. If there are some negative responses, there may be a need for a structural change, that is, to add a formal management position (Fig. 6.2). An alternative solution is to add a part-time PT to treat some of the owner's patients to give the owner more time for management responsibilities (Chapter 11). Figure 6.2 is a structure showing management having formal responsibility to the owner(s) for achieving the organizational mission through its employees. Management was hired to accomplish the organization's mission. The direct lines connecting management to owner(s) and employees to management indicate formal supervisor–supervisee oversight and communication relationships. In this structure, management speaks for, acts on the behalf of, and answers to the owner(s). Questions to ask about this arrangement might be:

Is there regularly observable organization-wide proof that the culture is as it should be?

Is the owner as informed about the operations as he or she ought to be?

How is the organization doing financially?

Are staff retention levels as expected?

Are all positions filled?

How do the customers feel about the organization?

Positive responses to these sample questions are indications that the operational configuration supports the mission and that the organizational values are being assimilated and used to guide behavior. There are several reasons for negative responses. It could be that there is management–employee strife. This may require mediation, discipline, or the transfer or discharge of management or employee personnel (Chapters 11, 12, and 17). Negative responses could also be an indication that there are too many managers issuing conflicting directives. Alternatively, there may not be enough managers to smooth the way for employees to complete their work. Figure 6.3 shows a physical therapy structure with managers for each of the organization's businesses.

The second part of structure is the legal designation assumed by an organization to meet its mission, and for tax, **liability**, and management reasons. The details about business law and choosing an organizational structure are discussed in Chapters 9 and 14, respectively. At this point, it is sufficient to know that for internal scanning purposes, the examination of structure is done to determine if the legal business designation is appropriate to the mission. For-profit businesses are concerned about taxes. Different legal structures are taxed at different rates. For example, profit made by a personal corporation is taxed at 35%. If the same business became a limited liability corporation, the rate is the same as for the owner's personal income level. When it comes to liability, all health service organizations, for-profit and not-for-profit, have the same need. The need is to separate the personal assets of owners or directors and senior managers from the assets of the business. This is done so that claims made against the business, its management, or its employees are limited to the assets of the business and not the personal assets of its members. This separation can be accomplished by becoming **incorporated**. In the examination of the legal structure of a physical therapy business questions of interest include:

Are owner's personal assets separate from the business assets?

Are there other legal business forms with better tax advantages?

Are the owners responsible for their own acts or are all owners liable for each other's acts?

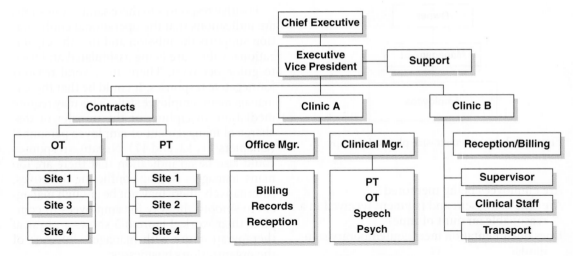

Figure 6.3. Large-size physical therapy organization.

Has our business outgrown or downsized so that our liability concern has changed?

Data for assessing the relevance of an organization's structure comes from various organizational sources. In a large physical therapy organization these sources can include legal counsel, upper, middle, and operational managers, risk management committees, and consultants. In a small organization, discussions between the owner(s), the business's accountant and attorney, and fellow private practice owners can be helpful in assessing internal structure issues.

Technology

An all-inclusive definition of technology is that technology includes ideas, equipment, methods, and anything else that helps expand human capabilities (Massachusetts Department of Education, 2007). In the workplace, the intent of technology is to facilitate human performance by:

Increasing knowledge (a video clip on a new balance challenging device, learning modules for a new management method)

Improving skills (a real-time teleconference with a master Pilates instructor or a management consultant group)

Allowing efficient, accurate, and timely communication (voice recognition software, Blackberry or wireless personal data assis-

tant device, system-wide mobile computer cart based documentation system)

Providing secure data collection, storage, and analysis (security cameras, billing and business intelligence software)

Helping create new knowledge (data aggregation, software for re-analysis of old data in new ways)

Having state-of-the-art equipment (recently approved cold laser device)

Improving integration across the continuum of care (accessible online medical records)

What technology does is change what is known, how things are done, what can be learned, and influence outcomes. A problem in health services in general is that technology is unevenly used (Porter and Teisberg, 2006). This comment applies to physical therapy organizations. Part of the problem is that technology development is an ongoing process. Once a purchase is made, the costs to keep the equipment up-to-date and working appropriately is expensive for technology users. One or more department members have to learn how to use the equipment and software, arrange for information technology support, and eventually deal with upgrades or new hardware and/or software. The salient point about investing in new technology is that if it is expected to improve organizational effectiveness, and funds are available, then the purchase should be made. Some physical therapy management examples of the decision to invest and the expectations for making the investment are:

Paying for online, transitional doctor of physical therapy courses for staff members to increase their knowledge.

Arranging for staff members to visit other physical therapy settings to learn how a particular technology works in that setting to help gauge how it might improve some aspect of their home workplace in a reasonable amount of time.

Providing Bluetooth-compatible smart phones with global positioning systems and services for home-health PTs so they can talk with patients before visits, find client's homes, access e-mail, schedule visits, complete their documentation, and see more clients in a day.

Having a pre-admission form on line for patients to complete before their initial visit.

Having online access to evidence-based evaluation and treatment guidelines, where such guidelines exist to enhance clinical outcomes.

Subscribing to a physical therapy benchmarking organization to obtain comparative outcome data to become a **preferred provider panel** member

Purchasing an evidence-supported whole-body vibration platform (Gusi et al., 2006) for the physical therapy department

Ideally, in a large health service organization, there is a chief technology officer. This individual oversees organization wide use of technology, including those used for measuring outcomes and costs throughout a cycle of care for targeted patients, identifying the methods used to bring about the outcomes and their costs, and aggregating appropriate patient demographic and diagnostic information to help determine what treatments are best for specific groups of patients. Such an information collection and dissemination infrastructure would facilitate sharing this meaningful information with potential customers so they can choose a provider based on value (Porter and Teisberg, 2006). Making such information publicly available to actual and potential customers would clearly be an organizational strength if competitors were unable or chose not to

provide equivalent information. See Additional Resources for a rehabilitation hospital example.

Authority

Organizational authority is formal power (McConnell, 2006). It has already been noted that an organization's authority map is its organizational chart. In addition, if the organization has become a state-recognized business entity, those who hold power are identified in the articles of incorporation. Authority also has a practical side: how power is disseminated, used, and the results of its use. In this section, the discussion of authority centers on examining the applied internal mechanisms used to pass power on through the levels of management. Mechanisms common to physical therapy settings are:

- Organizational **policies** and **procedures** (e.g., Support for advanced educational credentials will be provided; department managers will budget appropriately to meet their departments' needs annually)
- Department policies and procedures compatible with those covering the entire organization, (e.g., Full and part-time PTs and PTAs are eligible for up to $1,000 for tuition/year for work-related course that are part of a program terminating in a degree; submit applications three months before the starting date to the director of physical therapy for approval)
- *Job descriptions* that include decision-making authority, methods to coordinate work, responsibility for the work of others and organizational relationships (A physical therapy supervisor is responsible for the quantity and quality of work done by staff therapists and PTAs. A supervisor coordinates staff work and patient schedules with the director of nursing, the occupational and speech therapy supervisors, and the department scheduler. The supervisor reports to the director of rehabilitation services).
- Control over written communications: letters, memos, faxes, and e-mails that follow organization-approved format and content guidelines. Examples: an informative letter regarding a temporary change in the organizational management hierarchy whereby

the physical therapy supervisor becomes interim director of physical therapy; a memo from the director of physical therapy:

From: Director of Physical Therapy
To: Full and part-time occupational and physical therapists and certified occupational and physical therapist assistants
Subject: Discontinuation of per diem coverage contract
Message: The agreement with Everready Professional Services will not be renewed after its termination date of July 1. Current employees interested in working additional hours on a per diem basis are invited to contact the director of human services.
cc: [List]

To send correspondence with sensitive information, confirm reception-end security/privacy and be sure to include all senders' contact information and a standard security disclaimer clause on each page. Example text:

To: Walk-A-Mile-In-Our-Shoes, Inc.
From: Edmund Allen, Supervisor of Physical Therapy
Subject: Follow-up on sizing shoes for Johnny Walker, DOB 01/01/51
Message: This patient has had a great toe removed since the foot mold was made . . .

If the same message is sent via e-mail, ensure that the organization's security clause was included in the message. See example disclaimer in Additional Resources.

• Scheduled meeting minutes: Meetings are very common in all physical therapy settings. This is because when there are at least two people with a need to communicate on a work topic, and there is a need for a record of the discussion, a meeting is an ideal mechanism. For meetings to be relevant, efficient, and their results are shared there need to be some organizational guidelines regarding meetings. Recommended meeting guidelines are presented in Chapter 12. The current discussion of meetings is about authority associated with meetings. Man-

agement's view of the workforce impacts how much control is maintained over meetings and their proceedings. Authority issues related to meeting minutes include:

Who can authorize and who can cancel a meeting? A physical therapy manager consults with their manager if there is a potentially controversial topic, then calls the meeting.
Who can require attendance? Any manager may invite any employee who reports to them.
Who has control of the agenda? The manager who called the meeting
Who can participate in agenda formation? Ideally, all invited members
Who sets the meeting protocol for running a meeting and the process for taking minutes? Ideally, there are organizational standards
Who can limit the scope of decisions? Commonly, the manager above the one who called the meeting
The following are ideally performed according to the organizations standard procedures: How are decisions made? What will be recorded in the minutes? Who is responsible for dissemination of the unapproved minutes? What is the process for making corrections and signifying final approval of the minutes? Who determines who will see the approved minutes and how they will be shared? Where and how are minutes stored? Who has access to archived minutes? What is the process for gaining access to archived minutes?

Approved meeting minutes that are concise and accurate are invaluable for describing the views of individual meeting participants and the actions the group supports, rejects, or defers to another time. Giving meeting minutes access to the stakeholders affected by the actions taken by the meeting participants adds transparency to this part of the management decision-making processes. This is a double-edged issue. Letting people know what the decision is and who made it fosters openness in an organization's culture. It also can foster discontent and retaliation. Analysis of how this difficult issue of balancing transparency and maintaining order and similar difficult issues are handled, are indicators of management's perspectives about its work-force and of the organization's culture (Chapters 5 and 11).

Reports

Reports are another valuable source of internal information. In business there are two meanings of *report*. The first meaning relates to the organizational chart that identifies who is responsible for what and who answers to whom. All levels of managers below the **CEO** answer to or report to another manager. The second meaning of report is the more familiar one, a referenced document prepared for a specific purpose. Reports can be rich resources of information brought together from many segments of the organization: financial, human resource, marketing, strategic planning, legal, operations, and others. There are many similarities between what has been said about authority in the discussion of minutes and what can be said about authority related to reports. Reports are different from minutes in terms of depth of information and length. If sensitive information contained in reports were to be obtained by competitors, the organization's strategies for success could be jeopardized. For security purposes, authority to access reports with detailed sensitive organizational information is restricted. Authority to order the preparation of reports and who should produce them is also necessary because of the amount and duration of work they require. Reports may involve groups of people working for extended periods of time. Producing a report can impinge on the participant's availability to carry out other responsibilities. The authority issues related to reports are:

Who can order reports?
What is the standard format?
Who can contribute information for specific reports?
Who will have access to past reports?
Who will have access to complete new reports?
What security measures will be taken to limit unwanted exposure of sensitive information?
How will report recommendations be handled?

Reports integrate previous and current information. This consolidation can provide clearer indications of organizational or departmental strengths and weaknesses than other information sources. Physical therapy managers commonly produce reports for their managers. Samples of physical therapy department reports are:

Financial reports (expense and income budgets, **productivity**; Chapter 21)
Human resource reports (assessment process, actions taken, future needs; Chapters 16 and 17)
Marketing reports (new services, customer satisfaction, new equipment)
Occurrence reports (patient fall, employee back injury, theft; Chapters 8 and 16)
Strategic plans (space, equipment, new services; Chapter 13)

Strengths and weaknesses that a physical therapy organization manager gleaned from internal reports include determining:

If the department is achieving its mission and contributing to the organizational mission (Chapters 18 and 21)
How the department is doing compared to last year? (Chapters 16, 18, and 21)
Which department services have and which have not improved compared to last year? (Chapters 11 and 16)
What are the reasons for service shortcomings? (Chapters 11 and 16)
Who was responsible for performance improvements and performance shortfalls? (Chapters 11 and 16)
What areas have promise of becoming competitive advantages? (Chapters 5 and 18)

Talent

In the workplace, people with **talent** are those that possess a level of work-related competencies that enable them to excel at their job. Employees with talent are valuable resources to an organization. All organizations seek talented employees. The key question to answer about talent in an internal environment analysis: Is there enough talent in right places to fulfill the organization's mission for the foreseeable future?

An examination of talent has to be organization wide starting with the leadership (BOD and CEO) down through the organization. The official performance criteria are listed in job descriptions. However, it is common for job descriptions to have an open-ended statement to the effect that the employee will perform other tasks assigned by his or her manager or the BOD (Chapter 17). The assessment of the adequacy of the quantity and quality of talent throughout the organization is extremely difficult and complex because of the interaction and interdependency of the parts of the organization. Department managers and human resource staff collaborate on how and what to assess at the department level. External consultants are required to analyze the quality of the talent at the upper levels of management. The specific aspects of employee evaluation are covered more fully in Chapter 16.

Physical Therapy Talent

To discuss physical therapy talent it is helpful to develop a context. The first issue is that there are some basic differences between what employers expect of employees and what PTs and PTAs expect when they accept a job. With the lowest PT unemployment rate in a decade, employers have difficulty filling positions. Second, there is competition among employers for PTs and PTAs, particularly in home health and long-term settings (APTA, 2007d). Third, in this **seller's market**, anecdotal reports from human resource personnel and PT managers suggest that many applicants, new graduates and experienced alike, seem overly intent on serving their own interests rather than meeting the employer's needs. The list of personal interests include high income, flexible work schedule, low-cost health insurance, continuing education benefits, and guided growth opportunities in one or more clinical areas. Because of these contextual elements, it is quite appropriate to assess physical therapy talent where it starts, the recruitment process.

Most physical therapy organizations hire just enough staff to get the work done. With a finite number of employees, it is more likely that an organization will achieve its mission if every member works at maximum effectiveness and productivity. In other words, every-

one must get his or her work done right, in the least amount of time, and step in when others need help (Nosse et al., 2005). Ultimately, developing a talented workforce begins with recruiting the right people (Chapter 17). The right people are those that have work-related **competencies** and attitudes compatible with those of the organization (McConnell, 2006). Ideally, recruitment and selection efforts will produce a large number of qualified applicants, the best applicant(s) will accept the offer of employment, and they will perform as anticipated. Strategies to gather information to gauge the effectiveness of the recruitment-hire process include:

Examination of the recruitment process (advertisements, job descriptions, contact methods)

Examination of the selection process (criteria, paper review, interview, call-back, and follow-up processes)

Review of the performance records of recently hired personnel (criteria, strengths, weaknesses, remediation, advancement)

Review of disciplinary information (duration of employment, offenses, remediation efforts)

Analysis of exit interview information (reasons stated for separation, successes, failures, missed opportunities)

Criteria are needed to recruit and develop talent. The criteria are developed from the job description (Chapter 17). The selection group looks for matches between the job description and the applicant's background information. This matching process involves assessing a combination of information sources. For direct care positions these include

Applicant licenses/credentials/certifications
Formal, informal, and continuing education
Relevant experience
Peer recognition
Recommendations
And occasionally, demonstration of knowledge and skill

It is less common to explore a new graduate's knowledge and skill in management because they are usually interviewed for direct care positions. This may be a shortcoming of the recruitment process that becomes apparent later when *first-level manager* (supervisor) positions become available. A possible remedy is to include basic questions about management knowledge and skills in the interview phase of recruitment.

There is a set of evidence-based recommendations for the basic management knowledge and application skills for future PT graduates (Lopopolo et al., 2004; Schafer et al., 2007). These survey data from PTs in clinical and academic settings suggest that the management knowledge and skills new graduates should have can be distributed into six categories (Lopopolo and Schafer, 2004; Table 6.5).

These categories can serve as the framework for formulating management-related interview questions. Incorporating questions related to management in interviews can assist in assessing applicants' clinical and management knowledge and skills. The information can also be used to plan relevant management development opportunities. A complementary plan for current employees to enhance their management knowledge and skill has the potential to enhance employee retention, provide a flow of managers who have an understanding of the organization, and facilitate an employee's advancement within the organization's management structure. The absence of a plan for the internal preparation of the managers, particularly first-level managers, can be an organizational weakness. This oversight can foster an "us" and "them" culture within a physical therapy department. This is a culture where the clinicians perceive themselves as the good people and the managers as their antagonists. The lack of a management development program also leaves those interested in advancing their knowledge and skill in this area to find their own resources. General management preparation may or may not be applicable to an organization because of its organizational configuration, specialization, or other reasons.

The ability to attract talented and organizationally compatible members, develop them further, and retain them are all strengths that contribute to fulfilling an organization's mission. Long-term employees help sustain department continuity by example and through **mentoring**. Weaknesses in recruitment, retention, or development programs are serious because a high performing organization cannot function very long without a sufficient number of competent, growing, and committed employees. Retention of talented PT managers, professional staff members and PTAs, requires at least fair pay, clinical guidance, and opportunities for growth. The presence of these incentives is a department strength.

Uniqueness

The primary purposes of examining the internal environment of an organization are to determine its capabilities to deal with external challenges and to identify what customers think differentiates the organization from those offering similar services. This latter purpose is commonly referred to as defining the organization's **competitive advantage**(s). While strengths contribute to competitive advantages, they are something greater. They are what:

Table 6.5 Six Category Model for Management Knowledge and Skills Recommended for Physical Therapist Graduates by 2010

Category	Example Components
1. Finance	Cost control, reimbursement essentials, coding
2. Information	Sources, use of management data, record keeping
3. Networking	Professional development, consultation, negotiation
4. Human resources	Self-management, direct personnel, lead
5. Operations	Compliance, resource allocation, meeting management
6. Planning and forecasting	Sector analysis, competitor analysis, strategy analysis

Adapted from Schafer DS et al., Physical Therapy. 2007;87:274-281 with permission of the American Physical Therapy Association. This material is copyrighted, and any further reproductions or distribution is prohibited.

is unique to an organization that customers value

the organization continues to improve upon
   to maintain customers' perception of value
competitors lack, find difficult to duplicate, or
   are unable to develop a satisfactory substitute for (Hannagan, 2002)

A physical therapy competitive advantage may be lower cost, minimal paperwork,
or quality and consistency–all treatments
provided only by a PT and always the same
one. Table 6.6 is a template to be used to
bring together the information on strengths
and potential strengths uncovered by the
internal environment scan. The table can
help organize and summarize department
strengths that are or can become competitive
advantages.

The customer's view of what is valuable
about a physical therapy service encounter
is what counts when identifying strengths
or competitive advantages. In recognition of

this importance, customer satisfaction will be
emphasized in the next category and is continued in Chapters 16, 19, and 22.

Satisfaction

Health service customer satisfaction represents
the customer's emotional and cognitive evaluation of what they consider the important aspects
of their experience. The degree of satisfaction
is believed to be based on the extent of congru-
ence between the actual clinical experience and
what the customer expected the experience to
be like (Maciejewski et al., 1997).

The measurement of customer satisfaction
is important because it "is both an *indicator*
of quality of care, and a *component* of quality
care" (National Quality Measures Clearinghouse [NQMC], 2007, p. 1). Customer satisfaction has been found to be associated with
the following internal health service organization activities:

Table 6.6 Template for Identifying Strengths That Are or May Become Competitive Advantages				
What do we believe are our strengths?[a]	**Do we know customers value this?**	**Is this strength unique to us?**	**Can others copy us easily?**	**Can we change to hold/develop an advantage?**
1.	Yes No ?	Yes No ?	Yes No ?	Yes No ?
	Comments:	Comments:	Comments:	Comments:
Source/Date				
2.	Yes No ?	Yes No ?	Yes No ?	Yes No ?
	Comments:	Comments:	Comments:	Comments:
Source/Date				
3.	Yes No ?	Yes No ?	Yes No ?	Yes No ?
	Comments:	Comments:	Comments:	Comments:
Source/Date				
4.	Yes No ?	Yes No ?	Yes No ?	Yes No ?
	Comments:	Comments:	Comments:	Comments:
Source/Date				

[a]From internal environmental scan.

- Competitive position
- Employee retention
- Employee satisfaction
- Incidence of suits
- Profitability
- Accreditation
- Marketing strategy
- Quality of care (NQMC, 2007; Maciejewski et al., 1997)

The widespread internal influences of customer satisfaction make it very clear that a continual process for obtaining, analyzing, and reacting to customer perspectives can be good for an organization in many ways. Important as it is, customer satisfaction is only one of the areas that can be measured to improve the organization. The measurement of customer perspectives should be part of an overall outcomes measurement process that looks at clinical, technical or functional, and associated cost outcomes (Nosse et al., 2005). In addition, the level of satisfaction of stakeholders besides customers can impact the organization. These stakeholders include the BOD, upper management, professional employees, nonprofessional employees, vendors, visitors, and family members (Chapters 3 and 4). Satisfaction surveys can be broadly focused on the total organization (hospital), more narrowly focused on a particular unit or service level (physical therapy department), or focused on an individual (a PT; Maciejewski et al., 1997). Porter and Teisberg (2006) in discussing competition questioned the benefit of customer satisfaction surveys that focus more on the general service experience such as quality of meals, cleanliness, and friendliness than on the end result of the clinical service.

Satisfaction With Physical Therapy Services

There are several physical therapy-specific customer satisfaction measurement instruments that have had some level of reliability and validity testing for their use with patients treated in selected settings. Examples of these instruments were reported by Goldstein et al. (2007) and Roush and Sonstroem (2007) for use with outpatients in general. Beattie et al. (2007) reported on an instrument for outpatients covered by workers' compensation.

Typically, physical therapy-focused satisfaction surveys include questions that deal with:

Communication
Convenience
Cost/value
Customer–personnel interpersonal relationships
Making recommendations to others
Personnel responsiveness
Resources
Satisfaction with the direct-care personnel
Satisfaction with the overall physical therapy experience

The authors are unaware of a valid, physical therapy–specific, satisfaction instrument that has been tested for use in all types of settings and pointedly asks about the customer's level of satisfaction with respect to the problem(s) they were treated for. At this time satisfaction with the physical therapy experience is evaluated on a mixture of adjunctive criteria like demonstrated empathy, cost, customer interpreted expertise of the therapist, and "soft" questions about the outcome of the course of treatment. Ideally, satisfaction measurement is one part of a comprehensive outcome measurement system, and there is a strong and positive correlation between overall customer satisfaction and the clinical outcomes part of the outcomes evaluation process. High satisfaction and above average comparative clinical outcome ratings are significant physical therapy organizational strengths. Meeting or exceeding consumer expectations in outcome and cost is a value that is the ideal basis for competitive advantage (Porter and Teisberg, 2006).

The customer's opinion of the amenities, facility appearance, and customer service elements surrounding their physical therapy treatment certainly influences their satisfaction ratings (Beattie et al., 2007; Goldstein et al., 2007; Roush and Sonstroem, 2007). However, these items are relatively tangential to the question, "did you get better and how much better." The best that can be done at this time is to use a satisfaction instrument with known **reliabilities** and more than **face validity** (Finch et al., 2002). High satisfaction ratings based on data from inadequately tested survey instruments and less than average performance on comparative outcome measures is incongruent. This incongruence could become an internal weakness if made public by informed competitors.

Summary

This chapter reviewed the general principles of external and internal environmental scanning presented in Chapters 3–5 and applied them to the physical therapy field. The CORE STATUS mnemonic was introduced to assist remembering the major organizational categories to investigate in an internal scan. The letters represented an organization's culture/character, objectives, resources (tangible), excellence, structure, technology, authority, talent, uniqueness, and satisfaction. The individual components within each category were discussed in the context of generic health service/organiza-

---

CASE STUDY 6.1

Complete the External–Internal Environmental Analysis Process for Selected Physical Therapy Businesses

Overview

This case gives you the opportunity to integrate your environmental scanning and strategic planning knowledge and skill. The good news is that you have half of the work done. Your initial task will be to conduct a partial internal environmental analysis of the same three physical therapy businesses whose external environment you examined for the case study in Chapter 4. The parts of the internal environment you will examine will depend on which opportunities and threats you prioritized in the earlier case study. For example, say you found that a competitor was exploring a location for a new facility close to one owned by your chosen business. You determined that the potential impact on your organization would be severe and the likelihood of the competitor moving near you is high. By conducting an internal scan, you will determine your business' strengths for dealing with this threat as well as the shortcomings that limit your options. Combining work you did on the external environment in Chapter 4 with the internal environment information you gather for the current assignment, you will have the information you need to do a complete SWOT analysis, set priorities, and develop strategic plans, goals, and objectives.

Your Assignment

1. Conduct partial internal environmental scans of the three physical therapy busi-

nesses you examined in the Chapter 4 case study.
2. Choose any three of the CORE STATUS (Table 6.1) categories to investigate all three of your chosen businesses.
3. Gather whatever internal information is available on your chosen businesses. If there are significant voids, improvise (make up reasonable information).
4. Complete SWOT analyses for each of the three internal environment categories you chose for each of your businesses (i.e., 3 × 3 = 9 SWOTs).
5. Review your options based on the SWOT analyses and choose what you consider the most outstanding strength (an actual or potential competitive advantage) for any one of the businesses.
6. Review your options based on the SWOT analyses and choose what you consider the most glaring weakness of any one of the businesses.
7. Develop a strategic plan, including goals, and objectives, intended EITHER to improve the strength so it becomes or continues to be a competitive advantage OR to turn the glaring weakness into a future strength.
8. Reflect on what you did well in each of the parts of this exercise and identify what you feel you need to improve on if you were to complete an internal scan in the near future.

tions and selected physical therapy businesses. Four questions were asked or inferred in the discussion of all ten categories. First, do the category components constitute a strength that will help deal with external threats or benefit from external opportunities? Second, is this an area of deficiency such that offensive or defensive options are limited? Third, can strengths become competitive advantages? And fourth, can weaknesses be turned into future strengths? Competitive advantages were defined by three features: (1) they are the unique components of an organization that contribute to customer perceptions that the services provided and the processes surrounding the service are of value to them; (2) the organization has the ability to improve in the valued areas to maintain customer perceptions of value; and (3) competitive advantages are things competitors lack, have difficulty duplicating, or are unable to develop a satisfactory substitute for. Competitive advantages were melded into the discussion of measuring customer satisfaction because inquiring about satisfaction provides the primary means for gaining insight into what customer's value in their physical therapy encounters and how the experience matched their preconceptions. The necessity of pursuing customer satisfaction information was noted but with the caveat that many questions in physical therapy customer satisfaction measurement instruments focus on elements surrounding the actual physical therapy treatments. Somewhat indirectly, questions about the clinical results of the service are asked. It is suggested that the complete picture of how well a physical therapy department or clinic is doing should entail concurrent consideration of customer perceptions and other outcome measures.

REFERENCES

American Physical Therapy Association. Reimbursement, coding, and compliance for physical therapists. Available at http://www.apta.org/AM/Template. cfm?Section=Chapters&CONTENTID=30261 &TEMPLATE=/CM/HTMLDisplay.cfm. Accessed 6/09/07a.

American Physical Therapy Association. Get connected with APTA Connect. Available at http:// www.apta.org/AM/Template.cfm?Section=Info_ for_Clinicians&TEMPLATE=/CM/ContentDisplay. cfm&CONTENTID=36088. Accessed 6/11/07b.

American Physical Therapy Association. Professional resources. Available at http://www.apta.org/ AM/Template.cfm?Section=Ethics_and_Legal_ Issues1&Template=/TaggedPage/TaggedPageDisplay.cfm&TPLID=2&ContentID=36093. Accessed 6/11/07c.

American Physical Therapy Association. 2005 employment survey. Available at http://www.apta.org/AM/ Template.cfm?Section=Research&Template=/ MembersOnly.cfm&ContentID=27027. Accessed 6/20/07d.

Beattie PF, Pinto MB, Nelson MK, Nelson R. Patient satisfaction with outpatient physical therapy: Instrument validation. Available at http://www.ptjournal.org/ cgi/search?sortspec=relevance&author1=&fulltext =patient+satisfaction&pubdate_year=&volume= &firstpage=. Accessed 6/21/07.

Baldrige National Quality Program. Health care criteria of performance excellence. Gaithersburg, MD: Baldrige National Quality Program National Institute of Standards and Technology, Technology Administration, U.S. Department of Commerce. 2007.

Brooks Rehabilitation. Vision, mission, and values. Available at http://www.brooksrehab.org/why-brooks/ aboutbrooks/mission/. Accessed 6/15/07.

Care Connections. New and noteworthy. Available at https://www.careconnections.com/(S(u2f4fg45 mknmcw45as13fu45))/News.aspx?id=23. Accessed 6/15/07.

Centers for Medicare and Medicaid Services. Physician reporting quality initiative (Physical Therapy). Available at http://questions.cms.hhs.gov/cgi-bin/cmshhs. cfg/php/enduser/std_alp.php?p_sid=Db8o6TDi& p_lva=&p_li=&p_accessibility=0&p_page=1&p_ cv=&p_pv=4.968&p_prods=8%2C61%2C945%2 C968&p_cats=&p_hidden_prods=&prod_lvl1=8 &prod_lvl2=61&prod_lvl3=945&prods4=968 &p_search_text=physical+therapy&p_new_ search=1&p_search_type=answers.search_nl. Accessed 6/11/07.

Cleverley WO, Cameron AE. Essentials of health care finance, 5th ed. Gaithersburg, MD: Aspen. 2002.

Commission on Accreditation of Rehabilitation Facilities. Service providers. Available at http://www.carf. org/providers.aspx. Accessed 6/11/07.

Concentra. Mission, Vision, Values. Available at http:// www.concentrahealth.com/WhoWeAre/Mission-Vision-Values/. Accessed 6/07/07.

Connecticut Orthopedic Rehabilitation Associates. Our mission. Available at http://www.coraonline.com/ mission.htm. Accessed 6/14/07.

Darr K. Ethics in health services management, 4th ed. Baltimore, MD: Health Professions Press. 2005.

Davis MA. Survey of Texas physical therapy Facilities Benchmark Statistics. Available at http://www.coba. unt.edu/mgmt/Davis/PT/PT_FacilityReport.pdf. Accessed 6/11/07.

Deal TE, Kennedy AA. Corporate cultures: The rites and rituals of corporate life. New York, NY: Perseus. 2000.

Finch E, Brooks D, Stratford PW, Mayo NE. Physical rehabilitation outcome measures: A guide to enhanced clinical decision making, 2nd ed. Baltimore, MD: Lippincott Williams & Wilkins. 2002.

Focus on Therapeutic Outcomes. Products. Available at http://www.fotoinc.com/products.htm. Accessed 6/11/07.

Friesner D, Meufelder D, Raisor J, Khayum M. Benchmarking patient improvement in physical therapy with data envelopment analysis. International Journal of Health Care Quality Assurance Incorporating Leadership in Health Services. 2005;18:441–457.

Goldstein MS, Elliott, SD, Guccione AA. The development of an instrument to measure satisfaction with physical therapy. Available at http://www.ptjournal.org/cgi/content/full/80/9/853?maxtoshow=&HITS=10&hits=10&RESULTFORMAT=&author1=goldstein&searchid=1&FIRSTINDEX=0&sortspec=relevance&volume=80&resourcetype=HWCIT. Accessed 6/21/07.

Gusi N, Raimundo A, Leal A. Low-frequency vibratory exercise reduces the risk of bone fracture more than walking: A randomized controlled trial. BMC Musculoskeletal Disorders. 2006;7:92. Available at http://www.biomedcentral.com/1471-2474/7/92. Accessed 6/18/07.

Hannagan T. Mastering strategic management. New York, NY: Palgrave. 2002.

Joint Commission on Accreditation of Healthcare Organizations. Accreditation programs. Available at http://www.jointcommission.org/AccreditationPrograms/. Accessed 6/11/07.

Joyce W, Nohria N, Roberson B. What (Really) Works: The 4 + 2 Formula for Sustained Business Success. New York, NY: HarperCollins. 2003.

Longest BB, Rakich JS, Darr K. Managing health services organizations and systems, 4th ed. Baltimore, MD: Health Professions Press. 2000.

Lopopolo RB, Schafer DS, Nosse LJ. Leadership, administration, management, and professional (LAMP) processes in physical therapy: A Delphi study. Physical Therapy. 2004;84:137–150.

Lopopolo RB, Schafer DS. Re-conceptualizing the role of leadership, administration, management, and professionalism (LAMP) in physical therapy practice. HPA Resource. 2004;4(2):1–3.

Maciejewski M, Kawiecki J, Rockwood T. Satisfaction. In Kane RL, ed. Understanding health care outcomes research. Gaithersburg, MD: Aspen. 1997:67–89.

Massachusetts Department of Education. Science and technology/engineering curriculum framework. Available at http://www.doe.mass.edu/frameworks/scitech/2001/resources/glossary.html. Accessed 6/17/07.

McConnell CR. Umiker's management skills for the new health care supervisor, 4th ed. Boston, MA: Jones and Bartlett. 2006.

Middlesex Health System. Vision statement. Available at http://www.middlesexhealth.org/go/B18B091C-9096-AC88-60118E32760C3EBB/. Accessed 6/17/07.

National Quality Measures Clearinghouse. Medical practice satisfaction: Mean section score for "During your visit" questions on Medical Practice Survey. Available at http://www.qualitymeasures.ahrq.gov/summary/summary.aspx?doc_id=397&string=patient+AND+satisfaction. Accessed 6/20/07.

Nosse LJ, Friberg DG, Kovacek PR. Managerial and supervisory principles for physical therapists, 2nd ed. Baltimore, MD: Lippincott Williams & Wilkins. 2005.

Nosse LJ, Sagiv L. Theory-based study of the basic values of 565 physical therapists. Physical Therapy. 2005;85:834–850.

Porter ME, Teisberg EO. Redefining health care creating value-based competition on results. Boston, MA: Harvard Business School. 2006.

PRORehab. Mission, vision and core values statement. Available at http://www.prorehabpc.com/about/vision.asp. Accessed 6/14/07.

Providence Health and Services Alaska. Mission and core values. Available at http://www.providence.org/alaska/kodiak/values.htm/. Accessed 6/15/07.

Rehabilitation Institute of Chicago. Mission, vision & philosophy. Available at http://www.ric.org/about/mission.php. Accessed 6/07/07.

Roush SE, Sonstroem RJ. Development of the physical therapy outpatient satisfaction survey (PTOPS). Available at http://www.ptjournal.org/cgi/content/full/79/2/159?maxtoshow=&HITS=10&hits=10&RESULTFORMAT=&fulltext=patient+satisfaction&searchid=1&FIRSTINDEX=0&sortspec=relevance&resourcetype=HWCIT. Accessed 6/21/07.

Saco Bay Orthopaedic & Sports Physical Therapy. Vision statement. Available at http://www.sacobaypt.com/mission.htm. Accessed 6/07/07.

Schafer DS, Lopopolo RB, Luedtke-Hoffmann KA. Administration and management skills needed by physical therapy graduates in 2010: A national survey. Physical Therapy. 2007;87:261–281.

Shepherd Center. Code of ethical conduct. Available at http://www.shepherd.org/about/codeofethicalconduct.htm. Accessed 6/15/07.

Sherman SG. Total customer satisfaction: A comprehensive approach for health care providers. San Francisco, CA: Jossey-Bass. 1999.

Swayne LE, Duncan WJ, Ginter PM. Strategic management of health care organizations, 5th ed. Malden, MA: Blackwell. 2006.

Tenet. Our tenets. Available at http://www.tenethealth.com/TenetHealth/OurCompany/Our+Tenets.htm. Accessed 6/21/07a.

Tenet. Mission and values. Available at http://www.tenethealth.com/TenetHealth/OurCompany/MissionValues. Accessed 6/07/07b.

Thompson Reuters. 100 top hospitals. Available at http://www.100tophospitals.com. Accessed 1/10/09.

Valley Physical Therapy. Vision statement. Available at http://www.valleypt.net/. Accessed 6/07/07.

ADDITIONAL RESOURCES

Several years of annual reports from the APTA are available at www.apta.org. A 21-item online form developed by Richard S. Gallagher for conducting an examination of a business' culture is available at http://members.aol.com/rsgassoc/Assessment.htm. A more in-depth method of examining culture is offered by Jackson and Schmidt at http://jacksonandschmidt.com/cultureassess.html. Power Point presentations on the Physician Quality Reporting Initiative program are available at http://www.cms.hhs.gov/PQRI/30_EducationalResources.asp. The federal government also has a voluntary basic quality measurement program for hospitals that includes a patient satisfaction section (http://www.cms.hhs.gov/HospitalQualityInits/Downloads/HospitalHCAHPSFactSheet200807.pdf) and a financial incentive program for hospitals (http://www.cms.hhs.gov/HospitalQualityInits/downloads/HospitalPremierCal200512.pdf). A classic book that focuses on competitive advantage is Porter ME. Competitive Advantage: Creating and Sustaining Superior Performance. New York, NY: Free Press. 1985. The following is an example of a disclaimer for e-mail transmissions:

This message and attachments have been scanned for viruses and dangerous content, and is believed to be clean. Privileged/confidential information may be contained in this message and attachments. If you are not the addressee indicated in this message, or responsible for delivery of the message to such person, you may not copy, distribute, disseminate, or take action on any of the information. Delete this e-mail immediately and all of its attachments. The sender assumes no responsibility, expressed or implied, regarding inaccuracies or the consequences of any action taken as a result of the information provided herein.

An example of an online customer satisfaction instrument for an ortho/sports outpatient organization is accessible at http://www.coraonline.com/mission.htm. Samples of online forms for clinic, customer, and staff satisfaction are available at (http://www.keysurvey.com/search.jsp?cx=017444378259885321029%3Aq_siozrhwbm&cof=FORID%3A11&q=survey+samples#819). A scholarly review of the literature on patient satisfaction is the measurement of satisfaction with health care: Implications for practice from a systematic review of the literature. This report provides insights about developing, administering, and analyzing this type of survey information. The full text is available through http://www.hta.nhsweb.nhs.uk/project/1035.asp. An example of publicly available rehabilitation hospital outcomes information is available at http://www.brooksrehab.org/outcomes/.

PART II

Guiding Behavior: Values, Ethics, Jurisprudence, and Oversight Agencies

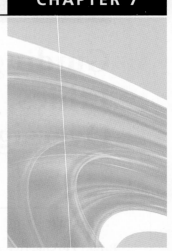

CHAPTER 7

BEHAVIORAL GUIDANCE: VALUES AND ETHICAL PRINCIPLES

LARRY J. NOSSE

Learning Objectives

1. In your own words, define and contrast the terms values, personal values, philosophical statement, mission statement, statement, moral, morality, ethics, and ethical.
2. Explore your personal value goal priorities.
3. Analyze and evaluate your personal values hierarchy and, based on your experiences, provide examples that reflect your prioritized value hierarchy.
4. Compare the fundamental documents of selected physical therapy- related organizations.
5. Analyze selected behavior related documents of the American Physical Therapy Association (APTA).
6. Initiate creating your own philosophical, mission, and vision statements (your fundamental documents).

Introduction

The macro view of general business **principles** applied to health service businesses was presented in the preceding chapters. Among the basic business principles discussed were those related to **environmental scanning** and **strategic planning**. Chapters 3–6 incorporated some information on *values*, **mission**, and **vision statements**. Together, these statements were called a business's **fundamental documents**. These documents are the written founda-

tion for the organization's strategic planning process (Swayne, Duncan, Ginter, 2006) as well as its organizational culture. Together the fundamental documents set boundaries, guide choices, and align actions throughout the organization (Darr, 2005).

The responsibility for formulating the fundamental documents is in the hands of **upper level management**. It was pointed out that it is important to have cohesion between values, mission, and vision statements in order to focus all efforts on fulfilling the mission and getting closer to realizing the vision.

From the two chapters on **internal environmental** analysis it is evident that reviewing the fundamental documents is essential to assure that direction, inspiration, and behavioral expectations are appropriately integrated with current practice and strategic efforts. The current chapter deepens the discussion on fundamental documents, particularly on the topics of values and *ethics*. A process for developing *organizational values* and ethics and vision statements is outlined. The process includes addressing values and ethics at personal, organizational, and physical therapy professional levels. This trilevel approach is taken because behavioral choices take place in all three contexts. A point reiterated is that values may be thought of as windows to goals that act as precursors to conscious actions (Sagiv and Schwartz, 1995; Schwartz, 1992; Seligman and Katz, 1996). The discussion of general life or personal values initially focuses on physical therapists (PTs) rather than on

Key Terms

Key terms, which are defined below, are bolded and italicized the first time they appear in the chapter. Other important terms are shown in boldface on first appearance and are defined by the context in which they are used. When either of these types of terms is used several times, its acronym will be identified and subsequently used in the chapter. Both types of terms are listed alphabetically in the online glossary with their definitions and (when applicable) their acronyms.

construct: a description that makes something more real that is otherwise difficult to define, like human values.

core values: the prioritized value goals of an organization stated in short form. Ideally, there is a philosophical statement that includes additional commentary.

ethics: also known as moral philosophy. The branch of philosophy focusing on morality which is what ought to be done in the ideal sense.

moral: following guidelines reflecting societal values for directing social interactions in ways that preserve peace and harmony.

moral ideals: in philosophy, those things which should be aspired to or what one should strive to attain.

moral oughts: in philosophy these are noncontingent, universal obligations.

motive goal(s): related to the Theory of Basic Human Values—the end(s) served by specific groups of value terms. In the theory, there are 10 motive goals that specific values reflect. Some of these goals can be pursued together (they have complementary goals) and others can not (they have antagonistic goals).

operationalize: put into action. Practical application.

organizational values: the values espoused by upper levels of management and shared with stakeholders for the purpose of identifying and aligning priorities. The ideals that drive actions.

philosophical statement: an organizational document identifying the values and principles reflecting the organization's view on what is morally right and not right or which behaviors are acceptable and which are not. This statement sets parameters within which the mission can be formulated.

philosophy: a systematic inquiry of questions such as the nature of reality (metaphysics), the justification of belief (epistemology), and the conduct of life (ethics).

self-view: a global cognitive construct representing what a persona or group believes about themselves. This includes motivations, moral will, ego, self-concept, and personality. Values act to maintain psychological harmony between choices and self-view.

value goal hierarchy: according to the theory of Basic Human Values this is the ordering of personal values by relative levels of importance.

values: in the theory of Basic Human Values these are consciously chosen goals that are not situational, vary in importance and function as guiding principles throughout life when making choices between competing options which are expected to fulfill priority-ordered goals.

win-win decisions: mutual benefits obtained in exchanges/transactions. Choices that lead to outcomes that balance benefits/losses for each party. Outcomes with no big winner or loser.

physical therapy organizations for good reason. Sometimes the terms **organizational values** are used to express what is important in an **organization's culture** (Chapters 5 and 6). However, an organization is an inanimate object. It is the people who are associated with the business that have value related goals, not the organization per se (Stackman et al., 2000). It is more accurate to say that organizational **value goals** are those that are espoused by upper level management. While organizations are made up of people who have

the same basic menu of values and goals that valued actions lead to, organizational members have different value goal priorities (Schwartz, 1994). Also, these priorities vary somewhat by context (Seligman and Katz, 1996). Another influence on behavioral choices is a person's moral or ethical perspective. Organizational members have their own personal systems of ethics (Harquail and Cox, 1993). Differences in value goal hierarchies and ethic systems are due mostly to variations in exposure to social influences (Brown, 1996; Laupa and

Turiel, 1995) and individualized interpretations of these experiences (Lent et al., 1996). The challenge for organizational leaders is to bring about an alignment of their value goal priorities and those of the other members of the organization. This is crucial for organizational success because when alignment occurs, everyone's efforts are focused on achieving the same prioritized ends (Chapters 3–6).

Whenever there are behavioral options, and choices must be made, values are involved. Choices involve identifying what is important, right, wrong, good, and bad. Whenever conscious decisions are made, personal values are involved. Personal values are clearly important. Understanding this point makes it logical to initiate the discussion with values before moving on to ethics, another important source of organizational behavioral guidance. This progression is based on the belief that to bring ethics into the decision-making process, one must first value making ethically defensible decisions (Kristiansen and Hotte, 1996).

It All Begins With What Is Important

In the social sciences it is generally assumed that behaviors are influenced by what people consider important (Braithwaite and Scott, 1991; Dawis, 1991; Feldman, 1999; Super, 1995). When something is considered important, it is valued. When people **value** something, they do so because the "something" meets one of three needs: biological need, a group coordination need, or a social need (Schwartz, 1992). A physical therapy example of a biological need is when a patient's need for relief of pain motivates them to seek physical therapy services. If an outpatient clinic is closed to consolidate physical therapy operations, this is an organizational coordination need. Participation in a balance screening event at a mall with other PTs and PTAs can fulfill a social interaction need. Valuing something provides an intrinsic motivational stimulus to select the path of action that is likely to result in fulfilling a need (Super, 1995). People make choices that serve their own prioritized needs (Feldman, 1999) and are also consistent with their *self-view* (Feather, 1995; Rokeach, 1973; Seligman and Katz, 1996). Simply put, what

people do (behavior) relates to what they need (value) and what they consider true about themselves (**self-view**) (Scheibe, 1970).

Personal Values

Personal values have been linked to a variety of behaviors from career choice (Super, 1995) to readiness for social interaction (Sagiv and Schwartz, 1995). A related group of studies has focused on testing a theory that there is a logical relationship among personal values. Validation studies on the theory and its measurement were carried out on more than 200 samples (Schwartz et al., 2001) involving more than 65,000 subjects from 65 countries including the United States (Schwartz et al., 1999). For these studies, values were defined as (1) desirable goals, which (2) apply to many situations, (3) vary in relative importance, and (4) serve as guiding principles throughout a person's life (Schwartz, 1992, 1994). There are 44 human value terms that have been recognized almost universally (Schwartz et al., 1997). These value terms are representative of ten different **goals** or ends that values serve. Each value term typically is associated with one of the 10 categories of goals. These value goals are logically and statistically related. Some of them are compatible. This means that they can be pursued concurrently. These same groups of value goals can be incompatible with, or antagonistic to, other groups of value goals. Incompatible goals cannot be easily pursued together (Schwartz, 1992; Schwartz and Bilsky, 1990). Figure 7.1 shows the general relationships among value goals. Table 7.1 adds the definitions of the common goals values served and lists the groups of value terms that are representative of each value goal.

Values that reflect fulfilling goals like benevolence and universalism (see Fig. 7.1) are compatible because they both focus on doing good for other people and things, respectively. As the distance between goals in either direction around the wheel increases, so does the degree of goal incompatibility. For example, in Figure 7.1 achievement and power which prioritize self-enhancement are directly opposite benevolence and universalism, goals which emphasize working for the welfare of others (Schwartz, 1992). It would be very difficult to honor both goals concurrently. Consider

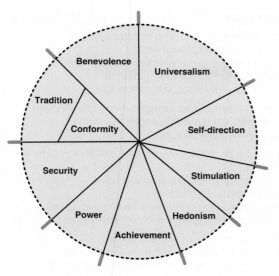

Figure 7.1. Boat steering model of the continuous relationships between compatible (nearby) and incompatible (further away) value goals. Adapted from Nosse LJ, Sagiv L. Theory-based study of the basic values of 565 physical therapists. Physical Therapy. 2005;85:834-850, with permission of the American Physical Therapy Association. This material is copyrighted, and any further reproduction or distribution is prohibited.

the PT who has risen within an organization to become a supervisor of multiple sites. As the supervisor, this PT is given bonuses and incentives for therapist productivity and efficiency. Operating under the mode of achievement and power with self- enhancing goals of more financial benefits with opportunity for more power, this supervisor may drive subordinates to practice in ways that maximize payment. For example, to treat multiple patients at the same time, limit therapist break times, insist on treatment regimes that can be carried out by a PTA or aide even when these tactics do not meet the specific needs of patients.

The theory provides a cohesive perspective on values. It categorizes values with the same general goal and it recognizes variations in the importance or hierarchy among the value goals. When all ten types of value goals are considered, a personal value importance hierarchy can be identified and compared. This hierarchy is what is important when talking about value driven behavior for it is a person's value goal priorities that influence choices rather than any single value term.

Table 7.1   Definitions of Value Goal Categories and Value Terms That Exemplify Them, Based on the Theory of Basic Human Values

10 Value Goals	*44 Value Terms*
Achievement: Personal success by demonstrating competence in accord with social standards	Ambition (hard-working, aspiring) Capable (competent, effective, efficient) Influential (having an impact on people and events) Successful (achieving goals)
Benevolence: Enhance and preserve the welfare of those one is in frequent contact with	Forgiving (willing to pardon others) Helpful (working for the welfare of others) Honesty (genuine, sincere, truthful) Loyalty (faithful to my friends, group) Responsible (dependable, reliable)
Conformity: Restraint of behaviors, inclinations, and impulses that are likely to upset or harm others, without violating social expectations or norms	Honoring parents and elders (showing respect) Obedience (dutiful, meeting obligations) Politeness (courtesy, good manners) Self-discipline (self-restraint, resistance to temptation)
Hedonism: Personal pleasure and sensuous gratification	Enjoying life (enjoying food, sex, leisure, etc.) Pleasure (gratification of desire)
Power: Attain social status and control or dominance over human and material resources	Authority (the right to lead or command) Social power (control over others, dominance) Wealth (material possessions, money)
Security: Personal, social, and societal relations that are stable, safe, and harmonious	Clean (neat, tidy) Family security (safety for loved ones) National security (protection of my nation from enemies) Reciprocation of favors (avoidance of indebtedness) Social order (stability of society)

(Continued)

Table 7.1   continued

Self-Direction: Independent thinking, acting and, decision making	Choosing own goals (selecting own purposes) Creativity (uniqueness, imagination) Curious (interested in everything, exploring) Freedom (freedom of action and thought) Independence (self-reliant, self-sufficient)
Stimulation: Excitement, challenge, and novelty	A varied life (filled with challenge, novelty, and change) An exciting life (stimulating experiences) Daring (seeking adventure, risk)
Tradition: Respect for, commitment to, and acceptance of customs and ideas of traditional culture or religion	Accepting my portion in life (submitting to life's circumstances) Devout (holding to religious faith and belief) Humble (modest, self-effacing) Moderation (avoiding extremes of feeling and action) Respect for tradition (preservation of time-honored customs)
Universalism: Appreciation, understanding, tolerance, and protection for the welfare of people and nature	A world at peace (free of war and conflict) A world of beauty (beauty of nature and the arts) Broad-minded (tolerant of different ideas and beliefs) Equality (equal opportunity for all) Protecting the environment (preserving nature) Social justice (correcting injustices) Unity with nature (fitting into nature) Wisdom (a mature understanding of life)

Reprint permission granted by the *British Journal of Social Psychology* to modify and publish Table 1 (page 7) of Schwartz SH, Verkasalo M, Antonovsky A, Sagiv L. Value priorities and social desirability: Much substance, some style. British Journal of Social Psychology. 1997;36 Part 1:3–18 and to reprint from from Nosse LJ, Sagiv L. Theory-based study of the basic values of 565 physical therapists. Physical Therapy. 2005;85:834–850, with permission of the American Physical Therapy Association. This material is copyrighted, and any further reproduction or distribution is prohibited.

Personal Value Goal Hierarchies of Physical Therapists and Student Physical Therapists

Several reports of the value goal priorities of PTs (Nosse and Sagiv, 2005), PT **managers** (Nosse, 1999, 2000), and student PTs (Nosse and Sagiv, 2000a, b) have been presented. The variables of interest have been differences in value goal priorities by age group and by job responsibilities. The relevance of these variables is that similarities and differences in value goal hierarchies can be related to the degree of commitment people have to giving their full effort to achieve certain organizational goals. In the workplace, a part of a good rapport between employee and employer is value goal compatibility. People whose most important value goals are compatible generally agree about which ends are worth pursuing. This can foster cooperative efforts. Alternatively, people who prioritize value goals that are antagonistic are at odds about what is important, and possibly, about degrees

of importance on things they agree are important. Individuals or groups whose most important value goals are incompatible are likely to cooperate reluctantly at best.

Even though PTs have essentially similar educational, clinical, and regulated practice backgrounds there are some differences among their goal importance hierarchies. Survey data from a large convenient sample of PTs is summarized in Table 7.2. The variable of interest was age. The context of the survey was the importance of value goals in life in general.

The table shows five value goals with subtle age-associated differences. The main points of Table 7.2 are:

- All age groups give primacy to benevolence values (e.g., regard for others)
- All age groups give their lowest importance to power values (e.g., control over others)
- Compared to the other age groups, the youngest therapists give significantly higher importance ratings to three value goals: hedonism (e.g., personal pleasure), achieve-

Table 7.2 Differences in Physical Therapists' Value Goal Importance Rankings by Age[a]

	Age Groups			
	Youngest (Y)	Middle (M)	Oldest (O)	
	≤31 Yrs	32–43 Yrs	≥44 Yrs	
	(n = 163)	(n = 209)	(n = 193)	
Value Goal	Rank Avg. (Rating)[b]	Rank Avg. (Rating)[b]	Rank Avg. (Rating)[b]	Significant Difference(s)[c]
Benevolence	5.97 (1)	6.03 (1)	6.05 (1)	—
Hedonism	5.39 (2)	4.92 (5)	4.40 (7)	Y > M and O; M > 0
Achievement	5.34 (3)	5.05 (4)	5.02 (4)	Y > M and O
Self-direction	5.32 (4)	5.30 (2)	5.31 (3)	—
Conformity	5.13 (5)	5.19 (3)	5.33 (2)	—
Universalism	4.65 (6)	4.83 (6)	4.98 (5)	Y < O
Security	4.53 (7)	4.52 (7)	4.76 (6)	Y and M > O
Stimulation	4.16 (8)	3.75 (9)	3.56 (9)	Y > M and O
Tradition	4.05 (9)	4.27 (8)	4.22 (8)	—
Power	2.55 (10)	2.58 (10)	2.65 (10)	—

[a]*Sources:* Nosse, 2000a; Nosse and Sagiv, 2005.
[b]Rating scale: 1 = not important to 8 = supremely important.
[c]$p = > 0.005$.

ment (e.g., competence related success), and stimulation (e.g., excitement)

- In addition, compared to the oldest therapist group, the youngest therapists give significantly lower importance ratings to universalism (e.g., respect all things), and security (e.g., stability) value goals
- Compared to the oldest therapists, the mid age therapists rated hedonism value goals more important and security value goals less important

For a manager or **supervisor**, the practical usefulness of recognizing age related value priority differences is that it can add an additional perspective on workplace dynamics. Known value goals can be considered when developing strategies for making work assignments or offering incentives for retention, job performance, or signing on. Value goal information as outlined in this discussion also provides a framework for understanding conflicts. For example, if staff members of widely different ages appear to avoid one another in the office or at meetings, it may be that there are issues related to the importance given to personal social experiences. Knowing the general age-related PT value hierarchy can also give direction to the

employment interview process. (Questions about job expectations will be presented in Chapter 17.) Asking what is desired in the workplace, or asking for self-descriptions, may offer insights into the interviewee's value priorities. The response provides the opportunity to estimate how the applicant might fit in with current staff members. When interviewing job applicants or staff members it is worth keeping in mind that the youngest therapists' overall value goal hierarchy pattern is very similar to the pattern reported for U.S. college students (Schwartz and Bardi, 2001) and for final year student PTs (Nosse and Sagiv, 2000a, b).

Personal Value Goal Hierarchy of Physical Therapist Managers and Supervisors

Another value goal hierarchy comparison with workplace relevance involves the similarities and differences between PT managers and supervisors and those whose work they oversee. Table 7.3 summarizes comparative data of PT managers and supervisors and PTs whose primary responsibility was to provide direct patient care.

Table 7.3 Value Goal Priorities of Physical Therapist Managers and Clinicians[a]			
Managers and Supervisors (n = 265)		**Clinicians (n = 258)**	
Value Goal	Rank Avg. (Rating)[b]	Rank Avg. (Rating)[b]	Significant Differences[c]
Benevolence	5.99 (1)	6.05 (1)	—
Self-direction	5.30 (2)	5.28 (2)	—
Conformity	5.22 (3)	5.21 (3)	—
Achievement	5.19 (4)	5.05 (4)	—
Hedonism	4.77 (5)	5.04 (5)	—
Universalism	4.72 (6)	4.91 (6)	—
Security	4.65 (7)	4.58 (7)	—
Tradition	4.24 (8)	4.17 (8)	—
Stimulation	3.69 (9)	3.89 (9)	—
Power	2.85 (10)	2.38 (10)	Managers > Clinicians

[a]*Source:* Nosse, 1999, 2000.
[b]Rating scale: 1 = not important, 4 = important, 8 = supremely important.
[c]$p = > 0.005$.

Both groups had members of various ages, but the manager/supervisor group was older. The median ages were ~44 and ~37 years for the managers and supervisors and PT clinicians, respectively or roughly, the middle and oldest age categories. These two groups' value goal hierarchies did not differ. Their ordering of the importance of the value goals was the same. This pattern is also what was observed for mid-age therapists in Table 7.2. The single unique finding was that managers and supervisors rated power values significantly more important than clinicians. Nonetheless, both groups ranked power the least important of the value goals (Nosse, 1999, 2000). Since working to achieve goals through others is the manager's job (Chapter 11), it is reasonable that power carries more intrinsic motivation for managers and supervisors than it does for those who **report** to them.

The relevance of these findings is that they provide a unique perspective on possible ways for a manager to deal with personal value-based differences in the workplace as well as to enhance their own self-understanding. The key points about the values theory related information for PT managers and supervisors are:

- A set of definitions to facilitate communication and understanding about personal values in terms of common value goals
- An empirically supported logic and structure for understanding value goals (motives) as an integrated system rather than as individual unrelated constructs

- A basis for gaining insight into behavioral choices and the possibility of predicting reactions better if values are not directly considered
- A foundation for analyzing causes of conflicts in the workplace
- An additional perspective on approaching conflict resolution based on starting discussions with the intent of establishing value goal similarities and exploring ways in which these prioritized common value goals can be fulfilled in the workplace (Nosse and Sagiv, 2005)
- Context affects personal value goal hierarchies (Elizur and Sagie, 1999; Kristiansen and Hotte, 1996) though there is contextual consistency (Rokeach, 1973).

While age and job responsibility group data provide general expectations, group data does not relate to an individual PT or student PT. This requires an individual assessment and comparison to norms. The case study provides some tools for self-assessment and Additional Resources contains more information on values assessment.

Philosophy First (When Possible)

In the real world, a new small business owner has an idea about what he or she will offer consumers and a vision sketch of the possibilities that could eventually be achieved by his or her efforts. The owner needs to describe

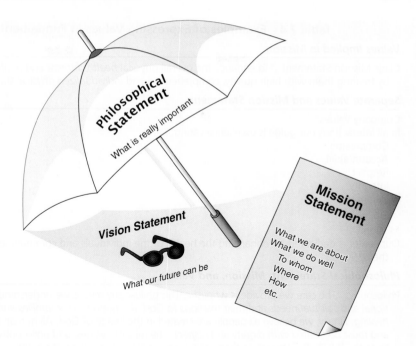

Figure 7.2. Overshadowing relationship of a philosophical statement to a mission and vision statement.

what the business does and its potential for sustainability to get financing (Chapter 22). What the business does is detailed in the mission statement (Fig. 7.2).

With a mission, and an idea about the future, the business owner goes to work hoping that they can bring in enough money to pay the business' bills and take a pay check to pay their personal bills on a regular schedule. The primary concern is, will there be adequate **cash flow** (Chapters 21 and 22). Ups and downs in cash flow impact on the amount of time that must be spent in income generating activities and, as the business evolves, how much time is left to consider philosophy, values, and refinement of the vision. Behavioral principles and values may have been implicit in the mission, but they probably were not explicitly expressed in a philosophical statement. The first example in Table 7.4 is a physical therapy organization's mission with value terms included. The middle example is more evolved. It has distinct values and mission components. The final example is more complete yet. It adds a formal philosophical statement that provides a background context for continuity among the mission and values documents. Developing and refining documents like these takes time and the thoughts of many mangers. The new business owner is likely to develop these documents when the

business provides financial "breathing room," or there is an incident involving inappropriate employee behavior, or a familiar physical therapy organization is charged with **fraud** (Chapters 8 and 9). Until one or more of these events occurs, talk of an umbrella philosophical statement is probably a low priority.

In an ideal world, the order of development of fundamental guiding documents would be as depicted in Figure 7.3. The first guiding document to be formulated would be a philosophical statement that includes the priority value goals and *moral* principles intended to guide behavior throughout the organization. The mission and vision would then be developed and refined within the context of the values and principles presented in the philosophical statement (Darr, 2005). These three statements formally express the official assumptions that are to guide the behavior of organizational members in their interactions among themselves and with stakeholders, and the future that can be attained by following the intent of these statements.

Building an Organizational Philosophy: Core Beliefs

In health services, philosophical statements or as some call them, core beliefs (Swayne et al., 2006), center around values, morals, and eth-

Table 7.4 Examples of Expressing Values in Fundamental Documents

Values Implied in Mission

Clinic Mission Statement: "To *enhance* the overall physical *health, fitness,* and *quality of life* of adults and children by treating them with high quality, comprehensive and *individualized* physical therapy services."

Separate Values and Mission Statements

Company Values:
In all interactions our guide is excellence caring, i.e.:
  Compassion
  Accountability
  Respect
  Integrity
  Neighborly
  Growth

Mission:
Our center is dedicated to enhancing the health of the individuals and communities we serve in partnership with them.

Philosophical Statement, Mission, and Values

Philosophy: "The care we provide is *wholistic.* This philosophy means we understand people have *physical, emotional and spiritual needs* and their *relations to God, themselves, their families and society* are vital to *health and healing.* Finally, we believe all people are created in the image of God. All human beings live under God's care and *must be treated with dignity and respect.* The mission, values, and philosophy of Advocate are often referred to as the 'MVP'. By integrating them into every aspect of the organization, these principles have strengthened the foundation of the Advocate culture in which we all work and *serve."*[a]

The mission of Advocate Health Care (2007) "is to serve the health needs of individuals, families and communities through a wholistic philosophy rooted in our fundamental understanding of human beings as created in the image of God."

Values: "Advocate exists to serve. The core values of compassion, equality, excellence, partnership, and stewardship guide our actions as we work together to provide health services to others in our communities."[a]

[a]Permission to reprint granted.

ics. The philosophical statement is a narrative that identifies and describes the value goals that organization leaders hold most important. From this statement *core values* are extracted and become a separate document for dissemination. The unique mix of social and economic value priorities contribute to making an organization's culture distinguishable from similar organizations (Swayne et al., 2006). Prioritizing the goal of positive relationships with stakeholders, including competitors, presents many difficulties (Chapter 5). In health

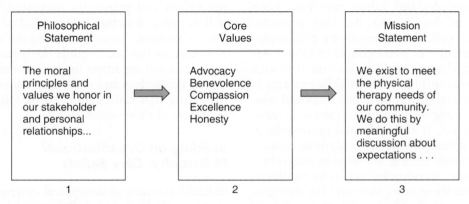

Figure 7.3. Idealized progression in the development of the philosophy, core values, and mission.

service business, serving one's own interests should be balanced with consideration of what is in the best interest of others because of the difference in health-related knowledge. There are societal morals that assist in making difficult **win-win decisions** that preserve a balance of benefits for all parties. Morals are universal guidelines reflecting societal value goals that foster peace and harmony (Purtilo, 1993). Morals also deal with duty and obligation (Omery, 1989). The branch of philosophy that deals with the morals of society is ethics (Hall, 1996). What ethics offers is systematic decision-making processes for evaluating competing options to determine moral rightness or wrongness (Veatch and Flack, 1997). The circumstances where moral issues commonly arise are whenever:

- The welfare of an individual or group is in question (Berkowitz, 1995)
- When justice or fairness is a concern (Veatch and Flack, 1997)
- When rights are in question (Purtilo, 1993)

Table 7.5 defines ethical principles with particular application to health service organizations.

None of the ethical principles is more important than any of the others. All are equally obligatory (Darr, 2005), which causes dilemmas. For example, a moral issue might arise if a PT is skilled in manual therapy (a professional interest) and believes this to be the appropriate treatment for a particular patient. To make this a moral issue, assume that the

patient says they are in so much pain today that they do not want to be touched. The main moral conflict is between the autonomy (of the patient) and beneficence (the therapist's knowledge and expertise). Personal value goals are involved here. They affect one's perspective when making judgments about viable alternatives. The point is, to make moral choices requires a commitment to taking actions that are likely to benefit key stakeholders (prioritizing conformity, tradition, benevolence, or universalism value goals [see Fig. 7.1]) at the expense of enhancing oneself (prioritizing security, power, achievement, hedonism, stimulation, or self-direction value goals [see Fig. 7.1]). Therefore, when there are moral conflicts, the examination of one's value priorities should be incorporated into the resolution process. Hall (1996) offers a clinically useful example of an ethical analysis process that incorporates this recommendation:

- Think about personal values: identify what is personally important to you in this situation
- Recognize that conflicts are based on value priority differences
- Consider what is important (personal values) to the stakeholder(s)
- Separate personal values and professional interests from stakeholder values
- Consider what the desired means and outcome should be from the perspective of the stakeholder
- Consider what the desired means and outcome should be from your perspective
- If there are differences, seek to determine if the conflict is related to a moral rule or an ethical principle
- If the matter relates to a moral rule or ethical principle determine, with help if needed, which principle is to be honored
- Review your choice to ensure that there has been impartiality throughout the process
- Act in accord with the outcome of the analysis process

The progression of thinking suggested by the preceding list is from personal values to philosophical principles. These are the basic components of a philosophical statement. A way to formulate a formal personal or group philosophical statement is presented in Table 7.6.

Table 7.5   Ethical Principles Applicable to Health Service Organizations

Principle	Definition
Autonomy	Respect the rights, decisions, and dignity of competent stakeholders
Beneficence	Do what is in the best interest of stakeholders
Fidelity	Keep explicit and implicit promises
Justice	Maintain fairness in allocation of good and harm
Nonmaleficence	Avoid harming others
Respect Life	Refrain from acts that will likely contribute to ending a life
Veracity	Tell the truth when it is known

Table 7.6 Philosophical Statement Template

Value Goals	Add Value Terms Intended to Reflect Goal
Achievement	
Benevolence	
Conformity	
Power	
Security	
Self-direction	
Stimulation	
Universalism	

Ethical Principles	Add Value Terms Intended to Reflect Principle
Autonomy	
Beneficence	
Fidelity	
Justice	
Nonmaleficence	
Respect life	
Veracity	

Instructions: Circle the most frequently used value terms. These can be considered the core values. If consensus is not reached on what is a core value, then replace the terms that have the least agreement and see if core values emerge with the new terms.

This table is a template for examining personal value goals and philosophical principles. The template can aid the development or revision of a personal or organizational philosophical statement. The value terms that are written most often can easily be identified. They can be considered core values. These core values publicly proclaim in a concise form what you or the organization stands for.

Ethical Principles in Management and Supervision Situations

Ethical principles reflect moral values, and as has been discussed, from values spring actions. Ethical principles are tools for systematically analyzing moral matters to determine the core issues, help weigh them, and aid morally defensible choices from among competing moral options. The choice to pursue fulfillment of a particular value goal is bolstered when ethical principles justify it. For example, when patient loads are down, some physical therapy department members may be

sent home. The day's **labor costs** are lowered if those are paid on an hourly basis. The department will lose income if everyone stays. The manager has to decide who will benefit from their decision. A sampling of ways this situation might be handled are:

Send no one home
Ask for volunteers to go home
Limit the pool of employees to be sent home to those who have not previously been sent home
Consider patient needs and limit the pool to department members least needed to meet the day's patient care needs
Send the most expensive staff home first
Ensure that staff are paid hourly versus salaried; sending salaried staff home will not assist the problem versus sending hourly staff home

There are several moral rules (Table 7.5) that might apply here. Retaining everyone harms the department's financial status. This could be seen as breach of the nonmaleficence principle. Asking for volunteers honors the entire staff 's autonomy. This option allows them to make their own choices. Restricting the pool to protect those who have been sent home before respects the principle of justice. Linking the decision to the needs of the primary **stakeholders** is an example of benevolence. This option may protect patients from harm, so this choice also supports the nonmaleficence principle. With all options ethically justifiable, the manager's decision will depend on their value goal hierarchy for this situation.

Managers have to be the moral exemplars. If they demonstrate exemplary behavior, others will recognize that managers act in the best interest of others as they carry out their responsibilities. This recognition can lead to managers being a resource for others where value goals and ethical issues are raised. The point is, to make moral choices in physical therapy requires a commitment to taking actions that are likely to benefit key stakeholders at the expense of enhancing oneself, the department, or the organization. Therefore, when there are conflicts among moral principles, the examination of one's value goal priorities should be incorporated into the resolution process. Hall

(1996) offers a clinically useful example of an ethical analysis process that incorporates this recommendation:

- Think about personal value goals and identify what is personally important to you in this situation
- Recognize that conflicts are based on value priority differences
- Consider what is important (personal value goals) to the stakeholder(s)
- Separate personal value goals and professional interests from stakeholder value goals
- Take the stakeholders perspective on what the desired means and outcome should be
- Consider what the desired means and outcome should be from your perspective
- If there are differences, seek to determine if the conflict is related to a ethical principle
- If the matter relates to an ethical principle, determine, with help if needed, which principle is to be honored
- Review your choice to ensure that there has been impartiality throughout the process
- Act in accord with the outcome of the analysis process

This analysis process is one example of a practical means of incorporating ethics into workplace decision making. Additional discussion of ethics is beyond the scope of this book. See the Additional Resources section for more sources of information on analyzing ethical issues.

Professional Ethics

A supplementary source of ethical guidance comes from professional organizations such as **APTA**. Ethical principles commonly associated with health service professionals focus on what ought to be in the ideal sense (Hall, 1996). Meeting moral ideals is in addition to meeting the noncontingent, universal, moral obligations discussed earlier. Professional ethics identify what shall be done (obligations) as well as what should be aspired to or what one should strive to attain (ideals). Professional

codes of ethics contain a blend of *moral oughts* and *moral ideals* (Gert, 1992). Failure to meet moral oughts results in professional condemnation (expulsion) because the obligations are universal for members. Not so for moral ideals. The moral ideals of a professional association are applicable to its members and reflect special concerns for the welfare of stakeholders and agreeable to the majority (Hall, 1996). The attainment of moral ideals is encouraged. However, failure to fulfill an ideal does not result in public punishment (Barker, 1992).

Behavioral Guides for Physical Therapists and Physical Therapist Assistants

For U.S. PTs and PTAs the moral oughts and ideals are contained in the APTA Code of Ethics (2007a) and Standards of Ethical Conduct for the Physical Therapist Assistant (APTA, 2007b), respectively, and are elaborated in the Guide for Professional Conduct (APTA, 2007c) and Guide for the Conduct of the Physical Therapist Assistant (APTA, 2007d). A companion document with moral ideals associated with professionalism is titled Professionalism in Physical Therapy: Core Values (APTA, 2007e). To bring together the author's perspectives of personal values, core values, ethical principles, and professional ethics, Table 7.7 was developed. The table shows that even when there are standardized definitions of terms and references to consult, there remains a great deal of subjectivity in determining which values and ethical principles apply to a statement. At the very least, Table 7.7 examines the APTA Code and associated Guide in an integrative manner. It makes practical use of the key concepts presented on value goals and ethical principles in this chapter. Finally, with the exception of Code principle 3, which deals with the obligation to be lawful, the table shows that APTA principles honor the self-transcending value goals of benevolence and universalism. The Code demands placing self-interest lower in the value goal hierarchy. This is very much in line with the value goal hierarchies reported for PTs and student PTs (Nosse and Sagiv, 2000a, b, 2005).

Table 7.7   Apparent Relationships Between APTA Code[a] and Guide[b] in Terms of Value Goals, Core Values of Professionalism[c], and Ethical Principles[d]

APTA Principles 1-11	Value Goals (Table 7.1)	Core Values of Professionalism[c]	Ethical Principles (Table 7.5)
1: … respect the rights and, dignity of all individuals …	benevolence, conformity universalism	compassion/caring, integrity	autonomy, beneficence, justice
2: … act in a trustworthy manner … in all … aspects of … practice	benevolence, conformity universalism	accountability, integrity	fidelity, veracity
3: … comply with laws …	conformity, tradition, security	integrity, social responsibility	all but respect life, i.e., advanced directives
4: … exercise sound professional judgment	achievement, benevolence, conformity, security, self-direction	accountability, compassion/caring, excellence	all but respect life, i.e., advanced directives
5: … achieve and maintain professional competence	achievement, benevolence, security, self-direction	accountability, excellence, integrity	beneficence, fidelity, justice, nonmaleficence
6: … maintain and promote high standards	achievement, benevolence, security	accountability, excellence, integrity, professional duty	autonomy, beneficence, justice, nonmaleficence
7: … seek only … remuneration … deserved and reasonable …	benevolence, conformity, universalism	altruism, social responsibility	beneficence, fidelity, justice
8: … provide … accurate and relevant information …	benevolence, power	accountability, compassion/ caring	autonomy, beneficence, fidelity, veracity
9: … protect pubic and profession from unethical, incompetent, illegal acts	achievement, benevolence, conformity, security, nonmaleficence,	universalism integrity, professional duty	beneficence, justice, veracity
10: … endeavor to address the health needs of society	benevolence, universalism	professional duty, social responsibility	beneficence, justice
11: … respect the rights, knowledge, and skills of colleagues and other … professionals	benevolence, conformity security, universalism	excellence, integrity professional duty, social responsibility	autonomy, beneficence, justice, nonmaleficence, veracity

[a]APTA, 2007a.
[b]APTA, 2007c.
[c]APTA, 2007e.
[d]Table modified from Nosse et al., 2005:96.

Behavioral Guides for Upper-Level Health Service Managers

Some PTs have advanced within organizational management structures and others are the owners of their own businesses. In the first case, they are upper level managers. In the second case, if they choose to retain and carry out significant management responsibilities, they too are upper level managers. There are additional ethical responsibilities for this level of mangers, in part, because they control financial resources. Excerpts from the codes of ethics of two health service professions are presented in Table 7.8 as exam-

ples for these additional business-related ethical obligations.

The Vision Statement

In the preceding values discussion, and in Chapters 5 and 6, it was noted that the vision is operationalized by the mission statement which in turn is bounded by the philosophical statement and the organization's internal environmental capabilities (Swayne et al., 2006). However, management of newer and small organizations is often occupied by reacting to

Table 7.8 Examples of Professional Ethics Requirements for Upper Level Health Service Managers	
American College of Healthcare Executives (2007)	*American College of Health Care Administrators (2007)*
Preamble: The purpose of the Code is "... to serve as a standard ... of ethical behavior for healthcare executives in their professional relationships ..."	*Preamble:* The Code's purpose is "... The preservation of the highest standards of integrity and ethical principles ... vital to the successful discharge of ... professional responsibilities ..."
Example Statements: "Avoid the exploitation of professional relationships for personal gain; Avoid financial and other conflicts of interest; Use this Code to further the interests of the profession and not for selfish reasons; ... ... Ensure ... a process ... to facilitate the resolution of conflicts ... when values of patients ... differ from those of employees ... Demonstrate zero tolerance for any abuse of power ... ... Ensure ... a resource allocation process that considers ethical ramifications; Lead the organization in the use and improvement of standards of management and sound business practices;" Create "a work environment that promotes ethical conduct by employees;" Ensure "a work environment is free from harassment ..., coercion ..., especially to perform illegal or unethical acts; and discrimination ..."	*Example Statements:* "Disclose to the governing body ... any actual or potential ... conflict of interest or have the potential to have a substantial adverse impact on the facility or its residents. Practice administration in accordance with the capabilities ... when appropriate, seek counsel from qualified others. Avoid partisanship ... provide a forum for the fair resolution of ... disputes which may arise in service delivery or ... management." Do not "defend, support, or ignore unethical conduct perpetuated by colleagues, peers, or students. Strive to provide ... quality ... services in light of resources or other constraints. Operate the facility consistent with ... standards of practice recognized in the field of health care administration. Inform the ... Ethics Committee of actual or potential violations of the Code of Ethics ... Take ... steps to avoid discrimination on the basis of race, color, sex, religion, age, national origin, handicap, marital status, ancestry, or any other factor ..."

unanticipated problems. There is little time to look or think ahead. Under such circumstances the organization's leadership may have verbalized in vague or general terms the hopes for the organization's future. These hopes get refined over time. Eventually, everyone in the organization has heard one or more versions of the organization's desired future. In time, the vision statement becomes a formal written document that is shared with stakeholders at every opportunity (Chapters 6 and 11). The task of formulating a viable vision statement is a difficult one. Those who are able to form and communicate a vision that others grasp, voluntarily accept, and are moved to act upon, are more than leaders, they are visionaries. Visionary leaders are able to create and market an idealistic image of a unique future (Kouzes and Posner, 1996) that others bring to life through their best work (Chapter 11).

Building a Vision

The process of building a vision for an organization has been called pathfinding (Mor-

ris, 1988). At some point in the pathfinding process the path to the future gets written down. A vision statement identifies the highly desirable future state of the organization when the mission has been accomplished. It expresses a long-term goal that serves to integrate and drive current efforts that are expected to measurably contribute to the ultimate goal of fulfilling the mission. A vision is dynamic in part because progress towards its achievement is made in steps over time. As the external and internal environments change, refinements are made to the vision (Swayne et al., 2006). The vision is something to aspire to, therefore, the vision needs to serve as both an inspirational and a motivational communication tool that guide efforts over an extended period of time (Hoyle, 1995). Because the end expressed in a vision statement does not exist, it must be given a reality through words. A vision statement is:

- Stated in terms to help the reader or listener form a clear and vivid image of what the organization can become (Clawson, 1999)

- Expressed in terms that stimulate diligence in working toward this idealized envisioned future (Darr, 2005; Swayne et al., 2006)
- Concise enough to be remembered by members at all levels of the organization
- Consistent with, and a logical extension of the philosophical and mission statements (Darr, 2005)
- Attainable, realistic given the organization's internal and external environments (Ginter et al., 1998)
- Repeated at every opportunity (Ginter et al., 1998)

Table 7.9 is a template for developing a vision statement as suggested by the preceding list. To complete the table requires concurrent review of the results of environmental scanning and the other fundamental documents. Wordsmithing is involved as precision in terms is sought.

Examine the mission first for words with impact. Another resource is to review terms used by similar organizations (see Chapter 6, Table 6.4). Additional possibilities include using a thesaurus, reading books on vision statements, and contracting a consultant.

Remember, the vision is formulated with knowledge of the organization's environments and is consistent with the philosophy, core values, and mission. These prerequisites are part of the reason the vision takes time to evolve from a hopeful sketch of the future to a strategy driven process to make the future a reality.

Markers of a Viable Vision

There are observable behaviors associated with a vision that "works." A vision encourages striving, i.e., doing more, better, creatively, taking some risks, to complete tasks that are expected to help achieve the imagined possibilities. When a vision statement is associated with personally prioritized value goals, it serves to motivate organizational members to exert effort willingly. When members "buy in" they do more than they have in the past, even exceeding their own expectations. They help move the organization closer toward the desired vision. When people direct the full force of their personal attributes for extended periods toward overcoming novel problems, they are inspired. A viable vision statement inspires. When people consistently give their full effort to achieve something that is out of reach now, they are aspiring to achieve the ideal organizational state. Finally, a viable vision is one that can be expressed by, and is believed possible, by those who carry out the mission.

Summary

This chapter provided the reader with comparative information about personal values, moral obligations, and ethical analyses. A theory was presented for understanding the role of personal values in influencing behavior. It was noted that personal values are associated with fulfillment of biological needs, group

Table 7.9   Template for Formulating, Analyzing, and Editing a Vision Statement

Element (future focus)	Key Term(s)	Possible Change(s)
Vivid verbal image of our future Our long-term goal What we aspire to become		

Element (behavioral focus)	Key Term(s)	Possible Changes(s)
What inspires us to maximum effort What we are motivated to become What we strive to accomplish		

Checks:

The statement is consistent with the organization's philosophy, core values, and mission.
The statement represents a realistically attainable future given the current environments.
The statement is concise enough that the key terms will have impact.
The statement is memorable enough for stakeholders to at least be able to paraphrase it.
The statement is consistent with strategic efforts and vice versa.

coordination needs, or social needs. The goals that personal values serve are logically organized. Some value goals can be met concurrently. Other value goals can not easily be met together. They cause conflict because they represent pursuit of antagonistic goals. This values theory provides information on the values of PTs. The value goal hierarchies of PTs of different ages and PT managers and nonmanagers were presented. Different age groups were shown to have some value goal priority differences, especially between the youngest and oldest therapists. The value goal hierarchies of managers and nonmanagers were reported to be the same, but managers placed significantly more importance on control over resources and other people. With knowledge of demographic-based differences in value goal priorities, a manager may be able to offer more precise incentives to facilitate staff cohesion, sustain adequate productivity levels, and improve the retention rate.

Organizations also have values. They are part of the culture. In an ideal case, the values of an organization are expressed in a philosophical statement before other behavior guiding documents. This philosophical statement elaborates on the core values to be honored and ethical principles to guide decision making where moral matters are involved. The philosophical statement sets the framework within which the mission and the vision statement are developed. Guidelines for developing the philosophical and vision statements were presented.

For PTs, there is an external source of values and philosophical guidance. The guidance is expressed in the APTA Code, Guide, and Core Values of Professionalism documents. These documents were analyzed in terms of their foundational value goals and philosophical principles, and discussed as they related personal value goals. Throughout the chapter it was pointed out how values, morals, morality, and ethical principles interrelate to influence PT managers, supervisors, and staff members in the choices they make in the workplace. Processes for value assessment and analysis of moral matters were described with applications pertinent to PTs. Managers are responsible for maintaining an ethical practice as well as for meeting mandated legal obligations. Managers are expected to be moral exemplars and law abiding practitioners and business persons.

While laws are the minimum guides to good behavior, they do not define ideal behavior (Hall, 1996). This difference is made clear in the next three chapters. **Jurisprudence**, the underlying philosophy of law, is discussed in Chapter 8. Business law is covered in Chapter 9, and government regulations is the focus of Chapter 10.

REFERENCES

Advocate Health Care. Available at http://www.advocatehealth.com/system/about/community/faith/mvp.html. Accessed 7/12/07.

American College of Health Care Administrators. Code of ethics. Available at http://www.achca.org/content/pdf/Code_of_Ethics25038.pdf. Accessed 1/12/09.

American College of Health Care Executives. Code of ethics. Available at http://www.ache.org/ABT_ACHE/code.cfm. Accessed 7/20/07.

American Physical Therapy Association. APTA code of ethics. Available from http://www.aptaorg/AM/Template.cfm?Section=Ethics_and_Legal_Issues1&CONTENTID=40904&TEMPLATE=/CM/ContentDisplay.cfm. Accessed 7/14/07a.

American Physical Therapy Association. APTA standards of ethical conduct for the physical therapist assistant. Available at http://www.apta.org/AM/Template.cfm?Section=Professionalism1&CONTENTID=40903&TEMPLATE=/CM/ContentDisplay.cfm. Accessed 7/14/07b.

American Physical Therapy Association. APTA guide for professional conduct. Available from http://www.apta.org/AM/Template.cfm?Section=Ethics_and_Legal_Issues1&TEMPLATE=/CM/ContentDisplay.cfm&CONTENTID=40901. Accessed 7/14/07c.

American Physical Therapy Association. Guide for the conduct of the physical therapist assistant. Available at http://www.apta.org/AM/Template.cfm?Section=Professionalism1&CONTENTID=40900&TEMPLATE=/CM/ContentDisplay.cfm. Accessed 7/14/07d.

American Physical Therapy Association. Professionalism in physical therapy: Core values. Available at http://www.apta.org/AM/Template.cfm?Section=Professionalism1&TEMPLATE=/CM/ContentDisplay.cfm&CONTENTID=39529. Accessed 7/14/07e.

Barker SF. What is a profession? Professional Ethics. 1992;1:73–99.

Berkowitz MW. The education of the complete moral person. Aberdeen, Scotland: Gorden Cook Foundation. 1995.

Braithwaite VA, Scott WA. Values. In Robinson JP, Shaver PR, Wrightsman LS, eds. Measures of personality and social psychological attitudes. Vol 1. The Measures of Social Psychological Attitudes Series. New York, NY: Academic Press. 1991:661–753.

CASE STUDY 7.1

Exploring Personal Value Goals

Overview

Recognition of your own value goal priorities is essential for self-understanding. The following exercises offer opportunities for exploring your own priorities in physical therapy contexts.

Self-Talk

In the workplace, the speed of life is often frenetic. Multitasking, unexpected obligations, and early and late patients are a few examples that call for immediate responses. There is little time to respond and thus, little time to think. Developing the habit of checking on why you make the on-the-spot decisions that you do can lead to consistent consideration of value priorities and better self-understanding.

A quick, simple, and private way to identify personal value priorities is to ask yourself and candidly answer for yourself the following questions.

- "If I do X (name your gut-driven choice), I expect Y (state your expectation) to happen."

- "If Y happens, what will that do for me?" Answer your own question and ask it again.
- "And, if that happens, what will that do for me?"
- Continue the self-questioning and answering process until you give the same answer several times in a row or when you realize that you have arrived at your likely motive goal.

After a few rounds of self-questioning and answering, the probable underlying motive goal will emerge. The final answer likely reflects the personal value goal underlying your decision. The last question to ask yourself is, "Will I be comfortable with doing what it takes to implement this choice?" If this answer is yes, you are probably going to be satisfied with your decision. If not, consider one or more additional options and repeat the process.

Identify Personal Values

Figure 7.4 summarizes a second way to identify prioritized values. This is a card sort method.

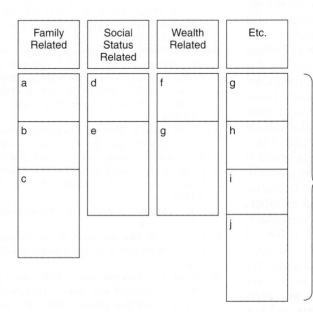

Step 3. Within each column, move the card with your most important value term on it to the top and the card with your least important value term on it to the bottom.

Figure 7.4. Value priorities determined by card sorting. From Nosse et al., 2005:337.

(Continued)

CASE STUDY 7.1

Exploring Personal Value Goals (continued)

Instructions

The first round of this exercise starts with you writing on individual note cards every single value term that you think is important to you, i.e., those things you would work hard to achieve or acquire. Security, substantive social interaction, desire to help others are example value terms. For example terms see Table 7.1. Place cards with terms that you feel are related in columns so you can read all of them. Related cards might be associated with gaining social power, sustaining culture, religion, family, or other common categories. Similar to the example in Figure 7.4, lay out as many columns as you need to organize related individual value terms.

For round two, go to your first column and find the most personally important value term. Move this card to the top of the column. Next, find the least personally important value term in the column. Move this card to the bottom of the column. Between the most important and the least important value terms place the remaining cards. When you finish, the cards in the column will represent the relative degree of importance you assigned to your personal values in that column. Repeat the process for the remaining columns. When you finish sorting, the top row of cards will contain your most important personal value terms, the bottom row of cards will contain the least important value terms, and the intermediate value cards will be ordered in terms of their greater or lesser personal importance. Number your prioritized value cards. In the future, you may wish to repeat the exercise to see if anything has changed. Also, knowing your value goal hierarchy will be helpful if you do the next engagement activity.

So ... What's Your Philosophy?

The preceding values identification exercises provided you with the value terms you can incorporate into your own philosophical statement. The task here is to look at your chosen life values and see if you can match them with the philosophical principles you think they reflect.

Instructions

You need three things: your list of life values and Tables 7.5 and 7.6. Use the descriptions of the philosophical principles to help you match principles to your value terms. Once you have done this, complete Table 7.6. When you are satisfied with your matching process, write a short philosophical statement and highlight your core values.

A Supervisor's Concern About Ethics

Overview

A physical therapy company has the contract for physical, occupational, and speech therapy in a large for-profit skilled nursing facility. The on-site supervising therapist is responsible for assuring that company policies are followed.

Many of the patients are Medicare beneficiaries covered by Medicare B. To assure that all employees understand Medicare rules, the therapy company provides training on its policies and procedures related to patients covered by Medicare. An important part of the training covers 1:1 treatment and group treatment. The training makes clear that this distinction is very important when treating patients with Medicare B benefits. There is a flat rate payment for treating two or more patients together. This payment is less if the patients were treated individually. The company policy is to avoid treating two patients together. This policy also applies to therapists co-treating patients. The basis for this policy is that only one of the therapists may charge for the service.

The Problem

Kay Tal, the speech therapist asked Benji Press to help her by facilitating a patient's head control as she worked on the patient's

(Continued)

CASE STUDY 7.1

Exploring Personal Value Goals (continued)

swallowing. The supervising therapist, Iona Piece-O'Daroc observed this. What are Iona's moral obligations? What are her ethically supportable options? To check the associated Medicare regulations for your own information go to http://www.cms.hhs.gov/TherapyServices/02_billing_scenarios.Asp.

Thinking About Professional Ethics and Core Values

A philosophical statement contains prioritized values and the philosophical principles that guide behavior. The practical use of a philosophical statement is that it is a reminder of what is important in human interactions and compatible with an individual or organizational self-view. This statement includes value goals and moral guidance derived from ethical principles. In this exercise you are being asked to examine a number of APTA documents to gain insight into the overall philosophical position of this professional organization. This exercise uses three internet accessible APTA documents and Tables 7.5–7.7.

Instructions

1. Access the APTA Guide for Professional Conduct and the Professionalism in Physical Therapy: Core Values.
2. Select any one of the 11 Code principles that interests you and read its associated conduct discussion.
3. Use Tables 7.6 and 7.7 to help you analyze your chosen Code principle and its associated Guide information for apparent value goals and ethical principles.
4. Now examine the core values document and compare the terms and definitions with those you derived from the other two documents.
5. Discuss your findings. What were the similarities and differences between your interpretation of the core values you identified in the Code and Guide and the core values of professionalism? If there were differences, what are some reasons you can think of?
6. What difference did this activity make (if any) on your understanding of professional ethics and the expression of core values?

Brown D. Brown's values-based, holistic model of career and life-role choices and satisfaction. In Brown D, Brooks L, and associates. Career choice & development, 3rd ed. San Francisco, CA: Jossey-Boss. 1996;337–372.

Cedarburg Physical Therapy & Sports Medicine. Clinic mission statement. Available at http://www.cedarburgpt.com/Philosophy.html. Accessed 1/18/09.

Clawson JG. Level three leadership: Getting below the surface. Upper Saddle River, NJ: Prentice Hall. 1999.

Crittenton Hospital Medical Center. Available at http://www.crittenton.com/?id=91&sid=1. Accessed 1/18/09.

Darr K. Ethics in health services management, 4th ed. Baltimore, MD: Health Professions Press. 2005.

Dawis RV. Vocational interests, values, and preferences. In Dunnette I, Hough MD II, Leaetta M, eds. Handbook of industrial and organizational psychology. Palo Alto, CA: Consulting Psychologists. 1991: 833–871.

Elizur D, Sagie A. Facets of personal values: A structural analysis of life and work values. Applied Psychology: An International Review. 1999;48:73–87.

Feather NT. Values, valences, and choice: The influence of values on the perceived attractiveness and choice of alternatives. Journal of Personality and Social Psychology. 1995;68:1135–1151.

Feldman JM. Four questions about human social behavior: The social cognitive approach to culture and psychology. In Adamopoulos J, Kashima Y, eds. Social psychology and cultural context. Thousand Oaks, CA: Sage. 1999:43–62.

Gert B. Morality, moral theory, and applied and professional ethics. Professional Ethics. 1992;1:5–24.

Ginter PM, Swayne LM, Duncan WJ. Strategic management of health care organizations, 3rd ed. Malden, MA: Blackwell. 1998.

Hall JK. Nursing ethics and law. Philadelphia, PA: WB Saunders. 1996.

Harquail CV, Cox T Jr. Organizational cultures and acculturation. In Cox T, ed. Cultural diversity in organizations: Theory, research and practice. San Francisco, CA: Berrett-Koehler. 1993:161.

Hoyle JR. Leadership and futuring: Making visions happen. Thousand Oaks, CA: Corwin. 1995.

Kouzes JM, Posner BZ. Envisioning your future: Imagining ideal scenarios. The Futurist. 1996;30:14–19.

Kristiansen CM, Hotte AM. Morality and the self: Implications for the when and how of value-attitude-behavior relations. In Seligman C, Olson JM, Zanna MP, eds. The psychology of values: The Ontario symposium, Vol. 8. Mahwah, NJ: Lawrence Erlbaum. 1996:77–105.

Laupa M, Turiel E. Social domain theory. In Kurtines WM, Gewirtz JL, eds. Moral development: An introduction. Boston, MA: Allyn and Bacon. 1995: 455–473.

Lent RW, Brown SD, Hackett G. Career development from a social cognitive perspective. In Brown D, Brooks L and associates. Career choice & development, 3rd ed. San Francisco, CA: Jossey-Boss. 1996:373–421.

Morris GB. The executive: A pathfinder. Organizational Dynamics. 1988;16:62–77.

Nosse LJ. Values and job satisfaction. Platform Presentation: American Physical Therapy Association Combined Sections Meeting. New Orleans, LA. February, 1999.

Nosse LJ. Understanding the connect between values and motivation: A study of physical therapists. Presented at the LAMP Summit III. Marquette University, Milwaukee, WI. June, 2000.

Nosse LJ, Sagiv L. Value structures of Wisconsin physical therapists and student physical therapists. Platform Presentation: American Physical Therapy Association Scientific Meeting and Exposition, Indianapolis, IN. June, 2000a.

Nosse LJ, Sagiv L. Value structures of Wisconsin physical therapists and student physical therapists. [Abstract] Values and job satisfaction. Physical Therapy. 2000b;80:Supplement:S67.

Nosse LJ, Sagiv L. Theory-based study of the basic values of 565 physical therapists. Physical Therapy. 2005;85:834–850.

Omery A. Values, moral reasoning, and ethics. Nursing Clinics of North America. 1989;24:499–508.

Purtilo R. Ethical dimensions in the health professions, 2nd ed. Philadelphia, PA: WB Saunders. 1993.

Rokeach M. The nature of human values. New York, NY: Free Press. 1973.

Sagiv L, Schwartz S. Value priorities and readiness for out-group social contact. Journal of Personality and Social Psychology. 1995;69:437–448.

Scheibe KE. Beliefs and values. New York, NY: Holt, Rinehart and Winston. 1970.

Schwartz SH. Universals in the content and structure of values: Theoretical advances and empirical tests in 20 countries. In Zanna M, ed. Advances in experimental social psychology. 1992;25:1–65.

Schwartz SH. Are there universal aspects in the structure and contents of human values? Journal of Social Issues. 1994;50:19–44.

Schwartz SH, Bardi A. Value hierarchies across cultures: Taking a similarities perspective. Journal of Cross-Cultural Psychology. 2001;32:268–290.

Schwartz SH, Bilsky W. Toward a theory of the universal content and structure of values: Extensions and cross-cultural replications. Journal of Personality and Social Psychology. 1990;58:878–891.

Schwartz SH, Lehmann A, Roccas S. Multimethod probes of basic human values. In Adamopoulos J, Kashima Y, eds. Social psychology and cultural context. Thousand Oaks, CA: Sage. 1999:107–124.

Schwartz SH, Melech G, Lehmann A, et al. Extending the cross-cultural validity of the Theory of Basic Human Values with a different method of measurement. Journal of Cross-Cultural Psychology. 2001;32:519–541.

Schwartz SH, Verkasalo M, Antonovsky A, Sagiv L. Value priorities and social desirability: Much substance, some style. British Journal of Social Psychology. 1997;36 Part 1:3–18.

Seligman C, Katz AN. The dynamics of value systems. In Seligman C, Olson JM, Zanna MP, eds. The psychology of values: The Ontario symposium, Vol. 8. Mahwah, NJ: Lawrence Erlbaum. 1996:53–75.

Stackman RW, Pinder CC, Connor PE. Values lost: Redirecting research on values in the workplace. In Ashkanasy NM, Wilderom CPM, Peterson MF, eds. Handbook of organizational culture and climate. Thousand Oaks, CA: Sage. 2000:37–54.

Super DE. Values: Their nature, assessment and practical use. In Super DE, Šverko B, Super CM, eds. Life roles, values, and careers: International findings of the work importance study. San Francisco, CA: Jossey-Bass. 1995:54–61.

Swayne LE, Duncan WJ, Ginter PM. Strategic management of health care organizations, 5th ed. Malden, MA: Blackwell. 2006.

Veatch RM, Flack HE. Case studies in allied health ethics. Upper Saddle River, NJ: Prentice Hall. 1997.

ADDITIONAL RESOURCES

Requests to use the values survey associated with the Theory of Basic Human Values may be directed to its author, Shalom Schwartz, Hebrew University, Jerusalem at msshasch@olive.mscc.huji.ac.il. The American Management Association published an excellent workbook containing practical exercises for exploring life values. See Weis DH. The Self-Management Workshop: Helping People Take Control of their Lives and their Work. New York, NY: AMACOM. 1999:29–75. A concise and very readable summary of moral philosophies and ethical principles targeted to health service professions is: Darr K. Ethics in Health Services Management, 4th ed. Baltimore, MD: Health Professions Press. 2005:15–35. The Realm-Individual Process-Decision Making (RIPS) model of ethical decision-making has been presented at recent physical therapy meetings and detailed in several articles in the physical therapy literature. See Glaser JW. Three realms of ethics: An integrative map of ethics for the future. In Purtilo RB, Jensen GM, Royeen CB, eds. Educating for Moral Action: A Sourcebook in Health and Rehabilitation Ethics. Philadelphia, PA: FA Davis. 2005:169–184; Swisher LL, Arslanian LE, Davis CM. The Realm-Individual Process-Situation (RIPS) model of ethical decision making. HPA Resource. 2005:5(3):3–8; Kirsh N. Ethical decision making: Terminology and con-

text. PT Magazine of Physical Therapy. 2006;14(2):38–40 and subsequent 2006 and 2007 articles by Kirsh. The APTA link to ethics information is http://www. apta.org/AM/Template.cfm?Section=Ethics_and_Legal_ Issues1&Template=/TaggedPage/TaggedPageDisplay. cfm&TPLID=2&ContentID=36093.

CHAPTER 8

JURISPRUDENCE ESSENTIALS

D. KATHLEEN LEWIS

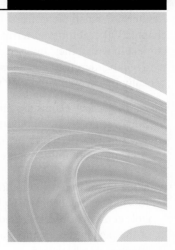

Learning Objectives

1. Define jurisprudence and its relevance to health service providers and managers.
2. Describe essential jurisprudence factors: practice acts, contracts, professional liability, and health service related crimes.
3. Discuss responsibilities of health service providers relative to jurisprudence factors.
4. Describe benefits of jurisprudence for self, your profession, and society.
5. Correctly apply legal concepts and principles to hypothetical cases.
6. Explore various consequences that may result from one incident or event and support your key points with information presented in this chapter.
7. Identify situations when health service providers and managers may engage in contractual relationships.
8. Explain risk factors related to common clauses in health service providers' contracts.

Introduction

Jurisprudence (Latin derivatives *iuris*, law, and *prudentia*, knowledge) means knowledge of law (Black, 2004). This chapter spotlights the recurring legal aspects of health care to prepare physical therapists (PTs) with a foundation of relevant laws and to arouse them to pursue expansion of their knowledge base, particularly since regulations related to providing health care services are undergoing rapid changes. The basic principles in this chapter will help readers recognize when they are approaching or encountering potential legal **risks**, enhance their desire to seek legal advice before an event ripens, and facilitate their abilities to communicate effectively with administrators, competitors, insurers, legal counsel, politicians, and vendors of goods and services. It is beyond the scope of this chapter to provide thorough coverage of the selected legal aspects, and is not possible to include individual states' application of related laws. This chapter includes common trends and highlights current issues that are unsettled among states. Information in this chapter is not intended to be used for legal advice. Specific legal concerns should be addressed by seeking legal counsel from an attorney who is qualified to practice in the individual's *jurisdiction*.

Changes in the Health Service Landscape

For centuries, the dominant ingredient in health care was sufficient clinical skills to treat the most acute conditions for survival. For example, malaria threatened progress along the Santa Fe Trail as evidenced by Sir Ronald Ross's exclamation, "Malaria fever is important not only because of the misery it inflicts on mankind, but also because of the serious opposition it has always given to the march of civilization. No wild deserts, no savage races,

Key Terms

Key terms, which are defined below, are bolded and italicized the first time they appear in the chapter. Other important terms are shown in boldface on first appearance and are defined by the context in which they are used. When either of these types of terms is used several times, its acronym will be identified and subsequently used in the chapter. Both types of terms are listed alphabetically in the online glossary with their definitions and (when applicable) their acronyms.

administrative law: claims are brought against individuals or groups by administrative agencies, e.g., licensing boards, which are created by the government to administer and enforce a particular set of statutes.

assault: a threat to touch another without consent. Touching without consent includes touching tangible items that are considered to be an extension of the person, for example a patient's clothing, crutches, or wheelchair.

battery: actual intentional touching of another without his or her consent.

civil law: claims made by individuals, groups, or the state to recover damages when a noncriminal act has been committed against a person or property.

contributory negligence: a legal concept related to torts, which holds that a plaintiff's own negligence had a causal part in their injury(ies).

criminal law: when an event is considered an act against society, the government, federal or state, brings criminal charges against the perpetrator(s).

damages: when a party who is owed a duty incurred damages, an award to remedy the damages is made by the court. Direct damages include lost earnings and current and future medical expenses. Indirect expenses may include a value for pain, emotional distress, and loss of consortium (those services performed by a domestic partner, for example—companionship, homemaking). Punitive damages may be added to an award when a provider's conduct was intentionally harmful or so grossly negligent that it was wanton and willful disregard for the standard of care.

defendant: the party accused of wrongdoing in a lawsuit or criminal proceeding.

joint and several liability: a civil law concept that allows a plaintiff to sue and collect damages from any of several jointly liable defendants.

jurisdiction(s): the legal power of a court to hear and decide on a case.

jurisprudence: the philosophy of law.

liability(ies): in accounting, this is the current and noncurrent financial debts. In law this is an actual or potential legal obligation, duty, or responsibility one is to do, pay, or make good. To be liable the plaintiff must show: (1) a duty was owed them, (2) the duty met, (3) they incurred damages, and (4) the breach of duty caused injury or there was a causal connection between the breach and the damages. If present in a contract indemnification clause, this is the part of the agreement that makes an organization liable for wrongs committed by agents or employees while performing their duties.

licensing board(s): the designated authority that grants permission to a qualified individual or entity to perform certain activities and acts as a judicial body in cases under its jurisdiction.

National Practitioner Data Bank (NPDB): a national database for health care malpractice settlements and judgments. A person who loses a health service related suit and pays damages becomes a named party in the database. Employers must check the database as part of the preemployment process for health service personnel.

negligence/negligent: omission (or commission) of an act that a reasonable and prudent person would (or would not) do under given circumstances.

plaintiff(s): the person or persons initiating a civil lawsuit. For example, a patient who claims to have been harmed by a physical therapist.

professional negligence: also called malpractice. Occurs when the alleged wrongdoer is a licensed professional and the requisite action is within the scope of practice, thus requiring the knowledge and skills of a professional.

regulation(s): a set of rules issued by the federal or state government bodies.

(Continued)

settlement: the resolution of a suit by the involved parties themselves without going to trial. Health service related settlements are not entered in the National Practitioner Data Bank.

states' rights: the Constitutional rights and powers held by individual states rather than by the federal government. Licensure to practice is a state's right.

summons: a written legal document given to the defendant(s) in a law suit which names the defendant(s), plaintiff, jurisdiction, and when and where the defendant(s) should appear.

tort: (French for "wrong"). An injurious act committed against a person or property or a breach of contract claim. A civil (private) wrong as opposed a crime.

no geographical difficulties have proved so inimical to civilization as this disease" (Hall, 1971, p. 82). Preventing death from disease and physical hazards was the utmost concern for pioneer health care providers. Since knowledge was limited, equipment was crude, and the number of trained care providers meager, many medical successes may have been due to sheer luck. Survivors were thankful to be alive, with or without loss of limbs, vision, or hearing. Later, the focus of medicine turned to research for prevention and treatment of diseases. Successes in research resulted in a knowledge explosion, development of high tech equipment, and advancements in clinical skills. Soon, education of providers and patients began taking center stage. During the 1966 Surgeon General's Workshop on Prevention of Disability from Arthritis, experts declared that too often, their care providers had advised patients that nothing could be done for their disease; subsequently, most of them passively went home and regressed (U.S. Department of Health Education and Welfare, 1966).

A primary recommendation from the surgeon general's workshop to increase funding for research and education on prevention of disabilities may have been a major turning point toward emphasis on research, education, and prevention of disabilities. In the mid-1960s, the health care industry began an era much like the Industrial Revolution, significant changes with many successes and failures. The Healthcare Revolution Age continues to the present. At the beginning of this era, the importance of management, legal considerations, patient involvement and education rapidly increased. Although some people claim that the increasing emphasis on legal aspects has been related to an emerging litigious society, research does not support

this claim. According to the Harvard Medical Practice Study (Bodenheimer and Grumback, 2002), only 2% of patients who suffer injury as a result of medical malpractice actually file malpractice claims and only half of those receive some compensation for their injuries. Legal considerations have become a major ingredient of health care because of consumer advocacy influences, demographics, different health problems, and economic, governmental, political, and technological advancements. These influencing factors have resulted in a proliferation of regulation of health care organizations and individual service providers. The following list of primary changes is not an exhaustive list, but a sample of major regulatory changes.

1. Proliferation of regulating occupations and professions from a mere handful in the early 1900s to more than 1,000 by 1990. In 1970, only 13 health-related occupations were regulated in all 50 states (Schmitt and Shimberg, 1996). Several studies report that one or more states license 800 occupations with certification or registration for the remainder (Cox and Foster, 1990).
2. Increased government funding for health services and products with corresponding regulation, e.g., Medicare and Medicaid.
3. Rapid increases in health care–related costs, which resulted in increased state and federal regulations to control costs (Chapters 2, 3, 9, and 10).
4. New and changing forms of business, e.g., managed care resulting in complex contractual arrangements (Chapter 21).
5. Increased emphasis on individual's rights resulting in regulations to prevent discrimination, e.g., Americans with Disabilities Act, equality of care for those with cultural

differences, and privacy of health records (Chapter 9).

6. Ethical issues related to rationing health care, right to life, and technological advancements in genomes.
7. The struggle to define quality of care resulting in increased accreditation requirements, peer review, performance review of individual workers, continuing education, specialty certifications, and pay for performance incentives (Chapter 1).
8. Computer technology has facilitated the ability to track organizations and individuals who provide poor quality of care and those who have committed **fraud** and **abuse**. Subsequently, government funding has been increased to enforce existing laws, the number of laws and regulations have increased, and published factual reports are readily available through the Internet.
9. The constant struggle between states' rights and the federal government regulation of health care matters cause political conflict and sometimes confusion.
10. Recent discussions by the media, politicians, and consumers about the economical impact the current *flailing* health care system has on the national economy and heated disagreements over optimal solutions (Chapter 1). Most of the proposed solutions involve some form of regulatory changes or additions.
11. Progression toward American Physical Therapy Association's (APTA) Vision 2020, e.g., changes in more jurisdictions' **practice acts** to allow direct access by PTs and strongly advocating that PTs should be "practitioners of choice" for musculoskeletal problems.

Today, health care may be one of the most regulated industries in our society; therefore, practitioners simply cannot afford to ignore the legal aspects of practice. Practice acts are changing to allow patients to be evaluated or evaluated and treated by PTs without a **referral** from a licensed prescriber, i.e., **direct access**, but many jurisdictions have limitations or conditions to these provisions. Practitioners must know and understand their practice acts to function within legal boundaries and to maximize opportunities to practice accord-

ingly. Due to rising costs for states to operate licensure boards, continuing increases in the number of professions desiring licensure, and concerns that boards are limited in their statutory abilities to ensure quality of care, states and consumer groups are recommending dramatic changes to licensure regulatory processes. Recommendations include standardizing language of practice acts and requirements for entry-to-practice among states, redesigning boards and their functions to ensure accountability of public demands and to reflect changes in health care delivery systems, changing processes to ensure continuing competence (e.g., time limiting certifications prior to re-examination), and passing federal laws to facilitate mobility and practice across state lines (Federation of State Boards of Physical Therapy [FSBPT], 2007a). Practitioners must monitor and be proactive as national and state regulatory changes are proposed. They can only be effective in this volatile state of health care affairs if they know and understand regulatory processes and related organizational and personal economic impacts.

Benefits of knowing basic legal aspects are much greater than those associated with potential or actual malpractice claims. Other benefits include:

1. Practitioners will be better negotiators with employment, business dealings, and other contractual relationships.
2. The number of jurisdictions requiring jurisprudence exams for initial licensure and/or renewal is increasing. (The section in this chapter on reading and interpreting practice acts will be valuable for those who are preparing to take jurisprudence exams).
3. Juries, judges, and *licensing boards* do not accept "ignorance of the law" as a defense.
4. Advocating changes with politicians, third party payers, and the public is much more effective when practitioners have at least a basic understanding of legal implications and are more adept at using appropriate terms according to the listener's knowledge base (Chapter 1).
5. PTs will be able to comply with Principle 3 of the **Guide to Professional Conduct**: "A physical therapist shall comply with laws and regulations governing physical therapy

and shall strive to effect changes that benefit patients/clients" (APTA, 2007a). Physical therapist assistants will be prepared to comply with Standard 4 of the **Guide for Conduct of the Physical Therapist Assistant**: "A PTA shall comply with laws and regulations governing physical therapy" (APTA, 2007b).

6. Practitioners will have a rewarding and lasting profession; otherwise, they are taking costly risks (economical, emotional, social, and family) of temporarily or permanently losing investments they and their families have made to become professionals.

In Figure 8.1, a Jurisprud-O-Meter is a suggested method for measuring your abilities to keep your profession within the safe zone of practice. The Jurisprud-O-Meter is similar to a tachometer, which measures the speed of an engine. It is important to monitor engine speed because running at excessively high rates or constant slow rates can drastically shorten engine life. Likewise, running your Jurisprud-O-Meter at excessively high speeds or constant slow speeds can shorten your professional life. Those who operate in the Slow Zone are generally ultraconservative and inefficient, slow to change, and have little knowledge about applicable laws. Those who operate in the Danger Zone make hasty decisions, are inattentive to details, rush to new opportunities without doing a SWOT analysis (Chapters 2–6), avoid seeking advice from qualified individuals, i.e., lawyers and accountants, justify actions by claiming that "others are doing it" as though observations of others are evidence of legal actions, and tend to make frequent changes with decisions. In contrast, those who function within the Safe Zone are attentive to detail, diligent, have a working knowledge of applicable law and **ethics**, use good judgment, modify actions and conduct to correspond with a particular set of facts, take precautions when necessary, use a degree of care required by the exigencies or circumstances, and seek advice from qualified individuals. What is your Jurisprud-O-Meter rating today? What do you want your Jurisprud-O-Meter rating to be in the future?

Jurisprud-O-Meter

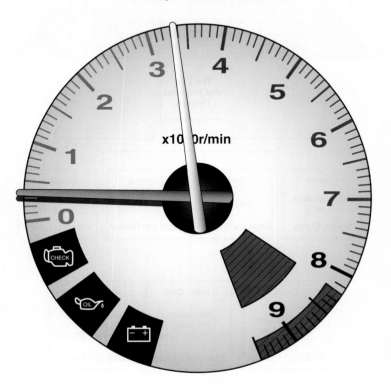

Figure 8.1. Jurisprud-O-Meter. Keep your Jurisprud-O-Meter intact. 0–3,300 is only for start-up and should not be kept constant; excessive operation in range 8,000–10,000 will shorten your professional life; 3,300–8,000 is the range for optimal operation and should involve changing speeds according to circumstances. Adapted with permission from D. Kathleen Lewis, Wichita, Kansas.

Overview of the Legal System

Before exploring particular legal concepts, it is necessary to have a basic understanding of the current legal system. Figure 8.2 shows the primacy of constitutional laws. The U.S. Constitution and the state constitutions supersede all other laws and regulations.

The U.S. court system is divided into three separate sections: *criminal law*, *civil law*, and *administrative law*. When an event is considered an act against society, the government, federal or state, brings criminal charges. Civil law claims are brought by individuals, groups, or the state to recover damages, e.g., when a *tort* (French for "wrong") has been committed against a person or property or a breach of contract claim. Administrative law claims are brought against individuals or groups by administrative agencies, e.g., licensing boards, which were created by the government to administer and enforce a particular set of statutes. Criminal, civil, and administrative law violations can coexist with any one set of facts (see Fig. 8.3). For example, a practitioner who has been charged with fraud and abuse of Medicare may face civil, criminal, and administrative charges.

This practitioner may be found legally accountable in one or two of the charges but not for a third charge. How can this happen? First, the burden of proof in a criminal case, where one's liberty and perhaps one's life are at stake, is much greater than when one's finances and license are at stake. In criminal cases the burden of proof is beyond a reasonable doubt; whereas, civil and administrative cases require only a "preponderance of" or "substantial" evidence. If death is a result of negligent care, it is possible that a practitioner could be charged with negligent homicide or manslaughter (criminal—for loss of liberty), malpractice (civil—for monetary damages), and licensure violations (administrative law—for limited or total loss of practice privileges.)

Administrative Law: Licensure, a Fundamental Requirement

With few exceptions, health service providers must be licensed to provide reimbursable

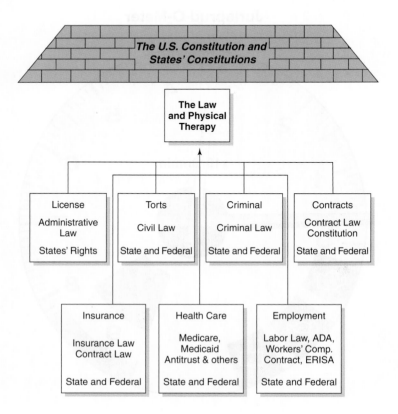

Figure 8.2. Constitutional laws supercede all other laws and regulations. Adapted with permission from D. Kathleen Lewis, Wichita, Kansas.

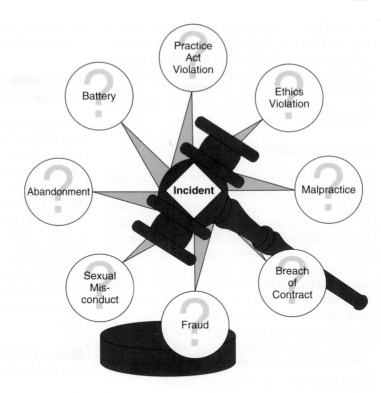

Figure 8.3. One incident, multiple legal concerns. Adapted with permission from D. Kathleen Lewis, Wichita, Kansas.

clinical services. A license is evidence that the state has given qualified individuals a privilege to practice within certain parameters as written in the state law (practice act). No one is guaranteed a license; qualified individuals (as defined in the practice act) must apply for a license and show evidence that they have met the state's qualifications. (Unless otherwise stated, use of the terms license, licensed, and licensee in this chapter include state granted registration and certification). After a license has been granted, a licensee must meet his/her responsibilities as stated in the practice act and corresponding regulations. When a licensee fails to meet those responsibilities, the privileges to practice may be limited, temporarily suspended, or permanently withdrawn (revoked).

Practice Acts: Enactment and Enforcement

Each state reserves the right to pass laws for protection of residents within the state (constitutional provisions for *states' rights*). Licensure laws are enacted through each state's legislative process to protect residents within

the state from incompetent and unscrupulous health service and other practitioners. Health service providers may influence laws that govern their respective practices by persuading legislators to sponsor legislative changes or defeat unfavorable bills (Chapter 1). However, legislators, as the lawmakers, ultimately control changes in the law by voting for or against licensure related **bills**. Typically, a governing board is granted authority in the practice act to issue and renew licenses to qualified individuals, discipline licensees who have not complied with the practice act, and adopt **rules** and *regulations* necessary for administration of the practice act. Rules and regulations have the same effect as the law (practice act); therefore, these should be reviewed and followed with as much diligence as the practice act.

Enforcement of practice acts is unlike civil and criminal law procedures, in which either a jury or a judge decides the case. The state boards follow administrative law procedures, which allow decisions to be made by a hearing panel, generally composed of health service professionals and public representatives. Administrative law procedures do not provide the same degree of protection for the accused party: strict **rules of evidence** are not required; courts will not overturn a board's decision unless the hearing panel has violated fundamental rights or the regulation may be unconstitutional; and the accused licensee may waive appeal rights simply by failing to submit timely responses.

Responsibilities of Licensees

Licensees are responsible for reading and understanding the practice act and its associated rules and regulations. Table 8.1 may be copied and answered as an easy reference for detailed information. Practice acts for all jurisdictions and some regulations may be accessed at www.fsbpt.org, www.apta.org, or www.washlaw.edu. The practice act, rules, and regulations must be studied for accurate and thorough completion of Table 8.1.

Although practice acts vary dramatically among jurisdictions, these are common responsibilities for individual licensees:

- Be truthful to the licensing board
- Meet requirements for licensure renewal and submit evidence according to board requirements
- Pay required application and renewal fees
- Practice within parameters of the law (practice act and corresponding regulations)
- Renew license by the specified deadline whether or not notice of renewal has been received

- Send written notification to the board when personal mailing address changes

Responsibilities of Department Managers

The department manager should not assume that employees have complied with licensure requirements (Chapter 17). The manager should implement procedures to ensure that personnel they are responsible for are practicing in accordance with licensure requirements of accrediting agencies, third party payers, other regulating agencies, and the organization's own policies. With numerous requirements and deadlines, the task can be onerous. Table 8.2 provides a general checklist for broad assessment of a department's tracking and use of licensure information.

Responsibilities of the Licensing Board

All licensing boards are responsible for protecting the public against incompetent and unscrupulous practitioners. They are granted statutory authority to deny a license when an applicant does not meet the required qualifications and to take disciplinary action against licensees who have violated the practice act or rules and regulations. The following examples present a variety of disciplinary actions and

---

Table 8.1　A Quick Reference to Licensure Details of Your Jurisdiction

Name of licensing board
Address of licensing board
Telephone and fax numbers of licensing board
URL of the board's website
Licensure renewal date
Renewal requirements: number of continuing education units and time frame; jurisprudence examination fees
Direct access: special requirements and limitations
Required supervision ratio of physical therapists to physical therapist assistants
Type and definition of supervision requirements for physical therapist assistants
Type of supervision requirements for aides and other ancillary personnel
Type and definition of supervision requirements for special circumstances, e.g., temporary licenses, graduate students
Practice privileges with additional requirements or limitations, e.g., 2 years' experience to supervise one who has a temporary license or proof of additional training for electromyography
Specific required clinical responsibilities, e.g., examination of patients performed only by physical therapists
Specific limitations or exclusions
List grounds for denial or disciplinary actions
Other important information

Table 8.2 Licensure Checklist for Managers		
Criteria	*Yes*	*No*
All physical therapists have a valid license from the jurisdiction of the clinic.		
All physical therapist assistants have a valid license from the jurisdiction of the clinic (if licensure is available in the state).	☐	☐
All temporary personnel, e.g., contract therapists, have provided a copy of a valid license and appropriate measures have been taken to verify authentication of the license.	☐	☐
Copies of all departmental licenses are displayed in a public place. (Essential if required by the practice act or an accrediting agency. Advisable for marketing if not required.)	☐	☐
Job descriptions for therapists and assistants are congruent with the jurisdiction's practice act. It is recommended that the job descriptions include limitations as well as responsibilities.	☐	☐
Job descriptions for ancillary personnel (e.g., aides, massage therapists, athletic trainers, exercise physiologists) are congruent with the jurisdictions' practice act. It is recommended that the job descriptions include limitations as well as responsibilities.	☐	☐
There is a mechanism to track licensure renewal requirements.	☐	☐
Performance appraisal instruments and mechanisms are congruent with licensure requirements and limitations.	☐	☐
Other	☐	☐

corresponding sanctions administered by state licensing boards.

1. The board suspended a PT's license for 12 months because the board found that the therapist had "falsified patient records, failed to provide appropriate supervision of support personnel, rendered billing and charges for treatments not performed, and failed to maintain appropriate documentation" (North Carolina Board of Physical Therapy Examiners, Summer 2006). That same year the board sent another PT a letter of reprimand for entering "misleading information" in patients' records (North Carolina Board of Physical Therapy Examiners, Winter 2006).

2. Documentation is not a favorite task of many professionals; however, failure to meet *documentation standards* can result in disciplinary actions by licensing boards. Arizona is one of many boards that has disciplined PTs for failure to provide adequate and accurate documentation (Arizona State Board of Physical Therapy, 2004).

3. Several PTs who were working in **unregistered facilities** had their licenses suspended for several months (Texas Board of Physical Therapy Examiners, 2001).

4. A PT was received a -year suspension for having engaged in "excessive use of alcoholic beverages" (Kentucky State Board of Physical Therapy, 2006).

5. At the time of this writing, the California Board of Physical Therapy had a final decision pending against a licensee for both *aiding and abetting* a person to violate the physical therapy practice and aiding and abetting the unlawful practice of physical therapy (California Board of Physical Therapy, 2007).

6. When the board found evidence that a PT allowed aides to treat patients "without supervision," the therapist's license was suspended for 45 days and the therapist was required to take a number of tutorial education hours (Texas Board of Physical Therapy Examiners, 2001).

7. In separate cases, a board determined that a PT and a PTA had practiced in a manner detrimental to public health and welfare when their respective patients suffered burns from "negligent application of modalities" (Texas Board of Physical Therapy Examiners, 2001).

8. When the FSBPT learned about widespread cheating efforts by U.S. physical therapy students in preparation for taking

the licensure exam, two individuals were denied access to sit for the National Physical Therapist Exam and a third individual's license was withheld pending further investigation (FSBPT, 2002).
9. In one jurisdiction where the law limited the number of times an applicant could take the licensure exam, the board refused to allow a PT assistant who had failed the licensure exam three times to sit for the exam a fourth time. The board's decision was upheld by this state's appellate court (American Health Lawyers Association, 2002a).

Regulating Professional Conduct

Although practice act may change slowly, grounds for disciplinary actions eventually change as the health care industry and society change. Examples of these changes over several decades are regulation of **moral** conduct, advertising, consumer rights to information about practitioners, and licensees' rights throughout investigations, hearings, and appeals. In the early 1900s, practice acts had strict codes of moral conduct. About mid to late 1960s, moral conduct outside the workplace came to be considered personal, and many references to such personal matters were stricken from regulations. In recent years, society has recognized problems of sexual misconduct by health care practitioners. In response to societies' dismay and concern, practice acts and codes of professional conduct have been revised to prohibit sexual relationships and activities between licensees and their clients. The following are examples of regulations about professional conduct:

- APTA Guide for Professional Conduct 2.1.C, Patient/Physical Therapist Relationship. A PT shall not engage in any sexual relationship or activity, whether consensual or nonconsensual, with any patient while a PT/patient relationship exists (APTA, 2007a).
- APTA Guide for Conduct of the Affiliate Member 2.1.E. A PTA shall not engage in any sexual relationship or activity, whether consensual or nonconsensual, with any patient entrusted to his/her care (APTA, 2007b).

- Texas Rules §322.4 (b) (8) states that "engaging in sexual contact with a patient/client as the result of the patient/client relationship" is one of 15 actions that are considered to be Practicing in a Manner Detrimental to the Public Health and Welfare according to the Texas Practice Act Sec. 453.351. (a) (7).
- Arizona Practice Act: 32-2044 Ground for Disciplinary Action (10): "Engaging in sexual misconduct. For the purpose of this paragraph 'sexual misconduct' includes: (a) Engaging in or soliciting sexual relationships, whether consensual or nonconsensual, while a providerpatient relationship exists; (b) making sexual advances, requesting sexual favors or engaging in other verbal conduct or physical contact of a sexual nature with patients; (c) intentionally viewing a completely or partially disrobed patient in the course of treatment if the viewing is not related to patient diagnosis or treatment under current practice standards."
- California: Section 2660.1: "A patient, client, or customer of a licentiate under this chapter is conclusively presumed to be incapable of giving free, full, and informed consent to any sexual activity which is a violation of Section 726." The commission of "any act of sexual" abuse, misconduct, "or relations" with a "patient, client, or customer" constitutes unprofessional conduct and grounds for disciplinary action for any person licensed under this division, under any initiative act referred to in this division and under Chapter 17 (commencing with Section 9000) of Division 3.

During the past two decades, society has influenced legislative changes related to use of drugs and alcohol. Professional licenses are affected by these regulatory changes and boards are acting accordingly. When a licensee has a driving under the influence felony conviction, the Texas Physical Therapy Board has suspended licenses for approximately 30 days with 5–6 years probation (Texas Board of Physical Therapy Examiners, 2001). The California Court of Appeals upheld the Medical Board of California decision to revoke a physician's license. The court stated that the two misdemeanor convictions for reckless driving involving alcohol were conclusive evidence of unprofessional conduct. Furthermore, the court found substantial legal authority that conduct occurring outside the practice of medicine may reflect on a licensee's fitness and qualifications, thus forming the basis for disciplinary action (American Health Lawyers Association, 2002b).

Additional Consequences to Licensure Disciplinary Investigations and Actions

Reverberations of a complaint against a licensee (see Fig. 8.2) may result in additional predicaments, ranging from effects on future employment to criminal investigations. Sometimes additional legal concerns arise when a board's investigation reveals issues other than those described in the initial complaint against the licensee. In *Cohan v. Duncan-Poitier*, a patient complained to the Dental Board of New York that Cohan, a dentist, refused to provide the patient with his treatment charts and x-rays. In addition to finding evidence to substantiate the patient's complaint, the board's investigation revealed that the dentist had also submitted false and fraudulent insurance claims and had failed to retain patients' records for the legally required time.

Another reverberation is the impact from laws, other than the practice act, requiring licensing boards to report certain information about licensees. In response to consumers' demand for easy access to information about licensed professionals, a few states passed laws requiring boards to post licensure and disciplinary actions on the Internet. The type and amount of information about licensees is quite different from state to state. In the near future, more states will probably be posting licensure information on the Internet. Although the legislative intent for posting licensure information is to protect the public, practitioners should be proactive when their state is considering legislation to provide profile information to the public. In particular, the legislation should include procedures for ensuring that information is accurate and mechanisms are available to correct errors. To see what a few states currently post about licensed PTs and PTAs who have been disciplined access several jurisdictions websites via www.fsbpt.org/Licensing or www.prairienet.org/~scruffy/f.htm. Some

jurisdictions list actions in a downloadable newsletter, some post a listing of licensees and the boards' corresponding sanctions, some boards require visitors to give the name of a particular licensee, and others will list a telephone number for inquiries about qualifications. Disciplinary action taken by the APTA Ethics and Judicial Committee is published in the *Magazine of Physical Therapy* (2005).

Current and Future Changes to Licensure Regulation

Numerous external and internal factors are likely to result in licensure regulatory changes of PTs, PTAs, and other health related providers. Some jurisdictions will be affected sooner than others, so licensees who are observant about legislative changes and trends in other jurisdictions will be prepared to advocate for effective legislative changes and to oppose less effective legislative changes in their respective jurisdictions (Chapter 1).

Temporary Licenses

Since licensing boards have been able to expedite issuance licenses with the advent of electronic administration and scoring of examinations, the FSBPT is encouraging all jurisdictions to eliminate temporary licenses. Some states have eliminated temporary licenses while many others are waiting for more favorable times before opening their practice acts to make this and other changes.

Continuing Education Versus Continuing Competence

Proponents of continuing education requirements for licensure renewal claim that continuing education is the best available method to ensure that practitioners practice according to current research and technology. Jurisdictions that require continuing education for licensure renewal have not been able to show conclusive evidence that passive learning activities is sufficient evidence that practitioners remain competent in their respective areas of practice (Finocchio et al., 1998). Continuing competence is a topic that most people agree is important for every health service provider; however, few agree on a fair, valid assessment method because the topic has an abundance of onerous issues (Swift, 1999). There is also the question of whether continuing competence should be pursued by state licensing boards, left to the APTA to determine means of assessment and standards, and how much the FSBPT should be involved in providing means to achieve continuing competence (FSBPT, 2007c).

Sunset Laws

Some states have sunset laws that require state regulatory bodies to provide convincing data that the actual function of the regulatory body is a benefit to the public. Generally, sunset laws have provisions to eliminate boards that cannot provide convincing evidence that they are effectively protecting the public from incompetent practitioners. Boards and state APTA chapters who have experienced sunset review face the challenging review process with trepidation. In the mid 1980s, the physical therapy board in Colorado underwent intense scrutiny when it was reviewed by the legislature. Some regulatory changes resulting from Colorado's sunset review include: changes in board structures, establishment of an oversight body, more aggressive disciplinary activities, and increased budgets to provide boards with adequate support to improve effectiveness (Douglas, 1999).

Multijurisdictional Practice or Interstate Licensure

When licensees move to another jurisdiction, getting a new license is often cumbersome, time consuming, and expensive. Numerous influential people and organizations suggest that defects in the licensure system could be remedied by some type of national oversight or national legislation to facilitate professional mobility and practice across state lines (Pew Commission, 1998; Puskin, 1999). There have been numerous attempts at the federal level to allow practice across state lines, particularly to provide services to residents in remote geographical areas (Puskin, 1999). The National Council of State Boards of Nursing has successfully lobbied for states to enact legislation for mutual recognition compacts. These compacts allow nurses to have one license to practice in member states of the compact. By 2002, 14 states had enacted compact laws for nurses and five states had pending legislation. On July 18, 2002, Senate Bill 2750 was introduced in the 107th Congress to "encourage and facilitate the adoption of State provisions allowing for multistate practitioner licensure across State lines." On March 20, 2007, H.R. 1601 was introduced in the 110th Congress to address **telehealth** and the medically underserved. This bill also includes multistate practice: "(b) Conference—Within 2 years of the date of enactment of the Telehealth Medically Underserved and Advancement Act of 2007, the Secretary shall convene a conference of State licensing boards, local telehealth projects, health care practitioners, and patient advocates to promote interstate licensure for telehealth projects." Members of Congress and various consumer advocacy groups continue to resurrect this issue, making it more likely that multistate licensure in health care is possible. Other professions are also studying this issue. In January 2001, the California Supreme Court appointed an Advisory Task Force on multijurisdictional practice to assess whether and in what circumstances attorneys licensed to practice in other jurisdictions should be permitted to practice law in California. In the final report of January 7, 2002, the task force recommended that two categories of out-of-state attorneys should be allowed to practice law in California through a special registration process (California Supreme Court, 2002). The American Bar Association and state bar associations have established committees to study multijurisdictional practice (National Council of State Boards of Nursing, 2002). State laws are distinctly different from one state to another; whereas, standards for health care are arguably approaching national standards. If state bar associations eventually allow multijurisdictional practice under certain circumstances, will health care regulatory bodies do likewise?

Practitioner Profiles

Among regulatory **policy** changes suggested by University of California, San Francisco Center for the Health Professions, report cards on individual practitioners should be made public by allowing boards to cooperate with public and private organizations in collecting data to identify a standard health personnel data set (Gragnola and Stone, 1997). **Third-party payers** have been collecting profile data on health care providers for several years; however, data from these various resources have not yet been merged to one common data set.

Professional Liability Insurance for Licensure Renewal

In 2002 at least one state (Pennsylvania) passed a law requiring PTs to carry **professional liability insurance**. A few other states are currently considering this as a requirement for licensure.

The areas discussed represent only a few of the changes on the horizon about regulation of health care providers by administrative bodies. The key prediction can be made from this information is, regulatory changes will continue to occur in the near and distant future.

Civil Law—Torts

Society protects individuals from wrongful acts of others by allowing those who are wronged to file lawsuits and collect monetary awards as compensation for the damages or seek other remedies as permitted by law. There are two general types of torts: negligent torts and **intentional** torts.

- **Negligence** is defined as omission (or commission) of an act that a reasonable prudent person would (or would not) do under given circumstances. *Professional negligence*, also called **malpractice**, occurs when the alleged wrongdoer is a professional and the requisite action is within the scope of practice, thus requiring the knowledge and skills of a professional.
- Intentional tort is defined as an act that is intentionally committed knowing that harm is a likely result. The following examples are common intentional torts.

1. *Assault* and *battery*: Assault is a threat to touch another without consent; battery is intentional touching of another without his or her consent. Touching without consent includes touching tangible items that are considered to be an extension of the person, for example a patient's clothing, crutches, or wheelchair. The *plaintiff* does not need to prove injury (damages), as is necessary in a malpractice or negligence claim. Consent is a good defense to a battery or assault lawsuit.

2. **False imprisonment**: confinement of a person to the extent that there is no reasonable exit and physical restraint was not necessary. There are special regulations on use of restraints and most organizations have policies and procedures about use of restraints that should be heeded. The Nursing Home Reform Law (OBRA) of 1987, Medicare and **Medicaid** regulations 42 CFR §483.13(a) (1990) prohibit use of chemical and mechanical restraints. Care givers may not use mechanical restrains such as belts, gates, geriatric chairs, mitts, side rails, and vests for disciplinary purposes or for their own convenience. Judges will closely scrutinize defenses to false imprisonment claims: consent, necessity to protect the patient or others.

3. **Defamation**: communication to a third party or parties that holds a person up to scorn and ridicule. Oral communication is **slander**; written communication is **libel**. Defamation is an injury to one's reputation as a result of an untrue statement. Patients' charts are available to patients according to HIPAA and third parties (payers, government agencies, and other care providers) have access to patients' charts. Beware, writing anything in the chart that could be construed as defamatory about anyone is a publication—proof of one element.

4. **Fraud**: intentional misrepresentation in a manner that could cause harm.

5. **Invasion of privacy**: intentional deprivation of one's right to be left alone. For example, disclosure of private facts (diagnosis, treatment, prognosis) that a reasonable person would find private. Consent and complying with laws (public health, worker's compensation, criminal) are defenses to invasion of privacy claims.

6. **Infliction of emotional distress**: intentional actions or omissions that would cause a reasonable person to suffer emotional trauma.

Table 8.3 contains some case examples of negligence, intentional torts, and criminal violations.

Chapters 3–8, 16, and 17 in this book discuss the importance of ethical conduct and organizations' policies and procedures that strive for quality of care; they will also help avoid claims such as those represented in Table 8.3. Each of the potential causes of action in Table 8.3 require a **litigant** to prove specific elements; although, there may be sufficient overlap that one incident may provoke a litigant to file several causes of action in one suit (see Fig. 8.2) and to file suit against all potential defendants.

Negligence: Malpractice and Ordinary Negligence

Negligence consists of four elements, each of which must be proven by the plaintiff (the injured party). In contrast, the *defendant* (the accused party) only needs to disprove any one of the four elements to prevail.

1. **Duty:** There was a *duty* owed to a person. A legal duty is established whenever a health care facility or provider undertakes care or treatment of a patient. A claimant must be able to demonstrate that there was an active patient/therapist relationship at the time of

---

Table 8.3　Legal Actions and Examples

Legal Actions	Examples
Ordinary negligence	After aquatic therapy, a patient slipped on water in the dressing room resulting in exacerbation of back pain and a grade 3 sprained right ankle. Investigation revealed that the clinic had sound safety policies and procedures; however, clinic staff carelessly failed to follow them.
Malpractice (professional negligence)	Hot packs were applied to a patient who had impaired circulation and sensation. No additional precautionary measures were taken. Subsequently, the patient suffered a burn to the area of hot pack application. There was nothing documented in the patient's chart about assessing the patient's circulation and sensation.
Products liability	Treadmill "stop" switch failed to function properly causing a patient to fall and subsequently suffer an ankle fracture. An investigation revealed that the product was defective in the design or manufacturing process.
Premises liability	The railing on the steps of a pool stopped short (prior to the last two steps into the pool). While entering the pool, a patient slipped on the last step resulting in a back injury.
Battery	A patient was persistent with his/her refusal of treatment but the physical therapist or physical therapist assistant proceeded to stretch the patient's hamstrings. The patient did NOT suffer any physical harm.
Invasion of privacy and negligent and intentional infliction of emotional distress	A health care facility released all medical records of a patient to an attorney for the patient's defendant in an automobile accident case. Among the released records were several pages marked, "Confidential. Do NOT release without Specific Authorized Consent." These confidential records disclosed positive results of the patient's HIV tests and had no relevance to the auto accident case.
Defamation	A health care provider wrote in a patient's record that another health care provider did not return a call (libel). A health care provider told a patient that his/her physician was incompetent (slander).
Fraud	A health care provider promises that a certain care plan will cure a patient, but knows that it will not (intentional tort). A health care provider knowingly bills Medicare or another third party payer for services to a group of patients and those services were never rendered nor was there any intention to render those services (criminal).

the alleged incident. Employers of health care providers have a duty to supervise employees, hire qualified employees, and monitor employees' performance. Courts reasoned that these duties and the fact that employers can recover costs of lawsuits by increasing the price of goods and services would better serve public policy rather than having injured plaintiffs who may receive nothing for their damages. Two legal theories, *respondeat superior* (let the master answer) and **corporate liability**, were created from the courts' reasoning to allow an injured plaintiff to file suit against employers and supervisors.

2. **Breach:** The duty was not met, either by failure to act (an omission) or by failing to meet the standard of care for the circumstance at the time (commission). The standard of care is determined by what a reasonable professional would have done under like or similar circumstances. The Guide to Physical Therapist Practice (APTA, 2007a), classical textbooks, research that was known at the time, the organization's policies and procedures, and documentation about the patient's care are all scrutinized to determine the standard of care.

3. *Damages*: The party who was owed a duty incurred damages. Damages are generally divided into direct, indirect, and punitive. Direct damages include lost earnings and current and future medical expenses. Indirect expenses may include a value for pain, emotional distress, and loss of consortium (those services performed by a domestic partner, for example, companionship, homemaking). Punitive damages may be added to an award when a provider's conduct was intentionally harmful or so grossly negligent that it was wanton and willful disregard for the standard of care.

4. **Causation:** The breach of duty caused injury or there was a causal connection between the breach and the damages. Proving that there was a causal connection between the breach and damages can be tricky; however, a sympathetic jury may base its decision on some minor association.

Malpractice is a special type of negligence that occurs when the actions in question require the knowledge and skill of a professional. The same four elements are required for proof in a malpractice case; however, expert testimony is required because the ordinary person is not capable of determining what the professional standard of care should be. However, professional negligence (malpractice) is NOT:

- A bad result
- Choice of one treatment when another is available
- Failure to cure
- An error in judgment (hindsight is always 20:20)
- Intentional harm

The four elements are easier to understand if you review a hypothetical case (Table 8.4) that is based on an actual case.

In this case, Mrs. D, the plaintiff (the party who sues), bears the burden of proving all four elements. If she fails to prove any one of the elements, the defendant or defendants will prevail and avoid liability. Table 8.4 suggests that breach and causation are the primary elements on which the PT's attorney in collaboration with the defendant PT should focus defense efforts. The PT will attempt to prove that he or she did not breach the standard of care by having thorough, timely, objective documentation supporting the therapist's claim that interventions were appropriate for the patient in the given circumstances (e.g., the patient's rate of recovery and tolerance to the treatment regime). Evidence provided by an **expert witness** for the PT should be easy for the jury to understand, the expert's testimony should be credible, and information provided by the expert should indicate that the standard of care provided by the therapist was within acceptable professional standards for this patient at the time of the incident and considering all circumstances at the time care was rendered. The PT's testimony must be credible, for example, confident demeanor but not arrogant, testimony consistent with documentation and his or her deposition, the testimony truthful, and testimony reflecting that the therapist is competent. If the therapist can prevail at proving the standard of care was met, Mrs. D will have failed at proving one of the four elements (Fig. 8.4, second small diagram showing the missing "breach" element). If, however, the therapist did not meet the standard of care,

Table 8.4   Malpractice Case Example

Case Facts: Mrs. Doe and her husband Buck were seriously injured in a motorcycle accident. Dr. Hunter repaired Mrs. Doe's femoral shaft fracture by inserting a rod and stabilizing the rod with a plate and screws. Mrs. Doe was discharged from the hospital and received physical therapy at home. About eight weeks after surgery, she appeared to be progressing with a normal course of recovery. Dr. Hunter advised the physical therapist to be "more vigorous" with physical therapy. Shortly, thereafter, during one of her therapy sessions, she heard a loud "pop" when the physical therapist was forcefully bending her knee. Later, it was discovered that the rod broke when Mrs. Doe heard the "pop." Subsequently, she had to undergo another surgery when the surgeon removed the broken rod and replaced it with a larger rod.

Duty	Both the doctor and the physical therapist owed Mrs. Doe a duty as soon as the patient/provider relationship was established.
	Duty for the doctor and physical therapist is not an issue in this case because the patient had not been discharged from neither the doctor nor physical therapist according to the patients' records and depositions. Duty for employers of the doctor and physical therapist may be an issue.
Breach	Dr. Hunter may have breached his duty by performing substandard surgical procedures.
	The physical therapist may have breached his or her duty by performing substandard physical therapy. (In this case, the amount of force, the direction of force, the duration of force, and location of stabilization may attribute to substandard care.)
	Breach of a duty and who breached a duty are issues in this case.
Damages	As a result of the rod breaking, Mrs. Doe had to undergo a second surgery, which resulted in a significantly greater recovery time.
	The fact that Mrs. Doe had damages is not an issue in this case; however, the amount of damages will be an issue if Mrs. Doe prevails in her lawsuit.
Causation	Since rods do not ordinarily break, the manufacturer of the rod may have produced a defective product or the design of the rod may have been defective. If so, Mrs. Doe could not prove that any possible breach by either Dr. Hunter or the physical therapist caused the rod to break.
	If the surgical procedure was substandard, e.g., insertion of a rod that was too small for the patient, Dr. Hunter's breach may be the cause of the rod breaking.
	If the physical therapist did not meet the standard of care when applying force to Mrs. Doe's leg, the therapist's breach may have been the cause of damage to Mrs. Doe. Investigation of the facts may reveal that the patient was not ready for more aggressive therapy, or the doctor did not intend for the therapist to apply excessive force with stretching.
	A battle of the experts during trial may convince a jury that more than one defendant (Dr. Hunter, the physical therapist, and/or the product manufacturer) were partially at fault. Communication between the surgeon and physical therapist are critical factors.
	Causation is an issue in this case.

this is not yet a lost cause. For example, fractures can occur as a result of osteoporosis or in this case a defective rod or a negligent surgical procedure, so the therapist should also focus on causation of Mrs. D's damages.

If the PT does not present clear and convincing evidence that the standard of care was met, it will be a challenge to avoid liability. The therapist will need to prove that breaching the standard of care did not cause Mrs. D's damages. Many jurisdictions today will prorate fault when there are multiple defendants and each of these defendants has contributed to the damages. In this case, the PT may be found 51% at fault, the surgeon 49% at fault, and the manufacturer not at fault for

a $200,000 award. Some jurisdictions will prorate the damages based on the percentage of fault: the PT owing $102,000 and the surgeon owing $98,000.

Some jurisdictions will allow the prevailing plaintiff to collect all damages from a defendant who is 50% or more at fault (called *joint and several liability*). In this example, if the therapist had liability insurance in excess of the award, but the surgeon was under-insured or had no insurance, Mrs. D may collect the entire award from the PT. The surgeon would remain liable, but the PT would have to file a claim against the surgeon to collect the $98,000. Providers should be cautious about purchasing excessive limits of liability insur-

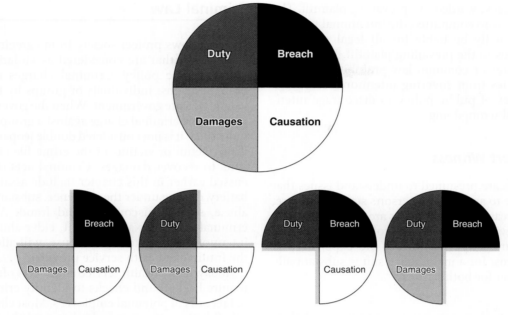

Figure 8.4. Elements that a plaintiff must prove to prevail in a negligence or malpractice case. If a defendant is able to disprove any one of the four elements, the defendant will prevail and avoid liability. Adapted with permission from D. Kathleen Lewis, Wichita, Kansas.

ance, particularly in jurisdictions with joint and several liability laws (Lewis, 1994).

In jurisdictions with *contributory negligence* laws, a finding that a plaintiff who contributes 50% or more fault will be barred from receiving any damages. The most credible and strongest resource of evidence when contributory negligence is an issue will be the patient's record; therefore, care providers should accurately and objectively document information such as missed appointments or other evidence indicating that the patient may contribute to damages.

Differences Between Intentional Torts and Malpractice

Malpractice suits often draw more attention from the media and health service practitioners than intentional torts. Newscasters focus on newsworthy reports, for example, multi-million dollar malpractice awards, a plaintiff who is considered to be "attention grabbing," or a case that represents a social issue. Health service practitioners should avoid devising practice decisions and actions based solely

on these featured stories. Those who do will tend to practice defensively and overlook other legal responsibilities. In many respects, the hazards and consequences of intentional torts are more detrimental than those of negligence. These are some differences between intentional torts and negligence.

Statute of Limitations

In many jurisdictions, the statute of limitations is longer (approximately 1 year longer) for an intentional tort claim than for negligence. If a potential litigant failed to file a malpractice claim within the statute of limitations and the facts could be construed to be an intentional tort, the statute of limitations cannot be used as a defense.

Liability Insurance Coverage

While professional liability insurance may cover legal costs to defend an intentional tort, the insurance carrier generally has the right to recover defense costs if the insured is found to have committed the intentional tort and the policy will not cover any damages awarded to a prevailing plaintiff. The party who committed the intentional tort will eventually be liable for all legal costs and awards to the prevailing plaintiff. Either state statutes or common law prohibits insurance policies from covering intentional torts as a matter of public policy to discourage intentional wrongdoing.

Expert Witness

Juries are presumed to understand issues that relate to an ordinary person's standard of care; whereas, expert witnesses are required to present evidence about the professional standard of care. Expert witnesses are expensive, so the cost for a malpractice suit is substantially greater for both parties.

Employers

Although an employer may be named as a defendant in an intentional tort claim, the employer may not be held liable for intentional acts of employees *unless* the employer knew or should have known about the intentional acts and failed to take remedial actions with the named employee. Employees who commit intentional torts in the course of their employment are subject to disciplinary action and possibly dismissal.

Elements to Prove

Each type of tortious act has different elements for the plaintiff to prove. For example, battery does not require proof that the plaintiff suffered physical harm. It simply does not matter whether or not there was physical injury. The plaintiff only needs to prove nonconsensual touching, the defendant intended to touch, and the touching was offensive to the plaintiff. Respecting patients' rights to refuse treatment and their rights to informed consent is more onerous than guides to professional conduct. Those who ignore these rights may be subjected to a variety of claims: battery, assault, false imprisonment, intentional infliction of emotional distress, and licensure disciplinary action.

Criminal Law

Criminal laws protect society from egregious acts or acts that are considered as violating strong public policy. Criminal charges are brought against individuals or groups by the federal or state government. When the government files a criminal charge against a group or individual, it is not considered double jeopardy if the victim or victims of the crime file civil suits to recover damages. Criminal acts discussed earlier in this chapter include assault, battery, driving under the influence, substance abuse, sexual misconduct, and fraud. Any criminal act, for example, theft, elder abuse, intentional failure to report abuse, will affect the future of a health service provider.

Today, many health service employers often require background checks to identify criminal records of potential employees. Most clinical affiliation sites require background checks on students. Licensure boards may refuse to issue licenses or may take disciplinary action against licensees who have been convicted of a felony.

Georgia's practice act is similar to those of many other states regarding the definition of conviction. It explicitly states that the criminal offense need not occur in the licensee's or applicant's jurisdiction. The statue reads,

> Been convicted of a felony or crime involving moral turpitude *in the courts of this state, the United States, or the conviction of an offense in another jurisdiction* which if committed in this state would be deemed a felony. For the purpose of this Code section, a '*conviction*' shall include a finding or *verdict of guilty, a plea of guilty, or a plea of nolo contendere* [Latin for I will not contest it] in a criminal proceeding regardless of whether the adjudication of guilt or sentence is withheld or not entered thereon pursuant to the provisions of Code Sections 42-8-60 through 42-8-64, relating to first offenders, or any comparable rule or statute.

Michigan's adult abuse law, like many other states' laws on abuse, recognizes the vulnerability of patients relative to health care provider's superior control. Michigan Adult Abuse Statute: § 28.342A(n)(2) states,

> caregiver or other person with authority over the vulnerable adult is guilty of vulnerable adult abuse in the second degree if the reckless act or reckless failure to act of the caregiver or other person with *authority over the vulnerable adult* causes serious physical harm or serious mental harm to a vulnerable adult.

Fraud and abuse in health care have been in the headlines since the False Claims Act (FCA) (also see Chapter 9) was significantly strengthened in 1986 to impose liability when one *submits or causes the submission of false or fraudulent claims* with "reckless disregard" or in "deliberate ignorance" of the truth or falsity of the claim. Congress has significantly increased the budget for the office of inspector general in support of investigation and prosecution of those who commit fraud and abuse in health care. Those who are convicted of Medicare or Medicaid fraud and abuse are excluded from participating in these programs, are subject to fines, and may be incarcerated.

Cost of health care in the United States is about 16.5% of the 2006 GNP or about $2.1 trillion. This trillion-dollar industry suffers annual losses from fraud amounting to millions of dollars, estimated between 3 and 15% of total health care expenditures (U.S. Department of Justice [DOJ] 2007; Federal Bureau of Investigation [FBI], 2006). Health care fraud is the second highest priority in the FBI's white-collar crime program (Ross, 2007). In 2006, this agency investigated 2,423 health care fraud cases resulting in 588 indictments, 534 convictions, and $2 billion in recoveries (FBI, 2006).

The most common fraud and abuse actions include falsifying diagnoses to bill for noncovered services, **upcoding** (charging a more expensive procedure than the one that was performed), double billing, billing for services provided by unlicensed providers, waiving **co-pays** or **deductibles**. Those involved in fraud and abuse include health care providers (doctors, PTs, podiatrists, and chiropractors), hospitals, nursing homes, durable medical equipment suppliers, pharmacies, and career

criminals (DOJ, 2007). Numerous federal and state laws can trigger investigations and accordingly impose sanctions. Examples include: The Anti-Kickback Statute 42 U.S.C. § 1320a-7b(b), The Stark Law 42 U.S.C. § 1395nn (Chapter 10), Mail Fraud—under 18 U.S.C. § 1341, Federal Bribery Statute, 18 U.S.C. § 666(b), False Claims Act ("FCA"), 31 U.S.C., and numerous individual state laws.

Why should every health service professional be concerned about fraud and abuse, which is a major factor of rising health care costs? Here are several reasons:

- Coverage of legitimate services have decreased as a measure to control health care spending
- Penalties for those who become involved range from licensure revocation, imprisonment, and fines
- Increased regulations to control fraud and abuse often result in additional paperwork with less time for direct patient care.
- An increase of about $200–300 per year per household are added to insurance premiums to offset insurance fraud

We are all health service consumers. Consumer issues related to fraud and abuse include:

- A percentage of personal and business taxes are spent to control and eliminate fraud
- Providers and their families may face critical, needless dangers such as unnecessary surgeries, unapproved prescriptions, and medical devices may be provided in kickback schemes
- Counterfeit prescription drugs may be issued
- Medical identity theft can result in changing the legitimate person's blood type, allergies, and diagnoses.

Many appalling cases are available at web sites for the FBI, OIG, HHS, and other government agencies (see Additional Resources). Every health service professional must help control and eliminate health care fraud to promote quality care and access to care for more consumers, decrease government costs of fraud control units, and support safe health care services.

Government initiatives to control and eliminate fraud and abuse are extensive. The FBI, the primary investigative agency, participates with CMS, DOJ, HHS-OIG, FDA, Bureau of Immigration and Customs Enforcement, Blue Cross Blue Shield, and others (FBI, 2006). Because fraud and abuse has been so prevalent in health care, the federal government advises Medicare and Medicaid beneficiaries to recognize or suspect fraudulent activities. Current federal law allows private persons (known as "relators") to file *qui tam* claims against health care providers. *Qui tam* is a Latin phrase meaning "one who sues for the king" as well as for himself. Rewards to relators include attorney fees plus as much as 30% of the government's ultimate recovery, which in some cases amounts to several million dollars (U.S. Department of Justice, 1998).

Individual health care providers can join efforts to control and prevent fraud and abuse. Some common ways are by following coding and reimbursement regulations, meeting professional documentation standards, seeking legal counsel for contract advice, particularly when agreements could be interpreted to include improper inducements, kickbacks, or self-referrals, and reporting any suspicious events.

Anatomy of a Malpractice Suit

Every **lawsuit** begins with a triggering event. The trigger may be as simple as a misunderstanding, a dissatisfied client, an unusual sign or symptom, an accident, or a clearly defined injury resulting from substandard care. The course of events in a lawsuit are depicted in Figure 8.5; however, additional events, such as appeals, lawsuits evolving from the original suit, and licensure or other regulatory investigation, can follow trial court decisions. From beginning to end, a lawsuit can last for 7 years or more, which often seems like an eternity to the involved parties. Clearly good practice and good ethics are worthwhile objectives for any health service provider, but even the best cannot be certain that they will never be sued. Some actions as depicted in Table 8.5 can deter lawsuits or decrease liability. As you read about the course of events in a lawsuit, consider dissecting a hypothetical case.

Table 8.5 Deterring a Lawsuit and Limiting Liability if a Suit is Filed

Event	Do NOT	Do
A patient reports a concern OR observation indicates a concern.	Ignore the concern—it is a *real* concern to the patient.	Address the concern ASAP. Document accurately, objectively, and thoroughly.
An official complaint has been filed OR a threat to sue has been made.	Discuss the complaint with friends, family, and colleagues. Alter the patient's record. Destroy any part of the patient's record. Distribute the original record.	Immediately, contact your insurer and/or personal legal representative. Contact your risk manager. Review the patient's record
You are being deposed during the discovery stage of a lawsuit.	Give more information than necessary to answer the question given. Answer compound questions. Use words like "always" and "never" in your answers.	Tell the Truth. Ask the deposing attorney to repeat or rephrase a question when you do not understand. Ask for a break if you become fatigued. Listen to your attorney's advice. Act professional and confident.
A settlement is being discussed.	Think that settlement is an admission of fault.	Cooperate with your attorney. Consider a jury that is sympathetic to an injured patient may award more than a settlement.
You are testifying at trial.	Show negative emotions. The same tips as being deposed apply.	Be alert, well groomed, and professional. The same tips as being deposed apply.

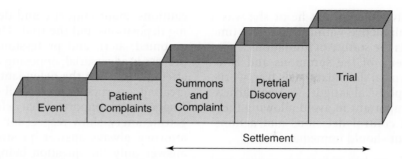

Figure 8.5. Anatomy of a lawsuit: As the suit progresses through these stages, legal costs increase, persona and professional stresses often increase, and more facts that may or may not be favorable are discovered. Adapted with permission from D. Kathleen Lewis, Wichita, Kansas.

A Physical Therapy Lawsuit Example

A month after diskectomy, a 39-year-old male reported to physical therapy for examination and treatment. Interventions were range of motion exercises, manual therapy, treadmill work, and instructions on a home exercise regime. Three days after his fourth visit, the patient called the clinic with concern about low back pain and radicular symptoms. The PT advised him to discontinue the exercises and contact his physician. The patient filed suit against the PT alleging severe disc herniation secondary to physical therapy interventions that were contraindicated.

The Event

As soon as an event occurs, the care provider should take immediate action to remedy the situation. Research shows that only 2% of patients who are injured as a result of malpractice actually file a claim and only half of this 2% receive compensation for injuries (Bodenheimer and Grumback, 2002). Dissatisfied clients are more likely to file a lawsuit than satisfied clients and they are more likely to return for care than dissatisfied clients. Taking appropriate actions immediately after an event is not only good risk management, it is good business.

In this case, the PT should have documented specific objective information about the patient's reported complaints and advice given to the patient. Subsequently, the therapist should have telephoned the patient's physician with this information and followed-up with a written memorandum to the physician (Lewis, 2002). The service provider should notify the clinic's risk manager and the provider's liability insurance carrier when:

1. A patient voices concern about an event.
2. A patient, family member, or an attorney places a phone call after treatment or after dismissal from care.
3. A patient, family member, or an attorney sends a letter to the clinic about the event.

Summons and Complaint

A lawsuit is formally initiated when two specific legal documents, a *summons* and a **complaint**, are filed with the court by the patient or his/her attorney. The summons names the defendant (or defendants), the plaintiff, the jurisdiction of the lawsuit, and when and where the named defendant should appear. The complaint gives detail about the case against the defendant and outlines the basis of the suit, including how the elements were fulfilled. Both the summons and complaint must be given to the defendant and filed in a court in the jurisdiction where the alleged malpractice occurred. Generally, these documents are delivered (called service of process) to defendant by a sheriff or other law official. The deadline (statute of limitations) for filing the summons and complaint varies from state to state, but is generally within 2 years from the date of the negligent action or omission and may be 3 years from the date of an intentional tort. Special circumstances, for example, if the patient is a minor or the plaintiff could not have known that he or she was a victim of malpractice within the 2-year time limit, extends the statute of limitations.

Upon receipt of the summons and complaint, the typical defendant feels fear, worry, mental and physical fatigue, and embarrassment. It is important to avoid allowing these emotions to control decisions and actions. The defendant should immediately:

1. Notify his or her insurance carrier and employer
2. Review all records
3. Preserve all records

The time limit for responding to the complaint, generally about 30 days, is not long considering that the defendant must meet with legal counsel and the attorney must prepare a response with plausible defenses. The defendant should NOT:

1. Distribute original records without advice from legal counsel
2. Make changes in the records
3. Converse about the case with colleagues, family, or friends

The plaintiff's attorney can **depose** (take testimony) anyone who knows about the case. Therefore, defendants who talk about the case with others risk the opponent getting access to unintended or misconstrued admissions or inconsistent statements.

Pretrial Discovery

During pretrial **discovery**, both parties to the suit (defendant and plaintiff), research relevant facts to be presented to the court. Discovery consists of oral depositions, written depositions (interrogatories), and requests for production of records including medical records, office calendars, diaries, correspondence, and personal notes. Oral **depositions** are taken under oath, in the presence of a court reporter. The plaintiff's attorney will attempt to gather admissions and inconsistencies that support the plaintiff's case. The deposed party will be given a transcript of the deposition to review, correct any errors, and sign. Once the transcript is signed, the document is a sworn testimony.

PTs and their assistants may be deposed as fact witnesses as well as when they are named defendants in a lawsuit. It is important to be cautious about etiquette and demeanor during depositions and the trial. That is, be well groomed, alert, and professional. The legal process is adversarial; opposing counsel often attempts to catch the defendant off guard by creating a particular emotional state to elicit responses. It is important that defendants avoid getting angry, show respect for the opposing attorney, always answer questions honestly, answer only the question being asked, and follow advice from his or her attorney.

The Trial

The trial begins with opening statements by attorneys for the plaintiff and defendant. These statements outline the case and respective arguments. The trial is adversarial, with each side trying to persuade the jury in its favor. Credibility of the parties and witnesses throughout presentation of the evidence can result in crucial turning points for or against the parties. If judgment is in favor of the plaintiff in a malpractice case, the defendant may face several consequences:

- Financial consequences: direct damages to the plaintiff for lost earnings and current and future medical expenses; indirect damages for pain, emotional distress and loss of consortium; punitive damages if the defendant's conduct was gross negligence. Punitive damages may not be covered by malpractice insurance.
- Employment consequences: unusual carelessness, intentional actions, or gross negligence may result in disciplinary action or dismissal.
- Licensure consequences: licensure boards may investigate and take disciplinary action, for example, **censure, suspension, or revocation.**
- *National Practitioner Data Bank (NPDB)*: The Health Care Quality Improvement Act (HCQIA) of 1986, which established the NPDB, requires that health care entities, insurance carriers, and state licensing boards report certain information to the NPDB.

Settlement

Settlement is an option until a case goes to trial. The defendant may fear settling a case, thinking that settlement is an admission of fault. A settlement is not an admission of fault. There are two primary advantages of settlement: (1) it is less expensive than paying for attorneys, expert witnesses, and court costs throughout a lengthy process, and (2) a settlement amount may be significantly less than a jury might award, particularly when there is a sympathetic plaintiff and/or the jury does not view the defendant's evidence as credible.

In the past, many PTs could function in the health care industry without clearly understanding his or her contract. Today and in the future, those who expand their knowledge and seek legal counsel on contracts will succeed in new ventures when their written agreements are clear and specific. They will feel secure when the final agreement does not include unnecessary risks. It is no longer a choice to ignore the subject. Practice acts across the country are changing to allow practice without referral, the number of PTs entering private practice is significantly increasing, and other professional groups are aggressively competing for the same clientele. Types of contracts that PT professionals will enter into include employment, lease of equipment or buildings, real estate property, insurance (health and liability), loans, networks, consultation, and third party payers (private and government).

Tragedies happen and 20-20 hindsight does not cover monetary and emotional losses. A PTA was recruited for a job; he gave appropriate notice to his employer and relocated to another state for his new job. When he arrived at the new clinic, the owner advised him that the clinic changed the staffing plan and no longer needed a PTA. A private practice PT, owner of multiple clinics, had PTs at two of the clinics give 24-hour resignation notice. This immediately created a staffing shortage for several months. Another private practice PT was given notice to repay thousands of dollars within a short time because the PT had signed a contract to reimburse the employer if third party payers eventually declined payment. The contract did not require the employer to provide regular accounting records or opportunities for the PT to make any legitimate corrections to patients' records. A PT testified at trial as an expert witness and was later sued over the testimony. Her professional liability insurance (a contract) did not cover this suit

because she had failed to add a rider to the standard liability policy (Reis, 2007).

Legal recourse is generally available in tragic events, but injured parties often opt not to take legal action because a clearly written contract is not available as evidence. A lawsuit is not a viable option when legal costs coupled with high risks of losing outweigh benefits. In contrast, a well-written contract can give injured parties sufficient evidence to make it worthwhile to file a lawsuit. For example, a contract between a small occupational therapy company and large corporate nursing homes prohibited the nursing homes from hiring the occupational therapy company employees. The occupational therapy company owner provided evidence that the nursing homes had blatantly breached the contract; the jury agreed and awarded $109,000 compensatory damages and $30 million punitive damages (Duffy, 2007).

Contract Basics

A contract begins with negotiations between two or more parties. According to van Dorne in an article about negotiating with insurance companies, PTs have little training and experience in negotiating but skills can be learned (van Dorne 2006). A skilled negotiator does not enter negotiations until he or she has developed a plan (identified what is optimally and minimally acceptable), learned about the other party and its goals, and prepared negotiation strategies. Unskilled negotiators should practice with a friend or colleague by role-playing a variety of strategies and communication styles.

A contract is formed when the parties have mutually agreed on terms. It may be an oral agreement or written and signed by the parties. Except in very specific instances required by law, oral agreements are enforceable but very difficult to prove if the parties later have a dispute or misunderstanding about the contract terms. PTs in private practice will encounter two of the exceptions when the law requires written agreements: contracts for sale of land and when fulfilling the contract takes 1 year or longer (e.g., leasing a building or long-term employment). The temptation to save money by using a contract template or copying a contract from a colleague and avoid seeking legal counsel to review contracts should be avoided. One size does not fit all (Shefrin, 2006). It is simply good business judgment and common sense to have agreements in writing.

Common Contract Clauses and Issues

Practitioners who are preparing themselves for the world of contracts are remiss if they do not understand some common contract clauses and issues.

1. **Integrated agreement clause**. Most, if not all contracts today include an integrated agreement clause, which states that the writing is the final representation of all agreed terms. If the parties agreed on terms that are not included in the writing, courts generally will not interpret what is not written. If any item is important enough to discuss, it is important enough to include in the contract.
2. **Illegal purpose**. Although the U.S. Constitution protects the freedom to contract, this right is not absolute. Courts will not enforce part or all of a contract with an illegal purpose.
3. **At-will employee**. This term or clause gives the employer the right to dismiss an employee with or without reason at any time (without advanced notice). Some contracts will simply use the phrase, "employee-at-will"; therefore, potential employees should carefully read employment contracts before signing. This term has advantages and disadvantages for each party; however, employees who do not understand or did not carefully read the contract may not be emotionally, professionally, and financially prepared for early dismissal.
4. **Restrictive covenants** or **noncompete clause**. This clause prohibits professional employees from working within a certain geographical area for a specified time period. These clauses are enforceable in many jurisdictions if the area and time limitations are reasonable. If these factors are not reasonable, courts often enforce the clause to protect the employer's business interests, but will alter the limitations to reasonable time and area. Some jurisdictions have statutes that prohibit restrictive

covenants; however, some of these state laws do not apply to PTs (Lewis, 2006).

5. **Indemnification** (hold-harmless) **clause**. The party offering a contract is attempting to have the other party agree to assume liability. This clause should be viewed as a "red flag" and definitely be reviewed by legal counsel. The clause may be overly broad by asking the other party to assume unreasonable liability. Another danger is that liability insurance will not cover incidents that are assumed under contract, because the insurance carrier is not a party to the contract. Always, discuss such clauses with liability insurance carriers prior to signing a contract with any wording that might be interpreted as assuming liability.
6. **Professional liability insurance**. Insurance policies are contracts and should be viewed with as much care as any other contract (Lewis, 2007). It is risky to assume that coverage is adequate, even after carefully reading the policy. Two examples have recently appeared:
   a. APTA announced in *PT Magazine* that standard professional liability insurance policies may not provide coverage for therapists who provide general health, wellness, and fitness-related services or perform management or other types of consulting (Healthcare Providers Service Organization, 2007).
   b. After serving as an expert witness, a PT was sued for her testimony and then discovered that her standard professional liability insurance policy did not cover services as an expert witness (Reis, 2007).
      Coverage for any circumstance is available. The professional needs to contact his or her insurance carrier, request a rider to the standard policy, and pay additional premiums. To avoid such unpleasant surprises, be sure to inform the insurance carrier about your practice and get the response about coverage in writing.
7. **Consultation Agreements**. There are unique legal issues with consultation agreements (Simons, 2007). The contract should clearly describe the services to be rendered, ownership of any intellectual property that arises out of the project, and responsibilities

of each party to the contract. Responsibilities may include such matters as delineation of who provides space and equipment. If the services are limited to consultation, the health care provider must avoid any temptations to provide clinical treatment. If the professional anticipates providing clinical services, at least occasionally, this should be specified in the contract.

Summary

Legal aspects of the health care landscape have dramatically increased in the past four decades, and practitioners are becoming progressively more accountable regarding their legal responsibilities. Licensure laws, as a fundamental regulation, either implicitly or explicitly incorporate most legal and ethical responsibilities. Individual licensees, licensing boards, department managers, and employers have responsibilities to protect the public from incompetent or unscrupulous individuals.

Federal and state health care regulations include civil, criminal, and administrative laws. When a practitioner is faced with a legal action (civil, criminal, or administrative) the consequences can permanently or temporarily paralyze his or her professional life. Responsible practitioners incorporate legal principles in their day-to-day clinical decision making as part of their best-practice standards. Lawsuits, however, can happen to anyone at any place and at any time. Thus, each practitioner and each clinic should manage risk while simultaneously striving to deliver quality care.

This chapter has provided a foundation of information to rate oneself on the Jurisprud-O-Meter (Fig. 8.1), identified what needs to be done to stay in the green zone, and cautioned about actions or failing to act that would position oneself in the red (risk) or yellow (caution) zones. Legal aspects must be closely integrated with business and clinical aspects of practice. Chapters 9 and 10 interweave business principles with laws and regulations demonstrating their close integration.

It is important to understand that there are nuances, exceptions, and additional legal aspects that are not included in this chapter and nothing in this writing should be viewed as legal advice for a particular question. The prudent practitioner will seek legal advice as needed from counsel who is qualified to practice in the jurisdiction of that practitioner.

CASE STUDY 8.1

Ready Access to Frequently Asked Questions on Licensure

Instructions

Locate the practice act and corresponding rules and regulations of a jurisdiction where you either have or anticipate getting a license at http://www.prairienet.org/~scruffy/f.htm. Using the items in Table 8.1, prepare answers in a word processing file and save the file in an accessible place. Be sure to include answers from both the practice act and rules and regulations. Discuss your answers with peers who choose different states' statutes.

- From the list of grounds for disciplinary actions, do you think that the list is thorough and clear. Why?

- Select one of the disciplinary actions described in "Responsibilities of the Licensing Board" earlier in this chapter. Do you think that the board in your chosen jurisdiction would be able to take disciplinary action? If yes, identify the statute and rule that support your answer. If no, explain why.

Risk Management Strategies

List risk management strategies that were included in malpractice case discussion in the Negligence: Malpractice and Ordinary Negligence section of this chapter.

(Continued)

CASE STUDY 8.1

Ready Access to Frequently Asked Questions on Licensure (continued)

Keeping your Jurisprud-O-Meter in Check

A middle-aged man was receiving physical therapy in a private practice clinic for a herniated lumbar disc with radiculopathy. The owner, a physical therapist, examined and treated the patient on the first visit. On the second visit, an aide, who did not understand or speak English well and was not licensed in the United States, treated the patient because the owner was out of the office at the time. The patient called 911 from the clinic with complaints of severe pain and alleged that the aide forcefully removed him from the treatment table. Subsequently, the patient had two surgeries—the first surgery resulted in nonunion. During discovery, the physical therapist owner stated that Medicaid would reimburse for services by an aide, but denied any knowledge that the state's licensure laws required a physical therapist to be in the facility to supervise aides.

Answer the following questions and discuss your answers with peers.

- What zone(s) of the Jurisprud-O-Meter was this physical therapist? (Refer to Fig. 8.1). What facts in the case support your answer?
- Identify legal actions that this physical therapist might encounter as a result of this incident. (Be sure to reference your jurisdiction's practice act as reference to some legal actions).
- Identify legal actions that the aide might encounter as a result of the above incident.

- List as many actions as you can that would represent what a prudent physical therapist would have done to avoid the above scenario or similar scenarios.

Impact of Contracts

Moe Kaching, owner of several outpatient physical therapy clinics, and Dr. Fox, physician and manager of the clinics, agreed to engage in a scheme to bill fraudulently Medicare and Medicaid. The scheme was to hire marketers who recruited elderly residents and offered to pay the marketers $100–$300 for each patient referral to the clinics. Dr. Fox would then misdiagnose these patients in order to receive maximum payments from Medicare and Medicaid and the clinic would bill for services that were never performed. According to the agreement, Dr. Fox was not required to directly supervise unlicensed aides for therapy performed. (These facts are based on an actual case: United States v. Jackson, No. 04-20600 (5th Cir. Mar. 2, 2007.)

- How does this case impact health care, the physical therapy profession, and society? Discuss your answer with peers.
- The agreement between Moe Kaching and Dr. Fox may have been oral or may have been written. Either way, assume that Kaching does not pay Dr. Fox the agreed amount, will the courts enforce the agreement for Dr. Fox to be paid the agreed amount? Why or why not?
- Discuss your answer with peers.

REFERENCES

American Health Lawyers Association. Missouri appeals court holds that statute barring candidates from taking PT assistant exam after three failed attempts applies retroactively. State Bd. of Registration for the Healing Arts v. Boston, No. WD 59989, 2002 WL 522631 (Mo. Ct. App. Apr. 9, 2002). Health Law Digest. 2002a;30(June).

American Health Lawyers Association. California appeals court says state law that defines physicians' convictions involving alcohol as unprofessional conduct is constitutional. (Griffiths v. Medical Bd. of Cal., No. B143674, 2002. WL 307761 Cal. Ct. App. Feb. 28, 2002). Health Law Digest. 2002b; 30(May).

American Physical Therapy Association. Guide to physical therapist practice. Available at http://

www.apta.org/AM/Template.cfm?Section=Ethics_and_Legal_Issues1&TEMPLATE=/CM/ContentDisplay.cfm&CONTENTID=14342. Accessed 7/20/07a.

American Physical Therapy Association. Guide for conduct of the physical therapist assistant. Available at http://www.apta.org/AM/Template.cfm?Section=Ethics_and_Legal_Issues1&TEMPLATE=/CM/ContentDisplay.cfm&CONTENTID=23731. Accessed 7/20/07b.

American Physical Therapy Association. APTA Ethics and Judicial committee disciplinary action. PT Magazine of Physical Therapy. 2005;13:(9):10.

Arizona State Board of Physical Therapy. Newsletter. January 2004;4:6–7.

Black's Law Dictionary, 8th ed. Eagan, MN: West Group. 2004:767.

Bodenheimer TS, Grumback K. Understanding health policy: A clinical approach, 3rd ed. New York, NY: Lange Medical Books/McGraw-Hill. 2002.

California Board of Physical Therapy. Citations and disciplinary actions. Available at http://www.ptb.ca.gov. Accessed 7/22/07.

California Supreme Court. Advisory task force on multijurisdictional practice. Final report and recommendations. Sacramento, CA: California Supreme Court. January 7,2002.

Cox C, Foster S. The costs and benefits of occupational regulation. Washington, DC: Bureau of Economics of the Federal Trade Commission. 1990.

Douglas B. Board and governance structure. Paper presented at the National Summit on State Regulation of Health Professionals in the 21st Century. Atlanta, GA: Council on Licensure, Enforcement, and Regulation. 1999.

Duffy, S. Retrial bumps $1.3 million punitive award to $30 million. 2005(Jan). Available at http://www.law.com. Accessed 6/25/07.

Federal Bureau of Investigation. Financial crimes report to the public: Fiscal year 2006. 2006. Available at http://www.fbi.gov/publications/financial/fcs_report2006/financial_crime_2006.htm. Accessed 8/1/07.

Federation of State Boards of Physical Therapy. Internet cheating: Physical therapist students. Federation News Briefs. 2002;4:1.

Federation of State Boards of Physical Therapy. Security watch. Data forensics. CSI? No, it's the NPTE. Federation Forum. 2006;21(2):14, 16, 17.

Federation of State Boards of Physical Therapy. Areas of focus. Available at http://fsbpt.org/about/focus.asp. Accessed 7/20/07a.

Federation of State Boards of Physical Therapy. FSBPT invalidates NPTEscores of 20 Philippines-educated candidates following forensic analysis of test results. Available at http://fsbpt.org/news/news.asp#FSBPTInvalidates20NPTEScores. Accessed 9/27/07b.

Federation of State Boards of Physical Therapy. 2007 annual meeting. Discussion on the floor of the FSBPT House of Delegates meeting on continuing competence (DEL-07-08). September 10, 2007c. Memphis, TN.

Finocchio L, Dower C, Blick N, Gragnola C. Strengthening consumer protection: Priorities for health care workforce regulation. Taskforce on Health Care Workforce Regulation. San Francisco, CA: Pew Health Professions Commission. October, 1998.

Gragnola C, Stone E. Considering the future of healthcare workforce regulation. San Francisco, CA: University of California San Francisco Center for the Health Professions. 1997.

Hall TB. Medicine on the Santa Fe Trail (Limited Edition to 1000 copies ed.). Dayton, OH: Morningside Bookshop. 1971.

Healthcare Providers Service Organization 2007. Certain You're Covered? PT Magazine of Physical Therapy. 2007;6(June):80.

Kentucky State Board of Physical Therapy Newsletter. January 2006;2.

Lewis K. Professional liability insurance: Are you covered? PT Magazine of Physical Therapy. 1994;2(July):49–54.

Lewis K. Do the write thing: Document everything. PT Magazine of Physical Therapy. 2002;10(July):30–33.

Lewis K. Employment contract: The tie that binds. PT Magazine of Physical Therapy. 2006;10(October):42–44.

Lewis K. "In"suring the best coverage. PT Magazine of Physical Therapy. 2007;5(May):40–44.

Long E, Helmstetter C, Martell L, Meyerhoff C. Occupational regulation: A program evaluation report. Legislative Audit Commission, State of Minnesota. 1999.

National Council of State Boards of Nursing. Nurse licensure compact. Available at https://www.ncsbn.org/nlc.htm. Accessed 8/24/02.

North Carolina Board Physical Therapy Examiners. Newsletter. 2006;36 Summer:3.

North Carolina Board Physical Therapy Examiners Newsletter. 2006;35 Winter:3.

Pew Commission. Strengthening consumer protection: Priorities for healthcare workforce. University of California, San Francisco, CA. October, 1998.

Puskin D. Board and governance structure. Paper presented at the National Summit on State Regulation of Health Professionals in the 21st Century. Atlanta, GA: Council on Licensure, Enforcement and Regulation. 1999.

Reis E. In my expert opinion. PTs who serve as experts in legal cases see many rewards and challenges. PT Magazine of Physical Therapy. 2007;5(May):54–57.

Ross, M. Lessons from Libby: Be prepared for government investigations. Health Lawyers News. 2007;11(August):20–24.

Schmitt K, Shimberg B. Demystifying occupational and professional regulation: Answers to questions you may have been afraid to *ask*. Atlanta, GA: Council on Licensure, Enforcement and Regulation. 1996.

Shefrin, D. Contracts: deal or no deal? PT Magazine of Physical Therapy. 2006;6(July):34–36.

Simons, G. The PT as consultant: Contract issues. PT Magazine of Physical Therapy. 2007;7(July):70–73.

Swift R. Continuing competence. Paper presented at the National Summit on State Regulation of Health Professionals in the 21st Century. Atlanta, GA: Council on Licensure, Enforcement and Regulation. 1999.

Texas Board of Physical Therapy Examiners. Disciplinary actions. Communiqué. 2001;Spring:4.

U.S. Department of Health Education and Welfare. Surgeon General's workshop on prevention of disability from arthritis. 1966. Available at http://www.sgreports.nlm.nih.gov/NN/B/C/H/O//nnbchg.pdf. Accessed 8/08/02.

U.S. Department of Justice. Health care fraud report fiscal year 1998. Available at www.usdoj.gov/03press/03_1_1. Accessed 10/23/98.

U.S. Department of Justice. Health care fraud. The United States Attorney's Office, Western District of Virginia. Available at www.usdoj.gov/usao/vaw. Accessed 8/1/07.

van Dorne E. How to negotiate with insurance companies. PT Magazine of Physical Therapy. 2006;12(December):52–57.

ADDITIONAL RESOURCES

Morrison R. Webs of affiliation: The organizational context of health professional regulation. Council on Licensure, Enforcement and Regulation. 2000. Morrison explains the history of healthcare regulation and discusses national and state issues about the relationship between current licensure processes and quality of care. The APTA has published a series of collections of articles on ethical and legal aspects of the profession. These collections are regularly updated to include evolving legal and ethical issues. Go to www.apta.org and look for publications entitled Ethics in Physical Therapy and Law and Liability. A licensed health care professional can check the information the National Practitioner Data Bank has about them or their organization at http://www.npdb-hipdb.hrsa.gov/. The APTA has endorsed a variety of insurance policies for individuals and professional business practices. Information can be found at http://www.apta.org and follow links to "Practice."

CHAPTER 9

REGULATORY ENVIRONMENT OF U.S. HEALTH CARE BUSINESSES

DEBORAH G. FRIBERG

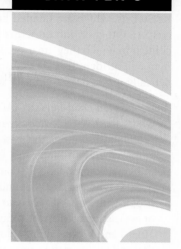

Learning Objectives

1. Describe the regulatory environment of U.S. health service businesses.
2. Become familiar with the source types of regulation impacting U.S. health service businesses.
3. Become familiar with management's role and responsibility in ensuring regulatory compliance.
4. Examine the possible elements of a corporate (regulatory) compliance program.
5. Become familiar with the major laws relevant to management of health care organizations and direct service providers.
6. Become familiar with the impact of regulatory noncompliance on health care organizations and service providers.

Introduction

Health care is often described as the most heavily regulated sector of the U.S. economy (Conover, 2002). The term *health care* encompasses individuals and organizations that are directly or indirectly associated with the provision of health services and health service products. Most aspects of health care are regulated in some way. **Regulation** starts with the formulation of a law (Chapter 1). Laws, also called **statutes**, governing the health services sector may originate from the federal, state, or local level. The legislative process of formulating Federal laws involves the U.S. Congress. This process is depicted in Figure 9.1.

Once enacted, a law must be implemented and enforced. This is accomplished through the promulgation of regulations. A regulation carries the force of the law issued by a federal or state agency (Nolan and Nolan-Haley, 1990) or independent regulatory bodies (Longest et al., 2000) (Chapter 8).

As was discussed in Chapter 1, health care is only one of the many competing concerns that elected legislators must consider when they exert their influence to shape **policies** and make laws. In democratic countries, public policies indirectly reflect voters' wishes. Voters vote to help get candidates of their choice elected. Once this is accomplished, constituents have the opportunity to engage their elected officials to express their views, and influence their elected representatives on issues of importance.

This chapter discusses the types of health service regulation and provides a sampling of pertinent laws that will affect health service businesses, their **boards of directors**, management, and individual health care practioners such as staff physical therapists (PTs). As businesses, health care organizations of all sizes and structures are subject to both general business regulations as well as those regulations that are specific to the health services sector. The chapter deals first with regulations applicable to the majority of employers regardless of their type

Key terms, which are defined below, are bolded and italicized the first time they appear in the chapter. Other important terms are shown in boldface on first appearance and are defined by the context in which they are used. When either of these types of terms is used several times, its acronym will be identified and subsequently used in the chapter. Both types of terms are listed alphabetically in the online glossary with their definitions and (when applicable) their acronyms.

Americans with Disabilities Act (ADA): in workplaces where there are 15 or more employees this act prohibits discrimination based on disability in employment, in state and local government, public accommodations, commercial facilities, transportation, and telecommunications. Protects people with a disability or who have a relationship or association with an individual with a disability. Titles I and V deal with employment discrimination and wire or radio communications (for hearing and speech impaired), respectively.

code of conduct: in business this generally is an organization's policy statement that defines the ethical standards underlying their behavior toward others. There are three ways: (1) through a compliance code that identifies prohibited behaviors, (2) through corporate credos that are broad statements of commitments to stakeholders, values, and objectives, and (3) upper management formed philosophy statements that formally stipulate how the organization deals with others.

corporate compliance program (CCP): an organizational program designed to help mitigate risks of intentional or unintentional regulatory noncompliance. A CCP is an organizational means of assuring that the members of the organization fully meet relevant laws, regulations, rules, standards, policies, and procedures.

Employee Polygraph Protection Act: bars most private employers (but not government employers) from using lie detectors on employees while permitting polygraph tests only in limited circumstances.

Employee Retirement Income Security Act (ERISA): amended by the Pension Protection Act of 2006 regulates employers who offer pension or welfare benefit plans for their employees. ERISA deals with fiduciary matters, i.e., the duty of trustees to act primarily for another's benefit. This act imposes a wide range of fiduciary, disclosure, and reporting requirements on fiduciaries of pension and welfare benefit plans and on others having dealings with these plans. Title I of ERISA is administered by the Pension and Welfare Benefits Administration (PWBA).

Fair Labor Standards Act (FLSA): sets standards for wages and overtime pay that affect most private and public employers.

Family and Medical Leave Act (FMLA): applies to employers of 50 or more employees. It requires employers to allow up to 12 weeks of unpaid, job-protected leave to eligible employees for the birth or adoption of a child or for the serious illness of the employee or a spouse, child, or parent.

Federal minimum wage: the lowest compensation an employer is allowed to pay an employee for hourly work. It is defined by federal and state laws. On May 25, 2007, FLSA was amended to increase the federal minimum wage in three steps: to $5.85 per hour effective July 24, 2007; to $6.55 per hour effective July 24, 2008; and to $7.25 per hour effective July 24, 2009. State laws may be more restrictive than federal law, and certainly may differ.

Health Insurance Portability and Accountability Act of 1996 (HIPAA): a five-part Act administered by CMS. Its varied purposes are to (1) improve portability and continuity of health insurance coverage in the group and individual markets, (2) combat waste, fraud, and abuse in health insurance and health care delivery, (3) promote the use of medical savings accounts, (4) improve access to long-term care services and coverage, and (5) simplify the administration of health insurance and for other purposes. The Administrative Simplification provisions required the HHS to establish national standards for electronic health care transactions and national identifiers for providers, health plans, and employers. It also addressed the security and privacy of health data.

Healthcare Fraud and Abuse Control Program (HCFAC): this program is intended to coordinate federal, state, and local law enforcement efforts to stop

(Continued)

health care fraud and abuse. It is under the joint direction of the Attorney General and the Secretary of the HHS acting through the Department's Inspector General.

Medicaid (Title XIX): this is a federal income-based program also known as Title 19 or T 19 of the Social Security Act. It is a jointly funded federal and state program that helps with medical costs for some people with low incomes and limited resources. Benefits and eligibility varies from state to state.

Medicare (Title XVIII): also known as Title 18 or T 18 of the Social Security Act. This is an age and disability related federal program. It is a fee-for-service health insurance plan that lets beneficiaries go to any doctor, hospital, or other health service supplier who accepts Medicare payment as the full payment and is accepting new Medicare patients. There are five parts designated by letters, A-D.

Occupational Safety and Health Administration (OSHA): assures the safety and health of America's workers by setting and enforcing standards; providing training, outreach, and education; establishing partnerships; and encouraging continual improvement in workplace safety and health through workplace inspection and investigation, compliance assistance, and cooperative programs.

Office for Civil Rights (OCR): is the part of HHS that protects Medicare beneficiaries rights, HIPAA PHI privacy, and provides assistance in complying with LEP matters.

overtime pay: FLSA requires employers to pay covered employees, who are not otherwise exempt, at least the federal minimum wage and overtime pay of one-and-one-half-times the regular rate of pay for hours worked beyond 40 hours per week.

personal health information (PHI): related to the administrative simplification portion of Title II of the Health Insurance Portability and Accountability Act of 1996 (HIPAA) dealing with privacy. This section of the law mandates security standards for electronic and physical health information and conditions under which PHI can be shared.

Stark Laws I–III: statutes regarding the regulation of physician self-referral. Named after the chief congressional sponsor, Pete Stark in the Omnibus Budget Reconciliation Act of 1989 (Stark I), and 1993 (Stark II and III).

Uniformed Services Employment and Reemployment Rights Act: an act that gives the right to certain persons who serve in the armed forces, such as those called up from the reserves or National Guard, to reemployment with the employer they were with when they entered service.

whistleblower(s): someone who informs empowered individuals or groups about organizational actions that are illegal, wasteful, unsafe, or restrain others from communicating about these activities.

---

of business. Health care–specific regulations then follow in this chapter and Chapter 10.

Important note: The intent of this chapter is to provide a starting point for PTs new to the practice and business of physical therapy. Readers should be aware that regulatory requirements might change frequently. Every health care provider and manager is responsible for being knowledgeable and compliant with the laws and related regulations that apply to their situation. Ignorance is not an excuse for noncompliance (Chapter 8). Organizations, their directors, managers, and individual providers need to stay current with regulatory requirements at all times. This can be accomplished through:

- Self-study
- Participation in professional associations or other networks of knowledgeable managers
- Consultation with available internal resources such as accounting, corporate compliance, human resources, internal audit, legal counsel, and risk management
- Consultation with external organizations or professionals in accounting, financial management, human resources, and law

An examination of the legislative and regulatory requirements to operate a health care business is part of the environmental assessment that management continually engages

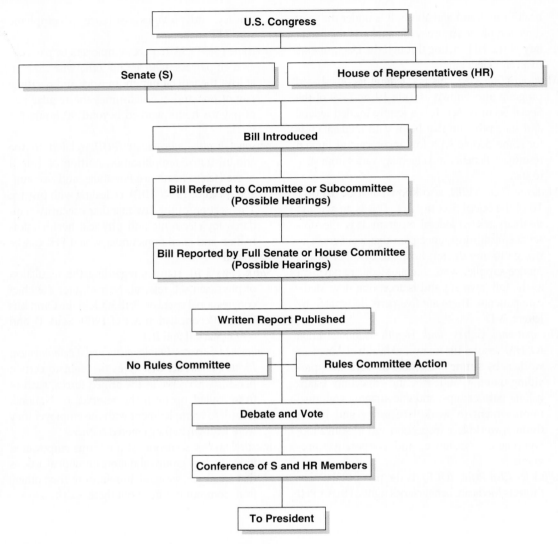

Figure 9.1. General process of formulating a federal law.

in to protect and advance the organization (Chapter 3). This chapter provides only the most basic sampling of information about business law. It is advisable for practicing managers and individual providers to seek the input of individuals with specific areas of legal expertise.

Corporate (Regulatory) Compliance

The risk of noncompliance to relevant laws is raised for health service providers treat-

ing beneficiaries of federal and state government–sponsored health care programs. For government-sponsored programs, almost any level of noncompliance with coverage and reimbursement guidelines represents substantial risk to the health care provider. Sanctions can range from recoupment of improper payments to imprisonment for owners and managers of businesses that engage in fraudulent practices. In addition to criminal and civil monetary penalties, health care providers found to have defrauded the federal health care programs may be excluded from future participation in these programs (Office of Inspector General [OIG], 2007).

We are in a current social environment that is focused on corporate responsibility. This responsibility for regulatory compliance rests with the board of directors (BOD) and the **senior leadership** (Chapter 5). The BOD has legal obligations to the

- corporation, stockholders, and its members, referred to as **fiduciary duties**;
- government; and
- people or organizations with whom the corporation interacts.

The BOD can delegate responsibility, but not the accountability, to meet these legal requirements to the **chief executive officer (CEO)** and senior leadership. However, all managers and employees must be knowledgeable of compliance requirements, risks, and how to avoid compliance violations. Health care businesses, to protect their organizations, must take an organized approach to regulatory compliance.

The stage for an effective *corporate compliance program* (CCP) is set within the **mission, vision,** and **values statements**. The importance of these as a foundation for a business's long-term success was discussed in Chapters 3 and 5 in the context of the strategic planning process. The mission statement defines the purpose for which a business exists, the vision statement defines its desired future state, and the value statements describe the forces that motivate a business and the behaviors it promotes in its employees (Jones, 2007). It is in the value statements that an organization can best define its commitment to honest and ethical business practices (Chapter 7). Periodic updating of value statements should be carried out to keep them in sync with business and regulatory changes.

In Chapter 2, regulatory requirements were identified as one external force that may require a rapid organizational change. In fact, a change in regulation may bring about a total revamping of business processes, a change in market position, and/or a change in business performance. Strategic planning needs to take into consideration the potential for rapid internal change. This is a key reason for adopting a cyclical strategic planning process that calls for the review and update of plans on an annual basis (Swayne et al., 2006).

Supported by organizational values that promote honest and ethical business practices and a strategic planning process that evaluates applicable regulatory requirements as an essential element of the internal environment, ongoing regulatory compliance can best be achieved through the establishment of a dynamic CCP.

A CCP is designed to help mitigate risks of intentional or unintentional regulatory noncompliance. In 1991, the **U.S. Sentencing Commission** adopted sentencing policies and practices for organizations found guilty of a federal **felony**. These guidelines reflect the principle that organizations with effective compliance and ethics programs will receive lower culpability scores, thus lessening the potential fines and penalties (Matyas and Valiant, 2006). In addition, having a compliance plan can act as evidence that any violations that might occur were truly inadvertent. The CCP must reflect a clear commitment on the part of the organization to know and comply with all applicable standards and regulations. This includes a plan to take action when violations are recognized (Reardon, 1997). The OIG (2007) recommends that health services businesses have in place a CCP that includes five elements: (1) an organizational structure for the program, (2) operational mechanisms to implement the program, (3) compliance infrastructure to assure leader's power to implement program, (4) measures to prevent violations, and (5) measures to respond to violations. The following implementation considerations may help in the CCP design process (Reardon, 1997; OIG, 2007):

1. A **code of conduct** "articulates the business's commitment of ethical behavior" (OIG, 2007). The code of conduct documents the principles, values, and actions related to compliance within the organization.
   Implementation Considerations: Stress the importance of ethical behavior and disseminate throughout the organization.
2. **Compliance-related policies and procedures** guide the organization's day-to-day management of high-risk activities.
   Implementation Considerations: Identify these areas and have regular consultations with legal counsel for regulatory updates.

3. Compliance infrastructure: The CCP is typically led by a designated **corporate compliance officer (CCO)** with the authority and accountability to manage all aspects of the organization's compliance program. The CCO should report on a regular basis to the senior leadership and the BOD, and should be supported by adequate organizational resources.
   Implementation Considerations: The CCO should have the ability and be expected to regularly report directly to the CEO and the BOD.

4. Measures to prevent violations should include:
   Organization-wide training on compliance **standards**, policies, and procedures
   Ongoing efforts to recognize and respond to regulatory developments
   Mechanisms to measure the effectiveness of the compliance program and adherence to related policies and procedures.
   Mechanisms to respond to identified compliance program weaknesses
   Implementation Considerations:
   Employees at all levels of the organization should easily understand training materials.
   Organization-wide training that defines employees roles and responsibility for regulatory compliance.
   Communication regarding the compliance plan should be highly structured, consistent, and ongoing.

5. Measures to respond to violations guide the organization in:
   Monitoring the organization to identify compliance violations
   Responding to suspected compliance violations
   Reporting suspected compliance violations
   Protecting employees who report compliance violations (**whistleblowers**) to the organization and/or outside regulators
   Policies to govern the reporting to the government of probable compliance violations
   Preserving relevant documents and information in the event of a violation
   Implementation Considerations:
   Compliance monitoring should be used including a well-publicized method for

employees to internally report any suspected fraud or abuse situations.
Organizations should make provisions to investigate and take corrective as well as disciplinary actions when necessary.
Any time a compliance violation is identified the organization must take steps to prevent similar violations in the future.
Prevention efforts should be documented.

These OIG (2007) recommendations can be used to assess a business's ability to protect against regulatory noncompliance. The measures to prevent violations are the assessment tools used to ensure that the compliance program is working and violations are avoided where possible or are recognized and corrected when they do occur.

Types of Regulation

Health care organizations and individual providers are subject to both general business and health care specific laws and regulations. Categories of regulations that should be of interest to health care managers are listed in Table 9.1.

Employment Regulation

The **U.S. Department of Labor (DOL)** is responsible for the administration of several federal laws related to employment and employee compensation, benefits, safety, health, and welfare. Many of the DOL-administered laws may impact health care organizations and their employees.

Fair Labor Standards Act (FLSA)

The FLSA sets standards for wages and *overtime pay* that affect most private and public employers. The FLSA requires employers to pay covered employees who are not otherwise exempt at least the *federal minimum wage* and overtime pay of one-and-one-half times the regular rate of pay. It also restricts the hours that children under the age of 16 can work and forbids the employment of children under age 18 in certain jobs deemed too dangerous for nonagricultural **operations**. For agricultural operations, it prohibits the

Table 9.1 General Categories of Regulations Relevant to Physical Therapist Managers	
Categories	*Examples*
Access	Emergency care, community service requirements
Employment practices	Pay practices, hiring, occupational health and safety
Environmental protection	Handling of materials used to clean up body fluids, cleaning of equipment
Facilities' regulations	Certificate of occupancy, building permit, environmental impact
Financial management	Medical records, fraud and abuse, taxation, securities and exchange
Food, drug and medical equipment manufacture, labeling, handling, sale and use	Sale of products, administration of unusual physical agents, topical medications
Quality	Accreditation/licensure, public reporting of clinical performance outcomes, Medicare program Conditions of Participation, NPDB

employment of children under age 16 during school hours and in certain jobs deemed too dangerous. Your intake interview may uncover violations that may be reportable to the agency responsible for this regulation, the **Wage and Hour Division of the Employment Standards Administration**.

Immigration and Nationality Act

This act enforces labor standard provisions that apply to aliens authorized to work in the United States under certain nonimmigrant visa programs. These standards could apply to the recruitment and employment of PTs or other difficult-to-recruit professional staff from other countries.

Occupational Safety and Health Act

The OSH Act regulates the safety and health conditions in most private industries. This also covers public sector employers. Employers have a general duty under the OSH Act to provide a workplace that is free from recognized, serious hazards. Employers must comply with the regulations and the safety and health standards promulgated by the *Occupational Safety and Health Administration (OSHA)*. OSHA uses workplace inspection and investigation, compliance assistance, and cooperative programs as enforcement mechanisms. An example of how OSHA impacts health care workers is in the requirements for **Material Safety Data Sheets (MSDS)**. MSDS provide information on the hazardous components, management of spills, and accidental exposure to chemical substances. The operators of health care businesses are required to prepare or have available to their employees MSDSs for any listed hazardous chemical found in the workplace.

Federal Employees' Compensation Act (FECA)

FECA is administered by the **Office of Workers' Compensation Programs (OWCP)**, establishes a comprehensive and exclusive workers' compensation program that pays compensation for the disability or death of a federal employee resulting from personal injury sustained while in the performance of their duty. The FECA provides benefits for wage loss compensation for total or partial disability; schedule of awards for permanent loss or loss of use of specified members of the body, related medical costs, and vocational rehabilitation. These resources pertain only to federal employees and agencies. Workers injured while employed by private companies, or by state and local government agencies, would contact their state workers' compensation board.

In addition to the FECA benefits there is the *Black Lung Benefits Act* which provides monthly cash payments and medical benefits to coal miners totally disabled from pneumoconiosis (black lung disease). The *Longshore and Harbor Workers' Compensation Act (LHWCA)* provides for compensation and medical care to certain maritime employees; and the *Energy Employees Occupational Illness Compensation Program Act*, which provides lump-sum payments and medical benefits to employees (or certain of their survivors) of the Department of Energy, its contractors, and subcontractors as a result of cancer caused by exposure to radiation, or certain illnesses caused by exposure to beryllium or silica incurred in the performance of their duties.

Other Acts

Another group of acts that PT managers should be familiar with are those that deal with post-retirement health benefits, labor unions, applicant screening, medical leave, hiring, pay, and employee military call-ups.

Employee Retirement Income Security Act (ERISA)

As amended by the *Pension Protection Act of 2006*, ERISA regulates employers who offer pension or welfare benefit plans for their employees. Title I of ERISA is administered by the **Pension and Welfare Benefits Administration** (**PWBA**). ERISA deals with fiduciary matters, that is, the duty of trustees to act primarily for another's benefit (Nolan and Nolan-Haley, 1990). It imposes a wide range of fiduciary, disclosure, and reporting requirements on fiduciaries of pension and welfare benefit plans and on others having dealings with these plans.

Comprehensive Omnibus Budget Reconciliation Act of 1985 (COBRA)

COBRA has several parts. Among its provisions, this law mandates that employers allow for the continuation of employee health care provisions (health care insurance) after termination of employment. The law does not address who pays the cost of continuing insurance coverage.

Labor Management Reporting and Disclosure Act of 1959

Also known as the Landrum-Griffin Act, this deals with the relationship between a union and its members. It requires labor organizations to file annual financial reports, requires union officials, employers, and labor consultants to file reports regarding certain labor relations practices, and establishes standards for the election of union officers thus protecting union funds and promotes union democracy. The act is administered by the **Office of Labor Management Standards** (**OLMS**).

Employee Polygraph Protection Act

This act, administered by the Wage and Hours Division of the Employment Standards Administration, bars most employers from using lie detectors on employees while permitting polygraph tests only in limited circumstances.

Family and Medical Leave Act (FMLA)

FMLA applies to employers of 50 or more employees. It requires employers to allow up to 12 weeks of unpaid, job-protected leave to eligible employees for the birth or adoption of a child or for the serious illness of the employee or a spouse, child, or parent. While this law has been a great benefit to employees, it can create a significant financial and operational hardship on employers who must often allow for the use of earned sick leave benefits or work shorthanded. The Wage and Hour Division of the Employment Standards Administration administers the provisions of the FMLA.

Immigration and Nationality Act

This act requires employers who want to use foreign temporary workers (less than a year) on H-2A visas to get a labor certificate from the **Employment and Training Administration** certifying that there are not sufficient, able, willing and qualified U.S. workers available to do the work. The provisions of this act must be met when recruiting PTs or other health care professionals from foreign countries. There are also visas for those who want permanent residency to work in the United States (Chapter 1). The Wage and Hour Division of the Employment Standards Administration enforces this law.

Acts Pertaining to Recipients of Government Aid

These three acts apply to recipients of government contracts, grants, or financial aid.

- The **Davis-Bacon Act** requires payment of prevailing wages and benefits to employees (laborers and mechanics) of contractors engaged in federal government construction projects.
- The **McNamara-O'Hara Service Contract Act** sets wage rates and other labor standards for employees of contractors furnishing services to the federal government.
- The **Walsh-Healey Public Contracts Act** requires payment of minimum wage and other labor standards by contractors.

Worker Adjustment and Retraining Notification Act (WARN)

WARN requires that employees receive early warning of upcoming layoffs or plant closings. Employees must be provided with severance pay that covers the required notice period if notice is not given. WARN is enforced through the federal courts.

Uniformed Services Employment and Reemployment Rights Act

This act allows for certain persons who serve in the armed forces, such as those called up from the reserves or National Guard, to have a right to reemployment with the employer they were with when they entered service. As with FMLA, this law is designed to protect the employee but may cause a significant impact on the employer and/or coworkers who may need to work short-handed while the protected employee is away from the workplace. The **Veterans' Employment and Training Service** (VETS) administers this act.

The Vietnam Era Veterans' Readjustment Assistance Act (VEVRA)

VEVRA requires covered federal government contractors and subcontractors to take affirmative action to employ and advance in employment specified categories of veterans protected by the act and prohibit discrimination against such veterans. The VEVRA was amended by the **Jobs for Veterans Act (JVA)** enacted in 2002 and became effective in September 2007. The JVA amendments raised the threshold dollar amount of the government contracts that are subject to the affirmative action provisions of VEVRA, changed the categories of veterans protected by the law, and changed the manner in which the mandatory job listing requirement is to be implemented.

Americans with Disabilities Act

This act has four parts:

1. Communications provisions
2. Employment provisions
3. Public accommodations
4. Transportation (ADA, 2007)

These four areas are enforced by several federal agencies including the Equal Employment Opportunity Commission, Department of Justices' Civil Rights Division, Federal Communications Commission, and Department of Transportation. Of particular importance to employers are the employment provisions that prohibit discrimination against a qualified individual with a disability when the discrimination is attributable to the individual's disability. In addition, an employer is required to make reasonable accommodation to facilitate the employment or continued employment of a qualified applicant or employee, respectively (Engel et al., 1996).

Section 503 of the **Rehabilitation Act of 1973** prohibits discrimination and requires employers with federal contracts or subcontracts that exceed $10,000 to take affirmative action to hire, retain, and promote qualified individuals with disabilities. All covered contractors and subcontractors must include a specific equal opportunity clause in each of their nonexempt contracts and subcontracts. This law is enforced by the Employment Standards Administration's **Office of Federal Contract Compliance (OFCCP)** within the DOL.

DOL's Office of Compliance Assistance Policy leads a variety of department-wide compliance assistance efforts, including its Web portal designed to provide businesses, workers, and others with the knowledge and tools they need to comply with DOL's rules. The DOL's Office of Compliance can be accessed at www.dol.gov/compliance/.

Financial Management

Financial management can be defined as "the process of managing the financial resources, including accounting and financial reporting, budgeting, collecting accounts receivable, risk management, and insurance for a business" (Small Business Notes, 2007). The effectiveness of these functions has a great impact on the success of the business. Many of these functions are evaluated as part of a **financial audit** of a business' financial statements and records (Chapter 21). An audit is an examination by an independent third party of the financial statements of a company that results in the publication of an independent opinion on whether or not those financial statements are relevant, accurate, complete, and fairly presented. The audit process will also look at the financial management policies, procedures, and practices of the business to assess whether the business is following **generally accepted accounting principles (GAAP)** (see Chapters 5 and 21).

All businesses, including health care organizations, are subject to regulation of their financial management and reporting practices. Ownership and legal structure (Chapter 5) will determine how existing regulations affect a health care organization. A number of major laws govern financial management and reporting.

Securities Act of 1933

The Securities Act applies to for-profit health care corporations whose stock is publicly traded and whose ownership is legally separate from its owners. Ownership or a percentage thereof is represented by stock (securities) that can be bought and sold to investors through the stock market. This law has two objectives: (1) to require that investors receive financial and other significant information concerning securities being offered for public sale, and (2) to prohibit deceit, misrepresentations, and other fraud in the sale of securities.

Securities Exchange Act of 1934

Created the **Securities and Exchange Commission (SEC)**, this act authorizes the SEC's broad authority over all aspects of the securities industry. Its authority includes "the power to register, regulate, and oversee brokerage firms, transfer agents, and clearing agencies as well as the nation's securities **self regulatory organizations (SROs)**. The various stock exchanges, such as the New York Stock Exchange, and American Stock Exchange are SROs" (SEC, 2007). The act also dictates acceptable and unacceptable conduct in the stock markets. It provides the SEC with disciplinary powers over regulated entities and persons associated with them. The act gives the SEC the power to require periodic reporting of information by companies with publicly traded securities.

Investment Advisers Act of 1940

This act, amended in 1966, regulates investment advisers. It requires advisers who have at least $25 million of assets under management or who advise a registered investment company to register with the SEC.

Sarbanes-Oxley Act of 2002

Enacted in response to events that involved allegations of misdeeds by corporate executives, independent auditors, and other market participants who have undermined investor confidence in the U.S. financial markets (Aguilar, 2002; Waggoner and Fogarty, 2002). This act effects sweeping corporate disclosure and financial reporting reform. It requires executive-level management of publicly traded companies to verify and sign the financial statements and other related information concerning the company they manage.

Food and Drug Regulation

The U.S. **Food and Drug Administration (FDA)** with enforcement through efforts of the **Drug Enforcement Administration (DEA)** is responsible for the administration of several statutes. According to the DEA (2007) these include:

- *Federal Food, Drug, and Cosmetic Act Public Health Services Act of 1944* allows for the regulation of drug and mental health related research, the effectiveness and efficiency of health care, regulation of biological materials, laboratories, blood banks, mammogram facilities, communicable disease control, animal research, and vaccine programs.

- *Best Pharmaceuticals for Children Act* amended the Federal Food, Drug, and Cosmetic Act to improve the safety and efficacy of pharmaceuticals for children.
- *Controlled Substances Act* provides the authority to control as well as set standards and schedules for all controlled substances.
- *Dietary Supplement Health and Education Act of 1994* amended the Federal Food, Drug, and Cosmetic Act to establish standards for labeling and safety of dietary supplements.
- *Mammography Quality Standards Act (MQSA)* established regulations and national quality standards for mammography services.
- *Medical Device User Fee and Modernization Act (MDUFMA) of 2002* establishes user fees for premarket FDA reviews for approval of new devices and technologies. The revenue obtained from these user fees allows the FDA to provide patients with earlier access to safe and effective technology, and more interactive and rapid review to the medical device industry. Reduced fees may be applied to small businesses.
- *Prescription Drug User Fee Act* establishes a user fee for premarket review for FDA approval of drugs and drug supplements.
- The *Public Health Security and Bioterrorism Preparedness and Response Act of 2002* (aka the Bioterrorism Act) was passed in response to the events of September 11, 2001, to enhance the security of the United States. The Bioterrorism Act addressed national preparedness for bioterrorism and other public health emergencies including enhanced controls on dangerous biological agents and toxins, protecting safety and security of the food and drug supply, and drinking water security and safety. The FDA is responsible for carrying out certain provisions, particularly the protection of food supply and the protection of the drug supply.
- *Project BioShield Act of 2004* amends the Public Health Service Act of 1944 to provide protections and countermeasures against chemical, radiological, or nuclear agents that may be used in a terrorist attack against the United States.

Environmental Regulation

There are several major laws that form the legal basis for the authority of the **Environmental Protection Agency (EPA)**. Many of these specifically impact health care organizations and providers including (EPA, 2007):

- *The National Environmental Policy Act of 1969 (NEPA)* establishes national policy to "encourage productive and enjoyable harmony between man and his environment; to promote efforts which will prevent or eliminate damage to the environment and biosphere and stimulate the health and welfare of man; to enrich the understanding of the ecological systems and natural resources important to the Nation; and to establish a Council on Environmental Quality" (The National Environmental Policy Act of 1969 [NEPA], 2007).
- *The Emergency Planning & Community Right-To-Know Act (EPCRA)*, also known as Title III of the *Superfund Amendments and Reauthorization Act (SARA)*, is the national legislation on community safety. EPCRA was designated to help local communities protect public health, safety, and the environment from chemical hazards. Broad representation on **Local Emergency Planning Committees (LEPCs)** by emergency response personnel, health officials, government representatives, community groups, industrial facilities, media, and local emergency managers ensures that all necessary elements for effective planning are represented. LEPCs have been increasingly active as part of the federal initiatives to improve homeland security.
- The Federal Food, Drug, and Cosmetic Act (FFDCA) regulates such health care activities as the use of investigational drugs or devices, clinical trials involving humans, pharmaceutical compounding, patient access to unapproved therapies and diagnostic procedures, dissemination of information about drugs, and devices of unintended uses.
- *The Pollution Prevention Act (PPA)* regulates pollution issues related to medical waste tracking and disposal as well as related health issues.
- *The Medical Waste Tracking Act (MWTA)* of 1989 requires the EPA to disseminate rules on the management of infectious waste.

Health Care

While many laws impact health care organizations and providers, those administered by the agencies of the **Department of Health and Human Services** (HHS) generally have the greatest impact on health care access, operations, clinical practice standards, and payment. The list of HHS-administered laws is extensive. Laws that may be of particular interest to health care consumers, organizations, and providers include the **Social Security Act**, the *Medicare Program Titles XVIII and XIX*), and the **State Children's Health Insurance Program** (**SCHIP**) (**Title XXI**) (Department of Health and Human Services [HHS], 2007a).

The Social Security Act established three health care insurance programs to guarantee access to health care for the young, the elderly, and the poor. The combined enrollment of these health insurance plans, including the Medicare program Title XVIII and XIX), and the State Children's Health Insurance Program (SCHIP) (Title XXI), has made the federal government the largest provider of health care insurance in the nation (Centers for Medicare and Medicaid Services [CMS], 2007a) (Chapter 2). Run by the CMS, the Medicare program covers nearly 40 million Americans at a cost of just under $200 billion (2007a).

The Medicare Program

This program provides health insurance to:

1. People age 65 or older
2. People under age 65 with certain disabilities
3. People of all ages with end-stage renal disease (permanent kidney failure requiring dialysis or a kidney transplant)

The Medicare program is divided into Hospital Insurance (Part A), which helps pay for inpatient hospital services, skilled nursing facility services, home health services, and hospice care, and Medical Insurance (Part B), which helps pay for doctor services, outpatient hospital services, medical equipment and supplies, and other health services and supplies (Chapters 1 and 2). Medicare enrollees or beneficiaries may have the choice of enrolling in the original Medicare **fee-for-service** plan or a Medicare managed care plan depending on what is available in their geographical area. Medicare **prescription drug coverage** is insurance covers prescription drugs at participating pharmacies. Private companies provide the coverage. Beneficiaries choose the drug plan and pay a monthly premium. This coverage is available to everyone with Medicare and may help lower prescription drug costs and help protect against higher costs in the future. Like other insurance plans, if a beneficiary decides not to enroll in a drug plan when they are first eligible, they may pay a penalty if they choose to join later.

The Medicaid Program

The Medicaid program is a health insurance program for certain low-income people (Chapters 1 and 2). It is funded and administered jointly by a state–federal government partnership. As a result of this partnership approach states are required to follow broad federal requirements for Medicaid but they have a wide degree of flexibility in the designing of their program. At a minimum, states must cover:

Inpatient and outpatient hospital services
Laboratory and x-ray services
Skilled nursing and home health services
Doctors' services
Family planning
Periodic health checkups
Diagnosis and treatment for children

States may establish eligibility standards, decide what benefits to offer and services to pay for as well as set payment rates. There are approximately 36 million people eligible for Medicaid who are certain low-income families with children, low-income people who are aged, blind, or disabled, low-income pregnant women and children, and people who have very high medical bills (CMS, 2007a).

SCHIP

SCHIP is run by CMS, along with the Health Resources and Services Administration (HRSA). This program is designed to help states expand health care coverage to uninsured children. Funding for SCHIP is assured only until March, 2009. As with the Medicaid program, states must follow broad federal guidelines, but they have the authority to determine eligibility and coverage. In all cases, enrollees must be low income, uninsured, and ineligible for Medicaid. Not all states choose to participate in the SCHIP program. Those that do participate must cover:

Inpatient and outpatient hospital services
Doctors' surgical and medical services
Laboratory and x-ray services
Well baby/child care, including immunizations

A Multivariate Act: Health Insurance Portability and Accountability Act (HIPAA)

Another act every PT manager and clinician and every PTA should be familiar with is HIPAA. HIPAA is administered by CMS. Its varied purposes are to:

"Improve portability and continuity of health insurance coverage in the group and individual markets
Combat waste, fraud, and abuse in health insurance and health care delivery
Promote the use of medical savings accounts
Improve access to long-term care services and coverage
Simplify the administration of health insurance and for other purposes" (HHS, 2007b).

There are five parts to HIPAA. The parts most relevant to PTs and PTAs are Titles I and II. Title I, Health Care Portability and Renewability, addresses the portability and continuity of health care insurance. Title II, Preventing Health Care Fraud and Abuse; Administrative Simplification; Medical Liability Reform, targets administrative simplification, waste reduction, fraud control, and privacy.

HIPPA—Title I

Title I, Health Care Portability, and Renewability protects health insurance coverage for workers and their families when they change or lose their jobs. This may help workers:

Increase their ability to get health coverage when starting a new job
Lower the chance of losing existing health care coverage

Maintain continuous health coverage when you change jobs
Buy health insurance coverage on your own if coverage is lost

HIPAA regulations accomplish this by limiting common methods health insurance plans have used to exclude some potential consumers. Prohibitions include: using preexisting condition exclusions, group health plans discriminating in coverage decisions based on past or present poor health, denying certain small employers and individuals the right to purchase health insurance, and guaranteeing that, in most cases, employers or individuals who purchase health insurance can renew the coverage regardless of any health conditions of individuals covered under the insurance policy.

HIPAA—Title II

Title II, Preventing Health Care Fraud and Abuse; Administrative Simplification; and Medical Liability Reform, set requirements for providers and health care organizations that are intended to reduce the costs and administrative burdens of health care. This is accomplished by making possible the standardized, electronic transmission of many administrative and financial transactions. Health information privacy is also a requirement of administrative simplification. Title II has had the greatest impact on health care organizations and providers in terms of time and resources. Rules to implement Title II have been categorized into three topics: security, electronic transactions and code sets, and privacy.

1. Security: The rule adopting standards for the security of electronic health information published in the **Federal Register** specifies "a series of administrative, technical, and physical security procedures for **covered entities** to use to assure the confidentiality of electronic protected health information. The standards are delineated into either required or addressable implementation specifications" (CMS, 2007a).
2. Electronic transactions and code sets: The rule adopting standards for the electronic

transactions and code sets for electronic health information establishes national standards that must be followed by all health care providers (including health care insurance plans) with the exception of retail pharmacies (CMS, 2007a). The goal is to establish a universal electronic language and a standardized health care information system that allows for the improved flow of information within and between organizations and thereby reduce the administrative costs of health care. The adoption of this rule impacted all health care providers, health plans, and health care **clearinghouses** that use electronic transmission for billing, collection of accounts, and/or communications involving health care information.

3. Privacy: The rule adopting standards for privacy applies to health information created or maintained by health care providers, health plans, and health care clearinghouses that engage in certain electronic transactions. These standards require covered entities to protect the privacy of individually identifiable health information referred to as *personal health information (PHI)* that applies to all entities. PHI is defined as all medical records and other individually identifiable health information held or disclosed by a covered entity in any form, whether communicated electronically, on paper or orally. Generally, the use of PHI is limited to health purposes only. General PHI use guidelines published by the *Office for Civil Rights (OCR)* (HHS, 2007c) advise that PHI can be used or disclosed by a covered entity only for purposes of health care treatment, payment, and operations. PHI disclosures must be limited to the minimum necessary for the purpose of the disclosure. This does not apply to the transfer of medical records for purposes of treatment. For nonroutine disclosures of PHI, patient authorization must be truly informed and voluntary. To ensure these requirements are met, covered entities are required to:

- Adopt written privacy procedures to include who has access to PHI, how it will be used within the entity, and when the information would/would not be disclosed
- Designate a privacy officer
- Establish grievance processes as a means

for patients to make inquiries or complaints regarding the privacy of their records
- Take steps to ensure that their **business associates** protect the privacy of PHI
- Train all employees to understand the new privacy protection procedures

The standards not only seek to control the flow of sensitive patient information but also to establish real penalties for the misuse or disclosure of this information. This latter rule gives patients new rights to understand and control how their personal health information is used. The OCR is responsible for implementing and enforcing the privacy regulation. According to the OCR (2007), the privacy rule has given patients the right to be educated about their rights related to privacy protection. Health care providers and health plans are required to provide each patient with written explanation of how they can use, keep, and disclose their health information. A signed acknowledgement receipt of this privacy notice by the patient or their authorized representative must be kept on record. The process entails the following actions:

1. Get copies of and request amendments to patient's records
2. Get a listing of all releases of their PHI. Covered entities must keep record of and be prepared to release information about most disclosures of a patient's PHI
3. Get consent in writing before PHI is released (health care providers are required to obtain patient consent before releasing PHI for treatment, payment, and health care operations purposes)
4. Obtain consent specifically for nonroutine uses and most nonhealth care purposes in a manner free from coercion for nonroutine disclosures
5. Complain to covered entities or the authorities about violations of any provision of the privacy rule (under HIPAA, covered entities that misuse PHI are subject to civil and federal criminal penalties)

Freedom of Information Act (FOIA)

FOIA impacts the availability of information. It is different from HIPPA in that it broadens access to certain types of government-generated information. FOIA stipulates that "any person can make requests for government information" (DOL, 2007b; Environmental Protection Agency, 2007). Persons requesting information are not required to identify themselves or explain why they want the information they have requested. All branches of the federal government must adhere to FOIA provisions. There are some restrictions for work in progress (early drafts), enforcement related confidential information, classified documents, and national security information. FOIA applies to government documentation related to health care facility licensure and quality of care reviews performed under the authority of the CMS. That means that any sanctions or performance deficiencies that are identified during government authorized health care facility or provider reviews/surveys are available to the public upon request.

Disadvantaged Minority Health Improvement Act

This act requires the **Office of Minority Health (OMH)** to enter into contracts to increase the access of **limited English proficiency (LEP)** persons to health care by developing programs to provide bilingual or interpreter services. Some states have also enacted laws that require providers to offer language assistance to LEP persons in many service settings (Office for Civil Rights, 2007).

The Omnibus Budget Reconciliation Act of 1989 (OBRA)

OBRA regulates **physician self-referral** as set forth in section 1877 of the Social Security Act. This law "prohibits physicians from referring Medicare patients for certain **designated health services (DHS)** to an entity with which the physician or a member of the physician's immediate family has a financial relationship—unless an exception applies" (Social Security Administration, 2007). Presenting or causing to be presented a bill or claim to anyone for a DHS, as a result of a prohibited referral is also not allowed. The provision for section 1877 was included in OBRA and is known as *Stark I*, named for its chief congressional sponsor,

Congressman Pete Stark (CMS, 2007b). The final rule that incorporated the physician self-referral prohibition as it applied to clinical laboratory services was published on August 14, 1995.

What has transpired since Stark I has become extremely complicated, as you will see in the next act, which deals with subsequent related legislation.

Omnibus Budget Reconciliation Act of 1993

This act expanded Section 1877 noted earlier. This 1993 Act included 10 additional DHS provisions related to the Medicaid program (Buto, 2007): These expanded provisions became known as *Stark II*. This legislation affected physician referral to businesses that provided the following services or equipment if they or a family member owned the business:

1. Durable medical equipment and supplies
2. Home health services
3. Inpatient and outpatient hospital services
4. Occupational therapy
5. Orthotics, prosthetics, and prosthetic devices and supplies
6. Outpatient prescription drugs
7. Parenteral and enteral nutrients, equipment, and supplies
8. Physical therapy (Chapter 22)
9. Radiology services
10. Radiation therapy services and supplies

In 1997, a provision was added to permit the Secretary of HHS to issue written advisory opinions addressing whether a referral related to DHS was or was not prohibited under section 1877. In response to this legislation, the CMS published regulations addressing the physician self-referral prohibition (Social Security Administration, 2007). The final rule covering the additional DHS services was published in two phases. Stark II, Phase I, 42 CFR Parts 411 and 424 Medicare and Medicaid Programs; Physicians' Referrals to Health Care Entities With Which They Have Financial Relationships; Final Rule was published on January 4, 2001. Stark II, Phase II, Interim Final Rule was published on March 26, 2004 (CMS, 2007b,c).

The Stark II, phase III final rule was published on September 5, 2007 and effective December 4, 2007. This final rule amends the regulations regarding physician self-referral, finalizing and responding to public comment regarding the Phase II final rule. While Stark II Phase III did include some changes, it did not include as many changes that health care industry **stakeholders** were expecting (CMS, 2007d; Sender and Watt, 2007). Among the areas not addressed in Stark III were:

A narrowing of the definition of in-office ancillary services that qualifies as an exemption to the self-referral prohibition
Compensation of faculty physicians
Determination of fair market value related to the lease of office space
Intra-family rural referrals
Nonmonetary physician compensation
Payment of physician productivity bonuses
Physician recruitment
Professional courtesy write-offs
Retention payments in underserved areas
See Additional Resources for Stark III updates. Chapter 10 will discuss additional referral for profit acts.

Ryan White Care Act

This provides HIV/AIDS primary health care treatment and support services for low-income individuals. It includes programs that provide medications to fight HIV. Ryan White funds go to eligible local communities hit hardest by HIV.

Health Care Fraud and Abuse

The *Federal False Claims Act* has been used by federal law enforcement to fight alleged cases of health care fraud. According to the American Medical Association (AMA), the False Claims Act provides for treble damages and mandatory fines of $5,000–$10,000 per claim and can result in payments of millions of dollars. Under the False Claims Act prosecutors do not have to prove intent to defraud federal programs (Reardon, 1997).

As mentioned earlier, HIPAA represents a consolidation of government efforts to fight health care fraud and abuse. The Act established a comprehensive program to combat fraud committed against all health plans, both public and private. The legislation required the establishment of a national **Health Care Fraud and Abuse Control Program (HCFAC)**. The HCFAC is under the joint direction of the Attorney General and the Secretary of the HHS acting through the Department's Inspector General (Department of Justice [DOJ], 2007). The HCFAC program is intended to coordinate federal, state, and local law enforcement efforts to stop health care fraud and abuse. The HCFAC is an active enforcement program that has returned more than 8.85 billion dollars to the Medicare Trust Fund. In the fiscal year 2005, the U.S. Attorney's office opened 935 new criminal health care fraud investigations and filed criminal charges in 382 cases (DOJ, 2007). State and local laws regulate health care organization and professional licensure, facility design and operation, and many other topics related to health care regulation.

Summary

This chapter focused on federal laws that are most relevant to health care organizations and providers. Many of these laws apply to all types of business organizations; others apply just to organizations in the health care sector. Health care organizations and providers are therefore subject to many regulations that cover almost all aspects of their operations. The areas of regulation that are of particular interest to clinical health care managers are related to: employment practices, financial management, environmental protection, food and drug manufacture, health care access, health care fraud and abuse, health care operations and clinical practice, and reporting and compliance practices.

In order to comply with regulatory requirements, health care providers must become familiar with the sources and types of regulation impacting the operations of their organization. There are many external and internal experts that can be of assistance. One of the keys to effective regulatory compliance is the adoption of a CCP. Failure to comply can result in loss of license to practice, exclusion from participation in government financed health care programs, or fines. The influence of state government in the practice of physical therapy was covered in Chapter 9 and will be discussed again in Chapter 10. With the amount of attention the authors have given to the legal aspects of being a health service pro-vider, manager, and organization it should be clear that legal business and clinical practices are crucial components of health care quality.

CASE STUDY 9.1

Getting Information from the Source(s)

An act is another term for a law. Acts that affect the health of the population, health care providers of services, goods and equip-ment, and payment for services, goods and equipment are continuously being enacted. The essence of this case study is for you to explore an act that has, does, or will affect you as a PT or PTAs. You should come to know more about your chosen act than your peers.

You will need to:

1. Identify a health care act that that inter-ests you as a clinician, manager/owner, researcher, educator, or consumer. This chapter discussed many of the impor-tant health care related acts but there are others you may be interested in.
2. Develop a progressive in-depth strategy to learn as much as you can about your chosen act in 4 hours of research. Start with written and electronic resources available from APTA sources. If you choose legislation after 1999, your cul-minating resource should be the original act as published in the Federal Register (http://www.archives.gov/federal-regis-ter/). If your act is older, your ultimate resource is likely to be documents pro-vided by the government agency respon-sible for administrating your chosen act, i.e., CMS documents (http://www.cms.hhs.gov/default.asp?) for the history of prospective payment regulations.
3. Implement your strategy.
4. Prepare a 2–5-page paper summariz-ing your information and your impres-sions about how various segments of the health care community and/or health care consumers were/are/will be impacted by the legislation.
5. Discuss your findings with your peers noting how this act relates to your pro-fession.
6. Respond to questions. If necessary, carry out additional research to formulate appropriate responses based on authori-tative references.

CASE STUDY 9.2

A Difference of Opinion

Background

The physician self-referral legislation includes discussion of physician supervision of and billing for services of ancillary per-sonnel. This has been termed billing "inci-dent to" physician services.

A few years ago, the National Athletic Trainer's Association made efforts to be included as ancillary personnel. This would allow physicians to bill for services provided by trainers they employed.

Your Tasks

1. Become familiar with the law. Consult governmental resources recommended in Additional Resources.
2. Become familiar with the issues. Consult the APTA and NATA websites.
3. Summarize your findings.
4. Based on this example, discuss how regu-lation affects clinical practice.

REFERENCES

Aguilar L. Scandals jolting faith of investors. Denver Post, June 27, 2002.

Americans With Disabilities Act. A guide to disabilities rights laws, August, 2001. Available at http://ada.gov/cguide.htm. Accessed 8/15/07.

Buto K. Testimony on physician self-referral regulations. Available at http://www.hhs.gov/asl/testify/t990513a.html. Accessed 8/15/07.

Centers of Medicare and Medicaid Services. Programs. Available at http://www.cms.hhs.gov. Accessed 8/10/07a.

Centers for Medicare and Medicaid Services. Physician self-referral: Overview. Available at http://www.cms.hhs.gov/PhysicianSelfReferral/. Accessed 10/26/07b.

Centers for Medicare and Medicaid Services. Federal Register, 42 CFR Parts 411 and 424 Medicare Program; Physicians' referrals to health care entities with which they have financial relationships (Phase II); Interim final rule. March 26, 2004. Available at http://www.cms.hhs.gov/PhysicianSelfReferral/Downloads/69FR16054.pdf. Accessed 10/26/07c.

Centers for Medicare and Medicaid Services. Phase III. Available at http://www.cms.hhs.gov/PhysicianSelfReferral/04a_regphase3.asp#TopOfPage. Accessed 10/26/07d.

Conover CJ. Health Care Regulation, A $169 Billion Hidden Tax. Policy Analysis, No.527, October 4, 2002. Available at http://www.cato.org/pubs/pas/pa527.pdf. Accessed 8/10/07.

Department of Health and Human Services. Department of Health and Human Services Organizational Chart. Available at http//www.hhs.gov/about/orgchart.html. Accessed 8/10/07a.

Department of Health and Human Services. Public Law 104-191. Available at http://aspe.hhs.gov/admnsimp/pl104191.htm. Accessed 8/15/07b.

Department of Health and Human Services. Testimony on physician self-referral regulations by Department of Health and Human Services and Office for Civil Rights. HIPAA Administrative Simplification. Available at http://www.hhs.gov/ocr/AdminSimpRegText.pdf. Accessed 8/10/07c.

Department of Justice. Department of Health and Human Services and the Department of Justice Health Care Fraud and Abuse Control Program Annual Report For FY 2005. Available at http://oig.hhs.gov/publications/docs/hcfac/hcfacreport2005.pdf. Accessed 8/15/07.

Department of Labor. Major laws. Available at http://www.dol.gov/opa/aboutdol/lawsprog.htm. Accessed 8/10/07a.

Department of Labor. Freedom of Information Act. Available at http://www.dol.gov/dol/foia/main.htm. Accessed 8/10/07b.

Drug Enforcement Administration. Homepage. Available at http://www.dea.gov. Accessed 8/15/07.

Engel DA, Calderone BJ, Lederman BG, Wesolik CJ, Warnick MP. Human resources issues. In Health

Insurance Portability And Accountability Act of 1996 Public Law 104-191 August 21, 1996. Available at http://aspe.dhhs.gov/admnsimp/pl104191.htm. Accessed 8/15/07.

Environmental Protection Agency. Freedom of Information Act. Available at http://www.epa.gov/foia. Accessed 8/10/07.

Jones J. The CEO Refresher. When is it time to rewrite your mission statement? Available at http://www.refresher.com/!jjmission.html. Accessed 4/13/07.

Longest BB Jr, Rakich JS, Darr K. Managing health services organizations and systems, 4th ed. Baltimore, MD: Health Professions. 2000.

Matyas DE, Valiant C. Legal issues in healthcare fraud and abuse: Navigating uncertainties, 3rd ed. Washington, DC: American Health Lawyers Association. 2006.

National Environmental Policy Act of 1969 (NEPA); (42 U.S.C. 4321-4347) 2007. Available at http://ceq.eh.doe.gov/nepa. Accessed 2/01/03.

Nolan JR, Nolan-Haley JM. Black's Law Dictionary, 6th ed. St. Paul, MN: West. 1990.

Office of Inspector General of the U.S. Department of Health and Human Services and The American Health Lawyers Association. Corporate responsibility and corporate compliance: A resource for health care boards of directors available at http://oig.hhs.gov/fraud/docs/complianceguidance/040203CorpRespRsceGuide.pdf. Accessed 4/15/07.

Reardon TR. Health care fraud and abuse update, report of the board of trustees of the AMA 25-I-97. 1997. Available at http://www.ama.org. Accessed 2/01/03.

Securities and Exchange Commission. Self-Regulatory Organization (SRO) Rulemaking and National Market System (NMS) Plans. Available at http://www.sec.gov/. Accessed 8/10/07.

Sender JP, Watt TN. Hospital law note: Stark II Phase III final rule. Health Care News. Smith Moore LLC., September 2007.

Small Business Notes. Definition of financial management. Available at http://www.smallbusinessnotes.com/glossary/deffinancialmanagement.html. Accessed 5/19/07.

Social Security Administration. Limitation on certain physician referrals. Available at http://www.ssa.gov/OP_Home/ssact/title18/1877.htm. Accessed 10/26/07.

State of Ohio. White Paper. Health Insurance Portability and Accountability Act of 1996 (HIPAA) Overview of HIPAA, Title I through Title V April, 2002. Available at http://hipaa.ohio.gov/whitepapers/overviewofhipaa.PDF. Accessed 9/29/07.

Swayne LE, Duncan WJ, Ginter PM. Strategic management of health care organizations, 5th ed. Malden, MA: Blackwell. 2006.

Waggoner J, Fogarty TA. Scandals shred investors' faith: Because of Enron, Andersen and rising gas prices, the public is more wary than ever of corporate America. USA Today, May 5, 2002.

ADDITIONAL RESOURCES

For physical therapy specific information on selected legal matters the website of the American Physical Therapy Association (http://www.apta.org) see practice and governmental affairs links.

An overview of visa information may be found at http://www.usaimmigrationservices.org. A web-based training course on Medicare and Medicaid fraud and abuse can be found through the CMS web site (http://www.cms.gov) to access http://cms.meridianksi.com/kc/ilc/course_info_enroll_lnkfrm_f1.asp?lgnfrm=wbt&table=crs&function=course_info_enroll&strBuildingID=5&strFunctionID=37&strFunctionPath=37.&strFrom=Search&topic=All&keywords=. Information about state and local health care regulation is available through official government websites that can be located through http://firstgov.gov and http://usasearch.gov/. Profiles of Health Care Compliance Officers can be found on the Health Care Compliance Association Website at http://www.hcca-info.org/Content/NavigationMenu/Compliance Resources/Surveys/Annual_Surveys.htm. The official regulations on hospital compliance programs can be found in the Federal Register, Vol 70, No. 19, Monday, January 31, 2005 available at http://oig.hhs.gov/publications/docs/press/2005/012705release.pdf. For more information on the administrative simplification portion of HIPAA, particularly covered entities, consult http://www.cms.hhs.gov/HIPAAGenInfo/06_AreYouaCoveredEntity.asp. Stark Laws can be located at http://www.cms.hhs.gov/PhysicianSelfReferral/. In addition, CMS publishes an updated "List of Codes" annually in the Federal Register (http://www.gpoaccess.gov/fr/) that lists the CMS **Common Procedure Coding System (HCPCS)** and **Current Procedural Terminology (CPT)** codes for four of the DHS that the physician self-referral prohibition applies. The List of Codes can be located at http://www.cms.hhs.gov/PhysicianSelfReferral/11_List_of_Codes.asp#TopOfPage.

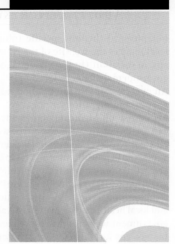

CHAPTER 10

EXTERNAL OVERSIGHT OF HEALTH SERVICE PROVIDERS

DEBORAH G. FRIBERG

Learning Objectives

1. Discuss the purpose of external oversight and examine the implications for health service providers.
2. Become familiar with the sources, forms, and implications of external health service oversight, including names, acronyms, and general authorities of oversight government agencies and private organizations.
3. Define trends in oversight regulations and examine the implications for health services providers.
4. Identify the most common government agencies that managers of health services are likely to have contact with on behalf of their organization.
5. Access information about oversight regulations and standards from Internet based sources.
6. Access sources of information about the practical implications of external oversight regulations and performance standards.
7. Correctly define and utilize common government health care related agencies' terminology in oral and written communications.
8. Examine the purposes and processes of risk management in health service settings.
9. Analyze the components of the risk management process.

Introduction

Many government agencies and departments were introduced and discussed in Chapters 8 and 9 to familiarize the reader with their names, general areas of health care involvement, and basic compliance requirements. This chapter builds on this background as it adds depth to the concepts of external voluntary and mandated health care *oversight*, compliance, and **risk reduction**.

Oversight is commonly defined as watchful care. The involvement of government agencies and private groups in oversight of businesses has proven to be one of the most effective techniques to protect the public from harm. Oversight can prevent waste and *fraud*, protect civil liberties and individual rights, accumulate information useful to lawmakers and education of the public, ensure compliance with laws, and critically evaluate performance (Department of State, 2007) (Chapter 9). As stories about corporate responsibility, health care costs, health care quality, and patient safety fill the headlines the attention on the external oversight of health service organizations has continued to escalate.

Oversight occurs when a party external to an organization reviews the activities of that organization for the purpose of evaluating their performance. As a result of this trend, the number and type of organizations engaged in the oversight of health care businesses, including individual clinical practice has

Key Terms

Key terms, which are defined below, are bolded and italicized the first time they appear in the chapter. Other important terms are shown in boldface on first appearance and are defined by the context in which they are used. When either of these types of terms is used several times, its acronym will be identified and subsequently used in the chapter. Both types of terms are listed alphabetically in the online glossary with their definitions and (when applicable) their acronyms.

abuse: misuse, hurt, or injure by neglect or harm. Typically the victim is someone who is vulnerable (aged, child, mentally compromised, etc.).

Agency for Healthcare Research and Quality (AHRQ): supports research designed to improve health care quality, reduce cost, improve patient safety, reduce medical errors, and improve access to essential services through the generation of evidence-based information on health care outcomes; quality, cost, use, and access.

The Commission on Accreditation of Rehabilitation Facilities (CARF): an international, independent, not-for-profit organization that promotes quality, value, and optimal outcomes of services through accreditation of human service providers.

Centers for Disease Control and Prevention (CDC): federal agency with the mission of promoting health and quality of life by preventing and controlling disease, injury, and disability. Among its responsibilities are national health statistics and workplace safety.

Department of Health and Human Services (HHS): the federal government department that oversees health related matters through 11 divisions: Administration for Children and Families (ACF), Administration on Aging (AoA), Agency for Healthcare Research and Quality (AHRQ), Centers for Disease Control and Prevention (CDC), Centers for Medicare and Medicaid Services (CMS), Food and Drug Administration (FDA), Health Resources and Services Administration (HRSA), Indian Health Services, National Institutes of Health, Substance Abuse and Mental Health Services Administration (SAMHSA), and U.S. Public Health Service Commissioned Corps.

fraud: intentional misrepresentation in a manner that could cause harm. For example, billing Medicare for services that were not provided.

General Accounting Office (GAO): exists to support the Congress in meeting its Constitutional responsibilities and to help improve the performance and ensure the accountability of the federal government for the American people.

Health Plan Employer Data and Information Set (HEDIS): a National Committee for Quality Assurance proprietary survey instrument used to measure managed-care plan performance in key areas like immunization and mammography screening rates. Used for comparing managed-health care plans' performance on standardized measures.

Health Resources and Services Administration (HRSA): funds more than 4,000 primary and preventive health service sites nationwide to assure services for poor and uninsured people living in rural or urban areas where health care is scarce. HRSA also oversees the national organ transplantation system.

Joint Commission (JC): formerly called the Joint Commission on Accreditation of Healthcare Organizations (JACHO). A nongovernmental, not-for-profit accreditation agency that develops professional standards against which the compliance of health service organizations is evaluated.

Medicare Payment Advisory Commission (MedPac): an independent federal body that advises the U.S. Congress on issues affecting the Medicare program. The members meet publicly to discuss policy issues and formulate recommendations to the Congress on improving Medicare policies. Issues addressed include payment for physical therapists and others.

National Committee for Quality Assurance (NCQA): a private not-for-profit organization that accredits managed-care plans (HMO, PPO, POS). Many private and government employers require that their health plans have NCQA certification making managed-care organizations seek NCQA accreditation.

National Institutes of Health (NIH): a medical research organization with the mission of science in pursuit of fundamental knowledge about the nature and behavior of living systems and the application of that knowledge to extend healthy life and reduce the burdens of illness and disability. It includes 27 separate health institutes, the National Center for

(Continued)

Complementary and Alternative Medicine, and the National Library of Medicine.

National Labor Relations Board (NLRB): an independent federal agency that administers the National Labor Relations Act, the primary law governing relations between unions and employers in the private sector. The Board grants employees the right to organize and bargain collectively with their employers or to refrain from all such activity.

Occupational Safety and Health Administration (OSHA): assures the safety and health of America's workers by setting and enforcing standards; providing training, outreach, and education; establishing partnerships; and encouraging continual improvement in workplace safety and health through workplace inspection and investigation, compliance assistance, and cooperative programs.

Offices of the Inspectors General (OIG): there is an inspectors general office in 57 of the 59 federal agencies. There is one for the Department of Human Services. OIG's central purpose is to prevent fraud and abuse. The OIG reports to the head of each agency and to congress.

oversight: watchful care. Private groups and government agencies provide oversight of health care businesses to: protect the public from harm by preventing waste and fraud; protecting civil liberties and individual rights; accumulating information useful to lawmakers and for educating the public; ensuring compliance with laws; and, critically evaluating performance.

risk(s): the probability of suffering harm or loss. In health services risk exists for the individual providing services, and if employed, the employer, and if working under a medical referral, the referring practitioner.

watchdog group(s): a private or government organization that watches for illegal or unethical conduct and alerts others of these acts.

proliferated. Oversight can come from governmental agencies, nongovernmental organizations operating under government contracts, or nongovernmental private organizations.

Historically, oversight that originates within private organizations has been voluntary while governmental oversight has been nonvoluntary. Today, many private oversight organizations are performing their oversight activities using publicly available data without or with only marginal involvement of the health service providers. Oversight has long been tied to a provider's ability to participate under private and governmental insurance programs. Another more recent trend in the clinical oversight arena has been to tie participation in oversight activities to payment rates. Health service providers who choose not to participate can be subject to lower reimbursement rates or participants can be subject to receive higher rates or performance bonuses. These types of oversight programs are often referred to as **pay for performance** (P4P). P4P programs are being used by both governmental and private insurance plans as an incentive for improved clinical practices. There is an expectation that many of the P4P programs will become nonvoluntary over time.

Oversight that comes from governmental agencies or nongovernmental organizations operating under government contract originates in and derives authority for enforcement of federal, state, or local laws. Government regulations are rules that carry the same weight as a law (Finkler and Ward, 1999). The U.S. health services industry, due to its size and importance, is one of the most-regulated industries in the United States economy. The attention to the health services industry comes in part from the government's obligation to protect the health and well-being of its citizens. This obligation is met through laws and related regulations that are designed to prevent illness or injury, provide access to health care services, and ensure that the available health care services are safe and effective (Chapters 8 and 9). The move toward increasing regulation is also driven by the financial realities discussed in detail in Chapter 2. Since the creation of the **Medicare** and **Medicaid** programs, the federal government has become the largest purchaser of health care services in the United States (Chapter 2). As the expense burden of providing health care to the sick, poor, and elderly (Chapter 1) continues to consume an ever larger portion of the tax dollar, more attention will be paid to eliminating payment fraud and *abuse* as well as controlling the quantity and quality of services provided.

The enforcement of the law is delegated to one or more governmental agencies, bureaus, departments, or offices. These government entities in turn formulate the rules or regulations to enforce the law. Oversight activities can be performed directly by the governmental entity or outsourced to another governmental or private oversight organization.

Those who are new to the health services industry are often surprised by the amount and diversity of the regulations with which health care organizations and providers must comply. It falls to the individual health service organization and/or provider to know and to follow all applicable regulations (Chapter 9). According to the **federal sentencing guidelines**, which set sentencing guidelines to eliminate disparity in how defendants are sentenced, the legal penalties for noncompliance can be significant to include (Matyas and Valiant, 2006):

- Loss of the opportunity to treat government-covered clients
- Loss of credentials to provide health care services
- Payment of one or more fines
- Recoupment of previous payments
- Imprisonment

The health services regulatory landscape seems to change almost daily. The amount, diversity, and frequent changes in regulations make **regulatory compliance** a real and costly challenge. It should be noted that ignorance of the law is generally unacceptable as a defense against a legal action. Regulatory compliance is best achieved through the adoption of an effective **Corporate Compliance Program** as discussed in Chapter 9.

Health service providers often turn to private oversight organizations to demonstrate the quality of their services and preempt the proliferation of nonvoluntary governmental oversight. Private oversight organizations may provide general and/or service specific accreditations, certifications, registrations, and recognitions to health service providers that meet specified standards of practice and/or performance. Under some circumstances, health services providers may choose voluntary participation in private oversight as an alternative to governmental oversight. This concept will be discussed in more detail under the topic of the *Joint Commission (JC)* formerly known as the Joint Commission on Accreditation of Health Organizations (JCAHO).

Note: Given the rapidly changing regulatory environment along with geographical and organizational differences, the information contained in this chapter should be verified for continued accuracy and applicability to an individual health services organization or provider. It remains the responsibility of the health care organization/provider to identify and comply with all applicable regulations. Much of the material in this chapter comes from various websites that readers can access on their own. The material in the chapter can be used as a guide to governmental and private oversight organizations.

Source of External Oversight

External oversight for health service organizations and individual providers can come from:

1. Governmental agencies
2. Nongovernmental organizations operating under government contracts
3. Nongovernmental private organizations acting independently of the government or the health service provider
4. Nongovernmental private organizations acting under agreement with the health service provider

Organizations that set performance standards and/or provide external oversight to health services organizations and individual providers are numerous and varied (see Chapter 16).

Government Oversight

Governmental oversight occurs at the federal, state, and local level as mandated by law. The enforcement of laws falls to government entities. Government entities are charged with the responsibility to (1) develop specific regulations to ensure the enforcement of the law and (2) either directly or in collaboration with other government entities ensure compliance with the regulations. It is not unusual for government agencies to contract with private review organizations to fulfill their responsibilities. For example the **Centers for Medicare and Medicaid Services** (**CMS**) contracts with several private insurance organizations to perform the role of **fiscal intermediary** to manage provider claims review and payments (Department of Health and Human Services [HHS], 2007a). A listing of all fiscal intermediaries can be found in the *Intermediary Carrier Directory* (CMS, 2007). The federal government also contracts with state and local governments for oversight services. Government regulations affect most of the service delivery, payment, and operations of health care providers including:

- Business and financial management practices
- Facility design, construction, and operation
- Organizational structure
- Patient accounts management
- Personnel practices
- Service delivery
- Service documentation
- Service evaluation

Full cooperation with the regulatory review process is mandatory. Failure to participate and/or cooperate could result in cancellation of a provider's **participation agreement** with government-funded health programs or loss of licensure to operate.

Federal Government Departments and Agencies Involved in the Oversight of Health Service Providers

Department of Health and Human Services (HHS)

HHS is the federal government's principal agency for the enforcement of laws related to protecting the health and providing essential human services to all Americans, especially for those least able to help themselves (HHS, 2007b). The department provides a broad range of services including more than 300 programs. The scope of HHS is far-reaching and best demonstrated by its organizational chart showing the 11 operating divisions in Figure 10.1. Its programs cover a broad spectrum of activities including:

- Assuring food and drug safety
- Comprehensive health services for Native Americans
- Health and social science research
- Health information technology
- Faith-based and community initiatives
- Financial assistance and services for low-income families
- Head Start (preschool education and services)
- Improving maternal and infant health
- Medical preparedness for emergencies, including potential terrorism
- Medicare (health insurance for elderly and disabled Americans) and Medicaid (health insurance for low-income people)
- Preventing child abuse and domestic violence
- Preventing disease, including immunization services
- Services for older Americans, including home-delivered meals
- Substance abuse treatment and prevention (HHS, 2007b)

HHS works closely with state, local, and tribal government agencies often working through these nonfederal government agencies or private sector contractors to deliver its services and for regulatory enforcement. HHS handles almost a quarter of all federal outlays, provides more grant than all other federal agencies combined. It is the nation's largest health care insurer handling more than 1 billion claims per year. In 2006, HHS employed 66,890 people and had a budget of $697.5 billion dollars (HHS, 2007c).

HHS administers its programs through 11 operating divisions that include eight Public Health Service agencies and three human service agencies. Health service providers can learn more abut any of these divisions and the services they provide by consulting the information provided online at www.hhs.gov.

Administration for Children and Families (ACF)

ACF has responsibility for 60 programs that promote the economic and social well-being of families, children, individuals, and communities including the state–federal welfare program and Temporary Assistance to Needy Families. ACF also administers the Head Start

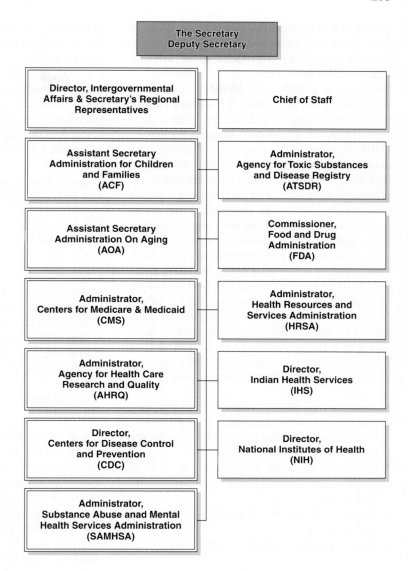

Figure 10.1. Department of Health and Human Services: Organization of 11 operating divisions. (Source: http://www.hhs.gov/about/orgchart.html.)

Program, provides funds to assist low-income families in paying for childcare, support state programs to provide for foster care and adoption assistance, and programs to prevent child abuse and domestic violence. In 2007, ACF employed 1,280 people and had a budget of $47.0 billion dollars (HHS, 2007).

Administration on Aging (AoA)

AoA is the advocate agency for older persons and their concerns. The AoA administers federal programs mandated under various titles of the Older Americans Act that help vulnerable older persons in their own homes. AoA funding provides supportive services, including

nutrition programs like home delivered meals (Meals on Wheels) as well as health enhancement programs. The AoA works with state and local agencies on aging to develop, plan, and coordinate community services that meet the needs of older persons and their caregivers. In 2007, AoA employed 115 people and managed a budget of $1.4 billion dollars (HHS, 2007).

Centers for Medicare and Medicaid Services (CMS)

Formerly known as the Health Care Financing Administration (HCFA), CMS administers the Medicare and Medicaid programs. The Medicare program provides health insurance for the elderly and some disabled individuals. It serves more than 43.8 million Americans. The Medicaid program is a joint federal–state program that provides health coverage for 49.1 million low-income elderly and children. CMS also administers the new **State Children's Health Insurance Program (SCHIP)** in collaboration with HRSA via state-based plans (Chapter 2). SCHIP is expected to provide health care coverage for a projected 4.2 million uninsured children. For more detailed information about Medicare, Medicaid, and SCHIP programs see Chapter 2. CMS is of particular interest to health care organizations and providers as it is the nation's largest health care payer. In that role, it sets many of the standards for health care delivery. CMS also regulates all laboratory testing (except research) performed on humans. CMS's stated mission is to assure health care security for beneficiaries. In fiscal year (FY) 2007, CMS employed 4,538 people and had a budget of $569.78 billion dollars (HHS, 2007). In administering the Medicare, Medicaid, and SCHIP programs, CMS:

- Assures that these programs are properly run by its contractors and state agencies
- Establishes payment policies for health care providers
- Conducts research on various methods of health care management, treatment, and financing
- Assesses the quality of health care facilities and services
- Takes action to enforce its regulations

Agency for Healthcare Research and Quality (AHRQ)

AHRQ supports research designed to improve health care quality, reduce cost, improve patient safety, reduce medical errors, and improve access to essential services. AHRQ-sponsored research provides evidence-based information on health care outcomes; quality; and cost, use, and access. Health care policy makers, leaders, providers, and patients can use this information to make more informed decisions about health care services. An example of AHRQ efforts was the introduction of a standardized survey, Hospital Consumer Assessment of Healthcare Providers and Systems (CAHPS), to be used in a CMS initiative

to measure patients' experiences with ambulatory and facility-level care. This hospital patient survey was requested by the CMS as a way to provide comparison information for consumers who need to select a hospital and as a way of encouraging accountability of hospitals for the care they provide (AHRQ, 2007). In 2007, AHQR employed 296 people and had a budget of $319 million dollars (HHS, 2007).

Centers for Disease Control and Prevention (CDC)

The CDC works with state and local government as well as other partners to provide a health surveillance system to:

- Monitor and prevent disease outbreaks (including bioterrorism)
- Implement disease prevention strategies
- Maintain national health statistics
- Provide for immunization services
- Provide for workplace safety
- Provide for environmental disease prevention
- Guard against international disease transmission

The CDC's mission is to promote health and quality of life by preventing and controlling disease, injury, and disability (CDC, 2007). Some examples offered by the CDC include the use of innovative "fingerprinting" technology to identify a food borne illness, evaluating family violence prevention programs, training partners in HIV education, and protecting children from preventable diseases through immunizations. In 2007, the CDC employed 8,823 people and had a budget of $6 billion dollars.

Agency for Toxic Substances and Disease Registry (ATSDR)

ATSDR helps prevent exposures to hazardous substances from waste sites considered to be a priority by the Environmental Protection Agency. The ATSDR is under the direction of the Director of the CDC (HHS, 2007).

Food and Drug Administration (FDA)

The FDA has the responsibility to assure the safety of foods and cosmetics, as well as the safety and efficacy of pharmaceuticals, biological products, and medical devices. These are products that represent 25 cents out of every dollar of U.S. consumer spending. In 2007 it employed 9,823 people and had a budget of 2.0 billion dollars (HHS, 2007).

Health Resources and Services Administration (HRSA)

HRSA provides access to poor and uninsured people living in rural or urban areas where health care is scarce. HRSA-funded health centers provide primary and preventive medical care serving 16 million patients each year at more than 4,000 sites nationwide in FY 2007. HRSA also works in partnership with state and community organizations, supports healthy mothers and children programs, and provides support services for people fighting HIV/AIDS through the **Ryan White Care Act** programs. HRSA also oversees the national organ transplantation system. In 2007, HRSA employed more than 1,487 people and had a budget of $6.4 billion dollars (HHS, 2007).

Indian Health Service (IHS)

The HIS operates hospitals, health centers, school health centers, and health stations in rural and urban areas that provide services to nearly 1.8 million American Indians and Alaska Natives of 560 federally recognized tribes. In 2007, IHS employed more than 15.331 people and had a budget of $4.09 billion dollars (HHS, 2007).

National Institutes of Health (NIH)

NIH is a medical research organization that supports more than 38,000 research projects for diseases like cancer, Alzheimer's, AIDS, arthritis, and heart ailments. NIH includes 27 separate health institutes, the National Center for Complementary and Alternative Medicine, and the National Library of Medicine. According to NIH (2007) its mission is science in pursuit of fundamental knowledge about the nature and behavior of living systems and the application of that knowledge to extend healthy life and reduce the burdens of illness and disability. NIH goals are to:

1. Foster fundamental creative discoveries, innovative research strategies, and their applications as a basis to advance significantly the nation's capacity to protect and improve health.
2. Develop, maintain, and renew scientific human and physical resources that will assure the nation's capability to prevent disease.
3. Expand the knowledge base in medical and associated sciences in order to enhance the nation's economic well-being and ensure a continued high return on the public investment in research.
4. Exemplify and promote the highest level of scientific integrity, public accountability, and social responsibility in the conduct of science.

In 2002, NIH employed 17,216 people and had a budget of $29.2 billion dollars (HHS, 2007).

Substance Abuse and Mental Health Services Administration (SAMHSA)

SAMHSA was established to improve the quality and availability of substance abuse prevention, addiction treatment, and mental health services. It provides federal block grants to states to support and maintain substance abuse and mental health services. SAMHSA provides funding for hundreds of programs nationwide to increase the use of proven prevention and treatment methods through Knowledge Development and Application grants. In 2007 SAMHSA employed 558 people and had a budget of $3.3 billion dollars (HHS, 2007).

Department of Justice (DOJ)

The DOJ has a mission to "to enforce the law and defend the interests of the United States according to the law; to ensure public safety against threats foreign and domestic; to provide federal leadership in preventing and controlling crime; to seek just punishment for those guilty of unlawful behavior; and to ensure fair and impartial administration of justice for all Americans" (DOJ, 2007).

There are two DOJ initiatives that have specifically impacted health service organizations and providers. The first is a joint initiative between the **Antitrust Division of the DOJ** and **Federal Trade Commission (FTC)** related to the enforcement of antitrust regulation in health care (FTC, 2007). The second is the DOJ focus enforcement of federal regulations related to health care charge setting and billing practices. According to the Department of Health and Human Services, the FY 2008 Budget Request, designed under the joint direction of the DOJ and HHS, includes resources and legislation to strengthen program oversight and reduce improper payments in the Medicare and Medicaid programs (HHS, 2007b).

Department of Labor (DOL)

The DOL "fosters and promotes the welfare of the job seekers, wage earners, and retirees of the United States by improving their working conditions, advancing their opportunities for profitable employment, protecting their retirement and health care benefits, helping employers find workers, strengthening free collective bargaining, and tracking changes in employment, prices, and other national economic measurements" (DOL, 2007). In carrying out this mission, the DOL administers a number of Federal labor laws related to workers' rights to safe and healthful working conditions, a minimum hourly wage, overtime pay, employment discrimination, unemployment insurance, and other income support. Health service organizations and providers are subject to the regulations administered by the DOL.

Drug Enforcement Administration (DEA)

The DEA has a mission "to enforce the controlled substances laws and regulations of the United States and bring to the criminal and civil justice system of the United States, or any other competent jurisdiction, those organizations and principal members of organizations, involved in the growing, manufacture, or distribution of controlled substances appearing in or destined for illicit traffic in the United States; and to recommend and support non-enforcement programs aimed at reducing the availability of illicit controlled substances on the domestic and international markets" (DEA, 2007).

The DEA is responsible for enforcing the U.S. controlled substances laws and regulations. Examples of DEA responsibilities that pertain to health service organizations and providers include:

- Enforcement of the provisions of the **Controlled Substances Act (CSA)**as they pertain to the manufacture, distribution, and dispensing of legally produced controlled substances
- Investigation and preparation for the prosecution of major violators of controlled substance laws
- Investigation and preparation for prosecution of criminals and drug gangs

The DEA's **Office of Diversion Control** is responsible for the diversion of controlled pharmaceuticals and controlled chemicals. In enforcing the CSA, Title II of the **Comprehensive Drug Abuse Prevention and Control Act of 1970**, the DEA is involved in the regulation of the manufacture and distribution of narcotics, stimulants, depressants, hallucinogens, anabolic steroids, and chemicals that could be used in the illicit production of controlled substances.

Environmental Protection Agency (EPA)

The EPA has a mission "to protect human health and the environment. Since 1970, EPA has been working for a cleaner, healthier environment for the American people" (EPA, 2007). The EPA works with health service providers and biotech firms to:

- Reduce waste, including mercury use
- Encourage product stewardship.
- Evaluate waste management rules and policies that impact health service facilities.

Another example of the EPA's role in health care is the production of materials to encourage health care professionals to educate patients on the safe disposal of "sharps" (lancets, needles, and syringes) in hard plastic or metal containers with screw-on or tightly secured lids. In addition, the **Waste Tracking Act** of 1989 amended the **Solid Waste Disposal Act** to require the EPA to promulgate regulations for the management of infectious waste.

Federal Accounting Standards Advisory Board (FASAB)

The FASAB promulgates accounting principles for federal government reporting entities. The Board's website provides access to all publications issued by FASAB including exposure drafts, the volume of original pronouncements ("Codification"), newsletters, minutes, and meeting agendas (FASAB, 2007). Specific questions about state and local governmental entity accounting may be answered by visiting the **Government Accounting Standards Board (GASB)** website (GASB, 2007). Questions about nongovernmental entity accounting may be answered by visiting the **Financial Accounting Standards Board (FASB)** website (FASB, 2007).

Federal Trade Commission (FTC)

The FTC is responsible for the enforcement of **federal antitrust** and **consumer protection laws**. The FTC's consumer protection mission is to "prevent fraud, deception, and unfair business practices in the marketplace. The mission is accomplished by identifying practices that cause the greatest consumer injury, stopping these practices through law enforcement, and preventing consumer injury through education" (FTC, 2007). Simply stated, FTC efforts are directed toward stopping actions that threaten consumers' opportunities to exercise informed choice. The FTC's antitrust authority comes primarily from the **Federal Trade Commission Act** and the **Clayton Act**. The FTC's antitrust arm, the **Bureau of Competition**, seeks to prevent business practices that restrain competition. Competition results in lower prices and greater availability of products and services. As noted earlier under the DOJ, both the FTC's Bureau of Competition and the Antitrust Division of the DOJ enforce antitrust laws.

The FTC Bureau of Competition has developed expertise in a number of industries important to consumers, such as health care, other professional services, and other areas of consumer interest. As part of its consumer protection role, the FTC publishes a variety of consumer advisories on health care topics such as tips for buying exercise equipment, diet and fitness, aging, health clubs, weight loss, and sources of information about health care products and services.

General Accounting Office (GAO)

The GAO is the "audit, evaluation, and investigative arm of Congress. GAO exists to support the Congress in meeting its Constitutional responsibilities and to help improve the performance and ensure the accountability of the federal government for the American people" (GAO, 2007). GAO examines everything from the use of public funds to the performance of federal programs and activities. The GAO operates **FraudNET** for the reporting of allegations of fraud, waste, abuse, or mismanagement of federal funds including Medicare and Medicaid funding.

Internal Revenue Service (IRS)

The IRS administers the **Internal Revenue Code** enacted by Congress. The IRS is the nation's tax collection agency. Its mission is to "provide America's taxpayers top quality service by helping them understand and meet their tax responsibilities and by applying the tax law with integrity and fairness to all" (IRS, 2007).

Medicare Payment Advisory Commission (MedPac)

The MedPac is an independent federal body that advises the U.S. Congress on issues affecting the Medicare program. MedPac is made up of 17 members who have diverse expertise in health care financing and delivery. The members meet publicly to discuss policy issues and formulate recommendations to the Congress on improving Medicare policies. MedPac publishes its recommendations twice annually and in other reports periodically mandated by the Congress. Examples of the commission's publications and opinions relevant to physical therapists are: durable medical equipment payment system and the outpatient therapy services payment system published in September 2006 (MedPac, 2007). MedPac seeks and accepts input from professional and advocacy organizations on topics of current interest.

National Council on Disability (NCD)

NCD is another independent federal agency. The NCD makes recommendations to the President and Congress on issues affecting Americans with disabilities. NCD is composed of 15 members who are appointed by the President and confirmed by the U.S. Senate. It was an NCD proposal for a civil rights law for people with disabilities that lead to the signing of the **Americans with Disabilities Act (ADA)** in 1990. The purpose of the NCD is to "promote policies, programs, practices, and procedures that guarantee equal opportunity for all individuals with disabilities, regardless of the nature or severity of the disability; and to empower individuals with disabilities to achieve economic self-sufficiency, independent living, and inclusion and integration into all aspects of society" (NCD, 2009). NCD has undertaken a multiyear study on the implementation and enforcement of civil rights laws including the Americans with Disabilities Act.

National Labor Relations Board (NLRB)

NLRB is an independent federal agency that administers the National Labor Relations Act (NLRA), the primary law governing relations between unions and employers in the private sector. The NLRA gives employees the right to organize and bargain collectively with their employers or to refrain from all such activity. The NLRA applies generally to all employers involved in interstate commerce other than airlines, railroads, agriculture, and government. According to NLRB publications (NLRB, 2007) it has two principal functions:

1. To determine, through secret-ballot whether the employees wish to be represented by a union in dealing with their employers and if so, by which union.
2. To prevent and remedy unlawful acts, called unfair labor practices, by either employers or unions.

The NLRB does not act on its own, but reacts to charges of unfair labor practices and petitions for employee elections that are filed with one of its offices.

Occupational Safety and Health Administration (OSHA)

OSHA has a mission to "assure the safety and health of America's workers by setting and enforcing standards; providing training, outreach, and education; establishing partnerships; and encouraging continual improvement in workplace safety and health" (OSHA, 2007). OSHA does this through the administration of the Occupational Safety and Health Act of 1970 working in partnership with state and local governments, workers, and employers. With more than 200 offices throughout the country, OSHA and its state partners have inspectors, investigators, engineers, physicians, educators, standards writers, and other personnel who establish and enforce protective standards. OSHA also offers technical assistance and consultation programs to employers and employees (OSHA, 2007).

Offices of the Inspectors General (OIG)

The OIG has offices in several federal agencies. The HHS OIG has local offices in every state, Washington DC, and Puerto Rico (HHS OIG, 2009). This is a reflection of the amount of oversight focused on federally funded health care. The specific purpose of the HHS OIG (see Fig. 10.1), as mandated by Public Law 95-452 is to "protect the integrity of HHS programs, as well as the health and welfare of the beneficiaries of those programs" (HHS OIG, 2009). The OIG reports on program and management problems and recommendations to correct them to both the Secretary of HHS and the Congress. The OIG's duties are carried out through audits, investigations, inspections, and other related functions.

Office of Special Education and Rehabilitative Services (OSERS)

OSERS is part of the **Department of Education (DOE)** (DOE, 2007). It is committed to improving results and outcomes for people with disabilities of all ages. OSERS mission is to "provide leadership to achieve full integration and participation in society of people with disabilities by ensuring equal opportunity and access to, and excellence in, education, employment and community living" (DOE, 2007). It achieves this mission through support of programs that benefit children, youth, and adults with disabilities. OSERS is comprised of three program components: the **Office of Special Education Programs (OSEP)**, the **National Institute on Disability and Rehabilitation Research (NIDRR)**, and the **Rehabilitation Services Administration (RSA)**. OSERS programs provide support to parents, educators, and states in special education, vocational rehabilitation, and research.

Veterans Health Administration (VHA)

The VHA is a division of the **Department of Veterans Affairs (DVA)**. VHA provides a broad spectrum of medical, surgical, and rehabilitative care to enrolled and eligible veterans. It is the stated goal of the VHA to "serve the needs of America's veterans by providing primary care, specialized care, and related medical and social support services" (DVA, 2007). The VHA serves veterans through a health system that includes medical centers and outpatient care clinics. The Veterans' Health Care Eligibility Reform Act of 1996 resulted in the creation of a Medical Benefits Package—a health benefits plan generally available to enrolled veterans. Like other standard health care plans, the Medical Benefits Package emphasizes preventive and primary care, offering a full range of outpatient and inpatient services. The majority of non service-connected veterans and noncompensable 0% service-connected veterans need to complete a means test annually or they must pay the VA an applicable co-payment. The means test is based on their income and net worth. Based on the means test veterans may be required to make co-payments for VA medical services. Veterans must also provide health insurance information so that the VA can submit claims to insurance carriers for treatment provided for all non service-connected conditions (Library of Congress, 2007).

State and Local Government

State and local governments also have the ability to regulate the activities of health service organizations and providers. On occasion, the federal, state, and local government may

regulate the same health services activities. When that occurs, the health services provider must consider all applicable regulations to determine their course of action. Because each state and local jurisdiction has unique governmental structure, the names and source of regulation may vary greatly. For this reason, the many roles of state and local government in the regulation of health care is best demonstrated by examples. Table 10.1 is a sample of the services administered by the State of Wisconsin's Department of Health and Family Services (WI DHFS). Table 10.2 is a sample of the WI DHFS regulatory responsibilities. Table 10.3 is a sample of the WI DHFS data collection and reporting responsibilities. Table 10.4 lists the services provided by the Dane County, Wisconsin Department of Human Services. These examples clearly demonstrate that health care oversight comes from many sources at the state level and local level. Again it is up to health care organizations and providers to identify and comply with all applicable governmental regulation. To learn more about specific state and local agencies go to http://www.firstgov.gov.

Student Notes

Compliance with governmental regulation and nongovernmental standards of practice is a basic part of health care professional practice. It is incumbent on every health care provider to be familiar and compliant with all applicable regulations. The risks of noncompliance may vary but can be as significant as loss of credentials, fines, and/or legal prosecution. A portion of workplace orientation information should include a review of the organization's corporate compliance plan. Prior experiences, good and bad, provide employers with the appropriate background to choose the point of emphasis. Given the breadth of governmental oversight, and the volume of governmental regulations, new graduates should expect continual education regarding government involvement in health care. Most health care organizations provide ongoing employee education that addresses regulatory requirements as well as the organization's policies and procedures aimed at regulatory compliance. The

Table 10.1   Sample of Services Offered by the Wisconsin Department of Health and Family Services

Adoption services	HUD emergency shelter grant program
Aging services	Immunization
All-Inclusive Care for the Elderly, Program of (PACE)	Independent living services
Bioterrorism preparedness	Indian and Native American affairs
Birth to 3 Programs	Infectious diseases
Blind and visually impaired	Injury prevention
Children's services	Intergenerational programs
Child protective services	Lead regulation
Children and youth with special health care needs	Living will
Chronic disease prevention and health promotion	Maternal and child health
Community Options Program (COP)	Medicaid (Medical Assistance, MA, Title X1X)
Comprehensive cancer control program	Medicaid abuse/fraud
Congenital disorders program	Mental health
Dental/Oral health	Minority health
Developmental disabilities	Organ and tissue donor program
Diabetes prevention and control program	Physical disabilities
Early intervention program/Birth to 3 Program	Program of All-Inclusive Care for the Elderly (PACE)
Elderly services	Protective services—Adult
Emergency medical services	Public health
Emergency Response (DHFS/DPH) Health Emergencies (general)	Rural health
	Sexual assault prevention
Environmental / Occupational health	Sexual predator law
Farmers' Market Nutrition Program (FMNP)	Stroke, stroke network
Fish advisories/toxins	Supplemental Security Income (SSI)
Food safety	Supported employment
Forensic services	The Emergency Food Assistance Program (TEFAP)
Foster care	Tobacco prevention and control program
Hazardous event surveillance	Vaccines
Hearing impaired/mental health	Women-Infant-Children (WIC) Nutrition Program

Wisconsin Department of Health and Family Services. Programs and services; consumer information. Available at http://dhfs. wisconsin.gov/programs.htm. Accessed 9/03/07.

Table 10.2   Sample of Wisconsin Department of Health and Family Services Regulatory Responsibilities

Adult day care	Food certification, restaurant
Adult family homes, policy, regulation and funding	Groundwater standards
Air pollution and contaminant monitoring, residential	Group foster home licensing
Ambulance–Air ambulance licensing	Hazardous waste sites
Assisted living facilities, general	HIPAA—Privacy (Health Insurance Portability and Accountability Act)
Background checks	
Bed and breakfast licensing	Home health agencies regulation
Bodies, disposition of human corpse	Hospice regulation
Body piercing	Hospital regulation
Campgrounds	Industrial hygiene/air testing
Child and Family Services Review (CFSR)	Life safety code, survey/certification-acute
Child care licensing	Local health department reviews (HFS 140)
Child placing agency licensing	Lodging inspections
Child welfare licensing	Nursing home regulation
Community Based Residential Facilities (CBRFs)	Paramedic licensing
Complaints, provider	Plan reviews of health care facilities (Hospitals, nursing homes and CBRFs, FDDs)
Community health centers	
Durable medical equipment	Radioactive materials, licensing, agreement
Emergency medical technician licensing—Basic	Restaurant complaints/inspections
Entity background checks	Restaurant licensing
Facilities management	Rooming houses, hotels, motels and tourist licensing
First responders/EMS	Sewer gas

(Continued)

Table 10.2 continued	
Soil—chemical contamination	Trash burning
Spills, toxic	Vehicles
Superfund sites	Vending machines
Swimming pools	Water—chemical contamination
Tanning devices	Waterparks
Vehicles	Well contamination
Vending machines	Whirlpools
Toxics monitoring—general	X-Ray, registration and inspection

Source: Wisconsin Department of Health and Family Services. Listing of DHFS topics. Available at http://dhfs.wisconsin.gov/data/topicalaf.asp. Accessed 9/07/07.

topic of corporate compliance plans was discussed in detail in Chapter 4. Currently, government websites provide the most readily available information at no cost.

Nongovernmental Oversight

Private organizations that set performance standards and/or provide external oversight to health services organizations and individual providers are many and varied (Chapter 16). These include private organizations acting under agreement with the health service provider and private organizations acting independently of the government or the health service provider. Examples of these types of oversight organizations include:

- **Professional review organizations** that both set standards for performance and provide voluntary accreditation to ensure compliance such as the JC or *the Commission on*

Table 10.3 Sample of Wisconsin Department of Health and Family Services Data Collection and Reporting Responsibilities	
Ambulatory surgery data (for Wisconsin agencies)	Induced abortion report
Behavioral risk factor survey data	Infants and pregnant women (data profiles)
Birth and infant death data	Lead registry
Birth statistics	Maternal and child health—data
Cancer incidence and mortality	Marriage statistics
Census data	MDS statistics
Certified nursing assistant child abuse and neglect data	Nursing home data
Child welfare outcome data	OASIS statistics
Child welfare reports	Occupational health surveillance
Chronic conditions (data profiles)	Physician office visit data
Community Aids Reporting (CARS) Death Statistics	Population estimates
Demographic information	Quality assurance—COP Waiver/Elders/PD
Divorce statistics	Quality assurance, developmental disabilities
End stage renal dialysis providers, survey	Quality services review (QSR)
Environmental disease tracking	Radiological environmental monitoring
End Stage Renal Dialysis Providers (ESRD) survey	Records management (department)
Family health survey data	Rehabilitation services (outpatient) survey
Health insurance statistics	Terminations of pregnancy report
Health Professional Shortage Areas (HPSAs)	Time study (DDES, OSF, and DCFS)
Health statistics	Vital records, customer services/Record search
Home health agency data	Vital records, field Rep. (local office services)
Hospice data	Vital records, special records and preservation
Hospitals, emergency dept. data (for Wisconsin agencies)	Wisconsin Interactive Statistics on Health
Hospitals, inpatient data (for Wisconsin agencies)	Wisconsin Public Health Information Network
Human Services Reporting System (HSRS)	Youth tobacco survey (YTS)

Source: Wisconsin Department of Health and Family Services. Listing of DHFS topics. Available at http://dhfs.wisconsin.gov/data/topicalaf.asp. Accessed 9/07/07.

Table 10.4   Dane County Wisconsin Department of Human Services Programs and Services
Alcohol, tobacco, and other drugs
Children, youth, and families
Developmental disability related services
Food, Jobs, Shelter, and Childcare
Medical assistance
Mental health
Nursing home—Badger Prairie health care center
Physical and sensory disability related services
Public health
Senior services
Transportation

Source: Dane County Department of Human Services. Programs and services. Available at http://www.danecountyhumanservices.org/. Accessed 9/07/07.

Accreditation of Rehabilitation Facilities (CARF).
- **Professional organizations (associations)** such as the **American Physical Therapy Association (APTA)**, **American Medical Association (AMA)**, and the **American Hospital Association (AHA)**. The national associations are often focused on setting policy and performance standards while their local (state) level branches may provide direct oversight functions.
- Professional organizations that set standards for professional practice and performance such as the FASB. FASB is the designated organization in the private sector for establishing standards of financial accounting and reporting (FASB, 2007).
- **General and medical liability insurance carriers** also provide external oversight of health service organizations and providers. Carriers have the expectation that the insured health care providers are doing everything possible to reduce the risk of general liability or medical malpractice claims. To ensure that this happens the insurer may provide direct **risk management** support including direct observation to make sure that providers (1) follow commonly accepted **standards of care**, (2) comply with industry **standards of practice**, (3) have an active performance improvement program, (4) have an effective risk management program. Failure to meet these expectations or a poor claims history may result in higher premiums or even difficulty getting insurance coverage.

- Private **watchdog groups** and **performance-ranking services** are getting more involved in oversight activities. These are most often organizations that are acting independently of the government or the health service provider (Chapter 16).

Voluntary Accreditation

According to the Institute of Medicine (2001) an ideal accrediting entity would be:

- Autonomous, i.e., independent of any particular interest group
- Credible with stakeholders
- National in the scope of its interests and actions
- Possess extensive knowledge of stakeholders' needs

Accreditation is a rigorous and comprehensive evaluation process used by external organizations to assess how well a health care organization manages all parts of its care delivery system. Accreditation is based on consensus quality standards. Therefore, organizational providers who seek accreditation are subjecting their outcomes, structure, and processes to scrutiny by external examiners (Sandstrom et al., 2003). There are several important accreditation organizations that affect physical therapy services. The most notable are the JC, CARF, and the *National Commission on Quality Assurance (NCQA)*.

The JC is probably the best-known non-governmental accreditation organization. JC evaluates and accredits more than 15,000 health care organizations in the United States. Its mission is "to continuously improve the safety and quality of care provided to the public through the provision of health care accreditation and related services that support performance improvement in health care organizations" (JC, 2007a). JC is an independent, not-for-profit organization that develops professional standards against which the compliance of health care organizations is evaluated. JC offers accreditation to health care organizations of many types:

- Ambulatory care
- Assisted living
- Behavioral health care
- Critical access hospitals
- Health care networks
- Home care
- Hospitals
- Laboratory services
- Long-term care
- Office-base surgery

The JC is governed by a 29-member board of commissioners that includes a variety of clinical and administrative health care professionals including representatives of the American College of Physicians-American Society of Internal Medicine, the American College of Surgeons, the American Dental Association, the American Hospital Association, and the American Medical Association. JC accreditation has many benefits (JC, 2007b):

- Enhances staff recruitment and development
- Improves risk management and risk reduction
- May fulfill regulatory requirements in select states
- Provides a competitive edge in the marketplace
- Provides education on good practices to improve business operations
- Provides professional advice and counsel, enhancing staff education
- Recognized by select insurers and other third parties
- Strengthens community confidence in the quality and safety of care, treatment, and services

CARF is an international, independent, not-for-profit accrediting body. Its stated mission is "to promote the quality, value, and optimal outcomes of services through a consultative accreditation process that centers on enhancing the lives of the persons served" (CARF, 2007).

CARF accredits the following services:

- Adult day services
- Alcohol and substance abuse treatment
- Assisted living residences
- Assistive technology services
- Blind rehabilitation services
- Child and youth services
- Community services
- Continuing care retirement communities
- Day habilitation services
- Employee assistance programs
- Employment services
- Mental health services (also called behavioral health)
- Methadone treatment (also called opioid treatment)
- One-stop career centers
- Pain management
- Physical rehabilitation (also called medical rehabilitation)
- Stroke specialty
- Supported living (for behavioral health)
- Supported living (for community services)

There are more than 5,000 health care facilities with CARF accreditation. Accreditation service is offered by CARF in the United States, Canada, and Europe. CARF's standards are established to help health care providers measure and improve the quality, value, and outcomes of their services. To accomplish this, CARF engages persons receiving services, rehabilitation professionals, and purchasers of services in the development of its standards (CARF, 2007a).

CARF uses a peer review process to assess the performance of an organization in serving its customers. It is interesting to note that government or other third party payers may require an organization to obtain CARF accreditation as a condition for licensure and/ or reimbursement. The programs and services accredited by CARF have demonstrated that they substantially meet nationally recognized standards. The basis for meeting standards is an onsite survey conducted by knowledgeable, trained, surveyors who are active professionals in the field being surveyed. The survey offers the organization's personnel an opportunity to consult with CARF surveyors to enhance the delivery of quality services. Input from consumers is obtained during the onsite survey process. CARF accreditation acknowledges that an organization has made a major commitment to enhance the quality of its programs and services that focus on positive outcomes.

NCQA is the primary accrediting organization for **managed-care organizations (MCO)**. The NCQA began accrediting MCOs in 1991, in response to the need for standardized, objective information about the quality of these organizations. The NCQA accreditation program is voluntary, and has been recognized by purchasers, consumers, and health plans as an objective measure of the quality of MCOs including:

- Disease management
- Managed behavioral health care organizations
- Managed-care organizations
- New health plans
- Preferred provider organization plans
- Quality Plus program (new for commercial insurance plans)

NCQA's mission is "to improve the quality of health care" (NCQA, 2007a). The NCQA has a vision to transform health care quality through measurement, transparency, and accountability. According to NCQA, approximately 90% of all health plans measure their performance using the NCQA's *Health Plan Employer Data and Information Set (HEDIS)* (NCQA, 2007b). HEDIS is a proprietary tool used to measure managed-care plan performance in key areas like immunization and mammography screening rates. The HEDIS tool is a set of standardized performance measures designed to ensure that purchasers and consumers have the information they need to compare the performance of managed health care plans. In combination with information from NCQA's accreditation program, HEDIS provides a quality health plan that can be used to guide choice among competing health plans. HEDIS is intended to provide purchasers and consumers with an ability both to evaluate the quality of different health plans along a variety of important dimensions, and to make their plan related decisions based on demonstrated value rather than simply on cost. HEDIS has

several performance domains for which measures are in place (NCQA, 2007c):

1. Effectiveness of care: These are measures that assess how well the care that is delivered by a managed-care plan achieves the clinical results.
2. Access/availability of care: These are measures that permit assessment of whether care is available to members, when they need it, and in a timely and convenient manner.
3. Satisfaction with the experience of care: These measures provide information about whether a health plan is able to satisfy the diverse needs of its members.
4. Stability of the health plan: Health plan stability is important, because consumers make enrollment decisions that generally bind them for a year. Should the plan's network of providers change significantly, or should the plan become insolvent, the member's health care could be badly disrupted.
5. Use of services: How a health plan uses its resources is a signal of how efficiently care is managed and whether or not needed services are being delivered; it may also provide some information about where there are opportunities to improve both the effectiveness and efficiency of care. These measures assess patterns of service use across different health plans.
6. Cost of care: These are measures that compare health plans based on the economic value of the services they deliver.
7. Health plan descriptive information. These measures provide the varied elements of interest to consumers regarding plan management (including a description of selected network, clinical, utilization, and risk management activities).

Professional Organizations

A professional organization, also referred to as an association, a congress, or a society, is an organization, usually not-for-profit, that exists to further the interests of its membership. Members share common characteristics such as a common profession, business, or interest. Members can be individuals, organizations, or both. A health care related professional organization can be focused on the protection of the interests of it members, the protection of the public interest, or both. The balance between these two varies by organization and may be a matter of opinion. Ways in which a professional organization might act to protect the public is by establishing standards of training, professional practice, and ethics in their profession.

The AHA and the **American Association of Homes and Services for the Aging (AAHSA)** are examples of professional associations that represent the interests of similar businesses. The AMA and the APTA are both examples of associations representing the interests of a group of professionals. Professional organizations provide a variety of products and services on behalf of or for the benefit of their members. The role, products, and services that an association provides can be demonstrated by using the APTA as an example.

The APTA is a national professional organization representing physical therapists and physical therapist assistants. Membership is voluntary. The APTA's mission "as the principal membership organization representing and promoting the profession of physical therapy, is to further the profession's role in the prevention, diagnosis, and treatment of movement dysfunctions and the enhancement of the physical health and functional abilities of members of the public" (APTA, 2007a). As a step toward accomplishing this goal the APTA has developed a vision statement for 2020, "Physical therapy, by 2020, will be provided by physical therapists who are doctors of physical therapy and who may be board-certified specialists. Consumers will have direct access to physical therapists in all environments for patient/client management, prevention, and wellness services" (APTA, 2007b). This vision statement is an example of the APTA's leadership role. The APTA also provides many products and services including:

- Advocacy
- Career management
- Consulting services
- Credentialing/certification
- Education
- Group purchasing opportunities
- Job search
- Research

- Networking opportunities
- Professional standards
- Publications
- Risk protection products (e.g., insurance products)

The APTA also has a cooperative relationship with the **Commission on Accreditation in Physical Therapy Education (CAPTE)**. CAPTE grants specialized accreditation status to qualified entry-level education programs for physical therapists and physical therapist assistants (Chapter 1). The **U.S. Department of Education and the Council for Higher Education Accreditation (CHEA)** recognizes CAPTE as an accrediting agency (CHEA, 2007). The Commission has representation from the educational community, the physical therapy profession, and the public. Accredited programs meet established and nationally accepted standards of scope, quality, and relevance (APTA, 2007c).

Professional Organizations That Set Standards

There are many organizations that are involved in setting standards for industry practices. Most notable of these is the FASB. A newcomer to this list is the **American Health Information Community (AHIC)**.

FASB is the designated organization in the private sector for establishing standards of financial accounting and reporting (Chapter 21). The FASB's mission is "to establish and improve standards of state and local governmental accounting and financial reporting that will result in useful information for users of financial reports and guide and educate the public, including issuers, auditors, and users of those financial reports" (FASB, 2007). It is the FASB standards that govern the preparation of financial reports. Since 1973, the **Securities and Exchange Commission (SEC)** (Financial Reporting Release No. 1, Section 101) and the **American Institute of Certified Public Accountants** (Rule 203, Rules of Professional Conduct, as amended May 1973 and May 1979) officially recognized FASB standards as authoritative (Rutgers, 2007). The SEC has the authority to establish accounting and reporting standards for public companies under the Securities and Exchange Act of 1934. Accounting standards are necessary for the efficient functioning of the economy because investors, creditors, auditors, and others rely on credible, transparent, and comparable financial information.

AHIC started out as a federal advisory body. It was chartered in 2005 by the HHS Secretary to make recommendations on how to accelerate the development and adoption of health information technology toward the goal of providing Americans with access to secure electronic health records by 2014. AHIC will transition to a public-private partnership based in the private sector by Fall 2008. At that time the AHIC will be independent and sustainable and will bring together the best attributes and resources of public and private entities. According to AHIC, this new public–private partnership will develop a unified approach to realize an effective, interoperable nationwide health information system that supports the health and well-being of the people of the country (AHIC, 2007).

Insurance Carriers and Risk Management

Risk is the probability of suffering harm or loss. Chapters 8 and 9 introduced the concept of risk at the organizational and personal level as it dealt with professional and legal liability. Risk should not be a new concept because it is something we deal with on a daily basis. A good example is the risk of injury that might occur during a routine activity such as driving. To minimize the public risk, laws exist to establish regulations about the operation, use, and performance of vehicles; require training and licensure before we operate a vehicle; and designate oversight and enforcement authority. To minimize personal risk, drivers operate safe vehicles, comply with driving regulations, follow safe driving practices, and buy automobile insurance. The first three activities are ways the driver can avoid risk, or **risk avoidance**. The fourth is a way to transfer some of the financial risk to the insurer, or **risk sharing**. Before an insurer agrees to assume this risk they are going to want to put a value on that service. They will want to know the driver's personal profile (i.e., age, sex, education, and academic performance), vehicle make and model (i.e., performance, safety, and value),

vehicle location (i.e., traffic, crime rates), potential driving mileage (opportunity for an accident), and the driver's previous record. All of this information will be used to assess the risk of paying a claim. A track record of effective risk avoidance would be viewed favorably. Based on their assessment the insurer will determine if they are willing to share the driver's risk and how much they will charge for that service. Collectively, activities undertaken to avoid or sharing risk are referred to as risk management.

Health service organizations and individual providers also need to manage the risk of operating their business and/or providing care. To protect the community, public laws exist to establish regulations about every aspect of health services delivery, require training and licensure before services are provided, and designate oversight and enforcement authority. To manage business risk health services, providers operate safe facilities, comply with regulations, follow standards of practice, and buy business and medical liability insurance. To make sure that this is done effectively, most health service organizations have formal risk management programs. Risk management can be defined as "the process of systematically monitoring health care delivery activities in order to prevent or minimize financial losses from claims or lawsuits arising from patient care or other activities conducted in a health care facility" (Scott, 2000, p. 191). Risk management should be closely tied to the health care organization's quality improvement, communication, and accreditation efforts. Insurance carriers, as a condition of coverage may engage in active oversight activities as part of a collaborative risk management effort. As part of this oversight, insurance risk management representatives may perform onsite surveys, interview care providers, offer consultation service, provide comparative benchmarking information, and best practice resources.

The Management Process in Health Care Organizations

The **American Society for Healthcare Risk Management** (**ASHRM**) is a personal membership group of the American Hospital Association. According to ASHRM, it has more than 5,200 members from health care, insurance, law, and other related professions. It role is "to promote effective and innovative risk management strategies and professional leadership through education, recognition, advocacy, publications, networking and interactions with leading health care organizations and government agencies. Its focus is on developing and implementing safe and effective patient care practices, the preservation of financial resources and the maintenance of safe working environments" (ASHRM, 2007).

ASHRM defines the risk management process as the identification, analysis, and evaluation of risk and the selection of the most advantageous method of treating it. This means "identifying, addressing, preventing, and monitoring any situation that could result in injury, liability, financial loss, or regulatory in non-compliance" (Chubb, 2007).

According to Chubb Health Care, a leading global property and casualty insurance firm, the elements of an effective risk management program include the elements listed in Table 10.5.

An effective risk management program is supported by consistent practices that allow for the identification, correction, prevention, and monitoring of the risk management program elements to include (Chubb, 2007):

1. Formal risk management functions to include a risk management role description, organizational chart, incident reporting system, and claims management system.
2. A process to review and revise all policies and procedures ensuring consistency across the organization.
3. A process to ensure that all policies and procedures are followed consistently.
4. Maintenance of policy and procedure manuals and archives.
5. Processes for exposure identification including a review of prior claims, complaints, inspections, surveys, quality improvement programs, and environment of care reviews.
6. A formal standardized incident reporting process that utilizes legal protections of confidentiality and disclosure, is nonpunitive, and manages the information around incidents for maximal protection.

Table 10.5   Elements of a Risk Management Program

Safety/security programs
Occupational Safety and Health Administration (OSHA) requirements
Employee health program
Clinical Laboratory Improvement Act (CLIA) requirements
Infection control
Medicare/Medicaid patient rights requirements.
Informed consent procedures
Clinical standard of care/negligence
Property damage and property accessibility
Medical waste and needle disposal
Medical record documentation
Confidentiality policy and standards for release of medical information
Mandatory reporting requirements
Licensure requirements/Accreditation standards
Credentialing/privileging guidelines
Contract management
Monitoring of marketing/public relations/external representations
Complaint/grievance management
Claim investigation and management
Employment practices guidelines
Construction/physical plant requirements, permits, etc.
Regulatory compliance activities
Risk transfer and financing management
Retention of insurance policies
Insurance broker relations management

Table 10.6 Sources of Information Used to Manage Risk	
Committee reports	Complaints
Incident reports	Survey results
Medical staff	Expert consultant reports
Patients records	Insurance company
Previous claims	representatives
Quality assurance	Industry publications
Safety inspectors	

7. Processes for following up on individual incidents and incident trending.
8. Staff training and education.
9. Integration of organizational activities including: quality improvement, safety, administration, clinical operations, corporate compliance, and governance.

The risk manager has numerous sources of information to consult. Some data come from historical sources such as previous claims against the organization, information from insurance company representatives, incident reports, and other records. Other sources of information require more investigation but may be helpful in anticipating undesirable events before they occur. These additional resources are presented in Table 10.6.

Part of a risk management program is managing claims when they do occur. **Loss reduction** can be accomplished when the organization is prepared with complete documentation, has all records completed in reasonable time frames, informs staff about claims that have been filed, educates staff for the possibility of legal action, and revises procedures that have lead to occurrences. Each of these loss reduction suggestions is applicable to physical therapy departments.

Private Watchdog Groups and Performance Ranking Services

Private watchdog groups and performance ranking services are getting more involved in oversight activities. These are most often organizations that are acting independently of the government or the health service provider. **Enloe Watch** is an example of a watchdog group, created by the caregivers of Enloe Medical Center, to inform the community of the declining workplace standards and their impact on quality patient care (Enloe Watch, 2007). **HealthGrades**, an Internet based health services provider rating service, is an example of a performance ranking service (HealthGrades, 2007). While the health service provider can not control the activities of these organizations it can protect itself best by effectively managing its operations within standards of community practice and through its risk management program.

The Concept of Continuous Readiness

Oversight often takes the form of onsite surveys, documentation, and financial audits. Federal, state, and local governmental agencies or their representatives perform regulatory compliance reviews. Regulatory reviews can occur as a condition of participation in government-funded health care programs such as Medicare and Medicaid. They can also occur as a condition of continued licensure, operation, and/or reimbursement as a state or local government approved health care provider. Reviews performed as a condition of continued operation may involve annual reviews for continued licensure, facility safety inspections, or compliance with state licensure requirements for medical professionals such as nursing. The purpose of health care regulation is to protect the interests of the public. Independent professionals and organizations involved in the delivery of health care services are held accountable to the public through the enactment and enforcement of regulations that set **community standards** for health care service delivery.

Successful reviews lie in the efforts of management and individual providers to recognize and meet oversight requirements on a **continuous readiness basis**. This means being compliant with requirements at all times, not just when an oversight review is expected. More and more, oversight activities are conducted on an unannounced basis to force organizations into a continuous readiness mode of operation. Be reminded that compliance relates to meeting *minimal* standards for performance, whereas driving should meet the *optimal* standards for performance—the desire to be the best, to succeed, and to excel. Other roles and responsibilities do not relieve health service providers from the responsibility to know and comply with the regulations and accreditation standards that apply to business practices and health services service delivery.

Assistance in meeting oversight requirements whether voluntary or involuntary can be obtained from any number of professional organizations, oversight organization, and professional consulting practices that provide voluntary review related to accepted professional standards for performance such as financial audit or legal firms.

Summary

Health care providers have historically been subject to external oversight. The purpose of health care regulation is to protect the interests of the public. Oversight can come from governmental agencies, nongovernmental organizations operating under government contracts, or nongovernmental private organizations. Nonregulatory reviews are most often performed by private review organizations. Federal, state, and local governmental agencies or their representatives perform regulatory compliance reviews. Regulatory reviews can occur as a condition of participation in government-funded health care programs such as Medicare and Medicaid. They can also occur as a condition of continued operation as a state or local government approved health care provider. Reviews performed as a condition of continued operation include such things as annual reviews for continued licensure, facility safety inspections, or compliance with state licensure requirements for medical professionals such as nursing. Historically, oversight that originates with private organizations has been voluntary while governmental oversight has been nonvoluntary. Today many private oversight organizations are performing their oversight activities using publicly available data without or with only marginal involvement of the health service providers. Another more recent trend in the clinical oversight arena has the linking of participation in oversight activities to payment rates. These types of oversight programs are often referred to as pay for performance. There is an expectation that many

of the P4P programs will become nonvoluntary over time. To be compliant with oversight requirements, health service providers must become familiar with the sources, forms, and implications of external health service oversight including names, acronyms, and general authorities of oversight government agencies and private organizations. Information about oversight regulations and standards can be easily obtained from Internet based sources. However, assistance is often needed to understand and fully assess the practical implications of regulations and performance standards. Use of external consultants and professional organizations can be helpful but, ultimately, compliance with regulatory and accreditation requirements is the responsibility of every member of the health services organization with management taking the lead. Effective risk management is one of the tools that health service providers can deploy to minimize risk and move to continuous readiness.

REFERENCES

Agency for Healthcare Research and Quality. Consumer assessment of healthcare providers and systems (CAHPS). Available at https://www.cahps.ahrq.gov/default.asp. Accessed 9/03/07.

American Health Information Community (AHIC). Available at http://www.hhs.gov/healthit/community/background/. Accessed 9/03/07.

American Physical Therapy Association. Mission. Available at http://www.apta.org. Accessed 9/03/07a.

American Physical Therapy Association. APTA Vision 2020. Available at http://www.apta.org/vision2020. Accessed 9/03/07b.

American Physical Therapy Association. Commission on accreditation in physical therapy education accreditation. Available at http://www.apta.org/AM/Template.cfm?Section=CAPTE1&Template=/TaggedPage/TaggedPageDisplay.cfm&TPLID=65&ContentID=20194. Accessed 9/03/07c.

American Society for Healthcare Risk Management (ASHRM). About us. Available at http://www.ashrm.org/ashrm/aboutus/aboutus.html. Accessed on 9/03/07.

CARF-The Rehabilitation Accreditation Commission. About CARF. Available at http://www.carf.org/consumer.aspx?content=content/About/News/facts.htm. Accessed 9/03/07.

Centers for Disease Control and Prevention. Available at http://www.cdc.gov. Accessed 9/03/07.

Centers for Medicare and Medicaid Services. Intermediary-carrier directory. Available at http://www.cms.hhs.gov/ContractingGeneralInformation/Downloads/02_ICdirectory.pdf. Accessed 9/03/07.

CASE STUDY 10.1

Ask the Answer Man

Introduction

You are a physical therapist clinician and manager in a small department. The other department members are Holly Pēno, a physical therapist assistant (PTA), and two aides. Holly is an army reservist. She informs you that her unit will likely be called to active duty in 1–2 months. She wants to know where she stands with regard to her job in your department when she returns $1^1/_2$–2 years from now. You really want to reemploy Holly when she returns but you will also have to recruit a new PTA while she is on duty.

Gathering Information

You wonder what the laws are regarding reemployment and temporary hiring. Your Human Resources liaison would be a good person to talk with but she is busy doing interviews today and tomorrow. The immediate need is to get a start on learning what the law is regarding reservists and reemployment. You sit down at your computer and think to yourself, *where should I start? To yourself you say, this is an employment thing–so go to the U.S. Department of Labor and the state Department of Labor. It is also*

a military matter. This means I should check out the Department of Defense website also. Since this is a Veteran's issue I may go to the Veterans Administration as well. I'll start with the two sources and see what I can find out.

Record and Report Your Answers

Write down what you learned about the following:

Resources and links from the Department of Labor website
Resources and links from the Department of Defense website
Resources and links from other websites
Some difficulties you encountered in trying to find specific information
Some suggestions for navigating each of the websites you examined

What Can You Tell Holly?

About her rights
The position of your organization on returning reservists
What you will consult the human services liaison about
Where might she go for additional information

CASE STUDY 10.2

Risk or No Risk, That Is the Choice

Introduction

Risk has been defined as the probability of suffering loss or harm. Two options are available to readers in this case study. One is for readers who are not yet licensed and the other is for licensees.

Option 1: Student Physical Therapists or Physical Therapist Assistants

You have just begun your second internship. It is in a type of facility you have not had prior experience in. Members of the department include physical therapists, physical

(Continued)

CASE STUDY 10.2

Risk or No Risk, That Is the Choice (continued)

therapist assistants, athletic trainers, and aides. You are one of the four student interns. Each of you are supervised by several physical therapists who in turn report to a clinical coordinator of clinical education who integrates the information and does the formal evaluation and report.

Identify five areas of risk based on standards of care and five areas of risk based on standards of practice and one way to minimize risk for each of your identified areas. Discuss your responses with a peer.

Option 2: Licensee

From your clinical experience choose five situations involving coworkers that you perceived as potentially or clearly risky.

- Describe the situations
- Based on Table 10.5, identify the elements of a risk management program that each of your situations related to
- What were the prevailing policies and procedures regarding each of the situations?
- What were the potential or, if known, actual outcomes of the risky situation?
- How would you improve the risk management program you are most familiar with?
- Discuss your cases with peers to determine if there are commonalities in the risk management programs

CASE STUDY 10.3

Something You Always Wanted to Know

Introduction

Chapters 9 and 10 contained introductory discussions of dozens of nongovernmental and state and federal government groups, agencies, offices, and departments relevant to physical therapist managers and clinicians. This case is your opportunity to explore any of the covered nongovernmental and state and federal government groups, agencies, offices, and departments to add depth to your knowledge.

Just Do It

Scan Chapter 10 and identify one resource of interest. If none of the groups, agencies,

offices, or departments enthuse you, go to Chapter 9 and find a resource to investigate. Summarize the information about your chosen resource in 1 typed or 2 handwritten pages. Record the reference sources. Exchange your work with a peer to review and discuss each other's paper. Verify each other's work and interpretations as needed by going back to the original resource information.

Chubb Health Care. Effective health care risk management programs: Components for success. Available at http://www.chubb.com/businesses/csi/chubb1148.pdf. Accessed 9/03/07.

Council on Higher Education Accreditation. Specialized and professional accrediting organizations 2007-2007. Available at http://www.chea.org/Directories/special.asp. Accessed 9/03/07.

Dane County Wisconsin Department of Human Services. Home page. Available at http://www.danecounty publichealth.org/programs.htm. Accessed on 9/3/07.

Department of Education. About OSERS. Available at http://www.ed.gov/about/offices/list/osers/aboutus.html Accessed 9/03/07.

Department of Health and Human Services. Medicare glossary. Available at http://www.medicare.gov/Glossary/search.asp?SelectAlphabet=F&Language=English#Content. Accessed 9/07/07a.

Department of Health and Human Services. HHS What we do. Available at http://www.hhs.gov/about/whatwedo.html/Accessed 9/03/07b.

Department of Health and Human Services. Michael O. Leavitt, Secretary U.S. Department of Health and Human Services on Medicare health care fraud & abuse efforts. Available at http://www.hhs.gov/asl/testify/2007/07/t20070717a.html. Accessed 9/03/07c.

Department of Health and Human Services Office of the Inspector General. Office of investigations (OI). Available at http://www.oig.hhs.gov/organization/oi/. Accessed 1/14/09a.

Department of Health and Human Services Office of the Inspector General. About the office of inspector general (OIG). Available at http://www.oig. hhs.gov/organization.asp. Accessed 1/13/09b.

Department of Justice. About DOJ. Available from http://www.usdoj.gov. Accessed 9/03/07.

Department of Labor. Our mission. Available at http://www.dol.gov/opa/aboutdol/mission.htm. Accessed 9/03/07.

Department of Veterans Affairs. About VA home. Available at http://www.va.gov/about_va/. Accessed 9/03/07.

Department of State. Oversight powers of congress. Available at http://usinfo.state.gov/products/pubs/outusgov/over.htm. Accessed 9/30/07.

Drug Enforcement Administration. DEA mission statement. Available at http://www.usdoj.gov/dea/agency/mission.htm. Accessed 9/03/07.

Enloe Watch. March 19, 2007. Available at http://www.enloewatch.org. Accessed 9/03/07.

Environmental Protection Agency. About EPA. Available at http://www.epa.gov/epahome/aboutepa.htm. Accessed 9/03/07.

Federal Accounting Standards Advisory Board. Reports and documents. Available at http://www.fasab.gov/reports.html. Accessed 9/03/07.

Federal Trade Commission. Promoting competition, protecting consumers: A plain English guide to antitrust laws. Available at http://www.ftc.gov/bc/compguide/index.htm. Accessed 9/03/07.

Financial Accounting Standards Board (FASB). Homepage. Available at http://www.fasb.org. Accessed 9/03/07.

Finkler SA, Ward DM. Essentials of cost accounting for healthcare organizations, 2nd ed. Gaithersburg, MD: Aspen. 1999.

General Accounting Office. Serving the congress and the nation. GAO's strategic plan framework. Available at http://www.gao.gov/sp/frmwk2007.pdf. Accessed 9/30/07.

Government Accounting Standards Board. Homepage. Available at http://www.gasb.org. Accessed 9/03/07.

HealthGrades. About HealthGrades. Available from http://www.healthgrades.com/consumer/index.cfm?fuseaction=mod&modtype=content&modact=shop_about_hg_consumer. Accessed 9/03/07.

Institute of Medicine. Preserving public trust. Accreditation and human research. Participation protection programs. Committee on Assessing the Systems for Protecting Human Research Subjects. Washington, DC: National Academy Press. 2001.

Internal Revenue Service. The agency, its mission and statutory authority. Available at http://www.irs.gov/irs/article/0,,id=98141,00.html. Accessed 9/03/07.

Joint Commission. Facts about The Joint Commission. Available at http://www.jointcommission.org/AboutUs/joint_commission_facts.htm. Accessed 9/03/07a.

Joint Commission. Top stories. Available at http://www.jointcommission.org/. Accessed 9/03/07b.

Library of Congress. Veterans' Health Care Eligibility Reform Act of 1996. Available at http://frwebgate.access.gpo.gov/cgi-bin/getdoc.cgi?dbname=104_cong_public_laws&docid=f:publ262.104.pdf. Accessed 9/07/07.

Matyas DE, Valiant C. Legal issues in healthcare fraud and abuse: Navigating uncertainties, 3rd ed. Washington, DC: American Health Lawyers Association. 2006.

Medicare Payment Advisory Commission. Publications directory. Available at http://www.medpac.gov/document_search.cfm. Accessed 9/03/07.

National Committee on Quality Assurance. About NCQA. Available at http://web.ncqa.org/tabid/65/Default.aspx. Accessed 9/03/07a.

National Committee on Quality Assurance. HEDIS and quality measurement. Available at http://web.ncqa.org/tabid/59/Default.aspx. Accessed 9/03/07b.

National Committee on Quality Assurance. HEDIS 2007 summary table of measures and product lines. Available at http://web.ncqa.org/Portals/0/HEDISQM/HEDIS2007/MeasuresList.pdf. Accessed 9/03/07c.

National Institutes of Health. About NIH. Available at http://www.nih.gov/about/index.html#mission. Accessed 9/03/07.

National Labor Relations Board. Fact sheet. Available at http://www.nlrb.gov/about_us/overview/fact_sheet.aspx. Accessed 9/30/07.

Occupational Safety and Health Administration. OSHA's

mission. Available at http://www.osha.gov/oshinfo/mission.html. Accessed 9/03/07.

Rutgers. FASB and IASB agree to work together toward convergence of global accounting standards. Available at http://accounting.rutgers.edu/raw/fasb/news/nr102902.html. Accessed 9/03/07.

Sandstrom RW, Lohman H, Bramble JD. Health services policy and systems for therapists. Upper Saddle River, NJ: Prentice Hall. 2003.

Scott RW. Legal aspects of documenting patient care, 2nd ed. Gaithersburg, MD: Aspen. 2000:191.

Vaughn JR. National Council on Disability 30 years of disability policy leadership 1978-2008. NCD: 2008 United States Senate Special Committee on Aging Award Winner. Available at http://www.ncd.gov/ward/award_main.cfm>. Accessed 1/13/09.

ADDITIONAL RESOURCES

An example of a physical therapy billing audit "Review of Florida Physical Therapist's Medicare Claims for Therapy Services Provided During 2003" (A-06-06-00078) can be found on the OIG website at http://oig.hhs.gov/oas/reports/region6/60600078.htm.

Up to date information about the various federal government Internet sites noted in this chapter may be found at:

ACF at http://www.acf.hhs.gov.
AHRQ at http://www.ahrq.gov.
AoA at http://www.aoa.dhss.gov.
CDC at http://www.cdc.gov.
CMS at http://cms.hhs.gov/default.asp?
DOL at http://www.dol.gov.
FDA at http://www.fda.gov.
FTC at http://www.ftc.gov/ftc/consumer.htm.
HRSA at http://www.hrsa.gov.
IHS at http://www.ihs.gov.
IRS at http://www.irs.gov.
Medicare at http://www.medicare.gov.
MedPac at http://www.medpac.gov.
NCD at http://www.ncd.gov.
NIH at http://www.nih.gov.
NLRB at http://www.nlrb.gov.
OSERS at http://www.ed.gov/offices/OSERS.
OSHA at http://www.osha.gov.
SAMHSA at http://www.samhsa.gov.
VHA at http://www.nlm.nih.gov/medlineplus/veteranshealth.html.

PART III

Business Acumen: Managing, Communicating, Strategizing, Planning, and Decision Making

PART I (CH 1–6)

Broad Perspective on Providing Health Services

PART II (CH 7–10)

Guiding Behavior: Values, Ethics, Jurisprudence, and Oversight Agencies

PART III (CH 11–16)

Business Acumen: Managing, Communicating, Strategizing, Planning, and Decision Making

PART IV (CH 17–19)

Business Acumen: Human Resources, Marketing, and Selling

PART V (CH 20–23)

Business Acumen: Financial Awareness

CHAPTER 11

Leading, Managing, and Supervision

CHERYL ANDERSON

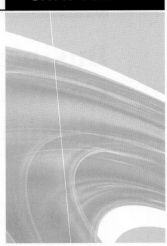

Learning Objectives

1. Compare and contrast leadership, management, and supervision in terms of scope, influence, personal attributes, skills, and knowledge.
2. Synthesize the similarities and differences among leadership, management, and supervision.
3. Investigate nonhierarchical management and leadership styles.
4. Determine appropriate methods for physical therapists (PTs) to acquire leadership, management, and supervisory skills.
5. Assess your own leadership, management, and supervision, knowledge and skills.
6. Apply management and leadership concepts in physical therapy-related scenarios.

Introduction

Management, **supervision**, and *leadership* are often used synonymously. However, each of these terms, denotes different responsibilities within an organization. The business world is replete with terms for levels of management within *organizations*. This chapter delves into the differences between the terms *management*, *supervision*, and *leadership*. Since management and supervision are integrated within the topic of leadership, most of the discussion is devoted to synthesis of management and supervisory techniques with some analysis of

leadership and the role of leaders. Understanding leadership and leaders helps to strengthen a PT's knowledge of management and understanding of why moving through the ranks from clinician to supervisor to manager does not guarantee that one is a leader.

There are as many definitions for these terms as there are writers and researchers in the field of business. However, there is a common thread throughout. Definitions for each usually include the person's concern for accomplishing organizational **goals** or **objectives** by working with and through individuals and groups.

The world of business, including physical therapy, which is a segment of health care businesses, is generally developed in hierarchical fashion. Though there is fervor surrounding the need for hierarchy and its companion, *bureaucracy*, most organizations, and facilities, nevertheless, have a **hierarchy** in place. This hierarchy allows for the *chain of command* policies and **procedures** to succinctly relate how employees should respond to or expect to act within the parameters of their work.

Traditional business hierarchy divides the ranks of management into three tiers. These include **lower level**, or **first-level management**, *middle management*; and **upper-level management**. The levels are organized in a pyramid fashion ranked in order of importance (Fig. 11.1). Most organizations have many more lower level managers (represented by the wide base of the pyramid) than upper level managers. Thus, the pyramid style reflects a gradually increasing level of responsibility for

Key Terms

Key terms, which are defined below, are bolded and italicized the first time they appear in the chapter. Other important terms are shown in boldface on first appearance and are defined by the context in which they are used. When either of these types of terms is used several times, its acronym will be identified and subsequently used in the chapter. Both types of terms are listed alphabetically in the online glossary with their definitions and (when applicable) their acronyms.

administrator: may be upper level generalist managers.

bureaucracy: an organizational system common in mid to large-size businesses that is mechanistic: clearly defined jobs, a clear hierarchical structure, and depend on the chain of command, or management structure, for work coordination. This type of organizational structure fits a top-down leadership style.

chain-of-command: the management structure of the organization related to decision-making power, supervision, direction, lines of communication, and others.

charismatic style: a style of management/leadership that relies on personality to lead and inspire employees. This style requires the ability to communicate well. Personality driven individuals may be well received by employees.

chief operating officer (COO): an upper level of corporate management who is responsible for managing the day-to-day activities of the corporation and who reports to the CEO or BOD.

direct report(s): a manager's subordinates. Employees whose performance a manager is responsible for and who must answer to or report directly to their supervising manager.

director of finance: an upper level manager, sometimes called the chief financial officer, responsible for planning, overseeing, and directing the department(s) that allocate and account for resources.

distributed leadership: seeing all members of the organization as experts in their own right—as uniquely important sources of knowledge, experience, and wisdom. Under Distributed Leadership, everyone is responsible and accountable for leadership within his or her area. Also called, shared leadership, team leadership, and democratic leadership.

laissez-faire: French for let the people do as they please. A leadership style with a light directive touch.

leadership: intentionally influencing the beliefs and actions of willing followers.

management: the formally recognized leadership of an organization. The act of realizing organizational goals through the efforts of others. The allocation of responsibilities and provision of resources to others so they can do the work that leads to fulfilling organizational objectives.

management style: the ways a manager chooses to respond in certain contexts based on their values, information at hand, experience, creativity, habit, constraints, and supervisee characteristics.

middle manager(s/ment): managers below senior and above lower levels of management.

organizational development(OD): the study of organizational leadership and how organizations are created, developed, mature, and end.

organization(s): groups of people brought together to achieve common purposes.

self-managed work team: teams that control their work, manage themselves within the context of the team and their usual work, distribute the work within the group, make operations-related decisions, actively seek help and resources from the organization, use their discretion to take initiative when problems arise, monitor their own performance, and seek candid feedback.

subordinate(s): those who are answerable for their work actions and results to an organizationally higher level individual.

Theory X: one of two parts of McGregor's conceptual framework for management style. Theory X assumes the average person inherently avoids work because he dislikes it, needs firm direction and threats to achieve work goals, lacks ambition so he needs direction, and values job security.

Theory Y: one of two parts of McGregor's conceptual framework for management style. Theory Y is the antithesis of Theory X. Theory Y assumes the average finds work a natural activity, there are various means other than punishment to get people to achieve work-related goals, job satisfaction is one of these means, given the opportunity, most people seek responsibility, and the ability to solve work-related problems is dispersed throughout the organization.

(Continued)

more and more people as one moves up the pyramid. In the hierarchy, staff report to lower level managers who report to middle managers who report to upper level managers. The level of authority, responsibility, and **scope** of control is the most expansive at the top. As one moves down the hierarchy, responsibility tends to lessen while the scope narrows.

Table 11.1 compares the levels of health care managers providing a frame of reference along with general duties found in each level.

What Managers Do

For decades, the literature on organizational management has often dealt with Fayol's (1949) concept of what managers do, e.g., control, coordinate, organize, and plan. Refining efforts to define the responsibilities and roles of managers were made by numerous business-focused authors (Mintzberg, 1973, 1975; Mintzberg et al., 1995; Yukl, 1994, 2002). Yukl melded information from management literature on

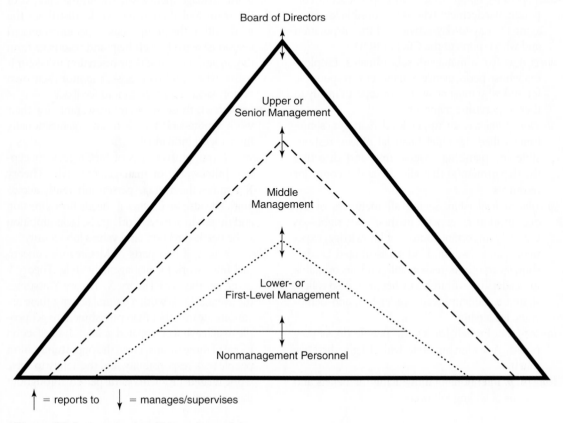

Figure 11.1. Organizational hierarchy model.

228

Table 11.1 Comparison of Health Care Managers: Frame of Reference and General Duties

Upper-Level Management

Frame of reference: the organization

Vision, values, mission

Coordination organization-wide

Integration

Dealing with the external environment

Long-term goals

Middle-Level Management

Frame of reference: various clusters of work groups and related work groups

Coordination of groups

A variety of operations

Relatively short-term goals

First-Level Management

Frame of reference: personnel in a department and functionally related departments

Coordination of individuals

Direct-care operations

Short-term goals

---

the work of managers at all organizational levels with his own observations of five small business executive officers. He identified ten roles managers fulfill. Yukl (1994, 2002) discussed nine areas of managerial responsibilities supported by survey data gathered over 11 years from more than 10,000 managers in 20 countries. For comparison, Table 11.2 presents these two lists of what managers do. The lists of the generic responsibilities of managers are aligned to indicate which terms have similar intent. Thus, there are several terms in the Mintzberg list that match Yukl's descriptive terms.

To *administrate* means to carry out activities such as formulating policies, analyzing data, and maintaining records. An *administrator* is a person at the upper level of an organizational hierarchy. The *consult* responsibility includes acting as a sounding board for others, maintaining current competence in technical areas, and offering expert advice. To *coordinate* means to share information with and bring about cooperative efforts among individuals who may not be directly under the control of

Table 11.2 Summary of Manager Responsibilities

Based on Mintzberg et al., 1995	Based on Yukl, 1994
Make decisions When critical unplanned events occur	**Make decisions** Quickly
When changes are needed	In unpredicted conditions
When resources are to be allocated	When resources are to be allocated
When negotiations must be carried out	When negotiations must be carried out When to stretch boundaries
Inform others About state of internal environment	**Inform others** About internal and external environment
External to the organization/department	External to the organization/department
About matters they would not usually know about	By sharing information
Interact with others As representative or organization/department	**Interact with others** As representative of organization/department
External to organization/department	External to organization/department
To motivate, inspire, lead	Administer policies, analyze data, record systems, etc. Develop subordinates: supervise, train, set performance objectives, etc. Coordinate efforts of others; solve problems, mediate, etc. Consult with others, for others, regarding new methods, etc. Control schedules, quality, effectiveness, etc. Organize and plan operational policies, procedures: short-, long-term plans, budget, etc.

the manager. *Control* over the delivery of services and production of goods requires analysis, scheduling, budgeting, and quality control. The responsibility of *decision maker* requires quick determination of what to do with resources and when to do it and resolving disagreements in the face of unique and unpredicted circumstances. All manager responsibilities involve decision making (Chapter 15). The *monitor* function is keeping an ear to the ground regarding the internal and external environments and assessing them in terms of their being threats to the organization/department or as opportunities to be seized. Monitoring involves developing broad networks and equitably exchanging information among network members. A manager must *organize and plan*. These responsibilities include making budgets, assessment of outcomes, resource utilization, and setting objectives and goals. Managers *represent* the organization/department to external **stakeholders** and others in ways that project a positive image toward the organization/department (Chapters 1 and 2). To *supervise* others involves assisting them to be able to self-assess what they do well and what they need to do to improve, the provision of technical training for them to meet their job related needs and assessment of their performance relative to defined objectives and goals (Chapter 17). More will be said about supervision later. It is worth noting that decision making and influencing could have been added alongside each of the responsibilities and roles (Table 11.2) to indicate that managers are always engaged in decision making (Longest et al., 2000) and opportunities to influence others (leadership) are ever present (Mintzberg et al., 1995).

A closer look at the identified responsibilities and roles of managers suggests that some condensing of the many terms used to describe what managers do is possible. Based on a review of the literature Yukl (2002) concluded that most manager activities fostered at least one of four general processes:

1. Building and maintaining relationships
2. Exchanging information
3. Making decisions
4. Influencing others

Similarly, Mintzberg et al. (1995) related their ten managerial roles to three higher order categories:

1. Decision making
2. Informing
3. Interacting

Comparison of these two perspectives on the responsibilities and roles are presented in Table 11.3 along with representative examples of managerial activities.

Of particular interest to new graduates and licensed therapists early in their careers is what to expect in the near future in terms of management responsibility as well as how to prepare for these responsibilities. The Standards of Practice of the American Physical Therapy Association (APTA, 2007a) and Guide (APTA, 2001) identifies ten management areas the leader of a physical therapy service should engage in:

1. Administration related to the service
2. Collaboration with other services
3. Development of departmental goals, mission statement, and purposes
4. Development of organizational plans
5. Development of policies and procedures
6. Development of the physical setting
7. Fiscal management
8. Quality of care and performance
9. Staff development
10. Staffing

The usual initial transition is from direct patient care responsibilities to a first-level

Table 11.3 Comparative Lists of the Responsibilities and Roles of Managers

Responsibilities (Yukl, 1994[a])	Roles (Mintzbertg et al., 1995)
Administrate	Monitor
Consult	Liaison
Coordinate	Disseminator, negotiator, liaison
Control	Resource distributor
Make decisions	Problem solver
Monitor	Monitor
Organize and plan	Entrepreneur, resource distributor
Represent	Figurehead, spokesperson
Supervise	Leader

[a]Adapted from Page R. The position description questionnaire. Unpublished paper. Minneapolis, MN: Con trol Data Business Advisors, 1985. Cited in Yukl G. Leadership in organizations, 5th ed. Upper Saddle River, NJ: Prentice Hall. 2002.

management position in which there are responsibilities for direct patient care along with management responsibilities. The initial transition could also involve assuming a first-level management position with infrequent or no direct patient care responsibilities. Yukl's (1994) description of management in terms of four general processes, i.e., relationships, information exchanges, decision making, and influencing others is useful to synthesize what first-level managers do and how to prepare to become a manager.

Lower-Level Management/ Supervisors

Supervisors are considered the lowest, or most junior-level of management positions. In a hierarchical system, supervisors are one step above a lead as in **lead PT**. Supervisors tend to be those employees who are more seasoned. This person may not have any formal training in management or supervising employees. To be a supervisor, one must have authority over at least one other worker. There is no magic validation as to what makes a supervisor or a mid-level manager. Though there are PTs with management degrees, there is no requirement or certification that states one may be a supervisor or manager.

First-level managers exchange information. They act as intermediaries between the staff and the next level of management. The information exchange runs up to the next level of management and down to the *subordinates/direct reports.* First-level managers usually have peer relationships, too. Thus, the exchange of information would also be a parallel relationship as well as moving upward (middle-level management) or downward (subordinates).

Since exchange of information is crucial to first-level, lower-level managers, the following are suggestions to foster communication (also see Chapter 12):

- Know the time constraints of the decision, of the people involved, of your own work needs.
- Actively listen to others; not just hear what is being said.
- Be genuine.
- Be prepared to objectively share information in a concise manner.
- Contribute to the discussion by offering actions, opinions, clarifications; help others to weigh options.
- Recognize your own nonverbal signs and reactions.
- Recognize nonverbal signs of interest, disinterest, disgust, belief, disbelief, sincerity, anxiety, and anger.
- Redirect unintended or undesirable reactions; attempt to maintain a problem-solving tone to communications.

More on Supervision: First-Level Management

To function as a manager requires overseeing others to assure a certain quantity of work is completed at an acceptable level of quality. Figure 11.2 depicts the relationship between performance and the components that influence performance.

Stated in words, this figure suggests that to have high levels of job performance a manager should hire the right people (ability, knowledge, and skill [Chapters 16 and 17]), meet their priority psychological needs (Chapter 7), prepare people to accept responsibility and delegate appropriately (empower [Chapters 16

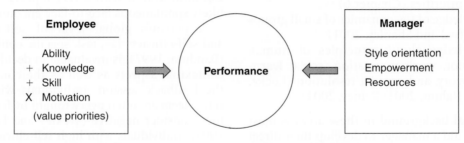

Figure 11.2. Employee and manager contributions to job performance.

and 17]) and provide the necessary tools, supplies, and systems to do the job (resources).

Supervision involves maintaining or improving the performance of direct reports by assisting them to develop the knowledge and skill to self-assess their strengths and weaknesses, and making available resources and opportunities for growth (Yukl, 2002). What this means for the first-level manager is addressed next.

Practicalities of First-Level Management

The distinguishing feature of first-level management is that the direct reports are not managers (McConnell, 2006). Commonly these direct reports include receptionists, clerks, secretaries, phone operators, volunteers as well as direct care staff. In health care settings, nonpatient care staff is often the first to be contacted by the public, e.g., customers, their family members and friends, and vendors. The core purpose of providing health care services is to meet customers' needs and expectations (Chapter 21). This places the first-level health care manager in an exceptionally strategic position relative to the success of a department or organization (Dunn, 1998).

To get the job done with and through others, the first-level manager requires knowledge of the jobs of direct reports. It is advantageous for a first-level clinical manager to be recognized as a competent clinical practitioner by their therapists because it intimates knowledge of their job and a tacit assumption that the welfare of patients will be a priority in the department. To foster getting the job done through others it is helpful if a first-level manager has:

- Self-understanding, i.e., knowledge of one's own values that shape his or her worldview (Bennis, 1994)
- Some knowledge of each direct report's value priorities (Chapter 6)
- Knowledge of the dynamics of small groups (Langfred and Shanley, 2001)
- Knowledge about principles of human behavior, work motivation, social learning theory, and conflict resolution (Locke, 2001; Rahim, 2001; Rainey, 2001)

Formal background in these areas is most likely to aid a manager to develop their direct reports when the knowledge is coupled with skill development opportunities and feedback from others on their performance.

Feedback

Knowledge of results is feedback on performance. Feedback includes criticism and praise or negative and positive feedback, respectively. Feedback is usually taken to heart if it relates to a prioritized goal of the individual whose behavior is being assessed (Locke, 2001). In the workplace, the first-level manager sets departmental goals in accord with organizational goals (Chapter 9). Direct reports need to have mechanisms to know how they are doing relative to departmental goals (Chapters 12 and 17).Therefore, to maximize performance to achieve goals, both the goals and feedback on performance must be paired. The goal(s) is/are the targeted end-result. The feedback is the degree of progress made relative to the goal(s). Some management opportunities to provide feedback are:

- Chance meeting
- E-mail
- Formal face-to-face meeting
- Group meeting
- Memo
- Phone call
- Post comparative data with personal identification numbers
- Reports
- Video conference

The choice of method depends on urgency, previous feedback, availability, personal preference, previous interactions with the person, and other situational variables (Chapter 12). While electronic means of communication are frequently used today, for the first-level manager, e-mail is likely to be used for communicating with peers and middle-level managers. Communication with direct reports is most likely spontaneous face-to-face encounters.

A person's global level of self-esteem and **self-efficacy**, i.e., task specific confidence (Bandura, 1997), is invaluable in deciding the contextual aspects as well as the content of the feedback session. Individuals with low self-esteem are often overwrought by feedback they consider negative (Wexley and Latham, 1991). Individuals with high self-efficacy will set high personal goals for that task, will pursue the goal with vigor, and will persist in the pursuit of specific goal achievement because they believe they have the ability to do what it takes to be successful (Peterson and Smith, 2000). A high level of self-efficacy may be developed by exposure to role models a person may identify with, mentor relationships, and public and private positive feedback. Feedback should be provided as soon as possible after a performance or at least within an interval that allows a clear connection between the behavior of interest and the outcome of the behavior. The comments should be specific and the volume of comments appropriate to the knowledge, skill, and experience of the direct report. New staff members usually benefit from the essential information while experienced staff members are often appreciative of the bigger picture.

In Table 11.4, the management responsibilities reflect a point of reference that targets "the here and now." The leadership list contains roles that reflect broader and future oriented judgments or the results of management decisions.

Change is inevitable. For health care managers, change is frequent, often unanticipated, and fraught with novel problems. In short, there are many opportunities for managers to influence others to deal with change in positive ways. The point is, those who influence others lead. Carrying out management responsibilities requires leadership. Management and leadership coexist.

Middle Management

Middle-level managers generally are responsible for at least two hierarchical levels of

Table 11.4 Comparison of a Managerial and Leadership Frame of Reference

Management	Leadership
Solve operations-focused problems	Solve change-focused problems
Short-term goals	Long-term goals
Predict tangible results	Offer a vision of the future
Maintain order	Communicate the vision
Establish structure	Establish strategies for change
Monitor results	Motivate and inspire

employees below them. This would include subordinates with no management authority, and lower level managers or supervisors. In the era of cost-efficiencies and productivity, many health care systems have eliminated hierarchical structures with three or more levels. Rather, the health care systems look for the "working" manager; that person who performs staff duties while maintaining a management position over other staff members. This is known as "flattening" of management levels. On an **organizational chart** there would be fewer management levels, therefore the height of chart is lower and flatter than one with more management levels. The loss of middle-level management has been a noted phenomenon across all business entities in this century. The advent of technologies such as computers and cell phones has taken away the need for many clerical or administrative assistant positions. Further, electronic medical records are allowing clinicians to document at the point of service negating the need to handwrite daily treatment notes or dictate progress notes. This has decreased need for transcription and filing or clerical help as these tasks are included in the daily functions of the clinician. The subordinate level of those who help a clinician is shrinking.

Management within physical therapy departments may be diverse. In a large physical therapy department, the head would likely be a middle manager. In a small department, a PT may be the department head and may have no lower level supervisors; often considered a working manager. In a private practice, depending on the size of the practice, there may be no middle management or even lower level supervisors. The employees would be considered subordinates with no supervisory level between themselves and the owner (Chapter 22). The owner would be the upper management executive. However, it should be noted that ownership is not necessarily synonymous with a level of management. Owners may not be involved in the practice at all or owners may be the driving force behind clinical care thus, hiring an **operations** person to manage the day-to-day details of the business.

Upper Management

Demarcations between middle management and upper management may be difficult to determine, too. Generally, upper level managers are at the top of the hierarchy. This may be a hospital administrator, **chief executive officer (CEO)**, *chief operating officer (COO)*, *director of finance*, and so on. Upper management drives the goals and strategies of the organization. Upper level managers may also be called executives (Chapter 9).

In many organizations, upper management also has a reporting structure to another level of management oversight through a **board of directors** or *trustees* of an organization. In cases with boards, the upper level managers do report to and are hired by the boards (Chapter 9). The boards hire upper level managers to operate the organization to meet financial goals, and oversee the operations of the organization.

Tiered systems of management appear to be neat and tidy. However, current practices reveal different systems in place across practice settings and in different areas of the country. The advent of interdisciplinary teams in hospitals, skilled nursing facilities, and home care has dissolved much of the hierarchy in health care systems. Interdisciplinary teams work in cooperative ventures in a process that best serves the client. This focus of patient-centered or client-centered care ignores the hierarchical structure followed by many organizations. The team members are generally professionals who collaborate in a fashion that does not require supervision, management, or leadership. More discussion on small groups will be provided later in this chapter.

Functional Categories of Managers

In addition to the tiered methodology for determining management responsibility, other terms may be used to denote a level of control or expertise within a certain area. Functional categories may be used to define managers responsible for functions within an organization. These include:

- Administrative managers are generalists who understand most of the functional areas of management; they have a broad understanding of the organization.
- Financial managers deal with the financial resources of the organization. These individuals are knowledgeable about reimbursement, cash flow, accounting, and investments.

- Human resource managers are responsible for employee hiring along with salary and benefits determinations. These individuals must ensure that all labor laws are closely followed and ensure that employees are educated about their employment rights.
- Marketing managers develop materials, strategies, and connections to promote an organization's products and services.
- Operations managers are responsible for creation and oversight of the systems that create an organization. In physical therapy, a hospital department head would be a type of operations manager. In a small private practice, the owner may also be the operations manager.
- Sales managers are responsible for selling the products or services to consumers. This position is generally outwardly focused toward how to serve customers or the public (see Chapter 19).
- Specialized managers are skilled in areas of special need. For example, risk management, compliance, public relations, or a technical skill area.

Skills of a Manager

Across all levels of management, generally there at least three skills needed to be a manager (Blanchard and Bowles, 2001). These include:

1. Technical skill includes the ability to use knowledge, methods, techniques, and equipment needed for the performance of specific tasks learned from experience or education. PTs have a technical skill set that includes the ability to understand and apply electrical modalities; evaluate and plan an exercise regime to assist an individual to improve in functional skills; or create a treatment plan to meet the needs of a patient.
2. Human skill is the ability to work with and through people; an understanding of motivation and application of effective communication, management, and leadership skills. PTs demonstrate human skills when working with patients to diagnose a physical disability; create a treatment regime; document progress; and collaborate with the patient and other health care practitioners to effectively treat the condition.

3. Conceptual skill is the ability to understand the complexities of the organization and where one fits within that organization. This is a higher level of functional thinking that allows a person to theorize and apply learning. PTs integrate conceptual skills when developing new programs for an organization. One must determine the need for a new service or product and then design a response to that need. Higher level, intellectual skills are needed to apply this new concept and help others understand the need and the response.

Management Process

The management process may be divided into four managerial functions. The functions central to any management discussion are:

- Planning
- Organizing
- Motivating
- Controlling

In the process of managing, multiple processes occur at the same time. As one sets out on a new task, planning begins by setting goals and objectives for the organization. Organizing becomes meaningful as the manager brings together resources—people, capital, and equipment—integrating each into the plan. With planning and organization comes motivating. Managers must effectively influence employees to complete tasks. Motivation may be part of providing direction while maintaining control and oversight of a project (Hersey et al., 2007).

The management process of planning, organizing, motivating, and controlling is a circuitous process, with each phase running into the next as the manager continues to develop, complete, or modify work tasks or projects.

Management Styles

Managers at all levels are in a position that has power or influence over a project, team of people, or work group. *Management styles* have been analyzed from the view of company success and employee satisfaction. Early in management theory development, two distinct management styles were identified through the work of McGregor (1960).

He created the now famous *Theory X–Theory Y* hypothesis. McGregor hypothesized that there were two management styles. The first was Theory X or an autocratic style. In this style, managers imposed their decisions on staff demanding compliance. The basic beliefs of this theory hold that employees are unmotivated, need to be told what to do, and value job security. On the surface, this belief might seem archaic or not relevant to today's environment. However, PTs will encounter subordinates who do require direct supervision with constant feedback. The subordinate may not wish to contribute as expected or may not have the education or experience to contribute to the organization. Thus, a type of Theory X approach may be needed.

McGregor's second hypothesized style was Theory Y, the *laissez-faire* or democratic style. This theory holds that decisions should be made by a consensus vote of the employees. Further, this theory assumes that people are self-motivated and may be self-directed and creative at work, if properly motivated. It would seem that Theory Y would be a favorable approach for managers to embrace. However, it too has its drawbacks. For example, not all decisions can be made in a democratic fashion. Some decisions need to be made and the process moved along. All employees cannot possibly have input into all decisions. The organization would be paralyzed with attempting to reach consensus on everything. Theory X–Theory Y attempted to define management into two divisions. It was a beginning to understanding management application to the modern business world.

In the years since McGregor's 1960s work, many books have been written about management styles. Many built onto the Theory X–Theory Y foundation pointing out the fallibility of each approach. One of the more modern concepts of participative management and leadership grew out of the work by Hershey and Blanchard (1982, 2007). These theorists developed a philosophy whereby a manager would provide the right level of cues and support depending on the need of the employee. Thus, in the physical therapy department, an administrative assistant may require more direction with set deadlines following a Theory X methodology. A staff PT may only require encouragement and can be asked for thoughts on new procedures or methods to improve the department function through the application of Theory Y.

Management style discussions have grown to encompass other attributes. These include:

- *Charismatic style* relies on personality to lead and inspire employees. Leaders who use this style communicate well. Personality driven individuals may be well received by employees.
- *Consultative style* considers the advice and feelings of others prior to a final management decision. This style makes employees feel included in decision-making processes.
- *Delegating style* allows staff to assume responsibility for decision making and problem solving through assignments from the manager. Asking a staff member to attend a meeting in lieu of oneself is a method of delegating. Delegating styles may be welcomed by employees where employees desire to increase their roles. However, delegating styles may be resented by employees where the manager appears to be shirking duties by assigning work to others.
- *Persuasive style* uses the power of persuading staff that the decisions already determined are the correct ones to implement. Persuading others may have a double-edged sword. Employees may feel little control or may feel taken advantage of by the manager who uses a persuasive style consistently.
- *Transactional style* denotes the manager who rewards staff with money, job promotions, or benefits in return for compliance. Bonus incentive programs for meeting productivity or efficiency standards are a type of transactional style application.
- *Transformational style* focuses on staff and attitude development. Providing continuing education formats and encouraging staff learning embraces a transformational style. Selecting and using the appropriate style for the right employee is one of the key strengths of an effective manager.

Another way to look at management styles was developed by Blanchard (1994). Blanchard focused on four basic styles of management:

1. Directing
2. Delegating
3. Supporting
4. Coaching

These styles are readily adaptable to physical therapy clinical practice as well as in management-type functions. Most PTs do have the opportunity to direct. PTs direct physical therapist assistants (PTAs) and therapy aides in completing tasks that assist the PTs. PTs also direct patients in how to complete treatment regimes.

PTs are part of the helping medical professions. As such, PTs support patients to improve rehabilitation potential through treatment planning and by providing an empathetic ear to the patient and their caregivers. PTs also support their colleagues and their work environment by participating in department and facility meetings, providing clinical care to patients, mentoring others, and through professional work in the community (Chapter 22).

Coaching is another management tenet that PTs may use in patient care and in professional interactions. Similar to providing positive direction to a team, a PT coaches patients to improve motivating through thoughts and actions. PTs may also serve as coach–mentors to other PTs and health care team members through participation in facility projects such as United Way Fund Drives, capital-building campaigns, and through positive feedback and exuberance in their environments (Chapter 22).

PTs need to positively delegate functions in both the clinical realm and in the professional realm. One cannot do everything in isolation. PTs need to work with others to sustain the profession and to improve patient care. Even the new graduate PT must delegate clinical tasks, such as patient transport, filing of forms, billing to third parties, and so on. PTs also must delegate the responsibility of getting healthier to the patient. The PT must design a client-centered care plan. However, the client has the ultimate responsibility to carry out the plan. The PT will support and even coach the patient in this plan. However, delegating the plan to the patient and directing its proper use will be of great benefit to all patients. Table 11.5 presents relevant examples of each of Blanchard's styles.

Alternatives to Hierarchy in Management

Circle of Influence and Seven Habits

There have been schools of thought that focus on doing away with management hierarchies.

Table 11.5 Blanchard's Management Styles Integrated With Physical Therapy Examples		
Management Styles	**When to Use**	**Examples in PT**
Directing—telling someone how to complete a task and when to do it.	Decisions need to be made immediately; there are few risks; staff commitment is irrelevant.	Assigning patients to therapists; Determining lunch or break schedules.
Delegating—the most challenging. Assigning task to others that might be considered beyond the scope of the employee.	When time commitments need to be kept; staff are eager to do more than what is required of their job function.	Asking a therapist to take a lead on a project; volunteer for a difficult patient; or when it appears the staff person needs a new challenge.
Supportive—collegial style for the manager to work alongside the staff. Supportive managers are concerned about "feelings."	Staff need motivation or more confidence. Requires the manager to be a good listener.	Mentoring students or staff; providing support for staff in new situations or changes in policy.
Coaching—combination of directing and supporting. Requires good two-way communication between staff and manager.	Staff desires to improve in a parameter or is willing to try something new.	Training a person in the use of a new modality; computer software; a different exercise regime.

Source: Blanchard, 1994.

One theory proposes a **circle of influence**, a concept promoted by Covey (2004a). The basic concept of the Circle of Influence calls for one to focus time and energy on the important things under one's own control. Further, through this Circle of Influence, one may enlarge the areas that they may influence thereby increasing the area of real influence. Covey's concepts allow for a proactive approach in management while purporting that all employees would be placed in a circular fashion with no one above the other.

Covey's work grew from his religious beliefs developed out of the Mormon faith. He became a national speaker and management guru promoting seven habits that he felt embodied effective people. Covey presents these behaviors as a progression from dependence to independence, and to interdependence. The habits are:

1. Be proactive based on principles of a personal vision.
2. Begin with the end in mind based on principles of personal leadership.
3. Put first things first based on principles of personal management.
4. Think win/win based on principles of interpersonal leadership.
5. Seek first to understand and then to be understood based on principles of empathetic communication.
6. Synergize based on principles of creative communication.
7. Sharpen the saw based on principles of self-renewal.

Recently, Covey has added an eighth principle—"Find your voice and inspire others to find theirs" (2004b, p. 3). It is hard to argue with Covey's positive view of becoming an effective manager and leader. However, critics do point out that the habits are overly idealistic and may be impractical in many difficult management decisions. Nonetheless, many of Covey's short phrased habits have become common management vernacular.

Matrix Management

Matrix management, also known as *dotted line responsibility*, is a second type of management system that does not use a hierarchical method. Matrix management recognizes that organizations are living organisms with managers who deal with multiple directives. Matrix management is commonly seen in project management or banking offices. Matrix management includes functional and operational managers, each having the same level of influence and responsibility, and each respected for an individual skill-set that contributes to the organization's goals. Based on concepts developed in the 1970s, new matrix management schemes implement horizontal maps, which detail work processes that require completion. The organization is managed by **steering councils** with horizontal governance to create strategic plans and missions (Gunn, 2007). Matrix management works best in project management situations or business process management systems. Inherent within matrix management is the philosophy of team-based methods. Team members do not report to the team leader, rather they rely on authority and a collaborative nature to complete tasks.

Matrix management may be an effective system for large physical therapy departments to consider. Given that there are few management or leadership positions available within large departments, matrix-developed teams might provide a way to nurture therapists to expand their management skill-sets while continuing to work within their designated patient care areas. Matrix management is a method of promoting professionalism by treating similarly skilled persons the same (Gunn, 2007). Well-functioning interdisciplinary teams may be a type of working matrix management. Each professional has multiple ways to communicate with others while maintaining control over one's own area or work. Matrix management is garnering attention in today's business world. Matrix management is occurring in physical therapy clinics across the nation, though it is seldom labeled "matrix management." Interdisciplinary teams operate in a matrix format. Each professional on the team has dotted line responsibility to others on the team. For example, in home care, matrix management is often used to provide the best services possible to homebound patients. A nurse or PT may be the person who starts or introduces the patient to home care services. By a thorough assessment, that person brings in other team members to assess and create an individualized plan for the patient. This may include occupational therapy, nursing, pharmacy, physician, and an array of home and community-based services. Each team member is responsible for treating or responding to specific needs of the client while maintaining communication channels with all of the other team members. There is no one person in charge. Rather, there is a group with a defined function working in home for the health of a client.

Matrix management may be used in large hospital settings, too. For example, large rehabilitation hospitals may have specialized areas of the department such as the neurological team or the orthopedic team. The neuro team may include a PT, occupational therapist, nurse, physician, speech language pathologist, and social worker. This team together evaluates the client and determines the treatment plan, discharge goals, and other needs. These teams are an excellent example of matrix management working in health care systems. Each team member and the patient rely on the others to do their professional best. Matrix management allows for professional growth of team members and a freedom from hierarchical structures that might have quashed creativity that matrix teams often enjoy.

Matrix management is also seen in private practice settings. Often private practices have several owners. One owner may be the operational manager, while another the financial manager, and yet another sales manager. This upper level management division of power may be a type of matrix management that works well for equal partnerships within a business structure.

Distributed Leadership

A third type of nonhierarchical management is *distributed leadership*. Spillane (2006) is the most prolific investigator into this type of management style. This researcher believes leadership happens in everyday practices through formal routines and informal interactions. Distributed leadership techniques look at the practices of leaders, followers, and the aspects of routines focusing on how responsibility may be divided among involved persons without resorting to a hierarchy of commands coming down from the top. Rather, individuals take responsibility and leadership in varying areas of the work environment. Most of the work in distributed leadership is in the educational environment. There is a paucity of this type of application in the health care arena yet there are similarities between groups of therapists and their managers and a group of teachers and their principle.

Small Teams

The organizational complexity of many health service organizations, e.g., acute care hospitals, skilled nursing facilities, and multi-service outpatient and home health enterprises, has led to increasing dependence on small teams to make meaningful decisions. For this discussion, a team consists of up to 12 members (Hiebert and

Klatt, 2001). Teams may be formally empowered to make decisions that were previously made by some level of management (Cohen and Bailey, 1997). Because of this empowerment, membership on a team offers opportunities to develop and fine-tune leadership skills. There are a number of different types of teams. Three generic types of teams are **functional operating team**, **cross-functional team**, and *self-managed work team* (Yukl, 2002). These types of teams differ in their membership, purpose, scope of influence, and means of designating the leader.

Membership of a functional operating team is relatively stable because the team is formed to deal with operational matters that are usually continuous. Moreover, the members come from the same organizational subunit. Management often appoints the team leader. The leader has considerable authority over internal operations and in representing the team to other subunits of the organization (Yukl, 2002). The tasks of the appointed leader of a functional operating team include:

- Motivating the members to work toward shared goals, i.e., sell the vision
- Communicating the message that the "team effort" can result in greater accomplishments than solitary efforts
- Building member confidence in the possibilities of the "team effort"
- Selecting members with relevant essential skills
- Assisting members to develop their team skills and an understanding of their role on the team
- Securing the resources necessary for the team to operate
- Representing the team positively to others

Functional operating teams are commonly formed to coordinate the delivery of services to various categories of patients. A manager may assign the group leader. In health care, an example of a functional operating team would be a departmental team made up of individuals whose jobs are specialized by license, yet organizationally similar, i.e., PTs, PTAs, and occupational therapists.

Another type is a cross-functional team. The purpose of a cross-functional team is to improve coordination between distinct but interdependent organizational subunits and

external stakeholders. The possible inclusion of members from outside of the organization is one of the differences from a functional operating team. Other distinctions include: the team is formed for a limited duration, it has a high level of autonomy over its work procedures, the members have diverse backgrounds, experience, and expertise, and the membership may change due to the changing nature of the teams' work (Yukl, 2002). The group leader may be assigned several ways: by management, a recommendation by the group for approval by management, chosen by the group, or on an alternating basis depending on the team's task. An example of cross-functional team is one made up of a home health PT, an occupational therapist, a nurse, a social worker, a case manager, a durable medical goods vendor, and a meals-on-wheels representative. A cross-functional team has a membership that is more heterogeneous than a functional operating team. This adds some challenges for the cross-functional team leader than for a functional operating team leader. For example, the leader may have more difficulty in scheduling meetings, reaching members, meetings may take longer due to communication lapses, technical jargon varies by discipline, and health care professionals may have greater loyalty to their functional unit than to the team. To counter the personal agenda issue, the designated leader needs to have recognized organizational power as well as support plus excellent human relations skills (Yukl, 2002). The success of the leader of a cross-functional team can be further bolstered by the ability to:

- Communicate about technical matters in ways all team members understand
- Plan, e.g., assign work appropriately, scheduling, and others
- Articulate strategies that support an expressed vision
- Resolve disputes, i.e., the ability to help the group formulate win-win decisions

A third type of team is called a self-managed work team. This type of team may be made up of any mix of individuals, but the members are typically from the same organizational subunit and have similar operational job tasks. Examples of self-managed team responsibilities are making hiring decisions, determining work schedules, and setting productivity goals. What makes a self-managed work team unique is that many of the responsibilities and the authority of one or more managers are, to varying degrees, turned over to the team. Langfred and Shanley (2001) characterize self-managing work teams as teams that:

- Control their work
- Manage themselves within the context of the team and their usual work, i.e., take responsibility for their work outcomes
- Distribute the work within the group
- Make operations-related decisions
- Actively seek help and resources from the organization
- Use their discretion to take initiative when problems arise
- Monitor own performance and seek candid feedback

Self-managing teams are autonomous or semi-autonomous in terms of direction and oversight. The members are from similar backgrounds, are assigned to the team for extended time periods, and deal with operational issues. These are also characteristics of a functional team. However, the common operational and professional backgrounds of the members and the ability of the team members to elect the leader, or to rotate the leadership role as circumstances change, gives a self-managing team much flexibility. The shared responsibility for the team's performance lessens the need for centralizing power in the position of team leader. To prepare team members to be contributors and leaders requires cross training. Cross training for these roles can enhance the skills of each member and impact positively on the team's performance. To help self-managing team members develop requisite knowledge and skills there is often a manager available to coach, consult, and teach the team members (Yukl, 2002). Yukl (2002) recommends that management fulfill the following conditions as a foundation for successful self-managing teams:

- Clear organizational objectives
- Demonstrable management support
- Meaningful, challenging tasks
- Significant authority
- Significant discretion within defined areas
- Access to necessary information
- Appropriate interpersonal skills
- Competent and committed coaching by managers

A challenge posed by shared leadership is the struggle to find a balance between individual and team leadership. Reports of how to achieve a balance have been contradictory. Successful self-managing teams have been found to have democratic leadership and active leader involvement in facilitating group participation (Stewart and Manz, 1995). However, others have found that leaders of self-managed teams more often than not controlled the decisions (Levi and Slem, 1995).

Leaders and Leadership

The field of *organizational development (OD)* devotes itself to understanding how organizations are created, developed, mature, and often times, end. OD also examines leaders and leadership. Popular authors such as Tom Peters, Kenneth Blanchard, Paul Hershey, Peter Senge, have devoted their careers and research expertise into dissecting leaders and leaderships as if there is a formula that one could swallow that would guarantee leadership. Not withstanding extensive research, the solution to what creates a leader and exactly what is leadership, remains elusive.

A Five-Level Leadership Proposal

There are various ways to examine leadership and leaders. Collins (2001) published seminal work investigating organizational leaders and what characteristics create a successful leader. Collins' work is interesting as it provides a dimension of leadership different from several popular authors. Collins' underpinning and theory is based on the belief that truly great leaders demonstrate humility and fierce resolve. He created a theory around five levels of leadership.

The five layers of this theory are arranged in a hierarchical fashion. Table 11.6 provides a visual summary of Collins' five levels along with attributes that may be found in each level.

Leadership begins at Level 1 with a highly capable individual. This person contributes to the organization through talent, knowledge, skills, and good work habits. Though in a leadership role, Level 1 leaders are not considered brilliant. This may be the PT that rose through the clinical career ladder, graduating into a

Table 11.6 Summary of Collins's Level 5 Leadership Hierarchy		
Level 5—Executive	Builds greatness through a combination of personal humility plus professional will.	This level is rare and may not be found in most organizations.
Level 4—Effective leader	Catalyzes commitment; stimulates others to high performance standards.	Administrator; CEO; or department head
Level 3—Competent manager	Organizes people and other resources toward the efficient completion of objectives.	Most department heads; many business owners; perhaps the Administrator or CEO, too.
Level 2—Contributing team member	Contributes to the achievement of group objectives; works well with others.	Most professional staff.
Level 1—Highly capable individual	Makes productive contributions to group efforts. Demonstrates good work habits.	All staff that remain employed because they get their job done well.

Source: Collins, 2001.

department head purely through seniority and ability to meet the organization's policies and procedures.

Level 2 is called the "contributing team member." Level 2 leaders contribute through group objectives. This person is effective in teams and works well in group settings. PTs who lead interdisciplinary teams are an example of a Level 2 Leader.

Level 3 leaders are termed "competent managers." These types of leaders are efficient at meeting or exceeding predetermined objectives. Level 3 leaders are able to organize people and resources. PTs who serve in operational capacities such as area managers, director of operations, etc., and who manage multiple groups or multiple facilities are a type of Level 3 leaders.

"Effective leaders" is the term given to Level 4 leaders. Level 4 leaders have integrated the power of personal influence. This type catalyzes commitment pursuing clear and compelling visions. These leaders stimulate others to perform at high standards. PTs who effectively run for State Chapter and/or APTA national offices often exemplify Level 4 leadership. These individuals are able to articulate their viewpoints and challenge others to follow. Level 4 leaders tend to be driven, positive-focused, and leaders who accomplish their internally set goals.

Finally, Level 5, the "Executive." This leadership style is at the pinnacle of the hierarchy. Level 5 leaders "build enduring greatness through a paradoxical combination of personal humility plus professional will" (Collins, 2001, p. 1).

Level 5 leaders are modest and willful, shy and fearless. This is a difficult concept to grasp as all other leadership styles focus on the outgoing charisma of the individual. Level 5 leaders, however, do not focus on personality. Rather, they appear to be internally driven to see great work done by others. Often times, outward modesty might seem to be a sign of inner weakness. Thus, finding a Level 5 leader is difficult.

Researchers find few in their reviews of countless organizations across the United States. Integrating a Level 5 leadership is an essential factor for taking a company from good to great. However, it is not the only one. There is a symbiotic relationship between these factors and the Level 5, humility-driven leader. Good to great leaders and companies constantly display three forms of discipline: disciplined people; disciplined thought; and disciplined action. When an organization has disciplined people, a hierarchy is not necessary; with disciplined thought, a bureaucracy is not necessary; with disciplined action, excessive controls are unnecessary (Collins, 2001). Combining a culture of such discipline with an underlying theme of entrepreneurship, a great performing team is founded.

There is controversy if one is born a Level 5 leader or if one may develop into such a person. However, the very things that create Level 1 through 4 leaders seems juxtaposed to the Level 5. There are few examples of Level 5 leadership. According to Collins (2001), of the thousands of companies surveyed, only 11 were found to have a Level 5 leader in charge, or in the management ranks. Thus, as PTs, we must be careful to watch for those instinctive leaders who do not seek adulation, who quietly perform; and who others look-up to for various reasons. These are the types of leaders that the profession should promote forward into positions and will provide insight and a clear vision while not being self-promoting. Level 5 leaders in physical therapy, like in other professions and businesses, indeed are a rare breed.

The Servant-Leader Theory

There are many divergent views of leaders and leadership. Germane to physical therapy, Gersh (2006) created a position paper that integrated the philosophy of servant-leadership with professionalism in physical therapy. Built on the work of Greenleaf (2002), Gersh explored the implication of a unifying matrix as a potential application to improving professionalism and leadership in physical therapy. Greenleaf's (2002) work asserts that leadership grows out of service to others. This theory emphasizes the leader's role as a *steward* of the organization's resources (human, financial, and assets). This theory encourages leaders to serve others while maintaining a results-oriented focus on the organization's values and integrity.

Gersh's (2006) work integrated the Code of Ethics (APTA, 2007b) and Guide to Professional Behavior (APTA, 2007c) with the servant-leader philosophy. The author noted that Principle 1—respect; compassionate care integrates with the servant-leadership characteristic of empathy. Principle 2—trustworthiness and Principle 9—protection of the public is comparable with the servant-leadership characteristic of stewardship/trust. Principle 11—respect for colleagues incorporates the servant-leadership characteristic of building community.

The servant-leadership characteristics of empowerment of those served and servant as leader are not specifically addressed in the APTA Code of Ethics (2007b). However, Gersh (2006) felt that the APTA Prin-

ciples of Professionalism, including the Core Values (APTA, 2007d) and Criteria for Standards of Practice (APTA, 2007a) did address these two characteristics. Gersh (2006) found that professionalism in physical therapy should be developed around instructing, nurturing, and empowering; or, in a word, serving. Servant-leaders in "physical therapy are those who envision dreams that unite people to move organizations forward" (Gersh, 2006, p. 15).

Physical Therapy Leadership, Administration, Management Preparation (LAMP)

Leadership in determining the interface between management and a clinical profession such as physical therapy was demonstrated by a section of the APTA.

In 1999, a taskforce of the Section on Administration (now Health Policy and Administration) created LAMP as an acronym for Leadership, Administration, Management and Preparation (Kovacek et al., 1999). From the taskforce seed, the LAMP concept has led to the development of a series of continuing education programs and research focusing for growing PT managers and leaders.

Seminal studies by Luedkte-Hoffmann (2002), Lopopolo et al. (2004), and Schafer et al. (2007) incorporated LAMP concepts and the visionary goals of the APTA, to focus on identifying the perceived needs of clinicians in the LAMP domains. The latter group concluded that the four basic LAMP tenets were interrelated and interdependent. These researchers therefore chose to make no distinction between leadership, administration, or management. Through a multiple-level survey, these investigators surveyed current physical therapy clinicians across a variety of practice settings to determine what administration and management skills the participants felt would be most necessary for new PTs to learn in their university education. The most salient findings from this study in order of rated importance are listed in Table 11.7.

The Lopopolo et al. (2004) and Schafer and associates (2007) studies initiated and refined the study of what physical therapy managers

Table 11.7 Analysis of Administration and Management Skills Required By 2010	
Skill Groups From Highest to Lowest Median Importance (Maximum 7, Range 6.5–4.29)	Examples of Specific Skills
1. Self-management	Verbal and nonverbal communication
2. Compliance	Documentation requirements
3. Ethics and culture	Professional ethics
4. Coding	ICD-9
5. Information management	Abel to access and use patient and clinical management data
6. Leading and directing	Leadership
7. Quality and risk management	Quality management
8. Practice analysis	Informed about profession
9. Personnel management	Performance appraisal
10. Networking	Consultation
11. Operational analysis	Process management
12. Operational management	Project management
13. Reimbursement review and analysis	Reimbursement sources
14. Strategic planning and marketing	Long-term planning
15. Financial analysis and budgeting	Profit and loss statement analysis
16. Environmental assessment	Community analysis

Reprinted from Schafer DS, Lopopolo RB, Luedtke-Hoffmann KA. Administration and management skills needed by physical therapist graduates in 2010: A national survey, with permission of the American Physical Therapy Association. This material is copyrighted, and further reproduction or distribution is prohibited.

expect their near future PT hires to know and be able to do in addition to providing quality hands-on treatment. Management and leadership knowledge and skill complement direct care skills. Demonstration of capability in these areas may magnify the worth of the individual to their employer and foster career advancement.

Summary

This chapter provided an overview of the roles and responsibilities of supervisors, managers, and leaders. Important characteristics, duties, knowledge, and skills of managers and leaders were discussed with examples presented in physical therapy contexts.

The chapter utilized a compare and contrast method to clarify how each level of management is viewed in the business world and physical therapy. Supervising, managing, and leading are distinct skill sets that are different from direct care hands on skill-sets. Given little attention in ear-

lier physical therapy educational preparation, management and issues surrounding people in management are becoming the focus along the continuum of age, degree type, and work environment. Recent research has provided a framework for educational preparation of PTs focusing on management knowledge and skill that is necessary in contemporary clinical practice. It was concluded that, to some degree, every clinician is a manager.

The next chapters in Part III will delve further into specific areas of management, which have been identified in recent research as important for clinicians of the near future. Chapter 12 provides principles for two areas reported to be essential for managers—communication and networking. Chapter 13 presents strategic planning in a relevant and practical way. Chapter 14 adds the foundation for organizational design to meet specific needs of a business. Chapter 15 deals with management decision-making processes. And, performance improvement is the focus of Chapter 16.

CASE STUDY 11.1

A Chance to Self-Assess Your Management Style and Knowledge

Background

You graduated from your physical therapy program last week and are beginning work in your first physical therapy position. The department works as a loosely defined self-directed team. Your team is three other physical therapists and a transport aide. On the second day in the facility, the therapy transport aide brought inpatients for the other three physical therapists. However, the aide refused to transport your patients.

Questions to Answer

What are the general rules of operation for a self-directed team?

What type of manager do you choose to be in this situation?

What type of management style might work best for you to remedy this issue?

Who will you involve as you work on this task?

What would you consider a successful management of this matter?

Share your work as your instructor has determined.

More on Styles

Examine your own management strengths and weaknesses.

Describe your own management style
Describe your leadership style

Respond to this question: are these styles that you may develop or change, or do you believe that once you have integrated a style of management or leadership, that style cannot be changed?

If you feel you need more information, locate, identify, and summarize three resources you found helpful.

Discuss your findings with a peer who knows you well enough to be able to compare your results of your self-evaluation with their observations of your management/leadership tendencies.

REFERENCES

American Physical Therapy Association. Guide to physical therapist practice, 2nd ed. Physical Therapy. 2001;81:9–744.

American Physical Therapy Association. Criteria for standards of practice for physical therapy, part 1. Available at http://www.apta.org/AM/Template. cfm?Section=Policies_and_Bylaws&CONTENTID =25762&TEMPLATE=/CM/ContentDisplay.cfm. Accessed 7/14/07a.

American Physical Therapy Association. Code of ethics. Available at http://www.apta.org/AM/Template. cfm?Section=Core_Documents1&Template=/CM/ HTMLDisplay.cfm&ContentID=25854. Accessed 7/14/07b.

American Physical Therapy Association. APTA guide for professional conduct. Available from http:// www.apta.org/AM/Template.cfm?Section=Ethics_ and_Legal_Issues1&TEMPLATE=/CM/Content Display.cfm&CONTENTID=40901. Accessed 7/14/07c.

American Physical Therapy Association. Professionalism in physical therapy: Core values. Available at http://www.apta.org/AM/Template.cfm?Section=Pr ofessionalism1&TEMPLATE=/CM/ContentDisplay. cfm&CONTENTID=39529. Accessed 7/14/07d.

Bandura A. Self-efficacy: The exercise of control. New York, NY: WH Freeman. 1997.

Bennis W. On becoming a leader. Cambridge, MA: Perseus. 1994.

Blanchard K. Leadership and the one minute manager. London: HarperCollins. 1994.

Blanchard K, Bowles S. High Five! The magic of working together. London: HarperCollins. 2001.

Cohen SG, Bailey DE. What makes teams work: Group effectiveness research from the shop floor to the executive suite. Journal of Management. 1997;23:239–290.

Collins J. Level 5 leadership: The triumph of humility and fierce resolve. Harvard Business Review. 2001;79:175.

Covey SR. The 7 Habits of highly effective people: Restoring the character ethic. New York, NY: Simon & Schuster. 2004a.

Covey SR. The 8th habit: From effectiveness to greatness. Minneapolis, MN: Tandem Library Books. 2004b.

Dunn RT. Haimann's supervisory management for healthcare organizations, 6th ed. Boston, MA: McGraw-Hill. 1998.

Fayol H. General and industrial management. Translated by C Stores. London, England: Pitman and Sons. 1949.

Gersh MR. Servant-leadership: A philosophical foundation for professionalism in physical therapy. Journal of Physical Therapy Education. 2006;2:12–18.

Greenleaf RK. Servant leadership: a journey into the nature of legitimate power and greatness 25th Anniversary Edition. Mahwah, NJ: Paulist Press. 2002.

Gunn MR. The matrix organization reloaded: Adventures in team and project management. London: Greenwood Press. 2007.

Hersey PH, Blanchard KH, Johnson DE. Management of organizational behavior: Using Human resources. Englewood Cliffs, NJ: Prentice Hall. 1982.

Hersey PH, Blanchard KH, Johnson DE. Management of organizational behavior, 9th ed. Academic Internet. Upper Saddle River, NJ: Pearson. 2007.

Hiebert M, Klatt B. The encyclopedia of leadership: A practical guide to popular leadership theories and techniques. New York, NY: McGraw-Hill. 2001.

Kovacek PR, Powers D, Iglarsh ZA, et al. Report of the task force on Leadership, Administration, and Management Preparation (LAMP). The Resource. 1999;29(1):8–13.

Langfred CW, Shanley MT. Small group research. Autonomous teams and progress on issues of context and levels of analysis. In Golembiewski RT, ed. Handbook of organizational behavior, 2nd ed. New York, NY: Marcel Dekker. 2001:81–111.

Levi D, Slem C. Team work in research-and-development organizations: The characteristics of successful teams. International Journal of Industrial Ergonomics. 1995;16:29–42.

Locke EA. Motivation by goal setting. In Golembiewski RT, ed. Handbook of organizational behavior, 2nd ed. New York, NY: Marcel Dekker. 2001:43–56.

Longest BB Jr, Rakich JS, Darr K. Managing health services organizations and systems, 4th ed. Baltimore, MD: Health Professions Press. 2000.

Lopopolo RB, Schafer DS, Nosse LJ. Leadership, administration, management, and professional (LAMP) processes in physical therapy: A Delphi study. Physical Therapy. 2004;84:137–150.

Luedtke-Hoffmann KA. Identification of essential managerial work activities and competencies of physical therapist managers employed in hospital settings [doctoral disseratation]. Denton, TX:School of Physical Therapy, Texas Woman's University; 2002.

McConnell CR. Umiker's management skills for the new health care supervisor, 4th ed. Boston, Mass: Jones and Bartlett. 2006.

McGregor D. The human side of enterprise. New York, NY: McGraw-Hill. 1960.

Mintzberg H. The nature of managerial work. New York, NY: Harper & Row. 1973.

Mintzberg H. The manager's job: Folklore and fact. Harvard Business Review. July-August 1975;53:49–61.

Mintzberg H, Quinn JB, Voyer J. The strategy process, Collegiate ed. Englewood Cliffs, NJ: Prentice Hall. 1995.

Peterson MF, Smith PB. Sources of meaning, organizations and culture. In Askanasy NM, Wildcromm CPM, Peterson MF, eds. Handbook of organizational culture & climate. Thousand Oaks, CA: Sage. 2000:101-116.

Schafer DS, Lopopolo RB, Luedtke-Hoffmann. Administration and management skills needed by physical therapist graduates in 2010: A national survey. Physical Therapy. 2007;87:261-281.

Rahim MA. Managing organizational conflict. Challenges for organization development and change. In Golembiewski RT, ed. Handbook of organizational behavior, 2nd ed. New York, NY: Marcel Dekker. 2001:365–387.

Rainey HG. Work motivation. In Golembiewski RT, ed. Handbook of organizational behavior, 2nd ed. New York, NY: Marcel Dekker. 2001:19–42.

Schafer DS, Lopopolo RB, Luedtke-Hoffmann. Administration and management skills needed by physical therapist graduates in 2010: A national survey. Physical Therapy. 2007;87:261-281.

Spillane JP. Distributed leadership. San Francisco, CA: Jossey-Bass. 2006.

Stewart GL, Manz CC. Leadership for self-managing work teams: A typology and integrative model. Human Relations. 1995;48:747–770.

Wexley KM, Latham GD. Developing and training human resources in organizations, 2nd ed. New York, NY: HarperCollins. 1991.

Yukl G. Leadership in organizations, 3rd ed. Englewood Cliffs, NY: Prentice Hall. 1994.

Yukl G. Leadership in organizations, 5th ed. Upper Saddle River, NJ: Prentice Hall. 2002.

ADDITIONAL RESOURCES

Emerald for Manager's is an internationally minded site for managers, students, and researchers. Emerald covers theory as well as discussions on various management-related issues including management styles, leadership, marketing, customer-relationship management, knowledge management, e-management. A free subscription is available at http://managers. emeraldinsight. com/info/site_changes.htm. A consulting organization that provides a free online management library with a focus on not-for-profit organizations if accessible at http://www.managementhelp.org/. This site provides short, clear discussions on multiple management, leadership, and supervision topics. The American Management Association provides abstracts of management books and they sell executive summaries of books (http://www.summary.com/cgi-bin/Soundview.storefront/ 471b9eeb00447c25271aac100b0d0643/UserTemplate/ 407?keyword=management&pub=AMACOM). A group of health manager toolkits, including some for leadership, are available on line at http://erc.msh.org/mainpage.cfm?fi le=96.0.htm&module=toolkit&language=English. The Free Management Library provides access to many management and leadership related resources at http://managementhelp.org/. The APTA sells business home study courses. See its professional development link. Combined Sections Meeting abstracts with health policy and administration content are accessible at http://www.aptahpa. org/. For Health Policy and Administration Section members, current LAMP updates and other physical therapist manager/leader materials are also available at this site.

CHAPTER 12

COMMUNICATING WITH SKILL

CHERYL RESNIK

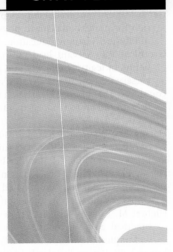

Learning Objectives

1. Define communication as a required skill of professional interactions.
2. Summarize the components of individual and small group communication.
3. Describe the essential components of successful interpersonal communication.
4. Explain methods to foster and enhance communication.
5. Describe common barriers to individual and group communication.
6. Describe the differences between formal and informal communication in the organizational setting.
7. Describe how to provide feedback for change.
8. Analyze generational differences that impact communication.
9. Describe networking give practical work-related examples.
10. Given communication-related scenarios, appropriately apply principles presented in this chapter to deal with the scenario issues.

Introduction

We all communicate in a variety of ways, in person, through electronic media, and through writing. However, how often do we think about *communication* as a process? How often do we analyze how and what we communicate to others? How often do we make efforts to improve our skills related to communicating our thoughts and grasping the messages expressed by others? This chapter addresses these questions about communication. Communication is defined and its various components discussed. The components specifically addressed are: the communication expression and reception processes, verbal and nonverbal communication, assessment of communication, and ways to improve workplace communications. Emphasis is on the verbal and nonverbal messages sent and received in workplace discourse.

Communication Is . . .

A common definition of communication between one or more message senders and one or more message receivers includes the following components:

- The act or process of communicating
- The imparting, transmitting, or interchanging thoughts, opinions, or information by speech, writing, or signs
- A document or message imparting news, views, information, and so on (Dictionary.com, 2008)

Liebler and McConnell (2004) also include an exchange of emotions as a component of communication. These authors write that, "in the broader sense, [communication is] the development of mutual understanding" (p. 496). In their definition, the development of mutual understanding is "dependent upon

Key terms, which are defined below, are bolded and italicized the first time they appear in the chapter. Other important terms are shown in boldface on first appearance and are defined by the context in which they are used. When either of these types of terms is used several times, its acronym will be identified and subsequently used in the chapter. Both types of terms are listed alphabetically in the online glossary with their definitions and (when applicable) their acronyms.

attentive listening: trying to grasp the sender's meaning most of the time and responding meaningfully to the message.

communication: the act or process of interchanging thoughts, opinions, or information by verbal and nonverbal signs/cues or through writing.

emotional intelligence/emotional quotient (EQ): according to Golman, EI is represented by a combination of personality characteristics and cognitive abilities that facilitate emotional self-awareness, self-control of emotions and emotional tendencies, social awareness, and relationship management.

empathic listening: according to Covey this entail making a sincere personal commitment to fully understand the speaker's frame of reference by attending to all aspects of their communication including the words, verbal changes, nonverbal signs, emotion, and others before planning a response.

goal(s): statement(s) of what is to be accomplished. The target toward which all efforts are directed.

networking: people engaging in collaborative interactions.

nonverbal communication: movements, postures, gestures such as head nodding, facial expressions that may reflect the feelings of the communication receiver, eye contact, and place of focus, touch, smell, space, distance, timing, and silence. Every nonverbal stimulus gives an intentional or unintentional message

open-ended question(s): if answered, this type of question requires the responder to provide more than a single or few word(s) as a response.

social capital: an economic idea that refers to the connections between social networks of individuals that include people who trust and assist each other and are an asset.

the sharing of whatever information each individual has about a specific subject and arrives at an agreed-upon meaning, whether that meaning is an opinion, a decision, or a course of action" (Liebler and McConnell, 1999, p. 468). The ultimate goal of communication is collaboration. Liebler and McConnell's refinement in the definition points to the critical importance of communication as a two-way process: message sending and message receiving. To be effective, managers and staff members need to be able to communicate effectively verbally, nonverbally, and in writing. Because communication is an exchange process, the generation and transmission of messages and their reception and processing for meaning are equally important (Chapter 19).

Process Components of Individual and Small Group Communications

A model of the communication process can be represented by six components: initiation, transmission, reception, processing, feedback, and environmental and mental noise or dis-

tractions. For communication to occur there needs to be a sender who begins the interaction. Sender initiation includes preparing both verbal and nonverbal messages. Transmission is next. This is the movement of messages from the sender to one or more receivers. Reception is the sensory impact of the message on the receiver. While dependent on the sender, reception is independent of, although influenced by, the sender. It is the receiver's perception that shapes the way in which a message is decoded and acted upon as verbal or nonverbal feedback. The receiver is now the sender who is acknowledging that the message has been received. It gives the sender some knowledge regarding the acceptance, suppression, or nonacceptance of the information (McConnell, 2002). Impacting throughout the communication is mental and environmental "noise." The cartoon Zits (Fig. 12.1) is a perfect illustration of the six components of communication and what happens too frequently between the sender and the receiver in the real world.

Let's look at an example, which at first glance appears to be an easy bit of communication. Dale, a physical therapist (PT), takes

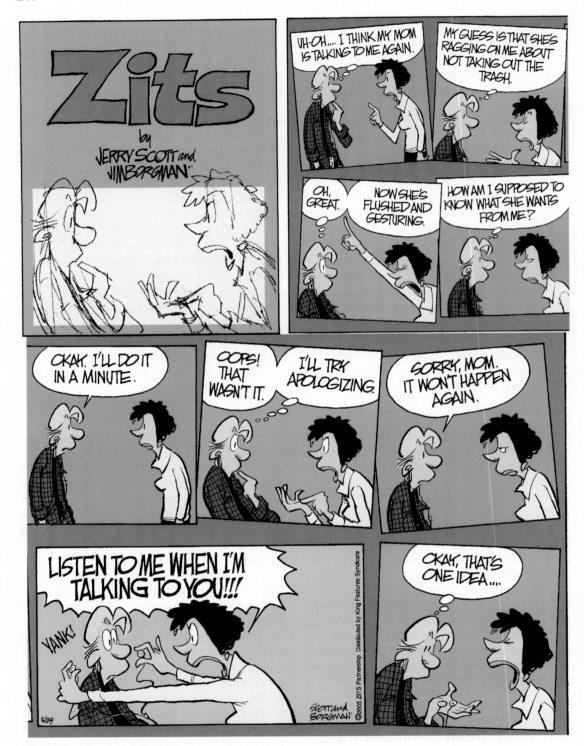

Figure 12.1. Hello! I'm talking to you! Reprint permission granted by Zits © Zits Partnership, King Features Syndicate.

a phone call from the ICU requesting a therapist to report to the unit and assist the team in setting up a patient with a newly acquired spinal cord injury in the newly acquired hospital bed specifically intended for patients who have sustained major trauma. Dale, the sender, walks up to the schedule board where all the staff are gathered to communicate the request. Dale is late for a meeting, so she makes a general announcement, the transmission, to the group about the request. A breakdown in communication is about to occur. Because Dale is in a hurry, while she may clearly communicate her message, the lack of an identified receiver provides the first potential for miscommunication. Potentially, no one will even hear the request because everyone is intent on their own task and the failure of Dale to identify a single receiver allows everyone at the board to assume she is not speaking to them. Add to this the fact that Dale's tone of voice, because she was in a hurry, was perceived as being rude. If her normal tone is a polite one, this difference may in itself cause the potential receivers to respond directly to Dale to identify what is really going on. If Dale always has an edge to her voice, she increases the probability that no one will listen because they are tired of jumping at Dale's edicts. The message may be clear, but the perception of the receiver is of paramount importance. Because she is late to her meeting, Dale does not confirm that anyone is taking responsibility for meeting the patient need. This absence of feedback ultimately results in no one going to provide the necessary care. It does not take much imagination to picture what happens among the staff members when the ICU staff follow up to find out why physical therapy failed to assist.

From this example, it is apparent that the backdrop against which communication occurs depends on the perceptions, past experiences, assumptions, age, gender, and culture of the individuals involved in the communication. All these features add a high degree of complexity to communication. It was discussed earlier in the section that communication also occurs on both the verbal and nonverbal level. There are three components of verbal communication: the voice, the content of the message and response, and the method used to transmit the information. Voice conveys emotions and impacts the response to the communication.

Emotion and intonation added to communication can add meaning to spoken communication. In the United States, raised voices usually communicate tension or aggression. In some black, Jewish, and Italian cultures, raised voices merely indicate an exciting conversation. Similarly, people who speak slowly or softly are often perceived as being inarticulate or disinterested when, in fact, they may be speaking a second language or speaking respectfully (Srivastava, 2007).

Communication = Words Plus

Verbal Communication

In verbal communications, voice modulations are used to add meaning to the message's words or signs. Voice modulations include: articulation, intensity, pitch, range, rhythm, tempo, and variation superimposed on the chosen words. The voice conveys the speaker's emotions by modal combinations of these speech variables. To pick up these sometimes subtle changes in face-to-face communications requires listening skill.

Listening Part of Communication

The message sent is not necessarily the message received. The fidelity of the reception and interpretation of a verbal message is dependent on how well the receiver is listening and attending to the sender's other signals. Effective listening is a skill. It is important to recognize that in interpersonal communication encounters most writers recommend listening more than speaking. This is critical when participants are mutually intent on discovering something from or about each other (Shonka and Kosch, 2002; Spector and McCarthy, 1995; Super and Gold, 2004). Covey (1990) suggests there are several ways listeners can deal with verbal input:

- Ignore the message—thinking about matters other than the sender's message
- Pretend to understand—hear the message, minimally process it, acknowledging the message was heard but without substantive feedback
- Selective processing—picking out and reacting to portions of the sender's message

- *Attentive listening*—trying to grasp the sender's meaning most of the time and responding meaningfully
- *Empathic listening*—making a sincere personal commitment to fully understand the speaker's frame of reference by attending to all aspects of their communication: words, verbal changes, nonverbal signs, emotion, and so on, before planning a response

This level of listening has similar core elements to what PTs do. We first seek to understand the client by giving our full attention to them and asking open-ended as well as closed clarifying questions. We provide physical therapy diagnosis when we clearly understand the client's input along with other information. We prescribe solutions through our plan of care. We strive to be understood by the client to gain compliance.

Listening Hints

Library, Internet, and academic and continuing education courses all have resources on how to improve listening skills. A sample of suggestions from several sources is presented in Table 12.1.

Table 12.1 Effective Listening Hints

Circumstances	Hints
Before interacting (Plan)	Commit your mental energy to understanding the speaker.
	If the environment will hinder your ability to hear, see or concentrate, move the conversation to a more appropriate place.
	Know your schedule. If you feel the discussion will not be completed before you need to be elsewhere, offer a better time to meet.
	Clear your mental chalkboard of presuppositions so the speaker can write on it.
During the interaction (Discovery)	Remind yourself that genuine interest in communicating requires focusing your senses on all aspects of the speaker's messages. This requires more energy than just being courteous or respectful.
	Key in on the content nuggets rather than the speakers idiosyncrasies or other distractions.
	Stay aware of all of the ways the message was sent.
	Verbal messages are conveyed in part through voice modulations. They may be intended for emphasis and level of emotion, by word choices as well as pauses and silence.
	Visual messages are in the speaker's eyes (eye contact and movement) focus, facial expressions, mouth and head movements, hand gestures, and leg movements.
	Physiological signs of emotional stress include pupil dilation, perspiration, perspiration odor, face/neck flushing, and dry mouth.
	Remember that all the above are affected by the context—noise, audience reaction, electronic problems, and environmental control.
Processing for understanding	What was the essential message?
	First and foremost, what were the key words/points?
	What were the salient words that emphasize the key points?
	What were the vocal cues that marked the important key words/points?
	What were the nonverbal cues that marked the important key words/points?
	Were their signs of physiological stress and if so, did they appear to be related to the important key words/points?
	Was there concordance between the verbal, nonverbal, and physiological cues and what you identified as the key words/points?
Feedback for mutual understanding	Based on your understandings, question the speaker about the key words/points. For example:
	Did I hear correctly that preplanning communications is related to effective message sending?
	I understand the word empathy, but I am not certain that I understand the derived term empathic listening. Will you say more about this?
	Does your point about concordance of verbal, nonverbal, and physiological cues relate to the discussion about trust?

Listening requires using your two ears, two eyes, and mental energy to minimize distractions and maximize the extraction of the sender's meaning. The benefit of genuine empathic listening is a clearer understanding of the communication partner's or partners' message or messages. When feedback reflects a clear understanding of the core message, the speaker or speakers can further advance their message. This adds depth to communication interchanges (Covey, 1990). For presentation purposes, the communication process was presented as if sending and receiving were somewhat independent components. They clearly are not. They occur concurrently as sender and receiver continuously exchange nonverbal cues even if only one is verbalizing.

Nonverbal Communication

Nonverbal communication is comprised of movements, postures, gestures such as head nodding, facial expressions that may reflect the feelings of the communication receiver, eye contact, and place of focus, touch, smell, space, distance, timing, and silence. Every nonverbal stimulus gives an intentional or unintentional message that impacts the response and, if noted by the sender, impacts the understanding of how the message may have been received (Liebler and McConnell, 1999). Nonverbal behavior is learned (in a culture) and involves shared understanding (Liebler and McConnell, 2004).

Continuing with the example with Dale, the major barriers to the communication on the nonverbal level consisted of the lack of eye contact or touch, which would have identified the target receiver, the lack of any kind of head nodding by the gathered staff indicating

receipt of the message, and the failure of Dale to note that there was really a nonresponse by the group to her communication.

The distance between communication participants is another nonverbal variable that influences the communication process. Hall (1966), in his seminal work on communication distance, identified four zones of social distance that are common for Americans.

1. The public zone
2. The social zone
3. The personal zone
4. The intimate zone

Regulation of the distance between people, who are communicating, provides the benefit of safety, ease of communication, affection as well a threat (Hall, 1966). Table 12.2 reflects Hall's general guideline for distance between American speakers that impact communication outcomes.

Nearly everyone has had an experience where they were being spoken to by someone who "invaded their personal space" by standing too close. People who are not aware that they have this tendency also fail to incorporate the nonverbal feedback they are being sent by the receiver who backs away during the communication. As the receiver moves back, the space invader continues to move forward. It is easy to see how this behavior may be interpreted as threatening.

This is a particularly important point for PTs, as the work requires extensive physical proximity to clients for treatment and communication (Chapter 8).

Dress is another nonverbal component of communication as many people judge others by their clothing, hairstyle, facial hair, jewelry, tattoos, and make up. In health care, conservative

Table 12.2 Summary of Hall's Culture and Human Space (Proxemic) Concept		
Zone	*Distance*	*Benefit/Message*
Public zone	>12 ft	Degree safety is felt as there is sufficient time and distance to react to any perceived threat and take appropriate action.
Social zone	4–12 ft	Distance allows for verbal communication but others are still at a safe distance. This is a comfortable distance for small group interactions
Personal zone	1.5–4 ft	Conversation is more direct. Good distance for two people to communicate earnestly.
Intimate zone	<1.5 ft	Arms length or less apart. Eye contact is easy. Can be used as nonverbal means of exerting power by threatening personal space.

Source: Hall, 1966.

attire is the norm. It is important to analyze the social norms in the organization (Chapters 7, 13, 14, 17, and 22) and make decisions regarding dress based on what is commonly seen.

Group Communication

The greater the size and complexity of the organization, the more difficult it becomes to ensure that two-way communication has occurred (Chapters 11 and 14). In group communication, the manager must be able to appraise the readiness or resistance of followers to move in a given direction and to know when dissension or confusion is undermining the group's will to act. Gardner (1990) describes this as social perceptiveness and, more recently, Daniel Goleman's writings have focused on *emotional intelligence (EQ)* (Goleman, 1995). He believes that emotional intelligence is a major factor in management success. Emotional intelligence consists of a combination of personality characteristics and cognitive abilities that facilitate:

Emotional self-awareness and the impact one's emotions have on their decision making
Self-control of emotions and emotional tendencies
Social awareness
Relationship management

See the Additional Resources section for more information on this topic.

Communication in Many Directions

PT managers tend to fall in the lower to middle levels of the organizational hierarchy (Chapters 11 and 14), and as such, are required to communicate multidirectionally. In the leadership role, managers have the primary responsibility to ensure that communication flows both upward and downward through the organization. Information, however, does not flow upward and downward with equal ease. Middle-level managers should recognize that they are dependent on information that has been filtered, analyzed, abstracted, sorted, and condensed by other segments of the organization. Following is a brief discussion of communication direction.

Downward Communication

Downward communication is facilitated largely through management's control of most of the means of communication (McConnell, 2002). The free flow of information from the manager downward, however, may result in those lower in the hierarchy blocking, filtering, or distorting the downward flow (Gardner, 1990). Such message changes can occur intentionally or because of incorrect interpretation of the original message. It is a reality that the further information needs to travel, the greater the distortion of the original message (Coiera, 2003). To reiterate earlier points, the perception of the receiver impacts the message. Without feedback to ensure the interpretation, the sender really has no idea of the receiver's understanding.

Upward Communication

Upward communication from subordinates to a superior is dependent upon the leader's ability to listen. "Good leaders listen, take advice, lose arguments, and follow" (Kouzes and Posner, 2002, p. 149). Managers do not work alone. By providing a safe atmosphere for employees to share their knowledge, the flow of upward communication is enhanced. Key to enhancing upward communication is establishing an atmosphere of trust. More will be said about trust in the section on enhancing communication.

The new manager also needs to become skilled at communicating upward to managers higher in organization than their immediate superior. In order to enhance upward communication the following techniques should be considered:

- Be selective in what you communicate. As a manager, a major positional responsibility is to problem-solve. Communicate upwards those issues that cannot be managed at your level.
- Prepare your communication by analyzing the problem, assessing its implications, preparing a few alternative solutions, and identifying your recommendation.
- Structure the communication to meet the time constraints of your superior. If this person is unavailable for a face-to-face meeting, communicate the issues in writing. Be available to meet at a time convenient for your superior on short notice. By identifying a mutually agreeable time, everyone's time is better utilized (McConnell, 2002).

Table 12.3 Example High-Impact Open-Ended Questions to Facilitate Understanding	
High-impact questions require the responder to reflect before responding and open-ended questions require the responder to provide a detailed response (Shonka and Kosch, 2002).	
If I want to get a clearer picture, who ...?	How would you have me do ...?
What do you think is ...?	How do you see ...?
Can you compare ...?	If ... is a problem, how would you ...?
When do you use ...?	Please review the order of importance given ...
If you were in my position ...?	What is your feeling about ...?
What has been the biggest ...?	At this point in time, what do you suggest ...?
What is next in ...?	What have others said about ...?

These same steps can be used when communicating with those you supervise. Asking questions, particularly the *open-ended* type, can add to your gaining understanding of the real problem, its implications, potential solutions, and staff's recommendations. Examples of open-ended questions are listed in Table 12.3.

By employing these suggestions, you model proactive problem solving and communication skill. Remember, the better the questions, the better the answers.

Lateral Communication

Lateral communications are between people at the same organizational hierarchy level. Critical to managing lateral communication is the understanding that this type of communication is based on cooperation between work groups. While a management position implies some organizational authority, this authority is positional only (Chapter 14). There is a tendency for component parts of organizations to create their own distinctive cultures and to establish less permeable boundaries than is optimal for communication across the organization. Some of these cultural differences are a result of professional designation (PT, OT, MD, etc.), "turf" issues (inpatient versus outpatient), or work group/service line divisions (pediatric versus adult orthopedic services). The example with Dale used earlier may be used to explore the issues of lateral communication. PTs are frequently viewed by other team members as "organic Hoyer lifts." If the communication between the ICU staff and the physical therapy staff is not optimal, the request for assistance with the new patient may

be seen more as a workload issue (PTs being the best to call on to move patients) than a request for a skilled intervention for optimal care for the patient. This scenario is played out on a daily basis in organizations where staffing is less than optimal and workload and patient acuity are high.

Whatever the cause, lateral communication may be facilitated by cross-boundary working groups collaborating to solve shared issues (Chapter 11).

Informal Communication— The Grapevine

No discussion on communication would be complete without a discussion of the informal communication network that thrives in every environment, the grapevine. The grapevine is the perfect description of the way rumors move through an organization; through branches that exist on all levels of an organization (Longest et al., 2000). Rumors spread quickly, uncontrollably and, once started, are often difficult to stop. Because rumors can harm both individuals and the organization itself, managers must consider how to deal with the grapevine. De Mare (1989) found that 70% of all organizational communication occurs at the grapevine level. The grapevine becomes active when the issues are perceived to be important and the situations are ambiguous. Additional research indicates that employees rely on the grapevine when they feel threatened, insecure, under stress, when there is pending change, and when they feel that communication from management is limited (Brownell, 1990).

The bottom line is, when formal communications are nonexistent or break down, the environment becomes more uncertain. These situations provide a basis for the grapevine and rumor mill to run rampant; therefore, maintaining open lines of communication at all times is a critical management strategy. Managers need to respect and understand employees' need to know and understand organizational issues. An informed employee is an asset to an organization. Communication needs to be planned to ensure that employees hear important information in a timely manner and that questions they have are answered. Additionally, planned communication offers the opportunity to get input and feedback from the workforce that results in increased teamwork and trust. Planned communication activities include:

Bulletin boards and newsletters
Communicating and clarifying organizational
    and individual goals and objectives
Dealing with dysfunctional conflict
Regular performance feedback to employees
Timely meetings (Crampton et al., 1998)

The grapevine can be useful to management as a downward information dissemination means that is faster than official channels of communication (Longest et al., 2000). This is one way to counter grapevine misinformation.

Barriers to Communication

Management manner and attitude have significant impact on how well information flows upward. A significant barrier to upward communication is erected if the manager adopts an attitude of "no news is good news." Frontline employees who are involved with day-to-day problem solving are invaluable sources of information that can assist the manager, but only if it is requested and the manager uses effective listening skills. One of the greatest inhibitors of upward communication stems from the manager's failure to respond to some earlier communication from a staff member (McConnell, 2002). It is not as important that the employee receive the response they expect to keep the upward lines of communication open; rather, it is more important to indicate to the employee that their message has been considered and provide them feedback on the matter. A more proactive management attitude would be a "no surprises" approach that is communicated by active solicitation of issues

that are occurring in the organization that may require intervention at some point. The earlier you, as manager, are aware of potential problems, the earlier a solution may be generated.

Not Just the Words

As discussed earlier, emotion is part of all forms of interaction. It is not just through word choices, but through tone of voice and body language that messages are communicated.

Body language is a series of conscious or unconscious postures that convey information to others. It is important to be aware that gestures are very culturally bound and it is best to check perceptions with the other person when interpreting gestures, expressions, silences, and body language (Liebler and McConnell, 2004). Emotional overtones may create barriers to successful communication. The level of stress is reflected in one's voice. The person receiving communication has no way to know if they are the source of the distress or something else is. Their interpretation may drive their response. It is as important to monitor your own nonverbal reactions to communications as it is to key into the reactions of the person to whom you are communicating. Words that do not have a negative connotation to you may cause unexpected emotional responses in others. Active listening and getting feedback are the only means to ensure that you are communicating what you really want to communicate.

When, Who, and Where

Time and place are also important considerations when communicating. Whether the information is on a one-to-one basis or to a group, what needs to be communicated needs to be analyzed to appropriately plan the interaction. Analysis includes determining:

- The level of confidentiality required
- Who needs to participate in the communication process
- What the potential reaction(s) may be
- How much time is to be allotted for the communication

Failure to plan adequate time and appropriate location for important communication will create unnecessary barriers and may increase resistance. Indicating what the policy is on sharing the communicated information with those outside of the group is important when decisions are not final. Representative stakeholders should participate in discussions that affect them. If you determine that you have misjudged the response to the communication, it is better to reschedule the conversation for a different time so that real collaboration may occur. More time should be allotted for contentious issues, larger size groups, first-time meetings, and when decisions have to be made in the near future. Let us return to the example of Dale's communication to the other staff members.

As the manager, you will be the one to receive the call from the ICU to follow up on why there is no one from physical therapy at the patient's bedside. Following up with Dale, the recipient of the phone call will probably result in your being told that she communicated to the whole group of the need. Talking to any of the other people involved will result in a myriad of responses: I didn't know she was talking to me; Dale doesn't carry her share of the load—who is she to tell us what to do; the ICU staffs are always calling PT to do their manual labor, and so on. It is obvious that there are barriers to communication present in this situation. You will need to determine how best to communicate future performance expectations to the group. What steps would you take here to ensure that there is a positive outcome to this situation?

Enhancing Communication

Two-way communication is essential to functioning in a leader–follower relationship. As the complexity of the organization increases, the amount of face-to-face communication between the leader and followers decreases (McConnell, 2002). Collaboration requires positive face-to-face interaction, the need for which increases with the complexity of the issue. People can achieve cooperative goals when information is shared, each other's ideas are listened to, resources are exchanged, and requests are responded to, all of which are key management skills.

Trust

While collaboration facilitates communication, collaboration is based on trust. Kouzes

and Posner (2002) and others (Covey, 1990) identify behaviors that a manager may take to promote trust. These include:

- Acknowledging the need for personal improvement
- Asking for feedback—positive and negative
- Admitting mistakes
- Avoiding talking negatively about others
- Being truthful
- Being willing to change your mind when others have good ideas
- Disclosing information about who you are and what you believe
- Inviting interested parties to important meetings (transparency)
- Listening attentively to what others are saying
- Openly acknowledging the contribution of others
- Saying, "We can trust them," and meaning it.
- Sharing information that is useful to others

People must feel safe to develop trust. Defensive communication strategies indicate that the participants do not feel secure at some level. To build a climate of trust, the listening-to-talk ratio has to be in favor of listening (Kouzes and Posner, 2002). People need to feel their voice matters and that their vote counts.

Communicating for Change

It has been well established that the majority of people find it difficult to make changes and some things are easier to change than others. Folkman (1996) offers a continuum of change which illustrates the ease or difficulty associated with those issues that are most commonly in need of change (Table 12.4).

Folkman's research suggests that people are unable to change multiple things at one time. Therefore, it is imperative to prioritize changes and manage them one at a time. The need for change by the person to whom you are providing feedback is affected by two perspectives:

1. A clear understanding of how the issue negatively affects the individual and their associates.
2. An understanding of the positive impact of making the required change.

Table 12.4 Relative Effort Needed to Change Selected Work Variables	
Variables	**Ease of Change**
Job skills	Easier
Organization and time	
Management	
Management of work	
Knowledge	
Attitudes	
Habits	
Traits	
Personality characteristics	
	Harder

Source: Reproduced with permission of J.R. Folkman (http://www.zfco.com).

Motivation to change is enhanced by concentrating on the benefits or value of making a change rather than the negative impact of the behavior to be changed (Folkman, 1996; Miller and Sankovitz, 2005).

To determine what change is most important it is necessary to distinguish between essential, necessary, and nonessential skills, knowledge, abilities, and activities. The second consideration is how much change is required; what level of competence is needed for a given task. As in any collaboration, another critical step is to put in place those strategies, structures and systems needed to support the required change (Chapters 11, 13, 14, and 16). The final consideration is to identify the specific change goal that is to be accomplished. Approaching change in this objective manner will assist in decreasing the defensiveness that frequently arises during performance feedback sessions.

Age and Communication

Significant study has occurred in the past 10 years related to generational issues. Differences in expectations about feedback can create generational conflicts. Lancaster and Stillman (2003) surveyed members of Generation X (born 1965–1980). They found that 45% of workers in this age group had never received training on how to give feedback and almost 65% had never received training on how to receive feedback. These findings are of importance to communication efforts for

these researchers concluded that the number one cause of turnover was a lack of feedback. The bottom line is that when different generations of workers cannot communicate with one another about performance, business suffers, morale suffers, and clients suffer.

Gender and Communication

Much has been written about the perception that there is a gender difference in communication style. However, research does not support that there is a substantial sex-based difference in communication behavior (Kirtley and Weaver, 1999). Norton (1983) identified nine different aspects of communication style that form a single continuum from a nondirective style to a directive style. These nine styles in a continuum from most autocratic to most democratic are labeled dominant, dramatic, contentious, animated, impression leaving, relaxed, attentive, open, and friendly. Both genders function along this continuum but there is a tendency for gender preference that appears to be based on Western sexual stereotypes. (Tannen 1990) Tannen's research showed that females exhibited a stronger tendency then men to be social, talkative, and to involve others when communicating. Males, on the other hand tended to be more dogmatic, pragmatic, and cerebral in their communication encounters. These differences may be due to cultural expectations of females as nurturers and males as decision makers. So, how does a new supervisor make use of this information? It is useful to pay attention to an individual's style and separate out your own potential gender bias when ascribing reasons for why a given person chooses to be a dominating, assertive communicator rather than a more socially oriented communicator.

Networking

Social capital is "the collective value of the people we know and what we'll do for each other" (Kouzes and Posner, 2002, p. 280). The successful leader cultivates social connections within and outside of the organization as they are the potential source of information, resources, and influence that is needed to get work done (Chapters 2, 4, and 11). For all members of an organization, the key to these relationships is the collaboration that is promoted through cooperative goals and trust building. Opportunities to form collaborative relationships are there in chance as well as planned meetings. Networking is most often associated with job hunting and in today's technology driven society, virtual relationships are established without ever meeting face-to-face. However, the most successful networking happens when there is a face-to-face component, so if the initial contact is virtual, a plan needs to be made to meet in person.

Using Social Capital

Spending your social capital successfully requires a plan, the proper place, advance preparation, and patience. Successful networking begins with setting your goals. Whether your purpose is to meet peers with other areas of clinical or management expertise or to ensure that those higher in the organization know who you are, you need to define what you want to accomplish. Determining your *goal* will not only help you identify why you want to network, it will also help clarify where you should network. Are they members of your own professional association or will you need to find another organization? Once an appropriate group or organization has been identified, you need to further identify which types of activities will best meet your needs. You probably do not have sufficient time to attend every gathering, so being selective will assist you with making the best use of your time.

Whether you are attending a wine and cheese event sponsored by a local organization or a series of workshops at a national health care conference, you need to be prepared. This means gathering background information about your intended **target** individuals or groups and preparing effective self or intermediary introductions for the targeted people. Networking is about building relationships. You cannot do that if you cannot initiate or maintain a dialogue. Work on your ability to make small talk. Before going to an event, select some topics to serve as icebreakers like current events, clinical concerns, mutual acquaintances, and so on. When the conversation turns toward your personal interest for which you are networking, be prepared to describe it. If you are not comfortable in new social situations, an excellent group to join is Toastmasters. Toastmasters is a **nonprofit** organization for developing public speaking and leadership skills through practice and feedback and has chapters in most cities (Toastmasters International, 2008).

One approach to networking outlines ten steps (Harris, 2003). For successful networking these steps are:

1. Network in places and at events that would attract your target audience. Don't choose venues and occasions where just your good friends hang out. Your friends may not have anything to do with furthering your business or career goals.
2. Sharpen your networking skills before attending an event. Have a few topics in mind to use as icebreakers. Ask open-ended questions to keep conversation flowing.
3. Set specific goals and stick to them. If your objective is to meet three new people at a local chat-and-chew make it a point to do that before you leave. Don't spend more than 10 minutes with one person when you're networking. If you find yourself spending more time than that, politely introduce that person to someone else and then move on.
4. Describe your business in 60 seconds or less. Create a concise and interesting way to let others know what you do.
5. Remember, it is a two-way conversation. Be willing to listen. Don't make the mistake of talking too much when attending a networking event. Ask questions of the person you're talking to and give them your undivided attention.
6. Relax. When networking, don't give out your business card seconds after you shake the person's hand. Create interesting dialogue first; that will begin the relationship-building process. Do give your card before you end the conversation.
7. Take notes. Whether you attend a conference, organization meeting, or have a personal meeting, gather information about person(s) with whom there is potential for collaboration and write it on the backs of their business cards. This will help you recall your conversations when it's time to follow up.

8. Look for people to refer. Sometimes the fastest way to get referrals is to give referrals, so pull your entrepreneurial peers into your discussions.
9. Follow up. After the event, do not throw all of the business cards you collected into a drawer. Follow up with a phone call, fax, letter, or e-mail. Invite them to your clinic or to another meeting that would be of interest to them.
10. Be patient. Making new connections through networking doesn't happen immediately. Stay focused, maintain contact with potential colleagues, and be graciously persistent.

Networking Plans B, C, and D

Not all networking contacts are fruitful. You may discover a targeted person really cannot provide you the useful information you anticipated. They may appear disinterested in engaging in discussion. They may ask to be excused to carry out other duties before the conversation gets substantive. These situations can challenge self-confidence but they can still yield benefits. Ask them to recommend one or more people that they think might be able to help you. If you get some names, ask for their permission to identify them as the source of the recommendation. Better yet, see if the targeted person is willing to contact the recommended key person to let them know you will be contacting them. If the targeted person is called away, quickly ask if you can contact them at a less busy time. Always assess your networking pluses and minuses. Analyze what you need to do to constantly improve your success rate and then implement appropriate strategies.

Summary

"What we have here is a failure to communicate" was a statement in the movie *Cool Hand Luke* that underscored the point that consequences for not getting the message can be severe. Similarly, failure to communicate in the workplace can have negative impact on interpersonal, inter- and intradepartmental understandings, and understandings among external stakeholders. Unlike the warden–prisoner culture of the movie, workplace culture should encourage communication at all levels of the organization.

The modes of communication are verbal, nonverbal, and written. Verbal and nonverbal means discussion. The meaning and interpretation of words, gestures, voice modulations, and other variables are influenced by many factors including: age, communication environment, ethnic background, experience, gender, intent, physical movements, and social culture. Since communication is an idea exchange process, fruitful communication requires message sending, message receiving, and processing skills.

The process of communicating involves one or more speakers and one or more receivers and it entails simultaneous sending, receiving, and mental processing activities among all parties. The keys to gaining understanding were presented from both the message sending and receiving perspectives. Skills for developing sending skills such as preparation, and effective receiving skills such as a commitment to understand, were discussed. Suggestions were offered for improving skill in both sending and receiving messages to facilitate mutual understanding.

CASE STUDY 12.1

Fighting Among the Staff

The Specifics

You have recently been promoted to the lead therapist position over outpatient rehabilitation. While walking by the waiting area you hear raised voices and go to investigate. At the front desk, in front of a waiting room full of patients and their families, Nikie Newcomber, a new graduate therapist, is having an argument with Robin Chirping, the receptionist who has been working at the clinic for more than 10 years. You step up to the desk and make the following statement:

(Continued)

CASE STUDY 12.1

Fighting Among the Staff (continued)

"I want you to both stop arguing immediately. What is the problem here?" Nikie begins to complain that Robin has double-booked his schedule and now he has two unhappy patients. You interrupt his comments defending the schedule. You know you don't want to have this discussion in front of patients and there are two patients waiting to be treated, so you offer to assist Nikie in getting both patients taken care of and indicate that you want to see both Nikie and Robin in your office at noon.

Your Tasks

1. Have you been in this situation in any of the roles?

2. If so, what was your reaction? Your coworkers' reactionS? Your supervisor's reaction? Now place yourself in the lead therapist's position.
3. How will you prepare for the discussion with Nikie and Robin?
4. Identify the issues that need to be discussed from a personal as well as organizational perspective.
5. What might you need to consider specific to the two employees involved; i.e., job title, age, gender, work history, experience, etc?
6. What would you consider a successful outcome to the counseling session?

CASE STUDY 12.2

The Grapevine

You are the head of rehab services. One of your staff members has approached you with the news "they overheard during a goodbye party for a member of another department" that the organization is in financial trouble and there are going to be layoffs in the near future. You know that everyone has been under pressure to increase productivity and you have already taken steps to improve the statistics generated by your division. You have had two valuable employees tender their resignation in the last month, neither of whom was very forthcoming about why they were leaving. Now you're wondering if their resignations have something to do with this news about the potential layoffs. You decide that you need to get to the bottom of the rumors and call the chief operating officer (COO) to schedule a meeting.

Your Tasks

1. What do you need to do about rumor control?
2. If your meeting with the COO cannot occur until the next week, what do you need to do immediately?
3. If there is a delay, who are some people to talk to in your network?
4. What information should you take to the meeting with the COO?
5. What nonverbal communication means will you be looking for in the COO?
6. Once you have had your discussion (improvise your own interpretation of the meeting), what will you share with the staff?

REFERENCES

Brownell J. Management: Grab hold of the grapevine. Cornell Hotel & Restaurant Administration Quarterly. August 1990;31:78–83.

Coiera E. Guide to health informatics, 2nd ed. New York, NY: Oxford University Press. 2003.

Covey SR. The seven habits of highly effective people. New York, NY: Fireside. 1990.

Crampton SM, Hodge JW, Mishra J. The informal communication network: Factors influencing grapevine activity. Public Personnel Management. 1998;27(4):569–584.

De Mare G. Communicating: The key to establishing good working relationships. Price Waterhouse Review. 1989;33:30–37.

Dictionary.com. Communication. Available at http://dictionary.reference.com/browse/Communication. Accessed 1/03/08.

Folkman J. Turning feedback into change. Provo, UT: Novations. 1996.

Gardner JW. On Leadership. New York, NY: Simon and Schuster. 1990.

Goleman D. Emotional intelligence. New York, NY: Bantam Books. 1995.

Hall ET. The hidden dimension. New York, NY: Doubleday. 1966.

Harris WM. Networking for success: It takes more than just handing out business cards. These days, entrepreneurs must use every resource available to develop and maintain professional relationships. Black Enterprise. 2003;34:4.

Kirtley MD, Weaver JB. Exploring the impact of gender role self-perception on communication style. Women's Studies in Communication. 1999;22:2.

Kouzes JM, Posner BZ. The leadership challenge, 3rd ed. San Francisco, CA: Jossey-Bass. 2002.

Lancaster LC, Stillman D. When generations collide. New York, NY: Harper Business. 2003.

Liebler JF, McConnell CR. Management principles for health professionals, 3rd ed. Gaithersburg, MD: Aspen. 1999.

Liebler JF, McConnell CR. Management principles for health professionals, 4th ed. Sudbury, MA: Jones and Bartlett. 2004.

Longest BB, Rakich JS, Darr K. Managing health services organizations and systems, 4th ed. Baltimore, MD: Health Professions Press. 2000.

McConnell CR. The effective health care supervisor, 5th ed. Gaithersburg, MD: Aspen. 2002.

Miller M, Sinkovitz J. Selling is dead. Hoboken, NJ: John Wiley and Sons. 2005.

Norton R. Communicator style. Beverly Hills, CA: Sage. 1983.

Shonka M, Kosch D. Beyond selling value: A proven way to avoid the vendor trap. Chicago, IL: Dearborn Trade Publishing. 2002.

Spector R, McCarthy PD. The Nordstrom Way: The inside story of America's #1 customer service company. New York, NY: John Wiley and Sons. 1995.

Srivastava R. The healthcare professional's guide to clinical cultural competence. Canada: Elsevier Mosby. 2007.

Super C, Gold RD. Selling (without selling). New York, NY: AMACOM. 2004.

Tannen D. You just don't understand: Women and men in conversation. New York, NY: William Morrow. 1990.

Toastmasters International. Home page. Available at http://www.toastmasters.org/. Accessed 1/09/08.

ADDITIONAL RESOURCES

A physical therapy related article that discusses the concept of social capital is: Peterson J. Board perspective. In league with others. PTMagazine. 2004;12(7): 22, 25–26.

Internet resources on communication include very practical articles, for example communication basics available at http://www.khake.com/page66.html to academic resources like ERIC at http://www.eric.ed.gov/ERICWebPortal/custom/portlets/recordDetails/detailmini.jsp?_nfpb=true&_&ERICExtSearch_SearchValue_0=EJ231844&ERICExtSearch_SearchType_0=no&accno=EJ231844. For more reading material on emotional intelligence include see Bradberry T, Greaves J. The Emotional Intelligence Quick Book. New York, NY: Simon and Schuster. 2005, and Cash-Padgett T. Virtuously emotional: The EI goldmine and how it works. Available at http://www.associatedcontent.com/article/449189/virtuously_emotional_the_ei_goldmine.html?page=2. To see more on emotional intelligence go to Danial Goleman's website, http://www.daniel-goleman.info/blog/emotional-intelligence/ei_reading/. Several free emotional intelligence tests are available online, for example http://www.queendom.com/tests/access_page/index.htm?idRegTest=1121. The University of the Pacific has a 7 module on-line resource that includes numerous thought stimulating self-quizzes and interactive exercises on cultural differences. It is available at http://www.pacific.edu/sis/culture/pub/Module_1_-_What_to_know_befo.htm. A free 20 module training manual for instructors and participants is accessible on line from the QA Quality Assurance Project at: http://www.qaproject.org/training.html#qiinhc.

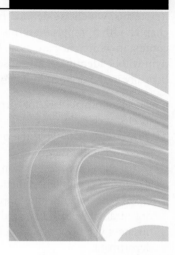

CHAPTER 13

STRATEGIC PLANNING

DEBORAH G. FRIBERG

Learning Objectives

1. Explain the relationship between strategic planning and business success.
2. Describe the common steps of a strategic planning process and the elements of a strategic plan.
3. Understand best practices and how to get the most value out of the strategic planning process.
5. Identify internal and external sources of information pertinent to the strategic planning process.
6. Describe the process of aligning strategic goals with business and market objectives and action plans.
7. State the differences between a strategic plan and a business plan.
8. Apply the major strategic planning principles and processes to formulate a strategic plan to guide you toward the fulfillment of your professional goals.

Introduction

The military, coaches, and business leaders use the same descriptive terms when they prepare for involvement in dynamic competitive endeavors that have potentially catastrophic penalties for failure. Generals want to win battles, coaches want to win championships, and managers want their organizations to succeed. These groups of leaders prepare ahead of time for dealing with their opponents by formulating **strategies**. Approaching planning in this way involves formulating the means to achieve goals and measures that determine success is the essence of the management philosophy known as **strategic management** (Swayne et al., 2006). The core components of strategic planning (Chapter 3)will be summarized here and expanded in subsequent parts of this chapter.

The Lexicon of Strategic Planning

Strategic planning is a tool that business leaders utilize to help them consider the questions of how and when a business should take action. Strategic planning is used to develop **strategic goals**, **strategic objectives** and, finally, specific **operational**, **action or tactical plans** that answer the how and when questions in detail (Kane, 2007). The tactical plan also addresses the question of responsibility and defines who will get the job done. The **strategic plan** documents the planning process and its results. In business, the strategic plan is the road map. Strategic planning is the process we go through to choose our destination and draw the map to that desired destination (Chapter 22). In preparing for the strategic journey, we must do our best to plan realistically and prepare for detours and unexpected road hazards along the way.

Chapter 3 introduced the elements of strategic planning. It explored the application of **strategic thinking** to address the questions of

Key Terms

Key terms, which are defined below, are bolded and italicized the first time they appear in the chapter. Other important terms are shown in boldface on first appearance and are defined by the context in which they are used. When either of these types of terms is used several times, its acronym will be identified and subsequently used in the chapter. Both types of terms are listed alphabetically in the online glossary with their definitions and (when applicable) their acronyms.

action plans: formal plans for carrying out actions to meet strategic objectives.

adaptive strategy(ies): what the organization will do to continue its vision quest. Options are total or partial expansion, contraction, or maintenance.

balanced score card: management tool to share and report outcome measures important to achieving organizational goals. Balanced score cards can be business wide or for a specific business unit or department.

business plan: a comprehensive planning document that clearly describes the developmental objective of a proposed or existing business. The plan is a written guide for starting and running a business successfully. Ideally, the information was gathered through a strategic planning process.

contingency planning: based on environmental scans, formulating likely scenarios and then implementing protective strategies.

continuous environmental scanning: regularly investigating a business' external environment to be able to quickly recognize and respond to unexpected external changes such as new technology, changes in governmental regulations, or new competitive challenges.

continuous strategic planning: cyclic strategic planning and analysis leading to decisions about strategic goals, objectives, and tactical action plans. Outcomes of tactical action plans are monitored and serve as the basis for the next cycle of planning and analysis.

directional strategies: upper management's view of what the organization wants to do as expressed by the mission, values, and philosophical statements.

director of planning: individual in charge of the strategic planning process.

operational strategies: implementation plans formulated within the functional unit that will carry them out.

planning schedule: timetable for annual strategic planning activities.

service mix: the various services offered to consumers.

smarter goal(s): (S)pecific, (M)easurable, (A)acceptable, (R)ealistic, (T)ime bound, (E)valuated, and (R)eviewed.

stretch goal(s): ambitious ends that are seemingly unattainable with current resources. Requires thinking outside of the box to approach the desired end.

---

what a business should be doing to fulfill its **mission** and achieve its **vision** for future success. Strategic thinking starts with the organization's **mission statement**, which defines the purpose of its existence. A **vision statement** defines its desired future state (Chapters 2, 3, and 7). Value statements describing the forces that motivate a business and the behaviors it promotes in its employees complement the mission and vision statements. Often, a business will have identified **critical issues**, internal or external factors that must be addressed (Chapter 3).

In an organization, a key responsibility of health service managers at any level is to understand the relationship between the strategic plan, business success, and the performance of the areas they lead. Understanding is facilitated by keeping in mind the

key characteristics of an effective strategic plan which are

- It is reality based
- Data driven
- Incorporates input from key **stakeholders**
- It is dynamic
- Shared throughout the organization
- Used daily.

In this chapter, we are expanding the foundational elements of strategic planning as we introduce the process of *continuous strategic planning*. Our goal is to provide sufficient motivation, knowledge, and skill to new graduates, inexperienced managers, and new practice owners so they will be able to create an effective strategic plan for their personal advancement, their department, and be able to contribute to an organizational strategic plan.

So Why Plan?

Why do organizations develop strategic plans? Because unlike Alice, during her famous adventures in Wonderland (Carroll, 1866), business leaders generally want to get somewhere specific. And they don't want to waste any time getting there. The hard part is determining where that "somewhere" is with enough specificity to figure out how to get there. For those who want to get to their destination faster and with fewer detours, a road map is advisable.

The strategic plan is that road map. Strategic planning is the process we go through to define our destination and draw our road map to that desired destination. A good strategic planning process will be dynamic enough to adjust for detours and unexpected road hazards along the way. Through the planning process, an organization's desired outcomes are identified and guidelines developed for making decisions about actions intended to better the organization's future (Swayne et al., 2006).

Strategic planning is applicable to any business endeavor. Whether a business is large or small, for-profit (Chapter 22) or non-for-profit, private or public, it makes no difference. The approach to planning may differ, but the value to the business is the same. First, businesses use strategic planning to answer three basic questions (MyStartegicPlan, 2007):

1. Where are we now?
2. Where are we going?
3. How will we get there?

In answering these questions, the strategic planning process serves to improve business performance in several ways.

Provides Focus—The strategic planning process serves to focus the thinking of an organization away from the day-to-day operations and toward the strategic concerns of tomorrow. This occurs throughout the process as management at all levels take in new, up-to-date information; assess the organization's mission, vision, and values; consider input from multiple sources; complete the external and internal assessment; and determine strategic goals and objectives (Chapters 5 and 7).

Sets Priorities—The strategic planning process can help a business prioritize efforts. Businesses are often faced with a multitude of opportunities to improve and expand. When a business lacks the resources to "do it all," the strategic planning process will help management determine which of the "good" opportunities are the "best" opportunities to ensure long-term success.

Provides the Road Map—The strategic plan is a management tool. Strategies are useless without effective implementation. Employees at all levels must be able to use the strategic plan as a guide for the implementation of detailed tactical action plans.

Aligns Effort—Strategic planning helps a business align efforts toward the achievement of common goals. It provides everyone in the organization with the same road map. Employees and business partners will be able to see how their efforts contribute to reaching the desired destination. Inclusion in the planning process can also serve to align employees' thinking and motivate them to support the strategic initiatives (Bourgeois and Brodwin, 1984).

Enables Rapid Response—Because the strategic planning process includes a **continuous environmental scan**—a review of the **external environment** (Chapters 4–6)—a business is better positioned to recognize and respond to unexpected external changes such as new technology, changes in governmental regulations, or new competitive challenges.

Enables Communication—The strategic plan is a communication tool for internal and external audiences. Internally, it can be used to communicate direction and alignment efforts. Externally, the strategic plan can be used to communicate the direction of the organization for the purposes of obtaining external funding from philanthropic sources or financial lending institutions. It may also be used to engage the community in cooperative dialogue or potential business partners in collaboration discussions.

Make Effort Worth the Investment

Strategic planning consumes management time and business resources. Businesses that invest in strategic planning should want to get the best possible return on that investment. For strategic planning, the bottom line is **outcomes**. No matter how good the plan, or how many activities management undertakes to achieve its goals, *results can be the only acceptable measure of success*. A strategic plan must guide the business in the right direction. For that to happen, the strategic plan must be:

Reality Based—An effective strategic planning process finds its foundation in the gathering and analyzing of information about the business itself. It is a plan that is based on a factual assessment of the organization's external **threats** and **opportunities** as well as internal **strengths** and **weaknesses**. An effective plan is based on an honest look in the mirror. It is sometimes difficult for management of a business to assess without bias. An external consultant or at a minimum, input from external stakeholders may be needed. A business that is unable to assess its strengths, weaknesses, opportunities, and threats will not produce an effective strategic plan.

Data Driven—To be maximally effective, decision-making should be supported by data-driven analysis including, wherever possible, comparative **benchmarking** (Chapters 6 and 16). After strategy is set and actions undertaken, available data must be used to assess whether the plan is producing the desired outcomes over time. The caution here is to avoid getting caught in the trap of analysis to the point of paralysis. Given the rapid rate of change in the health service industry, managers will never have all the information they would like to make a decision. Sometimes we must settle for making the best decision possible with the information available at the time.

Inclusive, but Not Too Inclusive—The best strategic plan is one that incorporates input from all appropriate internal and external key stakeholders (Chapters 6 and 7). This does not mean that everyone in the organization should be involved to the same degree or that all input needs to be weighted equally. It does not mean that the plan will meet all of the needs or expectations of the external stakeholders. It is likely that input from the **Board of Directors** (BOD) and **senior management** will be weighted more

heavily due to their broader viewpoint and experience. That should not negate the value of input obtained from **first-level** or **middle management**, who have better knowledge of daily operational demands and challenges (Chapter 11). The challenge is in getting the right mix of input from the right people (Zuckerman, 2005).

Dynamic—Health care is one of the most rapidly growing and changing business sectors in the United States economy. In most markets, it is highly competitive and faces frequent regulatory and reimbursement changes. An effective strategic plan must support the efforts of health care business leaders to adapt to frequent and rapid changes in the internal and external business environment.

Shared Support and Used—To be effective a plan must be taken off the bookshelf. In other words, it must be shared throughout the organization and used daily by management to guide and align the work of the organization. This happens most readily when the initiatives in the plan have the support of a broad contingency within the organization. Leadership must work to gather support as part of the planning process (Zuckerman, 2005).

The American Quality and Productivity Center's (AQPC) International Benchmarking Clearinghouse analyzed the strategic planning processes of 45 top companies including Alcoa, Deere & Company, Frito-Lay, and Xerox Corporation (APQC 1996). From this study, the authors were able to identify some of the best planning practices used by those businesses' leaders. These **best practices** included:

1. Use of **stretch goals**—goals that required a shift from business as usual to drive strategic out-of-the-box thinking.
2. Use of a "**continuous improvement**"— philosophy.
3. Formal communication of the strategic plan.
4. Emphasis on strategic thinking and business unit level action planning.
5. Business planning done within the context of the corporate vision or **culture**.
6. Recognition of the importance of strategic planning through links to other elements of the management system.

7. Stressed documentation of strategic thinking.
8. Diverse competencies were the basis for **competitive advantage** and new business development.
9. Although approaches vary, the framework of issue and option generation, prioritization, measurement, and reassessment were widely used.

Getting Started

Strategic planning should be approached as a continuous process. Figure 13.1 depicts a basic strategic planning cycle starting with information that is subjected to strategic analysis and interpretation. The strategic analysis leads to decisions about strategic goals, objectives, and tactical action plans. Interpretation of the analyses is enriched and modulated by experience, intuition, and creative thinking of those involved in the formation of strategies

(Helms, 2000). Once tactical action plans are deployed, the outcomes from these actions are measured for impact. If the impact moves the organization to its desired state, the actions continue. If not, the actions are modified and the cycle continues.

Getting started requires management to make some basic decisions about the planning process.

What Planning Approach Will Management Use?

The choice of a strategic planning model is dependent on the perspective of an organization's leaders, the upper level managers. As discussed in Chapter 3, the choice of a planning model is often driven by the style of the **chief executive officer** (CEO) with guidance from the board and senior leadership. The literature approaches the question of strategic planning models from two different perspectives. The first approach addresses the question of models

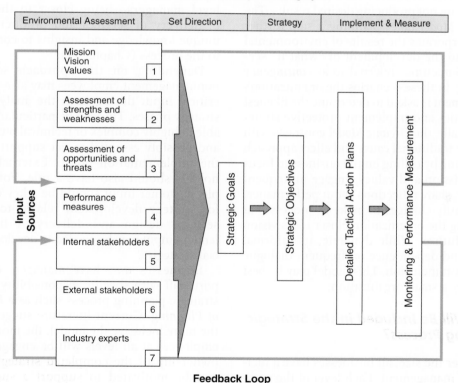

Continuous Strategic Planning Cycle

Feedback Loop

Figure 13.1. Continuous strategic planning cycle.

from the perspective of leadership and inclusion. Bourgeois and Brodwin (1984) describe five strategic planning models that find their basis in the style of the business' CEO. These models, described in some detail in Chapter 3, are really a continuum of inclusion. McNamara (2007) approaches strategic planning from the perspectives of scope and complexity. He describes five models from "basic" to "complex" that can build off each other depending on the needs of the business. McNamara's *Basic Model* is a simple top-down approach that is best suited to small businesses with little strategic planning experience; including only a few of the elements that make strategic planning effective. It may be best considered the first step in the development of an effective strategic planning process. McNamara's *Issue-Based Model* expands the basic model to include an assessment of internal and external factors, and identifies critical issues with corresponding goals and plans. Though still a basic model, it has all the key elements noted in Figure 13.1. The *Alignment Model* focuses on aligning resources to strategic initiatives and can be used to refine strategies that are not producing desired results. The *Scenario Model* takes planning a step further and incorporates the results of environmental scans into the development of "what if" scenarios. Sometimes referred to as *contingency planning*, in these scenarios the organization's management is asked to determine the likeliest possibilities and implement protective strategies. Finally, the *Organic Model* contrasts with the more traditional cause and effect approach to planning by calling on the business to focus on its mission and values, engage in frequent dialogue, share reflections about performance, and identify changes to make in process that will bring the organization closer to its vision for the future. While dynamic, its informal nature and dependence on frequent dialogue could limit inclusion. This model may be best for a very a small organization.

Who Will Be Included in the Strategic Planning Process?

No matter the size, all businesses have a hierarchy of management. Each level of the managerial hierarchy will have a different degree of planning responsibility (Chapter 11). As discussed in Chapter 3, most large, middle, and even some small businesses are legal **corporations**. Corporations are businesses whose operations have been legally separated from its owners. All corporations have a BOD, sometimes referred to as *trustees*. The BOD controls the corporation as a group and appoints the corporate officers who manage operations (Clarkson et al., 1995). The BOD is ultimately responsible for the success of the business and, in that capacity, has direct responsibility for strategic planning. Many corporations have a board level committee that is charged with responsibility to oversee the development and implementation of the strategic plan.

The board-appointed CEO is responsible for supporting the board in meeting this responsibility and should lead the strategic planning process while other top-level management may play a major role in organization-wide strategy formation. **Operational managers** should be involved as strategies evolve (Rouse, 2001). Managers lower in the hierarchy carry progressively narrower focused and more specific planning responsibility. Operational managers—middle- and **lower-level managers**—being closer to the point of delivery of services and products, have unique knowledge and insights to contribute to the process (Chapter 11).

Depending on the approach selected, nonmanagement employees may also provide critical input during both the analysis and strategy phases. This can be particularly valuable in highly complex or technical businesses and possibly essential to get support during the implementation phase. External stakeholders should also have a role. For example, customer input should be a key element for strategy development related to health services design and delivery. A financial lender's input may be needed to develop financial strategies.

Businesses may have managers or support staff with specific responsibility for the strategic planning process such as a *Director of Planning*. Current literature suggests that the more inclusive the model, the more likely employees at all levels will be engaged, take ownership of the completed strategic plan, and be motivated to support a successful implementation (Baldrige National Quality Program, 2007).

What Is the Scope and Time Frame of the Planning Effort?

Strategic plans may vary in **scope**. They can be written for an entire organization. However, some businesses are so large or diverse that a single plan is unusable. Strategic plans are written to address just the needs of a segment of the business. For example, a multisite physical therapy practice may undertake strategic planning both at the corporate and local site level. The corporate strategic plan might focus on regional market growth, financial, and managed-care contracting strategies while the local sites focus on local market development, customer satisfaction, employee retention, and expense management strategies. These planning efforts would be complementary, yielding alignment at both the corporate and local levels. The goal is to develop strategic plans that are meaningful and actionable.

Strategic plans may also cover variable time periods. Organizational size, complexity of *service mix*, **market**, and environmental volatility (Chapter 18) will all influence the time frame chosen. Given the speed and degree of change in the health care industry, it is hard to believe that any predictions greater than 3–5 years into the future will yield reliable outcomes (Center for Applied Research, 2007). This is a key reason for adopting a cyclical strategic planning process that calls for the review and update of plans on an annual basis (Swayne et al., 2006).

What Is the Planning Schedule?

A *planning schedule* defines the annual planning cycle that will be followed (Center for Strategic Planning, 2007) (Chapter 3). The planning schedule is the timetable for strategic planning activities to occur so that the annual financial planning process can be effectively linked to the desired strategic objectives and tactical action plans. Table 13.1 demonstrates the annual strategic planning cycle of activities, responsible parties, and linkage of strategic planning activities to the annual financial planning that might be used for businesses that follow a January –December fiscal calendar otherwise referred to as a **fiscal year**. The planning schedule should make allowances for unexpected changes in the internal or external environment that might require rapid response (Chapter 5).

What Resources Will Be Needed?

Support for strategic planning can come from a variety of internal and external sources. The availability of internal resources is dependent on the size and capability of the business. Businesses that lack internal resources may obtain planning support from external consultants, academic-based programs, or government-sponsored business services. Resources that may be required or prove to be of value include:

Table 13.1	**Annual Strategic Planning Cycle and Schedule**[a]		
Activity	**Responsible Parties**	**Start Date**	**Finish Date**
Implement annual plan	Management	January 1	December 31
Monitor/Measure outcomes	Decision support	January 1	December 31
Update and report balance score card	Decision support senior management	April 1 June 1 October 1 January 1	April 15 June 15 October 15 January 15
Evaluate current initiatives	Senior management	May 1	June 30
Review/Update strategic plan	Board of directors management	July 1	July 31
Prioritize initiatives	Senior management	August 1	August 30
Develop annual budget (aligned with approved initiatives)	Management	September 1	November 15
Plan and budget approval	Board of directors	November 15	December 15

[a]Based on a January 1 to December 31 fiscal year.

Management time—The most critical and sometimes the most difficult resource to obtain is management time. Health care managers are busy and their time can be easily filled with day-to-day operations. The flattening of organizational management hierarchies and the use of working manager roles (Chapter 11) just serve to increase the demands placed on a manager's time. Managers must take time to plan.

Process facilitation—The use of a facilitator to guide the planning process can be of great value. An effective facilitator can make the planning process more organized and efficient. They can pull in a variety of opinions while balancing any personal agendas or passionate positions of participants. Facilitators should be objective and neutral. Facilitators who are also content experts may have a tendency to discourage input and drive the process in a single direction. External facilitators may have a tendency to "know what is best" and should not be allowed to exclude input from within the organization.

Performance data gathering and analysis—The reader has learned that effective strategic planning is dependent on timely, complete, and accurate information about internal and external factors with the potential to impact performance. Accurate information about the current performance of the business is essential. This information may come from internal sources such as financial planning, clinical performance analysis, customer and staff surveys, or outcome measurement systems. Information may also be purchased from external rating and evaluation services such as industry performance benchmarking services (Chapter 16).

Market data gathering and analysis—Input from customers is essential. Market information may come from a variety of internal and external services. Types of information that may be of value include market trends, competitor analysis, performance benchmarks, customer feedback reports, and best practice benchmarks (Chapters 16 and 18).

Implementation support—First- and middle-level managers of clinical departments may have patient care skills that are stronger than their business skills. These managers may need support from nonclinical managers for implementation of tactical action plans.

Once the resources are in place, there are several organizational steps that, when taken together, can get the planning process off to the right start (Zuckerman, 2005). These include

1. Set and communicate planning objectives
2. Set and communicate the elements of the planning process
3. Define and communicate who will lead the process
4. Define and communicate who will support the process
5. Identify a planning facilitator
6. Set and communicate the planning schedule
7. Assemble relevant historical data
8. Review past successes and failures
9. Conduct orientation meetings
10. Prepare to stimulate future thinking
11. Set a future orientation
12. Resolve not to dwell on the past

The Planning Process

You are ready to get started. Referring back to Figure 13.1, the planning process starts with the **environmental assessment**. Information gained during this assessment is used to set strategic directions or goals. The goals lead to strategies or objectives that are actualized through tactical action plans. The results of actions taken are measured and the results used to continuously refine and update the plan.

The Environmental Assessment

The environmental assessment lays the foundation for the remainder of the strategic planning process. It starts with a confirmation of the business's mission, vision for the future, and the values or behaviors that the business will follow in reaching for that vision. The next steps involve the **internal assessment** of strengths and weaknesses and the **external assessment** to identify both opportunities and threats. This should include an honest assessment of current performance using benchmark comparisons and incorporate input from key stakeholders. A total assessment of both external (opportunities and threats) and internal (strengths and weaknesses) factors that have the potential to impact an organization's success is called a **SWOT analysis** (Learned et al., 1969; McConkey, 1976) (Chapter 3). Getting the information that is needed might require significant investment in time and financial resources. Input from experts both inside health care and from other industries should be incorporated whenever feasible. A guide to determining the scope of an environmental assessment required is to start with the known or anticipated factors that can be expected to have an effect on the organization's ability to carry out its strategic objectives (Dunn, 1998). When the environmental assessment is complete, the business should be in a good position to set direction for the future, develop strategies, and implement action plans. Performance measures will help management know if they are on track or need to make changes.

Mission, Vision, and Values

The first step in the environmental assessment is to affirm the mission and reach agreement on the vision for the future. The mission statement defines the purpose for which the business exists. As businesses grow and develop, their mission statements need to evolve with them. Mission statements should be short, to the point, and written in a way that will energize the business's internal and external audiences. The assessment of the mission, vision, and values statements should be done annually and updated as needed. The process should involve input from all levels of the organization and key stakeholders.

A Look at Some Physical Therapy Mission Examples

Private physical therapy practices provide a good source of examples. A scan of 15 private physical therapy practices from across the United States who advertise on the Internet found several common mission statement elements. All 15 practices described who they were. Some described their business, "a private physical therapy practice." Some answered "who are we?" from the perspective

of the owner(s) "a physical therapy practice owned by three experienced physical therapists." Some practices describe their customers very specifically, "adults with sports related injuries" while others left their customers undefined. All tried to describe what set them apart from the competition. Interestingly, most of the descriptions used in the mission statements to set practices apart were similar (Chapter 6). These included

- Advanced training and unique capabilities
- Best quality treatment available
- Convenient, friendly, fun care setting
- Patient-centered individualized care
- Premier, state-of-the-art, excellent services
- Quicker recovery
- Significant years of experience
- Specialized or scientific care
- Supportive environment
- Therapist delivered care

A notable absence from this list was any differentiation based on quantifiable outcome measures.

Vision statements, the defined ideal future state (Chapter 7), should clearly express what the quest is because the vision is the foundation for setting direction and developing strategic goals.

The vision for the future is typically considered at the beginning of the planning process and refined based on the results of the internal and external assessment. The online review of practices showed that only a few of the practices provided information about a long-term vision. However, practice values were more readily shared. Several practices cited education, the patient–therapist partnership, and compassionate care as values. Value statements complement the mission and vision statements by speaking to what behaviors or methods the business will employ. Some examples of value statements included, We will:

- Provide *compassionate* care with *respect* for the rights and dignity of the patients we serve.
- *Partner* with other health service providers in our community
- Be a *leader* in workforce development and employee satisfaction
- Take *pride* in our financial success

One method that can kick off the development of value statements is an employee survey. A survey can be designed to identify what the internal audience believes the business' values to be today and what they would like them to be tomorrow.

Internal Assessment: Strengths and Weaknesses

Internal factors are considered to be under the control of the organization (Chapters 5 and 6). Analysis of internal factors can reveal a business' strengths and weaknesses and raise key strategic questions including

How can our strengths be leveraged to achieve our goals?
How can our weaknesses be eliminated or, better yet, turned into future strengths?

Table 13.2 addresses the elements of an internal assessment, the areas for consideration when assessing each element, and possible assessment methods. An internal assessment is not intended to include every element, address every consideration, or use every method. Management must determine where and how much effort will be expended based on the characteristics of their organization and the scope of the planning activity.

Putting Things Together

Here is a physical therapy example that uses most of the strategic planning concepts introduced so far. The company is called Therapy First (TF). It is a hypothetical private physical therapy practice. TF is a moderately sized, owner-operated PT practice. The practice is a for-profit partnership. The owners are two PT partners and have ten employees. The mission of TF is to operate an "independent private practice providing the best available physical therapy services for adults experiencing acute or chronic back pain." Their internal assessment might start with a quick review of the mission. The mission should be updated any time it is out of sync with current business activities. This might occur if the practice has expanded to a new community, added a new service, or has a changed clientele.

Depending on the scope of activities, a review for regulatory compliance might include a review of the corporate compliance plan with related policies and procedures, a documentation audit, and an external financial audit to include a review of billing and collection practices. Governance and management may be the sole responsibility of the owner and therefore limited to a self-assessment of management skills and competencies. If the

Table 13.2	Internal Assessment	
Element	Considerations	Example Assessment Methods/Resources
Mission, vision, values	✓ Reflect current reality ✓ Send a clear and actionable message the business' employees ✓ Represent the needs of the customers	✓ Internal and/or External Stakeholder Surveys ✓ Assessment of current practices ✓ Customer feedback • Surveys • Focus groups • Complaints ✓ Service requests ✓ Community needs assessment ✓ Market image surveys
Regulatory compliance	✓ Health services delivery (licensure, registration, service regulations, etc.) ✓ Heath services coverage and reimbursement ✓ Employment ✓ Occupational health and safety ✓ Environmental impact ✓ Financial management and taxation ✓ Securities and Exchange	✓ Corporate compliance reviews ✓ Employee feedback ✓ Outside consultant reviews ✓ Annual financial audits ✓ Operational audits ✓ Compliance audits ✓ Compliance surveys ✓ Incident reporting and trends

(Continued)

Table 13.2 continued		
Element	Considerations	Example Assessment Methods/Resources

Governance and management	✓ Board Structure
	✓ Board Effectiveness
	✓ Management
	  • Demographics
	  • Diversity
	  • Structure
	  • Experience
	  • Effectiveness
	  • Stability
	  • Education
	  • Expertise
	✓ Culture and management style
		✓ Board
		  • Review of Board composition
		  • Performance assessment (external review or self-assessment
		✓ Management
		  • Review of structure and composition
		  • Performance assessment
		  • Assessment for skill and expertise requirements
		  • External management assessment
		  • Standardize testing
		  • Operating outcomes
		  • Leadership succession assessment
		  • Employee satisfaction/culture surveys
		  • Employee recruitment/retention trends

Organizational structure	✓ Alignment
	  • Work standardization
	  • Work control and direction
	  • Work coordination
	✓ Organizational
	  • Efficiency
	  • Effectiveness
	  • Change
	  • Size
	  • Scope of activity
	  • Geographical distribution
		✓ Span of control assessment
		✓ Alignment
		  • Mission with actions
		  • Global versus business unit goals
		  • Work responsibility with accountability
		✓ Organization performance against industry benchmarks
		✓ Review of organizational tools
		  • Organizational chart
		  • Job descriptions
		  • Employee competencies
		  • Policies and procedures
		  • Communication media

Operational performance	✓ Physical plant and facility infrastructure
	✓ Technology/ technology developments
	✓ Location and distribution
	✓ Resource availability
	✓ Workforce skill and availability
	✓ Key process performance
	✓ Process efficiencies
	✓ Critical success factors
	✓ Impact of emerging technologies on current market demand and business processes
		✓ Workflow/Time management
		  • Process flowcharting
		  • Cycle time measurements
		  • Service delays
		✓ Inventory/waste/errors
		  • Equipment utilization
		  • Supply utilization
		  • Resource productivity
		  • Error rates
		✓ Work environment
		  • Deployment of new technology
		  • Employee surveys
		  • Employment trends
		✓ Process Variation
		  • Performance outcome measures against industry benchmarks

Human resources	✓ Employees
	  • Right people
	  • Right number
	  • Right skill-sets
	  • Right schedule
	  • Performance
		✓ Assessment of employment trends
		  • Turnover
		  • Vacancy rates
		  • Compensation surveys
		  • Benefits surveys
		✓ Review internal practices
		  • Career/promotion opportunities
		  • Employment practices
		  • Competency assessment
		  • Work design
		  • Supervisory practices
		  • Performance recognition and reward
		  • Training and development resources

(Continued)

	Table 13.2	continued
Element	**Considerations**	**Example Assessment Methods/Resources**

		• Diversity management
		• Discipline and grievance procedures
		✓ Employee satisfaction measurement
		  • Employee surveys
		  • Employee focus groups
		  • Staff hot lines

Financial operations and resource availability	✓ Financial reserves ✓ Access to capital ✓ Financial performance ✓ Financial outlook	✓ Income from operations ✓ Financial statements ✓ Financial ratios ✓ Financial performance trends ✓ Capital reserves ✓ Financial Rating Agencies

Customer assessment	✓ Products or services purchased
	✓ Unmet needs
	✓ Satisfaction with current products and services
	✓ Rating of other providers of the same products or services
	✓ Customer loyalty
	✓ Customer willingness to refer
	✓ Market options customers would consider
		✓ Customer feedback
		  • Surveys
		  • Focus groups
		  • Complaints
		  • Service requests
		✓ Analysis of historical service trends
		✓ Demographic trends analysis
		✓ Blinded image surveys
		✓ Competitor assessment surveys

organizational structure is simple, with a **flat hierarchy**, an assessment may not be needed.

The vision for the future should be updated to reflect new interests or directions not yet achieved. If growth is expected, the need for supervision may exceed the owner's capacity and require a review of the organizational structure. Operational performance might be the heavy area for focus to ensure that

1. Facilities and equipment are adequate to ensure a smooth flow of patients in a safe environment as measured by such indicators as cycle times, service delays, equipment down time, and on time appointment starts.
2. Processes make efficient use of personnel and other resources as measured by such indicators as therapist **productivity**, supplies cost per visit, nonproductive time, waste, appointment cancellation rates, or other work environment factors.
3. Evidence-based care produces clinical outcomes that are comparable to industry benchmarks.

Human resource (HR)—related assessment should be driven by the business's current experience as well as projected workforce needs (Chapter17). If the business has low turnover, good recruitment experience, and minimum job

vacancies, HR might spend their time looking at long-term needs and industry trends. Poor current experience might steer the assessment toward a more thorough review of current practices such as a compensation survey, employee satisfaction survey, a review of job designs, and other employment practices. A review of financial performance including the sources and uses of capital would always be included as an element of the internal assessment (Chapter 21). Customer-related questions span both the internal and external assessment. The internal elements that would likely be assessed are those things under the control of the business including products and services offered, the customer experience, and service gaps. These usually need ongoing attention from management.

External Assessment: Opportunities and Threats

The information gained through an external assessment can assist with strategy development by raising key questions including

How can we take advantage of opportunities to achieve our goals?

How can we protect the business against potential threats?

The external assessment can be divided into (1) factors that have the potential to influence any organization in a community and (2) business-specific factors. The "relevant" community is defined by the business performing the assessment and could be local, regional, national, or international. Information about the external environment, particularly related to competitors or competitive services, may be difficult to obtain because most businesses try to limit access to sensitive information such as costs, litigation, competitive strategies, first to market technologies, and other future plans (Chapters 3 and 4). Some information is available because it is publicly circulated. Examples of source documents for publicly available information include annual reports, announcements in trade journals, public presentations to community stakeholders, and government reports.

Once again, it is not intended that an external assessment include every element, address every consideration, or use every method. Management must determine where and how much effort will be expended based on the characteristics of their organization and the scope of the planning activity. Continuing with our example of the moderately sized, owner-operated, and for-profit TF, the community would likely be defined as the local area and the state in which they operate. General environmental factors would include such things as local income and property tax laws or zoning requirements that apply to all businesses in their community. Tax and zoning laws can be favorable or unfavorable to business growth and development. Business-specific factors would include state licensure for physical therapy practice, **Medicaid** or locally-managed care reimbursement schedules, PT compensation rates, or availability of PTs and physical therapist assistants in the workforce. There are several models available for businesses to guide the analysis of external factors (Chapters 3 and 4). Among the most basic models are the **Political, Economic, Social,** and **Technological (PEST) analysis** (NetMBA, 2007). An alternative is to rearrange the word order to be **Social, Technological, Economic,** and **Political** or a **STEP** analysis (Hannagan, 2002). Both mnemonics make intuitive sense since pests can pose dangers and steps can be taken toward resolutions. A PEST/STEP analysis includes the following elements.

Political analysis—includes factors related to the type, stability, and regulatory activity of national, regional, or local governing bodies.

Economic conditions—includes factors that might have an effect on customer-spending patterns, business' operating costs, or access to investment capital.

Social conditions—includes information about the community population including their characteristics, living conditions, interests, attitudes, and preferences.

Technological developments—includes information about the business impacts of technology, both current and potential.

Table 13.3 provides a list of some examples of PERT assessment resources. Usually, there are external resources available for needed information. Some of this information will be readily available; some will come with a high price tag. Once again, management must decide what is needed and what price they are willing to pay for it. One of the most important resources is **best practice** benchmark data. Benchmark information is available for many aspects of business performance. Use of comparative benchmark data can be invaluable at driving performance improvement and improving a business's **competitive position**, that is, its distinctiveness.

Develop Strategies and Set Direction

Helms (2000) defines strategic goals as future related statements of desired ends that specify actions, means of discerning accomplishment, and time lines. Strategy decisions are informed decisions (1) based on management's analysis of current, accurate, and well-digested data and (2) interpreted by judgment that is supported by intuition, insight, gut feeling (Helms, 2000), and personal values (Mintzberg et al., 1995). Hannagan tells us that to be effective, strategic goals must be "**SMART**" (Hannagan, 2002). Others have expanded the acronym to "**SMARTER**" (Dolgoff, 2005). Strategic goals should be:

Specific . . . enough to be understood
Measurable . . . to see if it is working
Acceptable . . . to the people who have to make it happen
Realistic . . . to try
Timed . . . so management can target a completion date

Table 13.3   External Assessment Resources

Example Assessment Methods/Resources

✓ Publications
  - Federal government
  - Government regulations
  - Professional journals and trade magazines
  - Newspapers and magazines
  - Annual reports of competitors
  - Market surveys
  - Employment surveys
  - Customer feedback

✓ Websites
  - Government (see Chapter 10)
  - Competitors
  - Professional associations
  - Trade associations

✓ Trade associations
  - Chamber of Commerce
  - Professional associations
  - Advocacy groups
  - Purchasing groups
  - Investment groups

  - Business development groups

✓ External consultants
  - Audit firms
  - Legal counsel
  - Legislator offices
  - Academic personnel
  - Survey firms
  - Insurance brokers
  - Marketing firms
  - Human resource consultants
  - Diversity consultants

✓ Education sessions
  - Payer information sessions
  - Professional association sessions
  - On-line education
  - Continuing education courses

✓ Other publicly available data bases
  - Demographics
  - Health services utilization and outcome reports

Evaluated . . . by comparing current and desired outcome so changes can be made if needed

Reviewed . . . when goal achieved to determine what can be done to improve future goal setting processes

Strategic goal-setting should start with refinement of the vision statement. What do we want to become? How do we get there? Strategy needs to be directed toward that vision.

Returning to the TF practice, let us assume that the environmental assessment has confirmed some anticipated results and revealed some new information. The confirmations:

1. Cash reserves are very limited
2. Expenses per visit are up due to rising costs and low number of referrals
3. For the first time, we have been unable to fill a PT vacancy within 2 months
4. Managed care reimbursement rates have declined
5. Opportunities to grow business are somewhat limited due to our **niche market**
6. Our charges are the same or slightly higher than our competitors
7. Our patients are very satisfied and rate their experience as excellent
8. Patient referrals are off for the 3rd and 4th quarters (due to bad weather, holidays, and staff vacancy)

The surprising new information:

1. Market compensation for PTs has increased 10% over last year
2. Our private practice competitors have affiliated with larger provider groups
3. We have lost and our competitors have gained market share
4. Competitors now offer amenities, like free transportation, that will be hard to match
5. Competitors' rates have dropped, making our rates highest in the market
6. Even very satisfied self-pay patients are unwilling to pay higher prices

Analysis of TF Practice

Suddenly a mission to operate an "independent private practice providing the best available physical therapy services for adults experiencing acute or chronic back pain" does not seem as viable. TF owners see a challenging future unless they set a new direction. They need a vision. That vision could take them in one of many directions. While the reader may see many exciting opportunities to change course, let us presently assume that the TF partners are fiercely committed to the status quo. The only change they want to make is to find ways to increase referrals and decrease operating expenses while allowing them to remain in full control of their business. TF strategic goals might look something like this:

- Grow market share quarterly by 3%
- Improve fiscal performance quarterly by 5%
- Attract and retain the best workforce—new hire in one month

Deployment through Objectives and Action Plans

Once the direction is set it is time to begin setting strategic objectives, tactical plans, and assigning responsibilities. The outcome of these efforts should be tied to measurable performance outcomes whenever possible. Table 13.4 provides an example using the goals adopted by TF owners and how those goals could be expanded with a set of possible objectives, action plans, and related performance outcome measures. The action plans selected should reflect the competitive position and any competitive advantages of the business. The TF example reflects *adaptive* and *operational strategies* to adapt to changing external conditions in an attempt to maintain

the status quo. *Directional strategies* would be required if TF's owners were interested in changing their vision—for example, becoming affiliated with a larger private practice group.

Assessing Outcomes, Reassessing Strategy

Table 13.4 includes both time frames and examples of performance measures that might be used to assess the effectiveness of their objectives and action plans (Chapter 16). Are these efforts moving them toward their goals? A popular approach to collecting and presenting performance outcome measures is the *balanced score card* (Kaplan and Norton, 1996; Swayne et al., 2006) (also see Chapter 3). A balanced score card is a management tool that can be used to share and report outcome measures important to achieving an organization's goals. It can be business wide or focused on a specific business unit, department, or improvement initiative. A balanced score card (Table 13.5) is typically segregated into goal or topic areas. The balanced score

Table 13.4   Goals, Objectives, and Action Plans

1.–3. Goals (w/Responsible Party)

1.X – 3.X Objectives

1.X.X – 3.X.X Action Plan (w/Measures and Timelines)

1. Grow Market Share (TF Owner #1)

1.1. Expanded the number of managed care contracts
    1.1.1. Approach all area managed care plans with request for contract agreements (# of contracts/End 2nd Quarter)
    1.1.2. Set up competitive payment plans for self-pay patient market (% increase in self-pay patients / Ongoing)
    1.1.3. Accept Medicaid patients up to 8% of total business (% of Medicaid covered patients / Quarterly)
    1.1.4. Evaluate the addition of service amenities to attract additional referrals (Patients who say they came because of the amenities / Ongoing)

1.2. Build/strengthen relationships with new/current referral sources.
    1.2.1. Schedule outreach visits (# of outreach visits; % change in # of referrals / End 1st Quarter; Quarterly)
    1.2.2. Send follow up fax reports to every referring physician upon start of care, prior to each follow up visit, and at discharge. (End 1st Quarter; Quarterly)
    1.2.3. Send holiday gifts to all physicians referring 10 or more patients. (End 3rd Quarter)

1.3. Develop Medicare market by site visits to retirement and assisted living facilities.
    1.3.1. Establish contacts at local retirement and assisted living facilities.
    1.3.2. Develop resource materials and purchase logo items to give away during retirement and assisted living facility visits (# of site visits/# of referrals from retirement and assisted living facilities / End 1st Quarter; Quarterly)

1.4. Research market development strategies used by competitors and private practices in other markets (End 1st Quarter)

1.5. Maintain high customer satisfaction rating by continuing current strategies (Satisfaction ratings / Ongoing)

(Continued)

Table 13.4   continued

2. Improve Fiscal Performance (Business Office Manager)

2.1. Establish process to ensure prompt payment under all managed care plan contracts (Days in Accounts Receivable / End 1st Quarter)

2.2. Submit bills every 15 days and within 3 days of discharge (Days in Accounts Receivable End 1st Quarter)

2.2.1. Revise billing processes and ensure timely documentation completion (Ongoing)

2.3. Review supplies purchasing, distribution, and billing processes (Supplies cost per visit / End 1st Quarter)

2.4. Develop recommendations for PT salary adjustments for recruitment and retention of qualified personnel (See Goal #3, PT#1 Owner #2)

2.5. Evaluate move to less expensive facilities at end of lease (Potential savings / End 2nd Quarter)

2.6. Explore sources of external funding to provide cash flow needed to support business expansion/relocation (End 1st Quarter)

2.7. Evaluate joining a purchasing cooperative (Potential savings / End 1st Month)

3. Attract and Retain the Best Workforce (TF Owner #2) (; / Ongoing)

3.1. Review PT compensation and benefits programs against market (Turnover rates; Vacancy rate / End 1st Quarter)

3.2. Assess addition of flex and part time schedules (End 1st Quarter)

3.3. Assess expansion of business sponsored continuing education offerings (Turnaround on new hires / End 2nd Quarter)

3.4. Assess addition of clinical education program to attract PT and PTA students (Recruitment costs / End 3rd Quarter)

3.5. Assess addition of summer internships to attract PT and PTA students (Recruitment costs; End 3rd Quarter)

Table 13.5   Physical Therapist #1 Balanced Score Card

Goal	Performance Outcome Measures	Performance		
		Target	Actual	Status
Grow Market Share (Chapters 18, 19)	Number of managed-care plan contracts	5	3	▼—
	Percentage increase in self-pay patients	5%	0%	▼
	Percentage of Medicaid patients	8%	0%	▼—
	Percentage increase in new patient referrals	10%	−5%	▼
	Number of referrals from retirement and assisted living facilities	120	85	▼
	Percentage of patients who rate their experience as excellent	65%	80%	▲
Fiscal Performance (Chapters 20, 21)	Days in accounts receivable (AR)	80	120	▼
	Days cash on hand	95	65	▼
	Supplies cost per visit	$5	$6	▼
	Operating margin	6%	5%	▼
Attract and Retain the Best Work-force (Chapter 17)	Turnaround on new hires (days)	45	90	▼
	Turnover rates	10%	8%	▲
	Vacancy rate	0%	10%	▼

card format allows management to quickly see what is working and what is not. Table 13.5 provides an example of a balanced score card that might be used by TF's owners to keep track of their progress.

Summary

Strategic planning offers business leaders a tool to improve the performance of their organizations in several ways. A good strategic plan can be used to focus leaders on the future, prioritize their efforts, align the effort at all levels of the organization, incorporate environmental factors into their plans, communicate to internal and external audiences, and support the implementation of tactical action plans. In short, strategic planning can improve the odds in favor of a business, department, or an individual succeeding. Effective strategic plans share some common elements. Because strategic planning requires a significant commitment of the business' resources, management must understand best practices and how to get the most value out of the strategic planning process. Relevant information can be obtained many ways. Management must use good judgment in determining how much

of what information is needed to support the decision-making process. Once the environmental assessment is complete, management must use the information to set direction with strategic goals and use objectives and action plans to align the work across the organization, monitoring and measuring progress so they can adjust along the way. The bottom line for strategic plans is that results can be the only acceptable measure of success. The business plan and other tools needed to add depth to complete a comprehensive business plan are to be found in later chapters, particularly Chapter 22. Selecting an organizational structure for strategic purposes will be addressed in the next chapter, which blends strategic planning and the structuring of an organization to meet its mission.

REFERENCES

American Productivity & Quality Center. Strategic planning: Final report. Houston, TX: Author. 1996.

Baldrige National Quality Program. Health care criteria for performance excellence. Gaithersburg, MD: Baldridge National Quality Program National Institute of Standards and Technology, Technology Administration, U.S. Department of Commerce. 2007.

Bourgeois LJ, Brodwin DR. Strategic implementation: Five approaches to an elusive phenomenon. Strategic Management Journal. 1984;5:241–264.

CASE STUDY 13.1

Strategic Planning for Your Own Purposes

Introduction

In this chapter, you have seen example analyses of the guiding documents (mission, values, and vision) related to strategic planning of actual and hypothetical practices. You have also reviewed a schematic representation of the strategic planning process (see Fig. 13.1) and tables for gathering internal (Table 13.2) and external (Table 13.3) environment information. Table 13.4 was presented as a guide for stating what needs to be done to fulfill the mission and move closer to the vision. Using these informational resources to assist you, you have the opportunity to apply what you have learned about strategic planning.

Options

Individual PTs, like different organizations, have unique attributes and aspirations. In recognition of differences, you may choose the context that is appropriate for yourself for this case study assignment. You may approach this exercise from the perspective of a:

1. Student PT planning to look for their first physical therapy position
2. Licensed PT wishing to move into a first-level management position in their current workplace
3. Licensed PT aspiring to begin a private practice on a part-time basis

(Continued)

CASE STUDY 13.1

Strategic Planning for Your Own Purposes (continued)

4. Licensed PT manager in a health service organization with responsibility for increasing productivity within their current expense budget
5. A PT in private practice who desires to move the practice from the central city to a location closer to a suburb

Tasks For All Situations #1–5

Review Figure 13.1 and follow the seven steps:

1. Draft your personal mission, values, and vision statements (1/2 page maximum).
2. Assess your internal environment (what you bring to an employer, organization, employees, and your shortcomings in relationship to accomplishing your mission and vision).
3. Assess your external environment (where or what is/are the job(s) you want, who is/are your competitors, how do you match up?).
4. What metrics will you use to gauge your success (time, money, accomplishments, recognition, etc.)?
5. Who else needs to be intimately involved in your decision making (spouse, family, friend, etc.)?

6. Who else is interested in your success and can provide helpful information (faculty, former employer, acquaintances, etc.?).
7. What advice do experts offer to professionals in your situation? (career counselors, authors, websites, etc.?).

Continuing with the remaining four steps in Figure 13.1:

1. List your strategic goals (1–3-year career goals–stretch goals)
2. List your strategic objectives (e.g., shorter term, smaller step goals)
3. What do you have to do to achieve # 1 and #2?
4. What are the indicators that you will use/request to gauge how you are progressing toward #1 and #2?

The final step in this exercise is feedback. Hypothesize how you will respond if there are things that come up that are hindering your progress. Think about how you have historically responded to feedback experiences like scoring below class norms on exams, rejections, advisement sessions, performance reviews, etc. Give examples of when you responded to feedback in ways that led you to get closer to your goal(s).

Carroll L. Alice's adventures in wonderland. New York, NY: D. Appleton and Company. 1866.

Center for Applied Research. Briefing notes: A summary of best practice approaches in strategic planning processes. Available at http://www.cfar.com. Accessed 11/08/07.

Center for Strategic Planning. Outcome-based strategic planning approach for schools. Defining elements of actionable strategic plans. Available at http://www.planonline.org/planning/strategic/planningmodel.htm. Accessed 4/2/07.

Clarkson KW, Miller RL, Jentz GA, Cross FB. West's business law: Text cases, legal, ethical, regulatory, and international environment, 6th ed. Minneapolis, MN: West. 1995.

Dolgoff R. An introduction to supervisory practice in human services. Boston, MA: Pearson. 2005.

Dunn RT. Haimann's supervisory management for health-

care organizations, 6th ed. Boston, MA: McGraw-Hill. 1998.

Hannagan T. Mastering strategic management. New York, NY: Palgrave. 2002.

Helms MM, ed. Encyclopedia of management, 4th ed. Detroit, MI: Gale Group. 2000.

Kane M. The CEO refresher. The world of strategic thinking, it's not about time. Available at http://www.refresher.com/!mjkstrategic.html. Accessed 4/2/07.

Kaplan RS, Norton DP. Using the balanced scorecard as a strategic management system. Harvard Business Review. 1996;74(1):75–85.

Learned EP, Christensen CR, Andrews KR, Guth WD. Business policy text and cases, Revised ed. Homewood, IL: Richard D. Irwin. 1969.

McConkey DD. How to manage by results. New York, NY: AMACOM. 1976.

McNamara C. Basic Overview of Various Strategic Planning models. Adapted from the Field Guide to Nonprofit Strategic Planning and Facilitation. Authenticity Consulting, LLC. 1997–2007.

Mintzberg H, Quinn JB, Voyer J. The strategy process, Collegiate ed. Englewood Cliffs, NJ: Prentice Hall. 1995.

MyStrategicPlan. How to create a strategic plan. Available at http://mystrategicplan.com/strategic-planning-tools/how-to-create-a-strategic-plan.shtml. Accessed 4/2/07.

NetMBA. PEST analysis. 2007. Available at http://www.netmba.com/strategy/pest/. Accessed 1/04/08.

Rouse WB. Essential challenges of strategic management. New York, NY: John Wiley & Sons. 2001.

Swayne LE, Duncan WJ, Ginter PM. Strategic management of health care organizations, 5th ed. Malden, MA: Blackwell. 2006.

Zuckerman AM. Healthcare strategic planning, 2nd ed. Chicago, IL: ACHE Management Series Health Administration Press. 2005.

ADDITIONAL RESOURCES

A free trial of strategic planning software is available at http://www.Mystrategicplan.com and http://www.planware.org/strategicplansoftware.htm. An extensive descriptive template for strategic planning can be obtained at http://www.nsgic.org/hottopics/strategic_plan_template.pdf.

The American Physical Therapy Association (APTA) has an example of the continuous strategic planning process for educational strategies. The original 2006–2010 strategic plan and two updates with goals and objectives can be reviewed at ttp://www.apta.org/AM/Template.cfm?Section=Home&TEMPLATE=/CM/ContentDisplay.cfm&CONTENTID=43041. Examples of APTA state chapter strategic plans can be found at http://www.apta.org/AM/Template.cfm?Section=Leadership2&Template=/TaggedPage/TaggedPageDisplay.cfm&TPLID=2&ContentID=35514. Harvard University produces special series on business topics. A recent publication deals with marketing strategy as part of an overall organizational strategy. See Lucke R. Harvard Business Essentials: Marketer's Toolkit: The 10 Strategies You Need to Succeed. Boston, Mass: Harvard Business School Press. 2006. Another recent publication that expands on the material presented in this chapter especially analysis is: Elkin P. Mastering Business Planning and Strategy: The Power and Application of Strategic Planning. London, England: Thorogood. 2007. Interesting journal articles on the evolution of strategic planning include: Braker J. The historical development of the strategic management concept. Academy of Management Review. 1980;5(2):219–224; Mintzberg H. The design school: Reconsidering the basic premises of strategic management. Strategic Management Journal. 1990;11(3):171–195; Mintzberg H. The fall and rise of strategic planning. Harvard Business Review. 1994;72(1):107–114. Two articles on the balanced score card concept are: Inamare N, Kaplan RS, Bower M. Applying the balanced scorecard in healthcare provider organizations. Journal of Healthcare Management. 2002;47(3):179–195 and Wicks AM, St Clair L. Competing values in healthcare: Balancing the (un)balanced scorecard. Journal of Healthcare Management. 2007;52(5):309–323.

CHAPTER 14

ORGANIZING FOR BUSINESS SUCCESS

DEBORAH G. FRIBERG

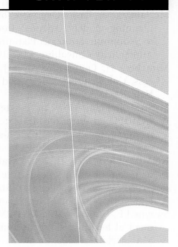

Learning Objectives

1. Compare the two component parts of organizational structure introduced in this chapter.
2. Analyze the relationship between organizational structure and business success.
3. Discuss how internal and external environmental factors influence management decisions about organizational structure.
4. Contrast four methods of coordinating work in a health care organization including the contexts each is best suited.
5. Integrate the concepts of organizational structure, coordination of work, and stages of organizational development.
6. Give examples of the impact of an organization's structure on its managers and staff.
7. Given an organizational chart, analyze the supervisory relationships, official communication patterns, and ability to respond quickly to changing needs.

Introduction

The term organization has many definitions. In Chapter 2, we discussed the concept of business organization from the perspective of ownership and legal structure. In this Chapter our focus will be on **organization structure**, **work coordination**, and *work design*. We will be approaching organizational structure in the context of relationships. These relationships are between the varied functions that contribute to the whole of the organization and the people that perform those functions. It is the "structure through which individuals cooperate systematically to conduct business" (American Heritage Dictionary of the English Language, 2003). In a business, whenever two or more individuals work together to accomplish a shared goal, there is a need to coordinate their efforts. Work coordination serves to create a common understanding of the work needed to achieve a desired outcome. It serves to:

- Assign roles and responsibility
- Communicate performance expectations
- Coordinate assignments between individuals
- Establish a work plan

The organizational structure provides the foundation for the coordination of the business. It defines authority, responsibility, and organization of decision-making relationships. Moreover, it is reasonable that as a business grows in size, the need for coordination will increase. An **organizational chart** is the graphic diagram of a business' structure.

Work design is the process of assigning content to jobs including training requirements, job duties, responsibilities, interactions, and work process. Work design is an inherent element of organizational structure (Mintzberg et al., 1995).

Management decisions about organizational structure, work coordination, and work design should be dynamic to accommodate growth,

Key Terms

Key terms, which are defined below, are bolded and italicized the first time they appear in the chapter. Other important terms are shown in boldface on first appearance and are defined by the context in which they are used. When either of these types of terms is used several times, its acronym will be identified and subsequently used in the chapter. Both types of terms are listed alphabetically in the online glossary with their definitions and (when applicable) their acronyms.

bureaucratic stage: this stage of organizational development is characterized by a high degree of reliance on work standardization, large, complex management structure, distinct operating departments divided by specialization (job specialists versus generalists), and large technical and general support service functions.

complexity: the degree of external environment variation among customers, services offered, regulations, and competitors. In such environments, managers must have in-depth knowledge and expertise to plan for the organization's future.

craft stage: basic stage of organizational development with little or no division of labor. The term craft is intended to describe the work of an organization in which all of the members can effectively perform all the tasks necessary to achieve the organization's common goal with little direct supervision.

divisional/divisionalized stage: a form of organizational development that breaks the company into two or more distinct business units called divisions.

entrepreneurial stage: early organization developmental state in which the division between management and staff occurs.

horizontal integration: expansion of an organization's current business (same type) into new markets.

hostility: unpredictable demands from multiple sources, for example, labor force, the government, the community, or competitors that make planning difficult.

life cycle: cyclic changes in sales and profitability of services and products over time. The cycle consists of the introduction stage, growth stage, maturity stage, and decline stage.

market diversity: the more products, services, and customers in a market, the greater the diversity.

A diverse market requires more organizational activities for coordinating work.

market expansion: broadening the scope of the business through diversification, vertical integration, market development, and penetration actions.

market integration: a market with few products, services, and customers.

output/outcome standardization: evidence-based ranges of results of treatment protocols with definitions, defined measurements, timelines, and resources used.

product(s): tangible and intangible items resulting from mental or physical labor. In the health industry, a new health related service could be called a new product even though it is a service. A service product has been used to describe such health related offerings.

product line model: an operational structure that shuns work-specific operating units like a physical therapy department in preference for product-based operating units like outpatient services.

skill standardization: for coordination purposes in delivering health care. This is accomplished through required education.

stability: the rate and predictability of environmental change. Slow and anticipated changes increase stability, the opposite decreases it.

vertical integration: business expansion through service or product diversification, whether by broadening services to the same market or by adding a new customer base.

work design: the process of determining the specific job duties of employees so there is a structure and a way to regulate work. Job descriptions, performance expectations, and reporting relationships are some of the outcomes of work design.

---

new service development, improve business performance, and accommodate changes in strategic direction. The responsibility for decision making about organizational structure, work coordination, and work design fall primarily to management. Responsibility for structure at the **senior management** level may fall, at least in part, to the **governing body**, the Board of Directors (**BOD**). In Chapters 3, 5, and 13, the discussions covered the elements of the **environmental assessment** including the **mission**, **vision** and **values**; **internal factors**; and **external factors** that drive the **strategic planning** process. It should not be surprising that many of these same elements might or should influence management decisions about the organizational structure. At the same time, managers must appreciate how decisions about the organizational structure, work coordination, and work design impact the organization's ability to perform under changing circumstances. As discussed in Chapter 13, the questions that management needs to answer in regards to the organizational structure are

Does it account for the scope and size of the business?
Does it align (coordinate) the work of the organization toward achievement of strategic goals?
Does it optimize operational efficiency and effectiveness?
Does it accommodate changes in direction?

A business's success depends on management's ability to maintain a productive work force that is prepared to adapt to continuously changing performance expectations (Worley and Lawler, 2006). For this reason, health services managers have a greater than average need to understand organizational structure and work design. The rapid rate of change in the health care industry environment can be readily observed. Increased market and competitive pressures in all forms of business have lead to increased organizational complexity (Worley and Lawler, 2006). Efforts to accommodate unremitting change have left many health care organizations in a state of continuous organizational restructuring. Every time the organizational structure and/or work methods change, the division and methods for the coordination of work will also change (McConnell, 2005). This can have a detrimental impact on performance. While management and employees learn new jobs and develop new relationships, work coordination and productivity can decrease. Under these circumstances, organizational performance becomes even more dependent on management's ability to understand, support, and assist the change process (Schneller, 1997).

Operating Structure

There are many ways to approach a discussion of organizational structure (Palmer et al., 2007). In Chapter 2, the concepts of legal forms of businesses and the implications of tax status were discussed. We will now address organizational structure from the perspective of its **operating structure**, which is the way an organization balances the division and coordination of work between employees. Operating structure sets the stage for a business's response to all of the environmental factors that influence its success. Mintzberg (1979) and associates (Mintzberg et al., 1995) have described the organization of human activity as the act of balancing two opposing requirements. The first is the division of work between employees. The second is the coordination of that work between employees to achieve a common goal. An organization's operating structure defines both work division and work coordination. There are innumerable ways to divide the work of the organization. Mintzberg (1979, 1983) suggests three methods to coordinate work between individuals:

1. Work standardization
2. Supervision
3. Mutual accommodation

Health care organizations use all three of these methods to coordinate the work of between employees. Management's decisions about operating structure are influenced by both internal and external environmental factors. There is no agreement in the literature regarding the relative importance and the interrelationship of any of these factors to any specific organization's operating structure (Brown and McCool, 1986; Liedtka, 1992; MacMillan and Jones, 1984). It is up to management to discern what operational structure and coordination methods will best fit their business *at a given point in time.*

Methods for Work Coordination

Work standardization reduces the need for direct **supervision** (oversight) and **mutual accommodation** (voluntary working adjustments) because it reduces the variation in the performance of employees. Standardization can be approached from three directions (Mintzberg, 1979).

1. *Work processes and task standardization* can be accomplished using such things as **policies**, **procedures**, work (treatment) **protocols**, or standardized work (treatment) plans. The adoption of evidenced **best practices** in the delivery of health care services is an example of work process standardization.
2. *Output (outcome) standardization* is on the rise in health care. A treatment protocol using mobility status and range of motion to determine the need for continued care or discharge is an example of outcome standardization.
3. *Skill standardization* accomplished through education, training, and licensure are fundamental elements for work coordination of health care organizations. The requirement that employees meet job qualifications, such as physical therapy (PT) licensure, experience, and/or postgraduate education are all examples of skill standardization methods. Skill standardization is most effective when accompanied by the application of on-the-job competency testing.

Supervision is the control and direction of the work of employees by another employee (Chapter 11). Supervision can be used to coordinate the work of the organization. For this to be effective, the supervisor must have direct knowledge of the work of a group of employees. The **supervisor** then directs employees to perform their work in a manner and time frame that complements the work of others in the work group.

Mutual accommodation is the simplest method of work coordination. Mutual accommodation results from the ongoing interaction between individuals. This interaction results in continuous adjustment between individuals toward the achievement of their shared goals. Common in simple organizations, this method of coordination may also be most effective in complex situations. Table 14.1 lists work coordination methods that are common to PT organizations of all types.

Creativity Versus Standardization

Consumers are demanding that health service providers improve outcomes, reduce errors, and provide a higher level of value (Porter

Table 14.1   Work Coordination in Therapy Practice

Production Technology	Work Standards	Supervision	Mutual Accommodation
Professional education	X		
Licensure requirements	X	X	
Advanced certification	X		
Advanced training	X		
Assessment practices	X		
Treatment algorithms	X		
Practice guidelines	X		
Treatment protocols	X		
Standardized care plans	X		
Clinical resource staff		X	X
Patient care conferences		X	X
Treatment teams			X
Policies and procedures	X		
Job descriptions	X		
Performance standards	X	X	
Flexible schedules			X
Staff schedules	X	X	

and Teisberg, 2006). These pressures are being exerted in an environment of reduced reimbursement and increased competition (Chapters 2 and 3). Clearly, health service providers need to encourage both creativity and innovation if they are to succeed and, in some cases, survive (Chapter 22). Standardization is, by definition, intended to reduce variation. A **standard** is something that has been developed based on experience and held up as a defined expectation for employees to follow. A standard "implies consistency and compliance" (Highet, 2007). While many see the conflict between the use of standardization to drive performance and the expectation of creativity and innovation, Kondo (1996) recognizes that both creativity and innovation are important and can be complementary if management can structure their organization to avoid conflict between the employees striving for standardization and those in charge of creativity and innovation. Land and Jarman (1992) speak to the growth cycle of organizations from birth through maturity and the importance of embracing continuous innovation and change even for established, highly bureaucratic organizations. It is up to management to determine which of the alternative methods of work coordination fit their business. The operating structure must support the adopted methods. Lack of attention to the methods of work coordination is likely to have a negative impact on business performance.

Internal Factors Influencing Operating Structure

Internal factors are those under the control of management (Chapters 5, 6, and 13). While many internal factors have the potential to impact operating structure some of the most significant include mission, **governance** and management, ownership, management style, regulatory requirements, current organizational structure, and operational requirements. Drilling down into these factors, **culture**, ownership, production technology, size, and age are of special interest.

Ownership

Ownership can be private, public, and governmental. All three types of ownership arrange-

ments are used in the health care industry. **Private ownership** means a business is owned solely by an individual, a group of individuals, or another privately owned business. **Public ownership** means that the stock representing an ownership interest is traded to members of the public through a stock exchange. Publicly traded business is owned by individuals (stockholders) who have invested in the business through the purchase of stock. **Government ownership** means that an organization is owned directly by a local, state, or federal government body (Chapter 2). As long as a business functions within the requirements of the law, it is accountable only to its owners. Adherence to ethical guidelines is a different matter focusing on doing the right thing for the right reasons for all stakeholders (Chapter 7).

Management Style

One system often used to classify organizations distinguishes between **mechanistic** and **organic** forms of organizational structure (Burns and Stalker, 1961). A mechanistic structure is the traditional **bureaucracy** common in mid- to large-sized businesses. As a bureaucracy, mechanistic organizations have clearly defined jobs, clear hierarchical structure, and depend on the chain of command, or management structure, for work coordination. This structure would fit with a management style that is more top-down, likes stability and control, and is focused on the status quo. An organic structure offers a flatter (see Chapter 11) and more open environment. There is more dependence on mutual accommodation and less on **chain of command**. Chain of command refers to the management structure of the organization. Here the management tends to have personal interactions with employees. This structure probably best fits the entrepreneurial manager who likes flexibility and encourages continuous change (Chapter 22).

Production Technology

Businesses can be differentiated based on the production technology systems they use. Production technologies include unit, mass, and process production systems (Woodward, 1965). **Unit production** is based on customer-specific requirements. This would include the production of prototypes or a customer-specific *product* designed to meet a specific customer's needs. Health care is provided on a patient-specific basis. **Mass production** describes a business that produces a large volume of similar product. Producers of health care products such as walkers or wheelchairs are good examples of mass production health care businesses. The description of mass production can also apply to some health services. Laboratory tests, radiology exams, even certain elements of therapy service, are mass-produced. Standardization is important to the production of mass-produced items. **Process production** describes the production technology of large quantities of liquid, gas, or other continuous flow products such as electricity. Process production technology has not been typically identified with health care delivery. Recently, health care providers have been more focused on patient flow as a way to compare and improve health care systems' service (reduced wait times), productivity, and other variables (European Observatory on Health Systems and Policies, 2007). Production technology will influence the type and division of the work to be performed. The division of work will determine the need for work coordination. Table 14.1 also provides examples of standardization and customized work coordination methods associated with unit and mass production that are common to therapy practice.

Culture

Culture (Chapter 6) is the term used to describe the patterns of social interaction that define the norm within the organization (Goffee and Jones, 1996). It reflects an organization's values in practice. Goffee and Jones (1996) describe two types of human relations: **sociability** and **solidarity**. Sociability measures the true friendliness between employees. Solidarity is a measure of an organization's ability to pursue shared objectives quickly and effectively. Culture is learned through formal and informal interactions among organizational members. The aspects of the job that are not formally described in the organization's **fundamental guiding documents** (Chapter 6) are transmitted to new employees by those who have experience and wish to share their experience. Solidarity reflects the ability of management to form a vision

and communicate it to those who provide the services. A **strategic plan** is one of the most effective tools that the management can deploy to achieve solidarity (Chapter 13).

Size and Age

Mintzberg (1979) provides several hypotheses regarding the relationship between the size and age of an organization. His observations indicated that as organizations age, size also increases, so does the division of labor leading to a larger, more complex management structure, differentiation of organizational subunits, and a more dominant organizational culture.

External Factors Influencing Operating Structure

External factors are things that originate or act from outside the organization (Chapters 3 and 13). There are numerous external factors that impact the operating structure of health care organizations. In Chapter 13, the external factors were considered under the categories of politics, economics, social trends, and technology. Drilling down into these factors, governmental regulation, economic climate and reimbursement, demographic trends, customers, competition, and technological innovation are of special interest. The impact of external trends on organizational structure can be understood by assessing the condition of the health care environment for *stability*, *complexity*, *market diversity*, and *hostility* (Schneller, 1997).

Stability is a reflection of the rate and predictability of environmental change. The faster rate of changes and the less predictable changes, together make the environment increasingly more unstable.

This type of environment challenges businesses to adopt rapidly new strategic directions. A mechanistic operating structure will be less flexible in meeting these challenges because of its layers of decision makers.

Complexity refers to diverse and ever changing expectations of customers, products, regulations, and competitors. A complex external environment is one where a high level of technical expertise and in-depth knowledge of all environmental factors is needed for success. Given the diversity of customers, products, and services, the highly technical nature of health care, the required levels and varied types of expertise needed to deliver care, the current health care environment is an example of a highly complex environment. A simplistic environment is one in which the demands of customers, products, regulations and competitors are homogeneous and therefore easily understood.

Market diversity is defined by the extent of *market integration*. An integrated market is one with few products and customers. The more products and customers in a market, the greater the diversity. A diverse market requires more diverse organizational activities requiring work coordination.

Hostility in the environment can arise from significant and unpredictable demands from multiple sources, for example, its labor force, the government, the community, or its competitors. The health care environment has and continues to face rapidly changing environmental demands, and the environment has been hostile for many years.

Common Organizational Structures

Every organization has three basic parts. Depending on the size of a business, owners and employees may function within one or more of the organization's parts. As the size of the organization increases, the division of labor will also increase.

Supervision: Management is the first division of labor in developing organizations (Mintzberg, 1979) (Chapter 11). With the addition of supervision, work performance is separated from work supervision.

Operating core is the part of the organization that actually performs the work.

Support services is separated into two groups, **technical support** and support services. Technical experts direct their efforts toward the development of work standards and responding to environmental complexity to enhance the performance of the operating core. A clinical lead or senior therapist

might fill this role in a PT practice. Support service personnel provide support that is not directly related to the work of the operating core. Marketing, the business office, the mailroom, and human resources are examples of support services.

Organizational structure defines the relationships among and between the parts of the organization. The right structure will facilitate performance, accommodate environmental factors, and position the organization to respond to external threats and opportunities. When considering the structure of a specific organization, management should ask if its form fits its function. Functions change during the *life cycle* of products (Zoltners et al., 2006) (see Chapter 18) when competitors change tactics, and for other reasons, so business forms or structures are not stagnant (Foss et al., 2007). Whatever the business structure, it must be able to deal with constant change (Drucker, 2006; Worley and Lawler, 2006).

The Organizational Chart

The organizational chart is a graphic representation of an organizational structure. Using boxes, lines, and occasionally other geometric shapes an organizational chart becomes a graphic representation of the parts of the organization. Typically, solid lines represent direct **reporting relationships**. Direct reporting relationships indicate both accountability and responsibility. Dotted lines represent communications and/or indirect control (MacStravic, 1986). An organizational chart can be used to depict any type of organizational structure. It may depict all or part of an organization's structure.

Organizational structures are most often pyramidal representing the hierarchy of the management structure (Chapter 11). In a pyramidal structure, the most senior management position would be placed at the pinnacle of the triangle. Subordinate positions and departments would follow in order of organizational position from high to low. Traditionally, the organizational chart describes the authority and responsibilities of positions within the organization. Occasionally, an organization will develop a structure that eliminates the typical management hierarchy. An organizational chart may be used to depict such a structure, but it may have little meaning outside of that organization. The organizational chart should represent the actual structure, not a desired culture or set of relationships.

Operating Structure at Progressive Stages of Organizational Development

The need for division and coordination of work will increase as an organization grows and develops. According to Mintzberg (1983) and Mintzberg et al. (1995), organizations will pass through five stages of development. These five stages of organizational development are

1. Craft stage
2. Entrepreneurial stage
3. Bureaucratic stage
4. Divisional stage
5. Adhocracy or Matrix stage

The Craft Stage

The *craft stage* is the most basic stage of organizational development. At this stage, an organization is small with little or no division of labor. The term "craft" is intended to describe the work of an organization where all members can effectively perform all of the tasks necessary to achieve the organization's common goal with little direct supervision. Supervision would most likely be provided by a working supervisor (Chapter 11) where that person commonly performs all the work of the organization alongside other organization members. The use of standardization as a method of coordination is largely dependent on the work of the craft organization. Mutual adjustment is more common than supervision at this stage. Figure 14.1 represents the organizational structure of the craft stage of development.

Small private therapy practices in which the organization consists of therapists who share

responsibility for the work of the organization would be at the craft stage. Work coordination would occur because of such things as professional education, licensure, practice standards, policies, procedures, and protocols. Mutual accommodation would be sufficient to coordinate the work shared by the therapists and other staff. If a practice expands, additional partners and/or employees would be needed. Eventually, they will need to expand both the supervisory and support functions of the organization. When that occurs, the organization will move into the *entrepreneurial stage* of development.

The Entrepreneurial Stage

The entrepreneurial stage of organizational development is represented in Figure 14.2. At this stage, mutual accommodation can no longer be relied on to coordinate the work of the organization. Additional supervision and support is required to increase efficiency. Alternatively, it may place the organization at a disadvantage as management layers lead to greater separation between senior management, employees, and the customers. More management can translate into a longer (slower) decision-making cycle. Increased standardization can decrease flexibility. These changes have the potential to make an entrepreneurial organization less responsive in a rapidly changing environment than a craft stage organization. Chapter 22 addresses the concept of entreprenurism, which is a different topic from the entrepreneurial stage of a business.

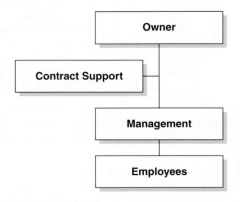

Figure 14.2. The entrepreneurial stage.

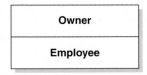

Figure 14.1. The craft stage.

The Bureaucratic Stage

As the entrepreneurial organization continues to grow, the demand for continued division of labor and a more complex work coordination system increases. At this point, the organization begins to move into the *bureaucratic stage*. Figures 14.3–14.5 illustrate various forms of the bureaucratic organizational structure. A bureaucracy is characterized by:

- A high degree of reliance on work standardization
- A large, complex management structure
- Distinct operating departments divided by specialization job specialists versus generalists
- Large technical and general support service functions

Bureaucratic organizations can be made efficient through high standardization and specialization and can be very successful in a stable environment. However, where the entrepreneurial organization is at risk from decreased flexibility, the bureaucratic organization would require even more effort to respond to environmental changes. Without special mechanisms in place (e.g., innovation teams or research and development centers), the lack of agility to respond to change, foster new ideas, and stay in touch with customers and employees could significantly interfere with the survival of a bureaucratic organization that finds itself in an unstable, hostile, and/or competitive market.

Recent and rapid changes in the health care industry have left many large health care organizations in exactly this dilemma. Having found success in a relatively unchanging, but growing market, bureaucratic health care organizations face continuous challenges in adapting to the new health care environment (MacStravic, 1986). Successful organizations are those that can adapt by developing a structure that can foster creativity to balance the impacts of growing bureaucracy (Land and Jarman, 1992).

An organization that continues to expand through **product diversification** and/or *market expansion* (Chapter 18) may move into the *divisional stage* (Fig. 14.4). This type of business expansion can be achieved through *vertical* or *horizontal integration* of the existing

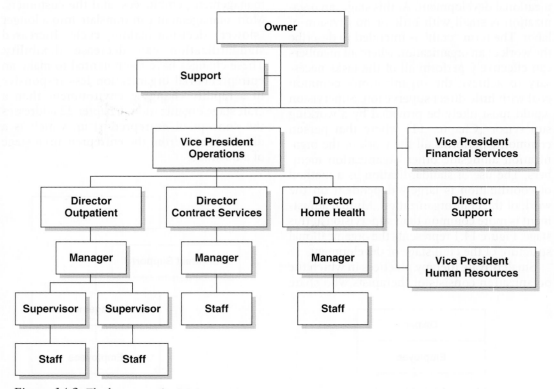

Figure 14.3. The bureaucratic stage.

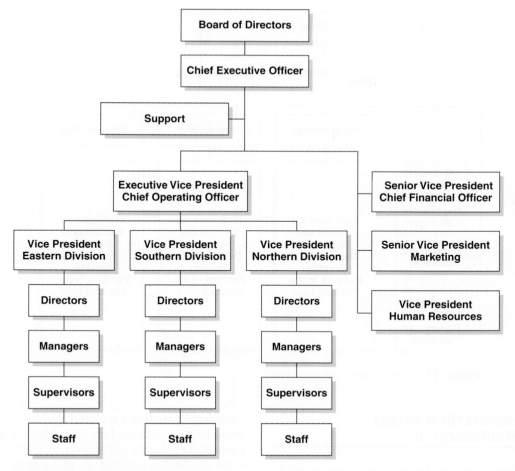

Figure 14.4. The divisional stage.

business with new or acquired businesses. On the other hand, a company might adopt a divisional structure due to a venture into a completely new line of business. The options for growth into a divisionalized structure involve vertical and horizontal integration.

Horizontal and Vertical Integration

Expansion of an organization's current business into new markets is called horizontal integration. A PT practice that acquires or develops additional PT practices to cover a larger geographical region is expanding to provide the same service to more customers. The addition of these similar business units is an example of horizontal expansion. Growth

in this manner would move the organization into a divisionalized structure.

Business expansion through product diversification, whether by broadening services to the same customer base or by adding a new customer base, is called vertical integration. A hospital that expands through the acquisition of a primary care physician practice, a long-term care facility, and a home care agency is expanding through vertical integration. Examples of environmental factors that may influence vertical or horizontal expansion include **demographic** trends, **third party** contracting and reimbursement, local economic trends, and the competitive environment. Organizations may have concurrent strategies for growth through both horizontal and vertical integration.

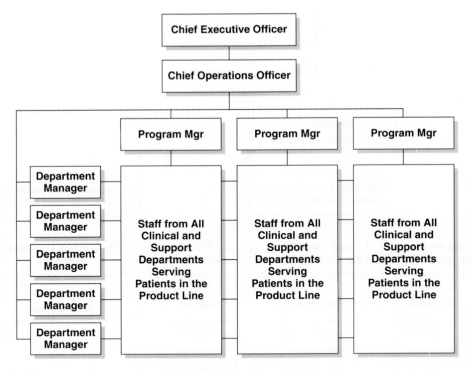

Figure 14.5. The adhocracy/matrix model.

Centralization Versus Decentralization

A key question for an organization at the divisional stage relates to the centralization or decentralization of responsibility and accountability for management and support functions. If decision making rests largely with management at the corporate (central) office or the BOD of a health care organization, the organization is **centralized**. Similarly, if support services are part of the corporate office and have authority over activities of other divisions, they would be described as centralized. To the extent that decision making and support functions are left to the divisions, the organization is **decentralized** (Longest et al., 2000). Full centralization or decentralization should be viewed as a continuum with most organizations resting somewhere between the extremes.

A centralized organization relies on supervision and standardization to coordinate the work between its divisions. Centralized standardization works well for **divisionalized** organizations whose success is tied to product

consistency, such as a regional health services provider or a national food franchise. In both cases, the customer will expect to receive the same quality of product at all locations. If, however, individual divisions must respond to local market demands or provide different products, centralization may decrease a division's flexibility and ability to respond to local market conditions. Performance could be impacted negatively.

Additional Operational Structural Models

In business, a product can be an idea, service, good, or a combination offered to a target market. The *product line model*, unlike the bureaucratic structure, is an operational structure that shuns work-specific operating units like a PT department. In this model, the preference is for product-based operating units rather than work-specific operating units (Litch, 2007). For example, a pain management program versus an occupational and PT department. Multiple approaches have been taken to product line structuring. One approach is to organize only a portion of the organization, such as the marketing department, along product lines. Alternatively, the entire organization may be aligned with specific products.

A hospital that maintains distinct centralized physical and occupational therapy departments, has managers for both departments with all therapists serving all patient types, would represent a work-specific department model. If the same hospital were to reorganize, assign physical and occupational therapy staff to distinct orthopedic, neurologic, and geriatric treatment teams, and eliminate the department management positions in favor of team supervisors, it would move toward a product line structure. A product line structure is more likely to use mutual adjustment than supervision as a method of work coordination. Standardization would still be used to coordinate work. Instead of department-based standards, however, you might see team care plans or other forms of product-specific standards of care.

The product line structure focuses the organization's attention outward toward the customer rather than inward toward specialized departments. Reasons that an organization might move to a product line model include multiple markets, diverse customers, or a large enough demand for a single product to commit dedicated resources. The use of a product line approach may attract additional customers in need of a specific product or set of products (Fottler and Repasky, 1988; MacStravic, 1986).

A **matrix model** is another operational structure (Fig. 14.5) that brings about centralization by function (Kaplan and Norton, 2006). This model provides an alternative to the traditional bureaucratic structure. A matrix structure is a hybrid between the traditional bureaucratic and the product line structure. It overlays a product line structure onto the department structure. The product line units and functional departments are organizationally equal. The matrix model allows an organization to respond to external factors while maintaining a high degree of internal efficiency. The work of a matrix health care organization is most efficient when it is coordinated through standardization and mutual accommodation with less reliance on supervision. The matrix model does create a dual system of responsibility and accountabil-

ity. Staff members working in a matrix structure are accountable to meet the expectations of both department and program management. This can become difficult should there be an adversarial relationship between the product manager and the functional (department) manager. Nonproductive conflict can be a difficult problem (Timm and Wanetik, 1983).

Reasons to Change Organizational Structure

In response to significant environmental pressures, health care organizations have undergone partial or total **reorganization** to improve the potential for continued success (Fottler and Repasky, 1988; Timm and Wanetik, 1983). Reorganization might be a way to improve business performance or change strategic direction. A fundamental change in an organization's purpose, vision, and/or strategic direction would be another reason for reorganization. Such a change often occurs when an organization is sold, changes its chief executive, or merges with another organization. Sometimes organizations change structure simply because reorganizing is a popular thing to do. Respected experts caution that even an imperfect but workable organizational structure is worth keeping because reorganization usually produces profound and often unpredictable organizational change (Drucker, 2006; Kaplan and Norton, 2006). A true reorganization entails an assessment (Chapter 11), and redesign of many organizational functions, such as:

- Division of work
- Employee relationships
- Employee skill needs
- Methods of work coordination
- Number and type of people employed
- Work group composition
- Work processes
- Work standards (policies, procedures, and protocols)

The planning required to implement a successful reorganization is significant. As a result, a poorly planned or implemented reorganization can hurt rather than help the organization (Roach, 1996). Reorganization should be undertaken to improve some aspect of organizational performance. However, performance problems that are significant enough to risk the initial disruption of reorganization are unlikely to be corrected by simply rearranging the structural elements of the organization. Reorganization should be one possible outcome of the strategic planning process (Chapter 13). It is not a goal to be achieved. Rather, it is tactical action plan to achieve a strategic business objective. For this reason, reorganization should be undertaken only after a comprehensive planning process has been completed.

Summary

Management has the responsibility for maximizing the performance of the organization. Organizational performance is influenced greatly by the organization of its parts into a defined organizational structure. The right organizational structure is essential for business success. Business structures have legal, tax, and operating structures that define an organization's function and form. Diverse internal and external factors influence the structure of a specific organization. Through a careful strategic planning process, management should look within and outside the organization at the factors that will impact the organization's success.

This information should be used to guide decisions about organizational structure and work design. Both should be dynamic, changing as the organization matures or changes its focus to meet internally and externally driven performance demands. Structure should be linked with and support the organization's service or product strategy. Structure includes the way that work is separated and coordinated within the organization. The dependence on supervision, standardization, and mutual accommodation will vary based on the structure of the organization. The organizational chart is the graphic representation of the organizational structure and can be used to understand supervisory relationships, official communication patterns, work flow, and even the flexibility of an organization.

In almost every chapter, it has been stated that management has the responsibility to make organizational decisions. Strategic management decisions are based on the analysis of internal and external variables. The next chapter will focus on analysis of relevant environmental variables and decision-making processes based on the analysis. The discussion includes the identification of key issues, ways to analyze them, and to formulate appropriate strategies to advance the organization.

CASE STUDY 14.1

It's Time to Change

Introduction

You are the manager in a not-for-profit community hospital that has a bureaucratic structure. You manage the PT department and treat patients when things get busy or someone is off. Over the past 3 years the department has grown from 5 to 31 employees. In addition to your position, the department has 12 staff physical and 6 occupational therapists, 5 physical therapist assistants, 3 certified occupational therapy assistants, 3 PT aides, and 2 receptionist/office personnel. The staff has evolved preferences regarding where they work most of the time: inpatient rehabilitation, acute inpatient, or outpatient. The three service settings provide 20%, 35%,

45% of the department's revenue, respectively. Mutual accommodation is the primary means of work coordination. Responsibility wise, everyone reports directly to you. While the staff like having this access, it has become overwhelming for you. You have to keep up on federal regulations that are different for each of the settings you manage. You have been serving on several institutional committees and are in line to become chairperson of one. In addition, you are enrolled in a distance learning MBA program.

You have made up your mind to establish one or more supervisory positions so you can delegate much of the direct clinical operation oversight. You need to flesh

(Continued)

CASE STUDY 14.1

It's Time to Change (continued)

out your reorganization plan to present to your manager for approval and later, to your staff.

Your Tasks

Answer the questions below and complete the indicated actions.

1. Why are you reorganizing?
2. What do you expect to accomplish?
3. How will the patients be better served/ how will value be increased?
4. What will the lines of communication be?
5. What structure will you choose?
6. What will the structure look like on paper (organizational chart)?

7. Hypothesize what changes will likely occur between staff members?
8. Hypothesize how staff members are likely to respond to the changes?
9. What are five concerns likely to be raised about the reorganization by your manager?
10. Formulate responses to these five concerns.
11. Once the above tasks are completed, discuss your work with a peer who has also completed the tasks. Question each other about your assumptions, concerns, chosen structure, and reactions of the stakeholders.
12. Based on peer discussion, incorporate changes to improve your plan.

REFERENCES

American Heritage Dictionary of the English Language, 4th ed. Boston, MA: Houghton Mifflin. 2003.

Brown M, McCool BP. Vertical integration: Exploration of a popular concept. Healthcare Management Review. 1986;11:7–19.

Burns T, Stalker GM. Management of innovation. London, England: Tavistock. 1961.

Drucker PF. What executives should remember. Harvard Business Review. 2006;84(2):144–152.

European Observatory on Health Services and Policies. HiT methodology and production processes. Available at http://www.euro.who.int/observatory/Hits/20020531_1. Accessed 12/06/07.

Foss K, Foss NJ, Klein PG. An entrepreneurial theory of economic organization. Organization Studies. 2007;28(12):1893–1912.

Fottler MD, Repasky LJ. Attitudes of hospital executives toward product line management: A pilot survey. Healthcare Management Review. 1988;13:15–22.

Goffee R, Jones G. What holds the modern company together? Harvard Business Review. November-December 1996;74(6):134–149.

Highet D. Innovation and Creativity versus Standards – Who is winning the battle in your company? Available at http://www.grizmo.com/management_news_200606.html. Accessed 11/08/07.

Kaplan RS, Norton DP. How to implement a new strategy without disrupting your organization. Harvard Business Review. 2006;84(3):100–109.

Kondo Y. Are creative ability and work standardization in contradictory relationship? Training for Quality. 1996;4:35–39.

Land G, Jarman B. Breakpoint and beyond: Mastering the future today. New York, NY: Harper/Collins. 1992.

Liedtka JM. Formulating hospital strategy: Moving beyond a market mentality. Healthcare Management Review. 1992;17:21–26.

Litch BK. The re-emergence of clinical service line management. Healthcare Executive. 2007;22:14–18.

Longest BB, Rakich JS, Darr K. Managing health services organizations and systems, 4th ed. Baltimore, MD: Health Professions. 2000.

MacMillan IC, Jones PE. Designing organizations to compete. Journal of Business Strategy. 1984;4:11–26.

MacStravic RS. Product-line administration in hospitals. Healthcare Management Review. 1986;11:35–43.

McConnell CR. Larger, smaller, and flatter: The evolution of the modern health care organization. The Health Care Manager. 2005;24:177–188.

Mintzberg H. The structuring of organizations. Englewood Cliffs, NJ: Prentice Hall. 1979.

Mintzberg H. Structure in fives: Designing effective organizations. Englewood Cliffs, NJ: Prentice Hall. 1983.

Mintzberg H, Quinn JB, Voyer J. The strategy process, Collegiate ed. Englewood Cliffs, NJ: Prentice Hall. 1995.

Palmer I, Benveniste J, Dunford R. New organizational forms: Towards a generative dialogue. Organization Studies. 2007;28(12):1829–1847.

Porter ME, Teisberg EO. Redefining health care: Creating value-based competition on results. Boston, MA: Harvard Business School. 2006.

Roach SS. The hollow ring of the productivity revival. Harvard Business Review. November–December 1996;74(6):81–89.

Schneller ES. Accountability for healthcare: A white paper on leadership and management for the U.S. healthcare system. Healthcare Management Review. 1997;22:38–48.

Timm MM, Wanetik MG. Matrix organization: Design and development for a hospital organization. Hospital Health Service Administration. November/December 1983;46–58.

Woodward J. Industrial organization: Theory and practice. Oxford, England: Oxford. 1965.

Worley CG, Lawler EE III. Designing organizations that are built to change. MIT Sloan Management Review. 2006;48(1):19–23.

Zoltners A, Sinha P, Lorimer SE. Match your sales force structure to your business life cycle. Harvard Business Review. 2006;84(7/8):81–89.

ADDITIONAL RESOURCES

A free trial of organizational chart templates is available from HumanConcepts at http://www.orgplus.com/products/orgplus-professional/index.htm?_kk=organizational%20chart&kt=e1771869-4397-42a9-aaba-361d904d12fe&gclid=CPnxv7y3nJACFVB1OAodhwQg8Q and Smart Draw at http://www.smartdraw.com/specials/context/Orgchart.htm?id=139815.

Four books that expand the discussion on organizational structure with more perspectives on the topic are:

Aldrich HE. Organizations evolving. Thousand Oaks, CA: Sage. 1999. This author provides an analysis of the key variables that affect contemporary organizations which include new knowledge and entrepreneurship.

Burton RM, DeSanctis G, Obel B. Organizational design: A step by step approach. Cambridge, England: Cambridge University Press. 2006.

Robbins SP, Coulter M. Management. Upper Saddle River, NJ: Prentice Hall. 2002. Chapter 10 is titled organizational structure and design. The information deepens the discussion in a complimentary manner to the introduction to this chapter.

Stroh LK, Northcraft GB, Neale MA. Organizational behavior: A management challenge. Mahwah, NJ: Lawrence Erlbaum. 2002. The authors nicely discuss managing individuals and groups, performance management, managing change and of course, organizational structure and design.

On the topic of organizational reorganization, Andersen challenges the connection between organizational function and form (Andersen JA. Organizational design: Two lessons to learn before reorganizing. International Journal of Organization Theory and Behavior. 2002;5:343–358). The concept of the evolution of organizations is the focus of an article by Djiksterhuis et al. Where do organizational forms come from? Management logics as a source of coevolution. Organizational Science. 1999;10:569–582. The breath of structural changes related to a successful example of mutual accommodation in a hospital oncology unit is discussed in: Buchanan DA, et al. Nobody in charge: Distributed change agency in healthcare. Human Relations. 2007;60(7):1065–1090.

CHAPTER 15

Management and Decision Making

DEBORAH G. FRIBERG

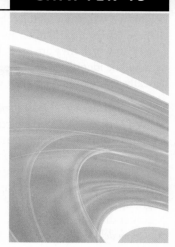

Learning Objectives

1. Give examples of the relationship between situational analysis, performance management methodology, performance management tools, and business success.
2. Demonstrate familiarity with a variety of management tools used in business for situational analysis, process improvement, and process design.
3. Be able to match the management tools used to improve organizational performance or design new business processes to selected business situations.
4. Appreciate the impact of an organization's approach to performance improvement or new business design on its managers and staff members.
5. Given a performance improvement or process design scenario, apply the concepts presented in this chapter to achieve the best outcome.

Introduction

In Chapters 2–6 readers learned why it is important to understand the internal and external environmental factors that can shape an organization and influence its success. In Chapters 7–10, the importance of ethical conduct and compliance with legal and external oversight requirements of business performance was reviewed. Chapters 11–14 addressed the role of management to lead, communicate, plan,

and organize to accommodate all the environmental factors in addition to the professional and legal requirements impacting their organizations. We are now at the point where the plan is set and the goals and overall performance outcomes are defined. The point where management needs to make things happen. However, managers must first understand that *business success is not measured in terms of how many things management does to reach a goal. Rather, a manager's effectiveness is measured by how well the goal is achieved.* In this chapter, the focus will be on providing managers with information about approaches, methods, and tools that can be used to analyze their current situation and make effective decisions.

What does management need to make the right decisions for their organization? Management's job is to direct organizational activities from the global plans to the details of performance, all to produce the best possible outcomes. Having support to make decisions is important whether looking at a new activity or current operations. Decisions support tools can help managers to

- Perform situational analysis—understand what is really happening
- Error proof processes—avoid mistakes
- Correct current process errors—avoid rework
- Improve process efficiency—reduce cost
- Improve process effectiveness—improve outcomes
- Engage process stakeholders—enhance employee commitment

Key terms, which are defined below, are bolded and italicized the first time they appear in the chapter. Other important terms are shown in boldface on first appearance and are defined by the context in which they are used. When either of these types of terms is used several times, its acronym will be identified and subsequently used in the chapter. Both types of terms are listed alphabetically in the online glossary with their definitions and (when applicable) their acronyms.

business intelligence (BI) systems: software tools designed to analyze detailed business data to guide decisions. Business intelligence software is sometimes called decision support software.

cause analysis tools: tools to support management decision making such as cause and effect diagrams (Ishikawa diagrams), Pareto charts, and scatter diagrams.

change model: a Bourgeois and Brodwin's strategic planning model where upper management's style is to include multiple level managers in the process.

collaborative model: group oriented planning using techniques like brainstorming used by management to broaden thinking.

commander model: management style characterized by top-down thinking dominated by the CEO.

crescive model: (derived from the Latin term meaning "to grow") management style somewhat the opposite of the Commander model as this is a bottom-up approach that includes input from the direct service/clinical providers of the organization.

cultural model: management style that is collaborative and seeks input from all levels of the organization.

decision matrix: a situational evaluation tool used to narrow a group of choices to the best one, or to evaluate performance. A matrix facilitates evaluation and prioritizing numerous options.

decision support tools: aids to help make data driven decisions about what, when, where, and how work is performed to produce the best outcomes for the customer and their business. Example tools are software for data gathering and analysis, creativity stimulating activities, and management planning strategies.

idea creation: group development of new ideas, or organizing multiple ideas using tools like: affinity diagrams, benchmarking, brainstorming, and nominal group techniques.

innovation: two types of change actions. The first is improving, expanding, or extending something that is already being done (incremental innovation). The second is the creation of a significantly new implemental concept (breakthrough innovation). Innovation is a way to leverage an organization's assets to yield improved outcomes.

process analysis: objective examination of existing processes to evaluate how effective and efficient the processes are in meeting their objectives.

project planning: management tools associated with the oversight of new design or improvement projects and include Gantt charts and multistep improvement models such as Plan–Do–Check–Act cycle (PDCA).

quality improvement (QI): a management engineering concept for continuously improving health care delivery.

situational evaluation tools: used to narrow a group of choices to the best one, or to evaluate performance. Tool examples are a decision matrix and multivoting.

Six Sigma: six sigma refers to the standard deviations either side of the mean. Practically, it is a data-driven approach to reduce defects in a process or reduce production costs. It can also mean an organizational philosophy where operations are defined, in part, by fact-based information. As a methodology for improvement, it can be summarized by the mnemonic DMAIC (Define–Measure–Analyze–Improve–Control).

total quality management (TQM): statistically based measures are used to identify and minimize product variability in the manufacturing sector. It is an organization's system of planning and controlling all business functions so that services/products are delivered/produced that meet or exceed customer expectations.

Toyota production system/lean management: the goals of lean production are to get things related to production right the first time. This means that the right things have to be in the right place at the right time, the first time, while minimizing waste and being open to change.

- Set performance expectations—realistic targets
- Measure outcomes—validate performance
- Communicate—alignment and organizational commitment

Overall, decisions support tools can help make data-driven decisions about what, when, where, and how work is performed to produce the best outcomes for both their business and the customer. Once the "what, when, where and how" decisions are made, management will be in a position to effectively establish the plan of work, assign roles and responsibilities, and ultimately coordinate assignments between individuals. Management will also be positioned to communicate individual employee performance expectations, designing their work including training requirements, job duties, responsibilities, and interactions. They will also be in position to measure the effectiveness of the decisions that they have made.

As we consider the topic of decision making there are three areas of focus:

1. Methodology
2. Tools
3. Information

Methodology refers to how management will approach the decision-making process. When related to new activity, these activities are often referred to using terms such as **project management**, **operational planning**, or **business planning**. When related to current operations, decision-making activities are often referred to as **performance management or quality improvement or performance improvement** (see Chapter 16). In all cases, these activities refer to the management's efforts to understand the current situation and determine the best course of action. In Chapter 13, the approaches to planning and strategic decision making were discussed in some detail. We will detail several methodologies that a business can adopt to organize their project management and performance improvement efforts later in this chapter.

Tools are available aids to help managers with **cause and effect analysis**, **situational evaluation**, **process analysis**, quality improvement, data collection, idea creation, project planning and implementation, and innovation.

Regardless of structure, information will be needed to guide the decision-making process.

The quality and availability of information is a critical element for any business in its quest for success.

Terminology Used in Relation to Analysis for Decision Support

The terminology used to describe organizational efforts related to improving the performance of current operations or designing new operations encompasses a broad range of activities and is used interchangeably throughout the industry and the literature. The meaning of specific terms changes from one source to the other and one organization to another. While this section provides the reader with some common definitions it will soon be clear that the distinctions are often vague. For that reason, the common meaning of these terms is generally less important to a manager than the meaning of terms as they are used within that manager's own organization.

Some terms commonly used in relationship to performance analysis to support management decision making include:

Business Intelligence (BI): BI is a broad category of applications and technologies for gathering, storing, analyzing, and providing access to data to help enterprising users make better business decisions. BI applications include the activities of decision support systems (DSS), query and reporting, **online analytical processing (OLAP)**, statistical analysis, forecasting, and **data mining** (Ramki, 2009).

Data Mining: A "class of database applications that look for hidden patterns in data that can be used to predict future behavior" (Webopedia, 2008).

Decision Support Systems (DSS): DSSs are "any computer application that enhances a person or group's ability to make decisions." (Decision Support Systems Resources, 2009). They are "interactive, computer-based systems that aid users in judgment and choice activities" (Druzdzel and Flynn, 2008a, p. 1).

Online Analytical Processing (OLAP): A "category of software tools that provides analysis of data stored in a database. OLAP tools enable users to analyze different dimensions of multidimensional data. For example, it provides time series and trend analysis views. OLAP often is used in data mining" (Webopedia, 2007).

Performance Improvement (PI): Refers to the methodology used to improve performance of organizations and individuals within those organizations. PI is data driven, emphasizes human performance factors, and starts with a **root cause analysis** (Bornstein, 2001). A root cause analysis is "a technique used to identify the conditions that initiate the occurrence of an undesired activity or state" (GAO, 2007).

Performance Management (PM): A defined process for management by which an organization involves its employees, as individuals and members of a group, in improving organizational effectiveness toward the accomplishment of its mission and goals (Department of Commerce, 2007).

Quality Improvement (QI): Refers to use of data driven methodologies to define and close the gap between the current and expected performance outcomes using performance management to address system deficiencies that, according to Bornstein (2001), generates a broader range of interventions than PI. It emphasizes processes and takes a more flexible approach to situational analysis using tools such as **Ishikawa's fishbone diagram** (Bornstein (2001) called this because of its shape. The Ishikawa's fishbone diagram, developed by Kaoru Ishikawa, a Japanese quality control statistician, is also referred to as the "cause and effect" diagram (Office of Organizational Excellence, 2008). It is a problem analysis tool. Other specific analysis tools and their applications will be described in more detail later in this chapter and in Chapter 16, which deals with health care performance improvement initiatives of public and private agencies.

Quality Management (QM): The "use of a program to ensure the production of high-quality products" (BNet, 2008a).

Total Quality Management (TQM): Refers to an organization's system of planning and controlling all business functions so that products or services are produced which meet or exceed customer expectations. TQM is a philosophy of business behavior, embracing principles such as employee involvement, continuous improvement at all levels, and customer focus (BNet, 2008b).

Methodology

Management's choice of methodology or approach to decision making is guided by many organizational and management characteristics. Two elements of greatest impact are the organization's culture and management style. Both can have a great influence on an organization's willingness to change.

Culture is the term used to describe the patterns of social interaction that define the norm within the organization (Goffee and Gareth, 1996). It reflects an organization's values in practice (Chapter 7). Goffee and Gareth (1996) describe two types of human relations: **sociability** and **solidarity**. Sociability measures the true friendliness between employees. Solidarity is a measure of an organization's ability to pursue shared objectives quickly and effectively. The higher the sociability and solidarity, the more likely organization members can effectively implement change in the pursuit of common goals.

Management style and top-down commitment to change are essential to the success of any change methodology adopted by the organization. The type of methodology should be compatible with the leader's comfort with engagement of others both inside and outside the organization. As discussed in Chapter 3, Bourgeois and Brodwin (1984) describe five strategic planning models that are defined by the role the Chief Executive Officer (CEO) plays and/or the extent of involvement of others within the strategic planning process. This extends to the implementation phase of the planning cycle. These models include:

1. *Commander model*: characterized by top-down thinking dominated by CEOs.
2. *Change model*: behavioral science oriented. Multiple levels of managers engaged in the process.
3. *Collaborative model*: group-oriented. Techniques such as brainstorming used to broaden thinking.

These three models limit input from front-line workers. This often results in limited success, making implementation difficult.

4. *Cultural model*: this is the collaborative model plus. Input sought from all levels of the organization.
5. *Crescive* or *Grow model*: somewhat the opposite of the Commander model. A bottom-up approach that includes input from the direct service/clinical providers of the organization.

Both the cultural and crescive models require more planning effort but they are more effective during implementation.

To effectively select a method (a system) and tools (aids) for decision making the American Hospital Association Quality Center (Hospitals and Health Networks, 2007) recommends that management should also know the answer to four basic questions:

1. Rate of process variability
2. Rate of waste
3. Types of defects or errors
4. Rate of organizational variability

With this information in hand, management can best assess which methodologies will be the most effective. Many methodologies have gained a following in health care (iSix Sigma, 2007). The major four systematic methods are the **Malcolm Baldrige National Quality Criteria, ISO 9000,** *Six Sigma*, and *Toyota Production System/Lean Management*. Table 15.1 summarizes the key characteristics of these four decision-making methodologies used by health care organizations.

Table 15.1 Common Decision-Making Methodologies for Health Care Organizations

Fundamentals	Methods			
	Malcolm Baldrige National Quality Criteria	**Six Sigma**	**Lean**	**ISO 9000**
Origin	The Malcolm Baldrige Quality Award created in 1987 by U.S. National Institute of Standards and Technology. Awards are given in six categories including health care.	Developed by Motorola in the 1980s	Toyota Production Systems post WWII	Published in 1987 by the International Organization for Standardization, ISO 900 standards are used to guide quality improvement.
Premise	Outcomes driven performance management system with a basis in data, analysis, and knowledge. Baldrige criteria provide a framework with performance requirements to guide the structure and relationships of all organizational activities.	Data driven quality improvement methodology designed to minimize process variation.	Improvement of quality and efficiency through waste reduction from: Defects Excess motion Processing Overproduction Transporting Excess inventory Wait times	Provides a framework for organizations to fulfill customer specified quality requirements, meet regulatory requirements, and continuously improve processes.
Components	Leadership Strategic planning Patient, customer, and market Focus Measurement, analysis and knowledge Workforce focus Process management Results	Define Measure Analyze Improve Control	Flow charting Elimination of non-value added steps Allows any employee to fix a defect as it occurs	Customer focus Leadership Involvement of people Process approach Systems approach Continual improvement Data driven Mutually beneficial relationships

(Continued)

Table 15.1 continued			
Fundamentals	*Methods*		
Benefits	Management commitment Inclusive of all staff Customer driven Data driven Alignment Compatible with other methods (e.g., Six Sigma).	Decrease variation Reduce errors Improve processes Reduce costs	Quick identification and improvement of processes Reduced cost Improved flow Improved quality Improved productivity	Systematic approach Data driven Alignment Communication Constant improvement
Challenges	Resource intensive Major cultural change Extensive monitoring Long implementation	Resource intensive Significant investment Long cycle times	Worker engagement Leadership engagement Short cycle times	Time consuming High standardization Extensive training
Applications	Structure for oversight of overall organizational performance	All types of processes	All types of processes	Structure for oversight of overall organizational performance
Reference	Baldrige National Quality Program www.quality.nist.gov	Six Sigma. Available at http://main.isixsigma.com.	Going Lean in Health Care. Institute for Health care Improvement at www.ihi.org.	ISO Standards. International Organization for Standardization at www.iso.org.

Source: Hospitals and Health Networks, 2007.

Tools

Tools are available to support management decision-making efforts. According to the American Society for Quality (2008) and Sahni (2009), some of the most common tools and their uses include:

Cause analysis tools: used to determine the cause of a problem. Tools in this category include **cause and effect diagrams**, **Pareto charts**, and **scatter diagrams**.

Situational evaluation tools: used to narrow a group of choices to the best one, or to evaluate performance. Tool examples are a *decision matrix* and **multivoting**.

Process analysis: used to understand (or design) all or part of a work process. Included tools are: **flow charts, failure modes and effects analysis (FMEA)**, and **mistake (error) proofing**.

Quality improvement: seven tools that are commonly associated with improving quality are cause-and-effect diagrams, **check sheets, control charts, histograms**, Pareto charts, scatter diagrams, and **stratification**.

Data collection: most of the tools mentioned are associated with the collection and use of data: check sheet, control chart, **design of experiments**, **histogram**, scatter diagram, stratification, and **survey**.

Idea creation: to develop new ideas, or organize multiple ideas includes tools like: **affinity diagrams, benchmarking, brainstorming**, and **nominal group techniques**.

Project planning and implementation: tools associated with the management of new design or improvement projects include **Gantt charts** and multistep improvement models such as **Plan–Do–Check–Act** cycle **(PDCA)**.

Innovation: tools to encourage innovation include **collaboratives** (Chapter 16), **innovation teams**, and **networking** (Chapter 12).

It is evident that several of the commonly used tools have applicability in more that one category of efforts. In alphabetical order, a brief description of each tool is as follows:

- Affinity diagram: Allows large number of ideas to be organized by their natural relationships.
- Benchmarking: Use of comparative data to compare the performance or work practices of one business to other simi-

lar businesses or a "best" practice. This allows a business to identify opportunities for improvement.

- Brainstorming: A method for generating multiple ideas on a focused topic.
- Check sheet: Any prepared form that can be used to manually collect data. This tool varies in form and content and is customized for the collected information. The check sheet design may assist with data analysis or data collected may be entered into a more automated system.
- Collaboratives: A form of networking that refers to multiple groups with different experiences coming together to work on common goals or problems. The groups could be from different areas of the same business or different businesses (Chapter 16).
- Control charts: Give a longitudinal view of performance measures. They can be used to visualize how process measures change over time. Control limits (deviation standards in standard deviations from the mean) are used to demonstrate whether process variation is consistent (insider control lines) or unpredictable (outside control lines).
- Decision matrix: Used to evaluate and prioritize options. Can also be used to evaluate the importance of one option as compared to all other options. It involves the evaluation of each option against a list of pre-weighted criteria to come up with a ranking for each option. If multiple stakeholders do weighing independently, it can also be an effective method for gathering input from multiple perspectives.
- Design of experiments: A series of experiments that begins with a great many variables and through the series narrows the focus to the few critical variables.
- Failure modes and effects analysis (FMEA): An approach for identifying all potential points of failure in a design, current service, or product before they occur. The process often starts with flow charting to identify potential points of failure. Once potential points of failure are identified, it uses a decision matrix to rank the risk of each potential failure so the business can reduce or eliminate the potential failures in order of priority.
- Fishbone (Ishikawa) diagram: A tool for organizing possible causal factors into categories. It takes the visual structure of a fish bone. It is often used to document the results of a cause–effect brainstorming effort (see Fig. 15.1).
- Flow chart: A graphic representation of the steps of all or part of a process using different shapes to represent inputs and outputs, decision points, and people involved. It may include cycle times for each step and/or other process measures. It is a good way to identify true process variation or discrepancies in the understanding of a process between workers.
- Gantt chart: A horizontal bar chart that lists in detail the tasks of a project charted against time. The bars show when each task must start and stop relative to all other tasks and its current status.
- Histogram: Graphic representation of frequency distributions.
- Innovation teams: Groups of people within a business who are charged with the development of creative new ideas.
- Mistake-proofing: The use of any method that makes it impossible for an error to occur or to occur without being noticed.
- Multivoting: Used by groups to narrow focus from many to a few options. Can result in a favored option that is not the top choice of all to rise to the top. Can be used for consensus building.
- Networking: Putting together people with varied expertise, responsibility, and experiences to foster the development of new ideas.
- Nominal group technique: Group brainstorming activity to encourage contributions from all members
- Plan–Do–Check–Act Cycle (PDCA): A four-step model for carrying out change. *Plan* is the assessment and idea phase. *Do* is the pilot phase. *Check* is examination of the results phase to determine what went right and wrong. *Act* is the full implementation phase of a change initiative: adopt, abandon, redo.
- Pareto chart: Uses a bar graph to display the variable impact of when multiple causes contribute to the same effect.
- Scatter diagram: A graph of pairs of numerical data, one variable on each axis, to help assess the relationship between those variables.

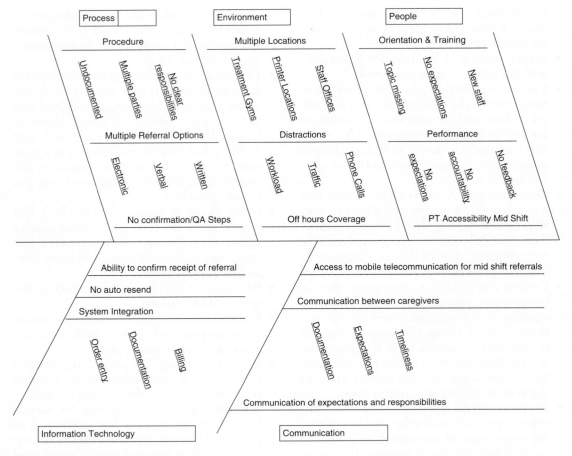

Figure 15.1. A Fishbone diagram.

- Stratification: Allows for the separation of data elements gathered from multiple sources to reveal patterns that might otherwise go unnoticed, for example, patients under 65 years of age.
- Survey: Data collected from specific groups of people (e.g., physical therapy outpatients) to obtain information about their opinions, behavior, or knowledge.

See Additional Resources section for more sources of information on these tools.

Information and Decision Support

Management's challenge is to make the right decisions at the right time to produce the best possible performance outcomes. We often think about decisions in terms of actions taken. Doing nothing, whether by design or default, is in fact a decision. At its simplest, decision

making is a process of selecting between alternatives. In their discussion of DSS, Druzdzel and Flynn (2008b) suggest that a more sophisticated view of decision making involves the search for alternative solutions when presented with a specific process. The most proactive view of management decision making is the process of searching for situations where decisions can or should be made. Druzdzel and Flynn recognize that as situational complexity and number of variables increases, the ability to evaluate and predict the outcome of alternative decisions might exceed human cognitive abilities. As a result, endeavors to develop *decision support tools* have been ongoing as seen from modeling tools developed by the fields of economics, statistics, operations research, and decision theory. They define DSS, otherwise known as knowledge-based systems, as systems that support decision making through:

- Financial analysis
- Modeling
- Reliability testing
- Statistical analysis
- Simulation

DSS is computer-based and can organize information, making it amenable to mechanized reasoning. DSS can be organization-wide or business unit-specific. It can be focused, like clinical DSS, financial DSS, or weather decision support (Hall, 2008). While such sophisticated DSS may seem inaccessible to all but the savviest user, anyone who has accessed Weather.com or the local traffic channel has used an automated DSS.

A barrier to the implementation of automated DSS is cost. Automated DSS requires

- IT applications to automate source data
- IT applications to integrate source data or pull data from disparate databases
- Personnel to manage the IT applications
- Personnel to manage the DSS system

The need for these resources may prevent small or financially marginal organizations from investing the resources needed to provide management with an automated DSS.

Options do exist that may not be as time efficient or powerful as automated systems but are generally available, can be run on a personal computer, and require moderate training to be used in the decision-making process. These include:

- Bubble forms
- Decision matrix
- Data collection forms
- Decision algorithms
- Graphing programs
- Spreadsheets

Using Decisions Support Tools

Decisions support tools may be used alone or in combination. The availability of automated data is helpful but not essential to the use of many of these tools. The following are scenarios that are designed to create an understanding of how these tools might be used in various health care delivery settings.

Scenario One

Situation

On 15 occasions in the past 45 days, a referral for physical therapy for a hospital inpatient was "missed." Despite good staffing ration, many more referrals have experienced delayed response times. While the missed referrals represent less than 2% of total referrals, the manager believes there should be zero tolerance for these types of errors. The reasons for the errors have been variable. Despite the department manager's ongoing feedback and direction to staff, this error continues to occur. Just when it seems to be fixed, another referral is missed. The impacts of this error are significant including delayed treatment ranging from 1 to 3 days, extended length of stay, patient and physician dissatisfaction, and additional cost to the organization.

An improvement team made up of department staff has been formed to determine why this error keeps happening and to make the changes needed to prevent its recurrence.

The Performance Improvement Process

The team meets to clarify their charge, agree on a goal, review their membership to make sure that all of the positions in the department that have a role in the patient referral intake process have been included on the team, and to decide how to proceed. An inpatient nursing unit secretary is invited to join the team. The group will use a four-step *PDCA model* to approach the problem. The first phase is *Plan*. In this phase, the group will analyze the problem and develop one or more alternatives to solving the problem of missed referrals.

To start their analysis the group performs a *cause and effect analysis* using a *fishbone diagram* to organize the outcome of their work. To get started, the team engages in a *brainstorming session* to identify possible causal categories. They use a *nominal group technique* to encourage equal participation in the process regardless of rank in the organization. In the nominal group technique, each team member writes down a specified number of potential reasons for missed referrals. The group then takes turns sharing their potential reasons one reason at a time. These are recorded and the process continues until all the reasons have been shared. Generic categories that help the group get started include methods, equipment, people, materials, measurement, and the environment (Tague, 2004). The group works together to assign each potential reason to a causal category. The fishbone diagram as demonstrated in Figure 15.1 helps the team organize its thinking and provides a pictorial representation of the group's work. The fishbone diagram is a great tool for documenting the situation and communicating to interested parties outside of the team.

The next step for the team is to develop a *flow chart* for the referral intake process. The flow chart will document all the steps of the current process. The team will use the flow chart to identify process variation, points for potential errors, people involved as well as process cycle times. A flow chart is a good way to identify discrepancies in the understanding of a process between workers.

The first step in developing a flow chart is to agree on the meaning of the symbols that will be used. Tague (2004) suggests the common flow charting symbols shown in Figure 15.2. Because delay times are a part of the problem, the team also used a *check sheet* to track and record cycle times for referral over a two-week

period. Using a sound sampling methodology, they were able to determine the time ranges for the steps and total referral intake cycle.

Figure 15.3 depicts a high-level flow for PT referral intake from referral to scheduling and corresponding cycle times. It identifies

1. Major process steps
2. Responsible parties
3. Variation where it is recognized
4. Steps were delays might occur
5. Steps where the team believes that the process might fail (gray)
6. Cycle time ranges at key steps and for the full process

Now that the team has a better understanding of the process, it is time to identify opportunities of improvement. Do is the pilot phase. By focusing on steps with the greatest opportunity to avoid "misses" and delays, the team can begin to test the impact of process changes. Obvious opportunities would be the standardization of referral input, integration of the order entry and PT scheduling systems, and centralized scheduling. Being able to reach the PTs during the day would also be helpful.

Check is the results checking phase to determine if the changes being tested have

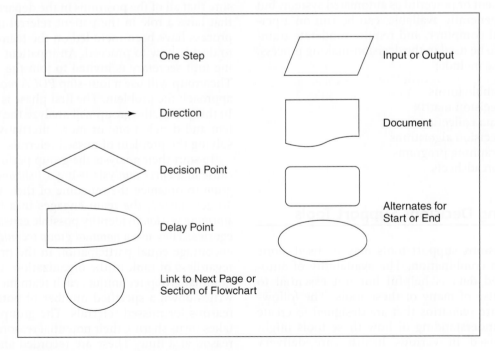

Figure 15.2. Common flow chart symbols.

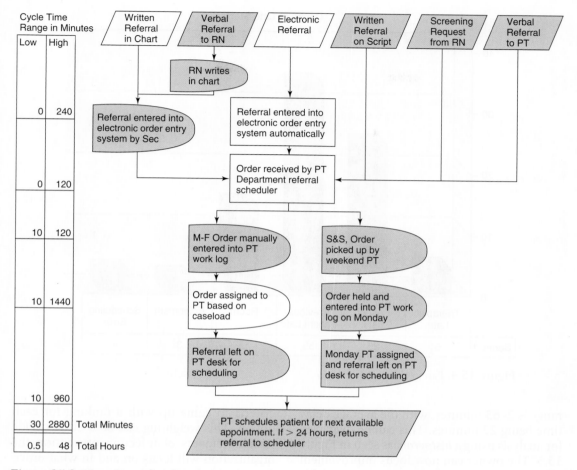

Figure 15.3. Flow chart referral intake process.

produced the desired results. The team will know by monitoring performance—in this case, the number of delayed or missed referrals. Act is the full implementation phase of a change initiative that has proven successful during the check phase.

Scenario Two

Situation

The owner/manger of a private PT practice has just completed a *survey* of patients to determine their level of satisfaction with her therapy experience. The leading complaint is "delayed start times." A quick review of the employee time sheets indicates that the majority of overtime pay is related to end of day appointments running over their scheduled end times. Given the impact on customer satisfaction and expense, the owner decides to dig deeper.

The Performance Improvement Process

Using a *check sheet* the practice owner collects information on late starts and related causes. The check sheet also collects information on late start appointment characteristics including

- Patient
- Therapist
- Scheduled start
- Scheduled end
- Scheduled length
- Actual start
- Actual end
- Actual length
- Reason for late start

Analysis of the data collected demonstrates that 35% of all appointments start 5 minutes or more after the scheduled start time. Using a *Pareto chart* (Fig. 15.4), the owner is able to rank the cause of delays by the impact. The

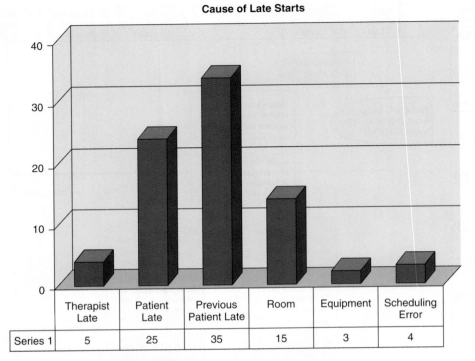

Figure 15.4. Pareto chart.

range is 2–65 minutes, with the average delay time being 22 minutes. This can be displayed for analysis using a *histogram* as seen in Figure 15.5. The owner can now focus improvement efforts on the causes that are most controllable or result in the longest delays.

Scenario Three

Situation

The risk of a health care-acquired infection is a major problems for patients. Avoidable infections are a leading cause of complications in patients and of waste in the health care system.

The Performance Improvement Process

Avoiding infections requires complex, multi-dimensional solutions. Avoiding infections is a problem that can be solved by tools such as an *FMEA*. Here potential process failures (e.g., failure to follow a hygienic hand-washing policy), and the related risk of spreading infections can be compared and prioritized using a *decision matrix*. A decision matrix compares each potential failure against a list of preweighted criteria to come up with a ranking for each option. This weighting can be used to decide which elements of infection prevention the organization will focus on and in what order. Criteria for an infection-prevention matrix might include ease of implementation, cost of implementation, likelihood of preventing infection, and number of patients impacted. The selection of performance improvement opportunities can be guided by *benchmarking* against other comparable organizations. Using industry benchmarks for hospital acquired infection rates would help an organization determine if they are outside the norm for best practice. If they are, that performance parameter is a good focus for improvement. Another way to address complex problems is through participation in *collaboratives*. This would involve *networking* between teams from multiple organizations who join together to share their different experiences and success related interventions to work on common goals or problems. The teams could be from different areas of the same business or different businesses.

All of these DSS tools have applicability in a variety of settings and situations. They can benefit the small practice owner as well as the

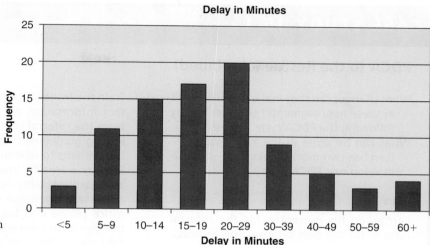

Figure 15.5. Histogram of delayed starts.

manager of rehabilitation services in a large multisite health care system. See Additional Resources section for more applications.

Summary

To successfully lead their organizations through times of change, managers need to have an appreciation for and knowledge of situational analysis, performance management, new process design, and business operations. Making the best use of the organization's information is a key element of maximizing performance. The knowledge needed to match the method and management tools used to the business situation will help managers make the best use of the resources of the organization and produce the best outcomes. The tools discussed in this chapter can help produce improvements in multiple operations from direct service delivery to payment. They can also inform strategic planning initiatives for developing and sustaining a competitive advantage.

There are additional free and proprietary tools for measuring and improving health care quality and a large number of agencies dedicated to quality/performance improvement. These tools and agencies are the core topics presented in Chapter 16.

CASE STUDY 15.1

PDCA to the Rescue

Background

Len Ahand is a final year physical therapy student. He is shadowing a preceptor in a physical therapy clinic located in a building owned by a family practice group. The group occupies three quarters of the building. At a recent staff meeting, Len listened as the five PTs complained about what they considered the low volume of patients that were being referred to them by the physician group from whom they rent their clinic space. Len asked his preceptor if he might look into this matter.

He remembered being exposed to the PDCA methodology and thought this might be an appropriate situation to apply it. Later, he went online (http://www.dartmouth.edu/~ogehome/CQI/PDCA.html) to refresh his memory. He made some notes:

What are they trying to accomplish? (Gain more referrals.)

How will they know that a change in volume is an improvement? (Increases in the number of referrals and revenue are the markers.)

(Continued)

CASE STUDY 15.1

PDCA to the Rescue (continued)

What changes can they make that will result in these improvements? (Answer this by following the PDCA cycle process.)

What can be done in the time available? (Len has two more weeks here—time to develop one PDCA cycle.)

Plan

Len asked his preceptor for the referral records for the past quarter. This included several types of patient referrals:

Patients who were treated

Patients who scheduled a visit, but did not keep it

Referrals that were phoned in or faxed, but the patients never scheduled a visit

Len used Excel® to organize the data. After entering the various types of referrals by medical specialty, Len found that 75% of the referrals came from orthopedists whose offices were around the PT clinic location. Fifteen percent of the referred patients were never scheduled or treated. Most of the referrals were for patients with low back and knee problems and most were issued on Mondays and Fridays. The smaller percentage of the referrals made by the family practice group most frequently were for patients with ankle sprains, low back or neck pain, and dizziness/loss of balance. The majority of the family practice referrals were written on Tuesdays and Thursdays. Len also noted that of all referrals received, 25% were phone or fax referrals that came in when the PT office was closed, after 5 PM or on weekends. He further found that referred patients often delayed scheduling an appointment until a week or more after the referral was issued. Len presented this information as graphs to his preceptor. Together they concluded that the practice might benefit from a change in its hours of operation and how they handled phone and referrals. The plan had five parts:

1. Have therapists stagger their starting times and rotate on Saturdays.

2. Train the front office staff to gather contact information on referred patients from the referral source, and then, following guidelines, make timely calls to the patients to schedule appointments.

3. Employ a Health Insurance Portability and Accountability Act (HIPAA) compliant answering service to receive off hour office phone and fax calls and contact the therapists who are starting early the next day so they can schedule visits in a timely fashion.

4. Initiate a marketing campaign targeting past referral sources to announce the extended hours and 24-hour scheduling service.

5. Hire Len to enter follow up data to complete the first PDCA cycle.

Do

The therapists met under the leadership of Len's preceptor. The therapists developed a 4-day week, 12 hours a day, week day schedule and split 3-hour shifts on Saturdays with therapists rotating weekly. A half-day training session was developed and held for the three office staff members who usually answer the phone. An in-Person answering service was contracted. A new trifold color flyer was produced and delivered in person to the targeted physicians' offices. The flyer identified the extended hours, rapid scheduling, and a summary of example programs for the low back, neck, knee, ankle, and balance problems. It was decided that the data would be collected for 2 months to determine the effect of the program on referral numbers and revenue.

Check

The therapy practice members were interested in changes in the number and type of referrals, as well as financial productivity. After 2 months of implementing the plan data was compared with those of the previous 6 months and the same 2 months of the previous year. The changes were:

(Continued)

CASE STUDY 15.1

PDCA to the Rescue (continued)

1. The number of orthopedic referrals was unchanged. However, the percentage of referred patients who did make and kept their appointments increased 15%.
2. The number of family practice referrals increased 10%. A quarter of the increase came from one physician who referred patients with balance difficulties. The increase in referrals from the remaining physicians was meager. The percentage of patients for whom phone or fax referrals were received who were scheduled and treated increased 10%.

By decreasing the referral to first treatment delay, responding quicker to phone and fax referrals, staying open longer, and treating more patients the practice profit was up 7% compared to the previous 6 months, and up 8% above the same time span last year. Further, although no formal metric for patient satisfaction was included in the plan, a few of the family practice physicians and several patients let the office staff and therapists know that the practice's quick response to referrals and extended hours were appreciated.

Act

Overall, the changes resulted in positive improvement. The therapists and office staff agreed to continue the work schedule, office procedures, and answering service for another 3 months. It was pointed out that a formal approach needs to be taken regarding patient and physician satisfaction during the next few months. Based on the responses, the next set of practice changes can be made and the PDCA cycle repeated. Since Len is gone, these tasks are left to you.

Your Tasks

1. Apply PDCA to patient and physician satisfaction. (A review of Chapters 5 and 6 can help you get started.)
2. For feedback on your work, follow the instructions of your instructor.

REFERENCES

American Society for Quality. Quality tools. Available at http://www.asq.org/learn-about-quality/quality-tools.html. Accessed on 1/05/08.

BNET Business Dictionary. Quality management. Available at http://dictionary.bnet.com/definition/quality+management.html. Accessed 1/07/08a.

BNET Business Dictionary. TQM. Available at http://dictionary.bnet.com/definition/Total+Quality+Management.html. Accessed 1/07/08b.

Bornstein T. Quality improvement and performance improvement: Different means to the same end? QA Brief. Spring 2001;9(1):6–12.

Bourgeois LJ, Brodwin DR. Strategic implementation: Five approaches to an elusive phenomenon. Strategic Management Journal. 1984;5:241–264.

Decision Support Systems Resources. Decision Support System (DSS). Available at http://www.dssresources.com/. Accessed 1/15/09.

Department of Commerce. Office of the Secretary: Office of Human Resources Management. Available at http://ohrm.os.doc.gov/Performance/prod01_001121. Accessed 12/30/07.

Druzdzel MJ, Flynn RR. Decision support systems. Available at http://www.pitt.edu/~druzdzel/abstracts/dss.html. Accessed 1/08/08a.

Druzdzel MJ, Flynn RR. Decision support systems. http://www.pitt.edu/~druzdzel/psfiles/dss.pdf. Accessed 1/08/08b.

Goffee R, Gareth J. What holds the modern company together? Harvard Business Review. 1996;74(6): 134–148.

Government Accountability Office. BPR Glossary. Available at http://www.gao.gov/special.pubs/bprag/bprgloss.htm. Accessed 12/30/07.

Hall M. Quick study: Decision-support systems. Computerworld. July 2002. Available at http://www.computerworld.com/softwaretopics/software/apps/story/0,10801,72327,00.html. Accessed 1/08/08.

Hospitals and Health Networks. AHA Quality Center. Which performance improvement method is right for your hospital? HHN Magazine. October 2007. Available at http://www.hhnmag.com/hhnmag_app/jsp/articledisplay.jsp?dcrpath=HHNMAG/Article/data/10OCT2007/0710HHN_FEA_Gatefold&domain=HHNMAG. Accessed 12/30/07.

Office of Organizational Excellence. Fishbone diagram: A problem analysis tool. Available at http://quality.enr. state.nc.us/tools/fishbone.htm. Accessed 1/22/08.

Ramki M. Business intelligence: Accelerate your performance. Available at http://ezinearticles.com/?expert= Ramki_M. Accessed 1/15/09.

Sahni A. Quality improvement: Seven basic tools that can improve quality. Medical Device & Diagnostic Industry Magazine. Available at http://www.devicelink.com/ mddi/archive/98/04/012.html. Accessed 1/15/09.

iSix Sigma. Six sigma and quality methodologies. Available at http://main.isixsigma.com/me/. Accessed 1/04/07.

Tague NR. The quality toolbox, 2nd ed. Milwaukee, WI: ASQ Quality Press. 2004.

Webopedia. Internet.com. Available at http://www. webopedia.com/TERM/O/OLAP.html. Accessed 12/30/07.

Webopedia. Internet.com. Available at http://www. webopedia.com/TERM/d/data_mining.html. Accessed 1/06/08.

ADDITIONAL RESOURCES

Key in any of the methodology or tool names at Bnet for concise additional information on the majority of terms used in this chapter (http://dictionary.bnet.com/ definition). Another site for definitions of many of this chapter's terms is http://strategis.ic.gc.ca/epic/site/stco-levc.nsf/en/h_qw00037e.html.

Baldrige National Quality Program. Health care criteria of performance excellence. Gaithersburg, MD: Baldrige National Quality Program National Institute of Standards and Technology, Technology Administration, U.S. Department of Commerce. 2007.

Institute of Healthcare Improvement. Going lean in health care. IHI Innovation Series white paper. Cambridge, MA: Institute for Healthcare Improvement; 2005. Available at www.IHI.org.

International Organization for Standardization. ISO Standards. Available at http://www.iso.org/iso/iso_catalogue.

A more detail description of the management decision making tools discussed in this chapter along with application examples can be found in Tague NR. The quality toolbox, 2nd ed. at the American Society for Quality Website: http://www.asq.org/learn-about-quality/quality-tools.html. An informative publication by Moyers H, Shaw JG, New W. is Choosing A Quality/ Performance Improvement Methodology: Methodology Comparisons: Six Sigma, Lean, Theory of Constraints and Customer-Inspired Quality available from Shaw Resources at http://www.shawresources.com/ artchoosingqualityimprovementmethod.html.

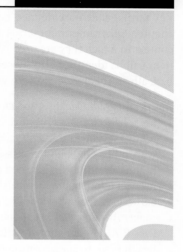

CHAPTER 16

STRATEGIES FOR HEALTH SERVICES PERFORMANCE IMPROVEMENT

CHERYL LaFOLLETTE ANDERSON

Learning Objectives

1. Define quality.
2. Provide an underpinning of current quality initiatives.
3. Highlight stakeholders in quality management.
4. Dissect the role of private versus public quality management efforts.
5. Investigate the role of multiple agencies and organizations.
6. Discuss quality management reporting organizations.
7. Identify quality management engagement strategies and best practices for physical therapists (PT).
8. Integrate performance improvement efforts with physical therapy.

Introduction

The current drive by governmental and private groups to quantify *quality management (QM)* and patient **outcomes** has been briefly discussed. The earlier chapters provide the background to complete the discussion on quality in this chapter. The discussions in Chapter 1 included identifying and comparing selected quality and safety differences found in health care systems worldwide. In Chapter 9, the approach to QM was focused on the perspective of federal and state regulations that health service managers and employers need

to be aware of from a risk management view. Chapter 10 added mandatory health care quality, safety, and legal oversight from the major governmental agencies involved in these endeavors. Private voluntary oversight and accrediting agencies were also introduced. Statistical and other management decisions support tools for multiple health care organization operations was the contribution of Chapter 15 to the theme of QM. The current chapter builds on the understandings developed in the preceding chapters. It sharpens the focus on health care QM by discussing how public and private efforts are at work in this area.

QM and health care quality is a broad topic area. This chapter will serve as an introduction to selected organizations and their formalized efforts to help clinical managers understand the breadth and depth of current QM efforts. This chapter integrates these broad foci with the role of the PT and PT manager by investigating ways that they may impact quality in their own clinical settings. Also noted are opportunities for PTs to become involved in health care quality and safety **policy** influencing bodies.

Terms

The term quality denotes a comparative level of excellence. QM, and the newer term, *performance improvement (PI)* (Chapter 15) are systematic ways of measuring and formulating ways to raise quality. These two terms are being promoted as the next wave in health care

Key terms, which are defined below, are bolded and italicized the first time they appear in the chapter. Other important terms are shown in boldface on first appearance and are defined by the context in which they are used. When either of these types of terms is used several times, its acronym will be identified and subsequently used in the chapter. Both types of terms are listed alphabetically in the online glossary with their definitions and (when applicable) their acronyms.

American Health Quality Association (AHQA): works on behalf of quality improvement organizations (QIOs). Through this association, QIOs network with other QIOs and professionals working in health care quality to share best practices and other relevant information. Membership is open to others besides those who work within or for a QIO.

Consumer Assessment of Healthcare Providers and Systems (CAHPS): an annual AHRQ survey used by health plans to assess consumer satisfaction with health plan and provider services.

Crossing the Quality Chasm: a 2001 Institute of Medicine report in which a comprehensive strategy and action plan to reinvent the U.S. health care system was presented.

external quality review organizations (EQRO): federally sponsored but private QIOs. QIO contractors are historically physician-directed groups that receive Medicare funds to foster quality health care services in hospitals, skilled nursing facilities, comprehensive outpatient rehabilitation facilities, and home health agencies. Recent emphasis is on quality through application of national, evidence-based guidelines.

failure modes and effects analysis (FMEA): an analysis tool that allows determining the likelihood of failures in a process and the potential impact of the failure.

Health Care Quality Improvement Program (HCQIP): a CMS program whose purpose is analyzing data from various sources and changing the patterns of care in targeted areas based on their public health importance and feasibility of measuring and improving quality.

health care triad: from the Institute of Medicine the triad is access, quality, and cost of care.

Health Plan Employer Data and Information Set (HEDIS): a National Committee for Quality Assurance proprietary survey instrument used to measure managed-care plan performance in key areas like immunization and mammography screening rates. Used for comparing managed health care plans' performance on standardized measures.

Institute of Medicine (IOM): a private organization associated with the National Academy of Sciences that serves as adviser to the nation to improve health.

Leapfrog Group: a voluntary health care quality improvement public reporting group of employers. This organization aims to mobilize employers' purchasing power by alerting the U.S. health industry that big leaps in health care safety, quality, and consumer value will be recognized and rewarded.

Medicare Quality Improvement Community (MedQIC): a CMS created and funded online resource of health-related quality improvement information for QIOs.

managed care: health care delivery systems that (1) strive to control the cost of services, (2) utilization of services, (3) regulate access to the services a particular health care plan offers and, (4) maintain or improve their quality.

peer review organization (PRO): an outcome focused QIO charged with reviewing quality and cost for care of Medicare beneficiaries.

performance improvement (PI): systematic ways of measuring and formulating ways to raise quality of ongoing operations. Decision-making activities related to current operations is often referred to as performance management (PM), or quality improvement (QI), total quality improvement (TQI), performance improvement, and quality management.

Physician Quality Reporting Initiative (PQRI): a voluntary, quality-reporting program that provides financial incentives for participation and for meeting certain criteria based on weighted calculations from the Medicare physician fee schedule. A form of pay for performance. Physical therapists are eligible to participate.

quality improvement organizations (QIOs): also called external quality review organizations (EQROs) or peer review organizations (PROs). QIOs are federally sponsored but privately operated groups that receive Medicare funds to foster quality

(Continued)

health care services in hospitals, skilled nursing facilities, comprehensive outpatient rehabilitation facilities, and home health agencies.

Quality Improvement Roadmap/Quality Roadmap: a Centers for Medicare and Medicaid Services (CMS) strategic plan for quality management (1) working through partnerships, (2) developing and providing quality measures and information, (3) developing payment means that reinforce a commitment to quality and cost efficiency, (4)

promoting electronic health systems, and (5) supporting efforts for rapid development and supporting evidence for new treatments.

quality management: emphasizes looking for improvements through statistical analysis of each step of a process.

Utilization Review Accreditation Commission (URAC): a leading, independent, nonprofit organization that promotes health care quality nationally.

---

management strategic initiatives. While improving quality is the goal of both, and both are quality improvement approaches to measure variations, they differ in focus. QM emphasizes looking for improvements through statistical analysis of each step of a process (Chapter 15). PI broadens the analysis to include human factors to determine what is needed to improve performance (Reproductive Health, 2008). Because of a lack of consensus at this time (Hillstrom and Hillstrom, 1998), in this chapter, these terms will be used synonymously.

Orientation

Health care QM from the federal government's perspective is distinctly different from QM encountered in the for-profit business sector. The difference is what is best for patients versus what is best for the shareholder/owner. For example, the **Institute of Medicine (IOM)** defines quality as, "The degree to which health services for individuals and populations increase the likelihood of desired health outcomes and are consistent with current professional knowledge" (IOM, 2008). As one of the leading agencies in health care quality, the IOM's definition has been the core of most health care quality work in the past decade.

Chapter 15 dealt with the essential QM tools and practices in the United States. These tools are derived from the original work of Deming, a statistician, who is often referred to as the father of the modern quality movement. Deming (2000) developed statistically based measures to identify and minimize product variability in the manufacturing sector. He called this process **Total Quality Management (TQM)**. Deming's efforts to identify and

correct variations in product quality eventually gave rise to multiple efforts to improve service delivery as well. TQM moved slowly from production business to health care business mainly through research and initiatives that began in earnest in the late 1980s (Laffel and Blumenthal, 1989). However, health care as an industry has been slow to advance efforts to define and measure quality. While progress has been made in the areas of ethics, leadership behavior, and corporate responsibility (Helms, 2006), quality clinical performance areas are in development. Difficulties in defining quality and developing meaningful prospective quality improvement and retrospective quality assurance measures are part of the problem (Booth et al., 2008). There are also arguments related to the "science" versus the "art" of medicine (e.g., professional autonomy) and the tug-of-war in the realm of **evidence-based practice** (e.g., primacy of randomized clinical trials) that have slowed progress in quantifying many clinical aspects of health care quality.

Underpinning of Current Health Care Quality Initiatives

Focused efforts to describe health care have hinged on the idea of a balanced **health care triad**. The IOM's staff and consultants (2001) have focused on a fundamental triad of interdependent goals for improving the U.S. health care system. The triad is

Access
Quality
Cost of care

Each part of the triad is considered equally important in contributing to the equilibrium of the health care delivery system. The three main quality initiatives are credited with bringing health care quality to the national agenda. Although access and cost of care are equally important as noted in Chapter 1, this chapter's concern is on the quality factor of the triad.

Governmental Quality Agenda Background

There are three recent governmental efforts to improve health care—the IOM's widely circulated report (2001), *Crossing the Quality Chasm: A New Health System for the 21st Century*, **Public Law 105-33, the Balanced Budget Act of 1997** (Government Printing Office [GPO], 2008), and a 2006 report to Congress titled **Improving the Medicare Quality Improvement Organization Program** (Leavitt, 2008). Together, these three initiatives have proved invaluable for advancing health care quality in the United States.

Following on the heels of their other provocative report, To Err is Human (Kohn et al., 2000), the IOM provided sound evidence that health care quality was lacking by quantifying the number of medical errors and resulting deaths that occurred each year. The public was astounded and dismayed. The public outcry motivated the IOM to continue its research efforts, which were published in Crossing the Quality Chasm (IOM, 2001). This report presented a comprehensive strategy and action plan to reinvent the health care system in the nation.

Crossing the Quality Chasm

Crossing the Quality Chasm articulated six aims for health care improvement. These aims for health care are that care is

1. Safe
2. Effective
3. Patient-centered
4. Timely
5. Efficient
6. Equitable

These six aims for improvement are built around the core need for health care to be safe. *Safe* means avoiding injuries to patients from the care that is intended to help them. The second, *effective*, is defined as providing services based on scientific knowledge to all who could benefit, and refraining from providing services to those not likely to benefit. *Patient-centered*, a popular term, denotes providing care that is respectful of and responsive to individual patient preferences, needs, and values, and ensuring that patient values guide all clinical decisions. *Timely*, the fourth aim, discusses reducing wait times and sometimes harmful delays for both those who receive and those who give care. *Efficient* is described as avoiding waste, including waste of equipment, supplies, ideas, and energy. Finally, *equitable* means providing care that does not vary in quality because of personal characteristics such as gender, ethnicity, geographic location, and socioeconomic status (IOM, 2001).

These six aims continue to be the cornerstone in health care quality initiatives. For example, the **white paper**, Engaging Physicians in a Shared Quality Agenda (Reinertsen et al., 2007), places emphasis on each aim discussing ways that physicians may be involved in changing the dynamics and directions of health care quality. The idea of **medical home** grew out of this concept. Medical home essentially is caring for patients as you would a respected friend or family member 24/7 (American Academy of Pediatrics, 2008). It is touted as the patient-centered method that physicians and other care providers should move toward. However, an alternative viewpoint held by some physical therapy leaders is that a "medical home" managed by physician providers keeps the physician in a patriarchal role overseeing the work of other professionals thereby creating a method to interfere with interdisciplinary processes and the goal of increased autonomy for other health care professionals including PTs (PT Bulletin Online, 2007). The American Physical Therapy Association (APTA) leaders are grappling with this concept at the time of writing, seeking to create a white paper that accurately represents the view of PTs while promoting QM through an interdisciplinary mode. A plausible complement would be PTs pursuing opportunities to serve on IOM committees and becoming participants in the national dialogue. As we all stretch ourselves to integrate quality, have we considered participating in these types of high-level discourse? There is certainly a role for PTs to be part of the volunteer expert force that is helping meld this nation's health policies. See Chapter 1 for suggestions for becoming politically involved.

Public Law 105-33: Balanced Budget Act of 1997

A watershed of legislated mandates occurred with enactment of Public Law 105-33, the Balanced Budget Act of 1997 (GPO, 2008). This act is often referred to as BBA97. Two effects of this act were reimbursement reductions and quality improvement mandates. The act legislated payment and reimbursement changes that became detrimental to many areas of health care including medical education and employment of PTs and physical therapist assistants particularly in skilled nursing facilities. It also mandated increased attention to performance monitoring and quality assurance in major governmental health-related programs. BBA97 had a beneficial effect on health care quality. Title IV, the part of the act that contained Medicare, Medicaid, and Children's Health provisions, established new requirements for PI and quality. Since the passage of that legislation, *managed care* health plans covering Medicare beneficiaries have dealt with a formalized method of measuring quality among its beneficiaries. Health plans are required to complete multiyear, formalized research that meets stringent criteria. These are called **performance improvement projects** (**PIPs**) (Leavitt, 2007). The challenge to the health plans is that each year requires a minimum number of PIPs to be developed while still working to sustain the PIPs from previous years. The PIP methodology demands measurable, positive change to be sustainable for at least 3 years before a plan may discontinue its efforts defined in that PIP. It is easy to see how the PIP efforts have snowballed into multiple projects creating a confusing complex for the plans and providers. Further, each health plan has its own PIPs. Thus, many providers must deal with multiple PIPs with different foci from different plans. This has created a situation of current contention between plans and providers. Providers desire that plans have a common theme and work on similar strategies while plans are focused on meeting their contractual requirements with federal bodies, accrediting organizations, and employer-based health plans. This dissension is likely to continue to grow as performance measurements and outcomes continue to push forward.

PT PIP Example

PIP development offers a unique opportunity for PTs to interact with health plans in effecting consumer or beneficiary change. An enterprising group of Minnesota (MN) PTs began development of a PIP in 2005. After receiving a competitive grant from the MN Department of Human Services (DHS), a work group with the MN Chapter of the APTA attempted to create a model falls program that could possibly be used as a PIP for one or several health plans in MN. The development of PIPs is a long process. Generally, PIP development begins as a **focus study** where the plan tries out different efforts to attempt change. With this knowledge in hand, the MN APTA work group created a systems-change project termed Stand Up and Be Strong (Anderson et al., 2007). This was a community falls project that would be used by one small health plan in rural western and south-central parts of the state. The intent of Stand Up and Be Strong was to:

1. Create a community-based system where fall risk assessment and prevention are routinely available to older adults.
2. Enable individuals to assess their risk of falling due to lower body weakness.
3. Enable individuals to take action to decrease risk or maintain a low risk level.

This is one example of how PTs may begin to discuss QM initiatives with payers and for therapists to consider their own unique skills applied to a population-based project. For more information on this PIP project see the Additional Resources section.

Centers for Medicare and Medicaid Services (CMS): A Driving Force for Quality

The Medicare program, administered by CMS, is the most significant driving force in quality in this nation as this department is the largest single purchaser of health care in the United States (Wood, 2007). With its sheer size and volume, and entitlement foundation, Medicare represents one of the most powerful policy forces in the American health care environment. CMS is taking an active role in moving health quality forward through the creation of the CMS *Quality Improvement Roadmap* (CMS, 2007a) and the newly re-defined roles of *Quality Improvement Organizations (QIOs)* (CMS, 2008a). Embracing technology, and working toward information dissemination, CMS created the *Medicare Quality Improvement Community (MedQIC)*, an online resource of quality information (MedQIC, 2008a). More will be said about QIOs and MedQICs. CMS supports multiple quality initiatives including those that focus on hospitals, home health, nursing homes, physicians, and patients with end-stage renal disease (IOM, 2007). Physical therapists have likely been impacted by CMS quality initiatives because of their impact on facilities where physical therapy services are provided.

CMS Quality Roadmap

CMS (2007a) developed a strategic plan in QM termed the CMS Quality Roadmap. This plan articulates five strategies for the federal government to support quality improvement in all areas of health care. The five strategies are:

1. Work through partnerships within CMS, with Federal and State agencies, and especially with nongovernmental partners, to achieve quality goals.
2. Develop and provide quality measures and information as a foundation for supporting more effective quality improvement efforts.
3. CMS and health plans must pay for care in a way that reinforces a commitment to quality while helping providers and patients to take steps to improve health and avoid unnecessary costs.
4. Promote electronic health systems that are believed to support quality improvement.
5. Support efforts that work toward more rapid development and better evidence for new treatments.

Through this Roadmap, CMS is actively working with health care **stakeholders** to identify health care efficiency measures, to address opportunities for improvement in health care quality, and to consider policy approaches for reducing the currently observed regional variation in quality and efficiency. Roadmap projects offer an opportunity for provider organizations to be involved with national quality initiatives. Given the newness of the Roadmap and the desire of the federal government to effect change, PTs have opportunities to become active in Roadmap initiatives. An excellent first step is to investigate the local or state QIO.

Agency for Healthcare Research and Quality (AHRQ)

AHRQ is one of the most important federal agencies focused on improving health care quality (AHRQ, 2008a). It is a visible force in the area of research and quality. AHRQ's strategic goals are emulated by many organizations. These goals are:

- Safety and quality
- Effectiveness
- Efficiency
- Organizational excellence

The first three goals are similar to those listed for the IOM. However, the fourth, organizational excellence, is different. AHRQ efforts include looking at systems and organizations that impact quality. In addition to the research grants and projects, AHRQ is involved with Medicare, Medicaid, and health plan efforts in quality. The grants have focused on quality improvement interventions that target either or both health policy environments and health care delivery organizations (AHRQ, 2008a).

As part of payer quality efforts, AHRQ is responsible for the *Consumer Assessment of Healthcare Providers and Systems (CAHPS)* surveys (AHRQ, 2008b). Through collaboration with the National Committee for Quality Assurance (NCQA), CAHPS surveys are examples of federal and private collaboration for quality reporting. CAHPS surveys are used by health plans yearly to assess consumer satisfaction with health plan and provider services. Questions include those that ask about patient wait times, the ability to see a specialist, and satisfaction with provider contacts. There are surveys that assesses pediatric care and two that are for adults ages 19–64 and 65 and up, respectively. All large health plans, most health maintenance organizations, and many state Medicaid programs use CAHPS surveys. CMS requires Medicare health plans and Medicare Part D sponsors to complete CAHPS annually and report on those findings.

AHRQ has many other initiatives aimed to assist providers and to survey patients. Of interest to health care managers is the agency's efforts to facilitate the transformation of research into practice in the areas of cost reduction, organizational excellence, and business processes.

Government Sponsored but Private

Health care quality and the measurement of health outcomes have become very broadbased. The reader should understand that the accurate measurement of health outcomes and the constant move toward evidence-based practice is here to stay. There is a diverse group of professionals involved in such issues. Physical therapists with an interest in the integration of clinical practice and outcome measurements will find helpful information and support through the additional organizations discussed next.

QIOs

Several CMS Roadmap initiatives have been directed toward Medicare Quality Review Organizations, often called QIOs. Other names for QIOs include *External Quality Review Organizations (EQROs)* or *Peer Review Organizations (PROs)*. Federally sponsored but private, QIO contractors are historically physician-directed groups that receive Medicare funds to foster quality health care services in hospitals, skilled nursing facilities, comprehensive outpatient rehabilitation facilities, and home health agencies (CMS, 2007b). They deal with many types of issues including review of beneficiary complaints and appeals, Medicare billing accuracy, and application of quality standards in care delivery. In the contract period 2002–2005, there were 41 organizations holding 53 QIO contracts covering all 50 states, the District of Columbia, Puerto Rico, and the Virgin Islands. 38 of the 41 are organized as not-for-profit organizations (Leavitt, 2007).

Since 2006, the focus of QIOs and the government contracts that they hold has shifted to an emphasis on quality through application of national, evidence-based guidelines. QIOs have broadened their focus from hospitals to nursing homes, physician practices, home health agencies, and health plans. QIOs are playing an increasing role in quality in all areas of health (IOM, 2007). We should be paying close attention to QIOs that monitor the practice areas and plans in our own geographical areas.

QIOs represent a unique opportunity for organizations. Forging partnerships with QIOs will help bring quality initiatives more quickly to your organization. Cooperating and collaborating with a QIO means you have increased your consulting staff in the area of quality without increasing your costs. As physician-driven organizations, QIOs offer you the chance to change or modify provider practices toward current quality discussions.

Several QIO work plan projects have included restraint reduction and wound care in skilled nursing facilities, and admission and discharge criteria along with patient "dumping" issues in acute hospitals. QIOs have promoted health literacy programs throughout their regions and have provided monitoring of consumer grievances and complaints against health plans. PTs may be familiar with these types of quality project without realizing there is a government-contracted, local organization that actually is diligently working on these issues.

Medicare Quality Improvement Community (MedQIC)

CMS also created MedQIC to assist QIOs. MedQIC is federally sponsored through CMS and partners with the nonprofit **Institute for Healthcare Improvement** (IHI) in support of CMS's *Health Care Quality Improvement Program (HCQIP)* (CMS, 2008b). MedQIC provides an online, electronic format of information sharing in quality improvement (MedQIC, 2008a,b). This is an open, public format. MedQICs quality improvement frameworks are founded on community-based approaches. The knowledge-sharing formats may be worth investigating for application to organizations offering physical therapy or for sharing your own best practices. This is an opportunity for PTs to share evidence-based medicine research, best practices in physical therapy, and to provide input to other members on Listserves supported through MedQIC.

IHI

IHI is a leading authority on health care quality. Its revenue stream is mainly through fee-based program offerings and services though it is supported through contributions from foundations, companies, and individuals (IHI, 2008a). Its efforts are found throughout the health care environment as providers of multiple training opportunities and their significant publications, videos, audio tapes, and white papers on health care quality improvement. IHI also provides unique online tools such as the Improvement Tracker that allows individuals and organizations to track and measure efforts in topic areas supported by the IHI (IHI, 2008b). IHI's interactive, web-based tools include the:

Failure Modes and Effects Analysis (FEMA) tool
Trigger for Measuring ADEs (adverse drug events)
Physician Practice Safety Assessment

The FEMA tool determines the likelihood of failures in a process and the potential impact of the failure (IHI, 2008a). The FEMA tool has potential for PT managers because it can be used to analyze specific protocols, incidents, or outcomes. The environment seems ripe for therapists to integrate this particular tool into areas of risk analysis such as falls, balance issues, or even outcomes from different surgical procedures.

The Trigger for Measuring ADEs (IHI, 2008c). A trigger is a clue that helps identify adverse events related to medications. This tool allows practitioners to measure drug-related events in an organization and to track changes over time. The tool may be of value to PTs to foster collaborating with nursing in scheduling the timing of certain medications to minimize harm from loss of balance, reduced cognition, or other dangerous conditions during treatment times.

The third IHI tool, the Physician Practice Safety Assessment, is designed for use by physician groups to help practices measure safety and quality (IHI, 2008d). This tool addresses: medications, patient transitions of care, surgery issues, personnel qualifications and competencies, practice management and culture, and patient education and communication. These last three parts of the tool may be of use to PT managers, particularly those in private practice.

The most public effort currently underway through IHI is the 5 Million Lives campaign. Physical therapists employed by hospitals or hospital systems may be involved with this campaign which is to protect patients from 5 million incidents of medical harm in U.S. hospitals, for the period 2006–2008 (IHI, 2008e; McCannon et al., 2007).

The 5 Million Lives Campaign challenges hospitals to adopt 12 changes in care to save lives and reduce patient injuries. They are:

- Deliver reliable, evidence-based care for acute myocardial infarction
- Deliver reliable, evidence-based care for congestive heart failure
- Deploy rapid response teams
- Get boards on board
- Prevent adverse drug events
- Prevent central line infections
- Prevent harm from high-alert medications
- Prevent surgical site infections
- Prevent ventilator-associated pneumonia
- Reduce surgical complications
- Prevent pressure ulcers
- Reduce methicillin-resistant staphylococcus aureus (MRSA) infections

The 5 Million Lives Campaign is a type of systems change management. It is the largest improvement initiative undertaken by the health care industry. The changes are bold and the goals are enormous. The only non-clinical goal relates to management leadership. It looks at defining and spreading the best-known leveraged processes for hospital boards and leaders to create organizations that are more effective in providing care safely. IHI offers organizations and individual providers opportunities to participate in driving the course of quality agendas. Further, IHI provides e-newsletters and frequent webcasts that focus on specific topics of interest to leadership in health care organizations. Most of these webcasts and e-newsletters are free (IHI, 2008e).

A benefit of PT manager and staff participation in programs like the 5 Million Lives Campaign goes beyond benefiting patients. It is a means of gaining broader recognition of PTs within the organization. It can be a means of increasing the breadth of functional networks (Chapter 12).

The American Health Quality Association (AHQA)

Just as the American Physical Therapy Association (APTA) represents PTs and the interests of PTs, the AHQA works on behalf of QIOs. However, unlike the APTA, AHQA membership is also open to others besides those who work within or for a QIO (AHQA, 2008).

Through AHQA, QIOs network with other QIOs and professionals working in health care quality. This is a membership-driven organization that works on behalf of its members with major policy groups such as CMS, Department of Health and Human Services, the National Quality Forum, and the Medicare Payment Advisory Commission. This organization is open to other groups and individuals in addition to its major focus, QIOs.

The AHQA is one step removed from provider organizations. It may be difficult to discern AHQA's impact on specific organizations or facilities. However, membership is open to interested providers and health plans making it another opportunity for PTs to become part of the quality agenda in health care.

National Committee for Quality Assurance (NCQA)

NCQA is a private organization with a large impact on most provider organizations. Though membership is voluntary, most large health plans seek NCQA accreditation. Many large employers require that their health plans have NCQA certification. Most Medicaid health plans and smaller health plans are also required to follow NCQA guidelines. NCQA certified health plans experience rigorous credentialing and survey processes every 3 years, in order to remain certified (NCQA, 2008a). The surveys are dynamic, take more than a week to complete, and have a constantly changing nature due to the fast-paced change of the health care environment.

The organization's revenues are derived from membership dues, accreditation and certification programs, along with educational programming. The NCQA is extremely influential in quality particularly as it relates to the payer side of the health plan business.

Using the simple formula for improvement: measure, analyze, improve, repeat, NCQA has effectively built consensus around important health care quality issues working with large employers, policymakers, doctors, patients, and health plans to decide what is important, how to measure it, and how to promote improvement.

NCQA's best known product is the *Healthcare Effectiveness Data Information Set (HEDIS)*. HEDIS' success is noted for promoting evidence-based medicine through yearly analysis of health plan claims data; hybrid data collection measures using surveyors who abstract medical records at provider sites; and integration of patient satisfaction measures from the CAHPS program. The yearly analysis creates 71 quality benchmarks for health plans and providers. HEDIS' effect on plans, regulators, and providers is growing each year. Savvy PTs would become educated in HEDIS and their own facility's measurement scores (Note, that facilities will have many different sets of HEDIS scores.). Since each health plan is mandated to do HEDIS, the facility will have HEDIS scores specific to each health plan. This allows managers to look at HEDIS scores for patient types and compare measures in an apples-to-apples method.

The 2008 HEDIS measurements have four specific measures that are of interest to PTs. These four are:

1. Falls risk management
2. Osteoporosis testing in older women
3. Osteoporosis management in women who had a fracture
4. Physical activity in older adults

These four areas offer PTs the opportunity to work with physicians and specific clinics that deal with older adults on these issues. It is likely that effective physical therapy intervention will help improve HEDIS scores within these four measures.

In concert with HEDIS, NCQA is widely recognized for its accreditation, certification, and physician recognition programs. See Additional Resources section for accessing a complete listing.

Given all the programs and credentialing efforts, no health care organization can ignore NCQA's impact from the national level through the single provider level. Report cards on more than 600 NCQA accredited health plans (NCQA, 2008b) are available as is its physician directory (NCQA, 2008c).

NCQA's benchmarking activities include publications such as the **Quality Compass**—a document that contains commercial national, regional, and state averages and percentiles from HEDIS analysis and State of Health Care Quality—an aggregate report of national averages for the current year, as well as previous years' national averages for the selected measures.

Proactive organizations will recognize the value of NCQA's report card and resources. Sitting back and observing is most likely a disadvantageous position for most organizations. Physical therapists work in many NCQA organizations. Also, the NCQA physician recognition programs include patients with diagnoses by PTs. These facts suggest that familiarity with NCQA's programs and resources can lead to improved QM in physical therapy.

Utilization Review Accreditation Commission (URAC)

The Utilization Review Accreditation Commission is known simply as URAC (URAC, 2008a). It is an independent, nonprofit organization, and well-known leader in promoting health care quality nationally. Similar to NCQA, URAC has accreditation and certification programs for plans and providers. Through a multistakeholder process, URAC creates its accreditation and certification programs. Most program certifications are in effect for 3 years.

URAC's accreditation programs differ from NCQA's accreditation. For example, in 2006, URAC began work on Pharmacy Benefit Management accreditation after the implementation of the Medicare Part D prescription drug program.

Similar to NCQA, it is a proactive, forward thinking organization looking at ways to collaborate in QM. Their health provider credentialing program (URAC, 2008b) may be of interest to PTs as a quality related form of recognition. State chapters involved in third level chart reviews for payers may wish to seek accreditation as an accredited utilization management organization (URAC, 2008a).

Other Quality Improvement Public Reporting Groups

Consumers are clamoring for quality care that is accessible and affordable. Thus, organizations have developed to support those needs. As the quality agenda moves forward, many other organizations are being formed. Thus, this section looks at examples in five different types of public reporting outside the realm of the organizations discussed thus far.

Quality improvement public reporting is embraced by all sectors of health care including:

- Employers
- Health plan collaboratives
- State governments
- Physicians
- Consumers

Leapfrog Group

There is a growing array of quality improvement public reporting groups. Leading these initiatives are employer groups. One seminal employer group organization is the Leapfrog Group. This organization is a voluntary program aimed at mobilizing employer purchasing power to alert America's health industry that big leaps in health care safety, quality, and consumer value will be recognized and rewarding. Leapfrog supports employers and consumers and promotes the notion of incentives and rewards for providers who meet or exceed specific criteria. This is a growing organization with hospital data collection efforts going on in more than 33 states covering half of the U.S. population and at least 58% of all hospital beds in the country (Leapfrog Group, 2007). The Leapfrog Group is expanding its public reporting efforts. Physical therapists do need to stay abreast of this type of reporting for both hospital and outpatient clinic areas. Employers are basing health plan and employee health purchasing decisions based on efforts such as the Leapfrog Group.

MN Community Measurement

Health plan collaborative efforts are also working toward quality measures. One example of such a collaborative effort is MN Community Measurement (2007). This organization was created by major health plans in MN to publicly report on their health plans as well as report on provider measures. Most of this project's data is derived from health plan HEDIS data submitted to MN Community Measurement for further analysis. Through these types of collaboratives, health plans are gathering their mandated HEDIS data and comparing outcomes of large provider groups against the findings of the other plans for the same provider groups. If quality health care is provided at a large clinic, one would anticipate the same HEDIS score outcomes for the same diagnosis not dependent on payer. Thus, a person with Medicaid coverage should have the same health care services and the same outcomes as a person with the same diagnosis and a private pay, fee-for-service plan. Persons interested in quality of care and health care disparities are particularly interested in this type of public reporting.

HealthScope

Many states are also entering the public reporting efforts of health care quality by ranking plans or providers. A state example is HealthScope, California's rating of health maintenance organizations and medical groups (CA Office of the Patient Advocate, 2007). Through website access, consumers are able to compare health care quality rankings for physicians, hospitals, and nursing homes. Though physical therapy is not currently part of the comparative data available on state reporting websites, can it be far away?

CDPHP

Many physician groups have joined the public reporting of quality measures as well. An example is CDPHP, a not-for-profit individual practice association (IPA) model HMO in New York. Though not a pure physician model, as CDPHP is a type of health plan, its physicians are involved in the QM activities and are helping lead the organization in quality initiatives (CDPHP, 2007). Physician reporting may be done in response to health plan outcome gathering that some physicians feel may be unfair based on patient populations and diagnoses of patients served. However, physician group reporting remains positive

as physicians have entered into the national quality discussion by forming such research and reporting interests.

Consumer Coalition for Quality Health Care (CCQHC)

Various consumer groups also publicly report on health care quality. Located in Washington, DC, one vocal example is the CCQHC. The organization has been involved in lobbying and policy formation at the federal level including the Medicare Part D program (CCQHC, 2007). Consumer reporting demands continue to fuel efforts of organizations such as the Coalition.

The implication of information transparency through public measuring and reporting is staggering to health care providers and provider groups. Additional methods of gauging quality and wider dissemination of the results make it a wise decision on the part of individual health care providers and provider organizations to monitor these initiatives and seek methods to become engaged in the efforts to ensure that care and patient quality outcomes are truly reflected.

Modeling Physical Therapy PI

The practice and measurement of PI and quality outcomes in physical therapy is encouraged (APTA, 2008) but available instruments are limited in their scope. Well-known examples are Focus On Therapeutic Outcomes (2008) and Therapeutic Associates Care Connections Outcomes System (2008). This section will discuss more expansive initiatives currently underway in physician practices and how these model initiatives may be similarly applied to the practice of physical therapy.

Physician Quality Reporting Initiative (PQRI)

The Physician Quality Reporting Initiative (PQRI) (2007) is part of a very important current federal quality CMS effort. CMS was authorized under Title 1, Section 101 of the 2006 Tax Relief and Health Care Act of 2006 (TRHCA), to create the PQRI (CMS, 2007c). PQRI is currently a voluntary, quality-reporting program that provides financial incentives for participation and for meeting certain criteria based on weighted calculations from the Medicare physician fee schedule. This is a unique concept of a **pay-for-performance** method created by federal law that financially rewards physicians and others for meeting certain criteria.

PQRI includes 119 unique measures from Medicare fee-for-service claims based on diagnosis and procedural codes (CMS, 2008c). The system works through calculations of electronic claims data submitted by physician practices for covered Medicare services. CMS does provide a comprehensive PQRI Tool kit that highlights eight steps for success in this process (CMS, 2007c). This complex system will no doubt continue to grow and impact providers who work with Medicare patients. We all need to keep abreast of this particular CMS focus as it is an effort that may not be voluntary in the future. Further, considering that PTs also use the physician fee schedule for billing, it is likely that PQRI formats may move out to clinicians other than physicians.

Since the program began in May 2007, larger physician groups are moving to capture incentive dollars. These proactive organizations are working on PQRI now. The financial incentives may be enough to promote participation by large organizations. Reimbursement drives behavior. Paying for efforts in quality measures may change provider practices and organizational systems. PQRI is another example of how the federal government through CMS is driving the nation's health quality agenda.

Practical Applications for Strategic Quality Improvement

With the huge number of issues and organizations involved in health QM, it is natural to wonder, where does one start? To answer this question we will next look at ways to execute **strategic** improvements in health care. This section will investigate leadership leverage, the Wills–Ideas–Execution strategy, and system-wide approach methods applied to quality improvement.

Beginning with the top-down approach of organizational change, IHI's (Reinertsen et al., 2008) white paper publication on leverage

in leadership has excellent talking points to support leaders and their challenge to encourage innovative improvements in health care organizations. These points include:

1. Establish and oversee system-level aims
2. Align system measures, strategy, and projects in a leadership learning system
3. Channel leadership attention to system-level improvement
4. Get the right team on the bus
5. Make the Chief Financial Officer a quality champion
6. Engage physicians
7. Build improvement capability

Reinertsen et al. (2008) outlined a simple strategy for leadership working in QM. First, the leader must establish and oversee true system-level changes. Leaders need to be truly integrated into the quality agenda of their organization. Leaders should not focus on individuals or practitioner groups, rather the focus should be on systems and system strategies. Second, leaders need to align system measures and projects into a leadership learning system. Third, leaders should channel their own efforts toward system-level improvements. The fourth point is that leaders need to make sure they have the right team members involved. Put simply, this means get the right team on the bus. Practically speaking, systems changes and QM ought to make good financial sense, too. The fifth point engages the Chief Financial Officer as a quality champion. Point 6 recognizes that in health care organizations where physicians remain the thought influencers, organizational leaders have the challenge of engaging physicians in the change process. Finally, leaders are charged with building internal improvement capability. Leaders need to walk-the-talk in terms of QM and foster the organization's PI capabilities.

Quality is part of the strategic imperatives of an increasing number of health care facilities and organizations. Determining how to move an organization into the QM movement leads one to multiple initiatives with little direction on how to begin. Nolan (2007) suggests that keeping the thought process simple, is the best method to start. A simple mantra Wills–Ideas–Execution is one idea to do this. It denotes you have to:

Have the *will* to improve—be committed to QM

Have the *ideas* about alternatives to the status quo—engage in creative thinking to combat stagnation and complacency

Make it real through *execution*—plan, implement, measure, and do it again but better

The idea of will needs to be a top-down effort. Though all levels of a health care organization need to have the will to change; the will to improve; the will to participate; the will to remain positively focused; it is the leadership that needs to embrace such efforts. The process cannot be directed by an individual or single group (e.g., medical practice only); it must involve all levels of stakeholders with new and alternative ideas that may be measured, benchmarked, worked on, and re-measured.

Execution—the needed step for any process improvement must occur. Deadlines should be set and kept. A quality agenda should be a working document where deadlines and criteria are adhered to and then modified after an execution trial. We learn as much from our failures as we do from our successes. For examples and guides to assist an organization in implementing quality improvement efforts see Additional Resources section—improvement tracker.

The field of change management brings forth the idea of systems changes. To change a product or a service, a system must be modified or changed. Successful organizations recognize and understand their systems. The idea of systems changes and system-level improvement may also be applied to QM.

From more IHI work in strategic improvements, organizations need to adopt system-wide changes to support innovation and change. Three areas were highlighted by Nolan (2007) on the idea of system-level performance capabilities. First, the ability to consistently deliver on system-level aims aligned with strategic priorities by coordinating a portfolio of projects. Second, ubiquitous local management and supervision of activities aimed at stabilizing local performance, supporting or sustaining strategic aims, and providing an environment that promotes joining in the work. And third, continual development of a sufficient number of employees who are capable of leading initiatives to produce system-level results.

IHI's work also focuses on physician engagement in change and quality. Reinertsen et al. (2007) discussed ways to engage physicians in quality initiatives. This researcher group's simple strategy may also be applied to physical therapy and used by physical therapy managers in their own efforts for engaging rehabilitation staff in quality improvement efforts. Their framework of six primary elements consists of:

1. Discover a common purpose
2. Reframe values and beliefs
3. Segment the engagement plan
4. Use engaging improvement methods
5. Show courage
6. Adopt an engaging style

First, discover a common purpose. These purposes could be to improve patient outcomes; investigate a problem area; reduce hassles and wasted time; understand the organization's culture; and understand the legal opportunities and barriers. When considering the first element, physical therapy managers might investigate perceived barriers that staff routinely complain about in staff meetings. For an inpatient program this may be issues such as patients are not ready for therapy at their assigned appointment; or therapy orders are only called to the department at the end of the day; or one orthopedist has a protocol that appears to be dated in light of newer techniques. For the skilled nursing facility it might be that the facility is admitting mostly hospice patients into the Medicare A beds; or the therapy contract company rarely has a speech-language pathologist available; or dietary staff feel occupational therapists should routinely feed difficult patients at all three meal shifts every day. In a home care setting a common purpose might be expressed as difficulty negotiating the lengths of travel expected within the per diem rates; or the lack of any type of equipment for a therapist to bring to a home; or some patients do not speak English and most therapists only speak English making patient communication difficult. In the private practice setting, a common defined purpose to discuss may be the inability to find experienced PTs to fill vacancies; difficulty with payer reimbursement or lengthy prior authorization procedures; or competing for patients with local chiropractors.

The second element, reframe values and beliefs (Chapters 3 and 4) focuses on making clinicians partners, not customers of the processes. The idea is to promote both system and individual responsibility for quality (Chapter 17). For the physical therapy manager, this would mean asking a therapist team to help create the solutions. Try to see the issue from all angles and put together a formal thought process that frames the values and beliefs of the therapists.

Segment the engagement plan is the third element. This element is based on Juran's 80/20 general rule which proposes that 80% of difficulties are caused by 20% of the processes (Chiorazzi, 2008). The point is to seek to identify the true champions, educate and inform leaders, develop project management skills, and identify the 20% who are late adopters or "laggards" who may be barriers for practice/provider success. The physical therapy manager should include looking for the champions among the staff who will engage in the issues and seek to develop solutions. Often, managers will have the chief complainer or the "laggard" involved in the process. In an engagement process, that will not be the most positive way to begin. Thus, identify the champions and ask them to begin developing the solution to the problem. See Chapters 12 and 17 for additional views.

For the issues in the acute care hospital environment this may mean to consider the appointment system used now and either rework it or throw it out for a solution such as the therapist sees the patient at bedside and brings the patient to the therapy department, if necessary. For the skilled nursing facility perhaps the therapy staff needs to be more involved in the admission process making visits to discharging hospitals or creating an admission protocol for the facility. For the home care agency, it may mean that the therapists help the home care company determine what the maximum travel length allowed for any patient to be admitted for therapy services. In the private physical therapy practice, it may mean including the therapists in working on recruiting other experienced therapists.

The fourth element embraces the notion of using engaging methods. Seek to standardize only what can be standardized. Use the data sensibly. Make the right thing easy to try. Make the right thing easy to do.

The fifth element is show courage. Any successful strategy needs top-down support. The board must be behind innovation and change. The therapy manager must also be behind any new strategy. This can be done by expecting that QM suggestions and innovation will be tried and that they will work.

The sixth element deals directly with all clinicians. This principle states that clinicians need to be involved from the beginning. That one should work with the real leaders, the early adopters. One should choose messages and messengers carefully. Make sure that clinician involvement is visible. With respect to any quality initiative, there must be inherent trust. All communication should be candid and frequent.

Last, value each clinician's time as if it your own time. If you want staff to put in time related to quality activities, the therapy manager also needs to put in time by consistently demonstrating the importance of quality performance in all areas benefits the patients served, the therapy department, and the facility.

Facility Level Quality Assurance

Hospitals, nursing homes, and home health agencies generally have programs labeled "quality assurance." In addition, many outpatient centers and private practices do engage in principles of "QM." For hospitals, these programs are often lead by health information or medical records specialists. While in skilled nursing facilities and home health agencies, monthly committee meetings that focus on "quality assurance" are really data gathering meetings to discuss issues such as medication errors and falls. Certainly, the committees do take action to address these important safety issues, however, these types of "post event" foci have limited application to the greater work of "ongoing, real time" PI.

Similarly, quality assurance programs may be focused on documentation issues or improving forms. This type of quality assurance falls more into compliance. Ensuring that documentation is complete, timely, and accurately meeting the payer's specification is no longer considered quality assurance. These are expectations for any treating clinician. Thus, ensuring that documentation or billing is correct is compliance and does not meet the higher standards of addressing quality.

Physical therapists that have fallen into the "rut" of reporting or tracking issues for quality assurance committees or facility requirements should begin to look further than their own facility. Consider all the organizations and multiple national initiatives going on nationwide. From looking at HEDIS scores, becoming involved in the 5 Million Lives Campaign, or serving as a content/peer review expert for the IOM, PTs have an expanding role and impact on the nation's discussion with quality health care, PI, and quality outcomes.

Summary

Chapter 16 provided the reader with an overview of the fast-developing area of quality management/performance improvement. The key terms of quality, quality management, and performance improvement were defined. The major public and private organizations and various forces impelling improvement in health care were discussed. The unique foci of the various groups were identified along with the resources they provide.

Encouragement was given for PTs to be involved in the broader quality management discussion. To integrate the role PTs have in quality discussions it was noted how each agency or organization's resources could benefit PT managers. Opportunities for the involvement of PTs in health care quality focused organizations were pointed out. The chapter was capped off by a discussion on practical implementation strategies to improve quality management efforts at the individual, department, and facility or organization level.

Many variables contribute to being able to deliver health care services that consistently meet criteria defining a desired level of service excellence. One important variable is the people involved in the service delivery process. Quality attainment requires people who are capable and willing to pursue this goal. The next chapter deals with recruitment, selection, preparation, evaluation, and promotion processes involved in gaining and retaining personnel who cannot only deliver but also improve quality in health care settings.

CASE STUDY 16.1

Choose One

Introduction

As a newly licensed DPT, you are strongly interested in quality management and measurement of health outcomes. To add depth to your knowledge, consider all of the organizations discussed in this chapter. Now choose one to investigate further.

The Rest of the Assignment

1. What are you most interested in? (National or not, public or private, federal or state, general or narrow focus, for-profit or not-for-profit, department or organization focus, etc.)

2. What do you want to learn most? (Define health care quality or quality measures, or measurement instruments, physical therapy quality efforts, etc.).

3. Choose and investigate your organization and aspect of quality management.

4. What opportunities are there for you to learn more about this organization?

5. What opportunities are there for you to become involved in the quality agenda of this organization?

6. Summarize your findings in a page or less.

7. Share your information as determined by your instructor.

CASE STUDY 16.2

Using HEDIS

Introduction

You are the physical therapy manager for several outpatient physical therapy departments. They are connected to several groups of physician practices. It has been brought to your attention that HEDIS scores related to osteoporosis management in older adults are trending down (getting worse). The physician provider groups currently contract with six major health plans. Each reports similar findings for its members who are 65 and older. What would you do in this scenario regarding proposals to include physical therapy in the response for improvement for this group of patients?

Your Tasks

1. Review information about HEDIS
2. Explain what the HEDIS scores measure
3. Identify the resources you will need to develop an outline for a plan for the physical therapy departments to raise the HEDIS profile for the target patients.
4. Outline your strategic plan.
5. Who will you present your plan to for review?
6. Meet and discuss your plan
7. Improve your plan
8. Share your final plan as directed by your instructor.

REFERENCES

American Academy of Pediatrics. Children's health topics: Medical home. Available at http://www.aap.org/healthtopics/medicalhome.cfm. Accessed 1/15/08.

American Health Quality Association. About AHQA. Available at http://www.ahqa.org/pub/inside/158_670_2426.cfm. Accessed 1/06/08.

American Physical Therapy Association. Quality assurance and performance improvement. HOD P06-98-13-13. Available at http://www.apta.org/AM/Template.cfm?Section=Home&CONTENTID=25474&TEMPLATE=/CM/ContentDisplay.cfm. Accessed 1/19/08.

Anderson CL, Gjerde K, Gilchrist L, Noonan S. Stand up and be strong! Grant funded project that focused on community tests and outcomes. Gerinotes. 2007;14(6):17–20.

Agency for Healthcare Research and Quality. At-a-glance AHRQ facts. Available at http://www.ahrq.gov/about/ataglance.pdf. Accessed 1/06/08a.

Agency for Healthcare Research and Quality. CAHPS surveys and tools to advance patient-centered care. Available at https://www.cahps.ahrq.gov/default.asp. Accessed 1/06/08b.

Agency for Healthcare Research and Quality. Federal balanced budget act of 1997: Excerpts. Available from http://www.ahrq.gov/chtoolbx/fbba97.htm. Accessed 12/30/07.

Booth M, Fralich J, Bowe T. 2005 discussion paper. Home and community based services: Quality management roles and responsibilities. Available at http://www.cms.hhs.gov/HCBS/downloads/qmrolesdispaper.pdf. Accessed 1/16/08.

CA Office of the Patient Advocate. Health care quality report card: California's gateway to health care quality ratings. Available at http://www.opa.ca.gov/report_card/. Accessed 12/30/07.

CDPHP. Overview. Available at http://www.cdphp.com/aboutCDPHP/overview.aspx. Accessed 12/30/07.

Centers for Medicare and Medicaid Services. Executive summary. CMS quality roadmap. August, 2005. Available at www.cms.hhs.gov/CouncilonTechInnov/downloads/qualityroadmap.pdf. Accessed 12/30/07a.

Centers for Medicare and Medicaid Services. Quality initiatives: General information overview. Available at: http://www.cms.hhs.gov/QualityInitiativesGEnInfo/. Accessed 12/30/07b.

Centers for Medicare and Medicaid Services. Statutes/regulations/program instructions. Available at http://www.cms.hhs.gov/PQRI/05_StatuteRegulationsProgramInstructions.asp. Accessed 12/31/07c.

Centers for Medicare and Medicaid Services. Resources for quality improvement. Available at http://www.cms.hhs.gov/QualityImprovementOrgs/02_ResourcesforQualityImprovement.asp. Accessed 1/02/08a.

Centers for Medicare and Medicaid Services. Quality improvement organizations: Overview. Available at http://www.cms.hhs.gov/QualityImprovementOrgs/. Accessed 1/15/08b.

Centers for Medicare and Medicaid Services. Measures/codes. Available at http://www.cms.hhs.gov/PQRI/15_MeasuresCodes.asp. Accessed 1/18/08c.

Chiorazzi M. Books, bytes, bricks and bodies: Thinking about collection use in academic law libraries. Available at http://www.law.arizona.edu/Library/research/guides/paretoarticle.cfm?page=research. Accessed 1/18/08.

Consumer Coalition for Quality Healthcare. Consumer Coalition's 6 month report. Available at http://www.consumers.org/6month.htm. Accessed 12/29/07.

Deming WE. The New Economics: For Industry, Government, Education. Cambridge, MA: MIT Press. 2000.

Focus on Therapeutic Outcomes. Research at FOTO. Available at http://www.fotoinc.com/research.htm. Accessed 1/18/08.

Government Printing Office. Public and private laws: Browse 105th congress. Available at http://www.access.gpo.gov/nara/publaw/105publ.html. Accessed 1/14/08.

Helms MM. Encyclopedia of management, 5th ed. Detroit, MI: Thompson-Gale. 2006.

Hillstrom K, Hillstrom LC. Encyclopedia of small business, Vol 12. Detroit, MI: Gale. 1998.

Institute for Healthcare Improvement. About us. Available at: http://www.ihi.org/ihi/about. Accessed 1/06/08a.

Institute for Healthcare Improvement. Tracker tour. Available at http://www.ihi.org/ihi/workspace/tracker/TourImprovementTracker.htm. Accessed 1/06/08b.

Institute for Healthcare Improvement. Trigger tool for measuring adverse drug events. Available at http://www.ihi.org/IHI/Topics/PatientSafety/MedicationSystems/Tools/Trigger+Tool+for+Measuring+Adverse+Drug+Events+(IHI+Tool).htm. Accessed 1/06/08c.

Institute for Healthcare Improvement. Physician practice patient safety assessment: Office practices: Primary care access. Available at http://www.ihi.org/IHI/Topics/OfficePractices/Access/Tools/PhysicianPracticePatientSafetyAssessment.htm. Accessed 1/06/08d.

Institute for Healthcare Improvement. Protecting 5 million lives from harm. Available at http://www.ihi.org/IHI/Programs/Campaign/. Accessed 1/06/08e.

Institute of Medicine. Committee on Health Care in America. Crossing the quality chasm: A new health system for the 21st Century. Washington, DC: National Institute Press. 2001.

Institute of Medicine. Crossing the quality chasm: The IOM health care quality initiative. Available at http://www.iom.edu/CMS/8089.aspx. Accessed 1/12/08.

Institute of Medicine. Report brief March 2006. Medicare's quality improvement organization program: Maximizing potential. Available at http://www.iom.edu/Object.File/Master/35/322/Medicare%20QIO.pdf. Accessed 12/30/07.

Kohn LT, Corrigan JM, Donaldson MS, eds. To Err is Human: Building a safer health system. Washington, DC: National Academy Press. 2000.

Laffel G, Blumenthal D. The case for using industrial quality management science in health care organizations. Journal of the American Medical Association. 1989;262:2869–2873.

Leapfrog Group. About us. Available at: http://www.leapfroggroup.org/about_us. Accessed 12/30/07.

Leavitt M. Report to Congress: Improving the medicare quality improvement organization program. Response to the Institute of Medicine study. Available at http://www.cms.hhs.gov/QualityImprovementOrgs/downloads/QIO_Improvement_RTC_fnl.pdf. Accessed 1/10/08.

McCannon JC, Hackbarth DA, Griffith FA. Miles to go: An introduction to the 5 Million Lives Campaign. Joint Commission Journal on Quality and Patient Safety. 2007;33(8):477–484.

MedQIC: Background. Available at http://medquic.org/dcs/ContentServer?pagename=Medquic/MQGeneralPageTemplate&name=Background. Accessed 1/06/08a.

MedQIC. Welcome to MedQIC. Available at http://medqic.org/dcs/ContentServer?pagename=Medqic/MQPage/Homepage. Accessed 1/15/08b.

MN Community Measurement. Our community approach. Available at: http://www.mnhealthcare.org/~wwd.cfm. Accessed 12/30/07.

National Committee for Quality Assurance. About NCQA. Available at: http://web.ncqa.org/tabid/65/Default.aspx. Accessed 1/06/08a.

National Committee for Quality Assurance. Create report card. Available at http://hprc.ncqa.org/frameset.asp. Accessed 1/06/08b

National Committee for Quality Assurance. Physician directory and search. Available at http://recognition.ncqa.org/. Accessed 1/06/08c.

Nolan TW. Execution of strategic improvement initiatives to produce system-level results. IHI Innovation Series White Paper. Cambridge, MA: Institute for Healthcare Improvement. 2007.

Physician Quality Reporting Initiative (PQRI) coding and reporting principles. MLN Matters. MM5640. Available at http://www.cms.hss.gov/PQRI/31_PQRI-Toolkit.asp. Accessed 5/18/07.

PT Bulletin Online. PTs need to be involved in the evolution of "medical home" model. 2007;8(46). http://www.apta.org/AM/Template.cfm?Section=Archives2&Template=/Customsource/TaggedPage/PTIssue.cfm&Issue=11/06/2007#article44015. Accessed 12/18/07.

Reinertsen JL, Gosfield AG, Rupp W, Whittington JW. Engaging physicians in a shared quality agenda. Available at http://www.IHI.org. Accessed 12/30/07.

Reinertsen JL, Pugh MD, Bisognano M. Seven leadership leverage points for organization-level improvement in health care. Available at http://www.ihi.org/NR/rdonlyres/C84E1503-C05E-4D1B-B8D5-C74CEFE68F7F/0/LeadershipWhitePaper2005.Pdf. Accessed 1/06/08.

Reproductive Health. Frequently asked questions about performance improvement. Available at http://www.reproline.jhu.edu/english/6read/6pi/pi_FAQ.htm. Accessed 1/14/08.

Therapeutic Associates. Care Connections Outcome System (formerly TAOS). Available at http://www.therapeuticassociates.com/Tools/CCOutcomes.aspx. Accessed 1/18/08.

URAC. About URAC. Available at: http://www.urac.org/about/. Accessed 1/06/08a.

URAC. Health provider credentialing accreditation program overview. Available at http://www.urac.org/programs/prog_accred_HProvider_po.aspx?navid=accreditation&pagename=prog_accred_HProvider. Accessed 1/15/08b.

Wood DS. An expensive idea who's time may have come. Available at http://www.cnn.com/SPECIALS/2000/democracy/doctors.under.the.knife/stories/medicare.drug.benefit/index.html. Accessed 12/31/07.

ADDITIONAL RESOURCES

For more information on the Stand Up and be Strong program contact the Minnesota Chapter of the APTA at http://www.mnapta.org. Related to PQRI, CMS has tool kit to enhance the likelihood of receiving a 1.5% bonus available at: http://www.cms.hhs.gov/PQRI/31_PQRITool Kit.asp#TopOfPage. Also, the APTA has a discussion of PQRI and example forms. See http://www.apta.org/AM/Template.cfm?Section=Coding_Billing&Template=/

TaggedPage/TaggedPageDisplay.cfm&TPLID=343&ContentID=45337. A listing of QIOs by state is available at http://www.medqic.org/dcs/ContentServer?pagename=Medqic/MQGeneralPage/GeneralPageTemplate&name=QIO%20Listings.

For assessment forms related to PQRI see: http://www.apta.org/AM/Template.cfm?Section=Coding_Billing&Template=/TaggedPage/TaggedPageDisplay.cfm&TPLID=343&ContentID=45337. An article that includes several quality improvement initiatives involving PTs and PTAs is: Muir J. The quest for quality. PTMagizine. 2004;12(7):50–57. There are templates on the IHI website to assist with designing, executing, and documenting a quality management project. See http://www.ihi.org/ihi/workspace/tracker/.

PART IV

Business Acumen: Human Resources, Marketing, and Selling

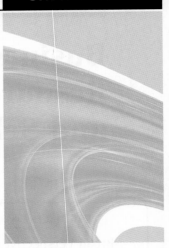

CHAPTER 17

EMPLOYMENT LAW

DEBORAH G. FRIBERG

Learning Objectives

1. Describe the U.S. regulatory environment impacting human resource management.
2. Identify the major federal laws impacting human resource management.
3. Summarize management's role and responsibility to ensure compliance with applicable employment law.
4. Describe the potential impact of regulatory noncompliance.
5. Describe some of the basic do's and don'ts impacting the management of routine personnel activities.
6. Apply legally supportable management principles in example personnel case studies.

Introduction

This chapter is a continuation of legislative actions that affect health care organizations and their employees. Chapter 8 dealt with administrative law with the focus on state licensure acts. Chapter 9 introduced the general process of the formation and implementation of laws and focused mostly on laws that apply to all businesses. Chapter 10 advanced the discussion by addressing oversight regulations associated with government health care programs, particularly those of the Department of Health and Human Services and its agencies especially the Centers for Medicare and Medicaid Services. The current chapter

focuses on federal and state laws that regulate the actions of management toward potential and current employees. These laws include those dealing with all aspects of employment and personnel matters such as equal rights, discrimination, and leaves of absence. This information is relevant to Boards of Directors, managers, and individual health care practitioners because breaches of personnel laws can result in huge fines.

The four chapters in this book dealing with legal matters underscore the authors' and others (Conover, 2002) belief that health services is one of the most heavily regulated sectors of the U.S. economy. The fact is, most of the activities of health care providers are regulated in some way. Employment practices are certainly no exception. Regulation of employment practices starts with the formulation of a law. Laws governing employment practices may come from the federal, state, or local level of government. The legislative process of formulating federal laws involves the U.S. Congress. This process was presented in Chapter 9, Figure 9.1. Once enacted, a law is implemented and enforced through the promulgation of regulations (Chapter 8). A regulation carries the force of the law issued by a federal or state agency (Nolan and Nolan-Haley, 1990) or independent regulatory bodies (Longest et al., 2000).

This chapter will discuss the types of regulations that govern the employer–employee relationship. Many of these regulations extend to potential employees as well as past employees. A sampling of pertinent laws that impact

Key terms, which are defined below, are bolded and italicized the first time they appear in the chapter. Other important terms are shown in boldface on first appearance and are defined by the context in which they are used. When either of these types of terms is used several times, its acronym will be identified and subsequently used in the chapter. Both types of terms are listed alphabetically in the online glossary with their definitions and (when applicable) their acronyms.

Age Discrimination in Employment Act of 1967 (ADEA): prohibits employment discrimination against persons 40 years of age or older applies to employers with 20 or more employees, employment agencies, employees and job applicants with respect to any term, condition, or privilege of employment, including hiring, firing, promotion, layoff, compensation, benefits, job assignments, and training federal, state, and local governments, and labor organizations.

Civil Rights Act of 1991: Title VII prohibits employment discrimination based on race, color, religion, sex, and national origin and provides for the recovery of compensatory and punitive damages in cases of intentional violations.

Comprehensive Omnibus Budget Reconciliation Act of 1985 (COBRA): a multipart act that includes a provision mandating that employers allow for the continuation of employee health care provisions (health care insurance) at cost after termination of employment.

disability: Titles I and V of the ADA prohibits employment discrimination against qualified individuals with disabilities. A person with a disability is one who has had a record of, or is regarded to have a physical or mental impairment that substantially limits one or more major life activities.

employment law: laws that deal with the rights and obligations that exist between employer and current employees, job applicants, and former employees. These complex relationships include issues as diverse as discrimination, wrongful termination, wages and taxation, and workplace safety.

Equal Employment Opportunity Commission (EEOC): a federally appointed five-member Commission that makes equal employment opportunity policy and approves most litigation.

Equal Pay Act of 1963: a part of the FLSA that prohibits sex-based wage discrimination between men and women in similar positions.

Glass Ceiling Act: this act is part of the Civil Rights Act of 1991 that amended the laws enforced by the Equal Employment Opportunity Commission and established the Glass Ceiling Commission to study the existence of artificial barriers to the advancement of women and minorities in the workplace, and to make recommendations for overcoming such barriers.

Occupational Safety and Health Act (OHS Act): regulates the safety and health conditions in most private industries and public sector employers. Employers are required to provide a workplace and work free from recognized serious hazards.

Older Workers Benefit Protection Act Of 1990 (OWBPA): amended the ADEA. It prohibits employers from denying benefits to older employees in most cases. In limited circumstances, an employer may be permitted to reduce benefits based on age as long as the reduction is not less than the cost of providing benefits to younger workers.

Pregnancy Discrimination Act: an amendment to Title II of the Civil Rights Act that prohibits discrimination on the basis of pregnancy, childbirth, and related medical conditions.

qualified employee or applicant with a disability: related to ADA. A person who, with or without reasonable accommodation, can perform the essential functions of the job in question.

reasonable accommodation: related to ADA. Qualified applicants or employees may request that an employer make some adjustments in the workplace such as: (1) making facilities accessible and usable, (2) job restructuring, (3) work schedule modification, (4) reassignment, (5) workplace modifications, (6) training, (7) accommodations for examination, for example, more time, and provide readers or interpreters.

Section 1921 of the Social Security Act (Section 5(b) of PL 100-93): is the Medicare and Medicaid Patient and Program Protection Act of 1987 that is related to the National Practitioners Data Bank.

sexual harassment: per Title VII of the Equal Rights Act prohibits workplace practices ranging from workplace conditions that create a hostile environment for persons of either gender. This includes same sex harassment to direct requests for sexual favors.

(Continued)

Title VII of the Civil Rights Act: prohibits employment discrimination based on race, color, religion, sex, and national origin and provides for the recovery of compensatory and punitive damages in cases of intentional violations.

Titles I and V of the Americans with Disabilities Act of 1990 (ADA): Titles I and V deal with employment discrimination and wire or radio communications (for hearing and speech impaired), respectively.

undue hardship: related to the ADA. An employer is required to make a reasonable accommodation to the known disability of a qualified applicant or employee unless doing so would cause significant difficulty or expense that would harm the operation of the employer's business.

Uniformed Services Employment and Reemployment Rights Act: an act that gives the right to certain persons who serve in the armed forces, such as those called up from the reserves or National Guard, to reemployment with the employer they were with when they entered service.

employers will be discussed. Employers of all sizes and structures are subject to employment laws but the impacts may differ based on the size and number of persons employed. In large health care organizations, the complexity of job-related legislation is best understood by organizational legal staff and the human resources department. The latter department is intimately involved with all departments' recruitment and hiring processes. Nonetheless, clinical managers and staff have many opportunities for informal and formal contact with potential employees. As will be discussed, there are very specific legal requirements that guide recruitment, interview, selection, and advancement procedures. In large health care organizations, a strong relationship between the departments of human resources and physical therapy will aid in complying with personnel laws. Failure to adhere to the law certainly has undesirable consequences for employers.

Important Note: The intent of this chapter is to provide a starting point for health care providers new to the practice and business of health care. Readers should be aware that regulatory requirements do change frequently. Every health care provider and manager is responsible for being knowledgeable and compliant with the laws and related regulations that apply to their situation. Ignorance is not an excuse for noncompliance (Chapter 8). Organizations, their directors, managers, and individual providers need to stay current with regulatory requirements at all times. This can be accomplished through

- Self-study
- Participation in professional associations or other networks of knowledgeable managers

- Consultation with available internal resources such as human resources, accounting, corporate compliance, risk management, internal audit, and legal counsel
- Consultation with external organizations or professionals in law, financial management, accounting, and human resources.

An examination of the legislative and regulatory requirements to operate a health care business is part of the environmental assessment that management continually engages in to protect and advance the organization (Chapter 3). This chapter provides a sampling of information about employment law relevant to physical therapist (PT) managers, practice owners, and those they manage or employ, respectively. When there are employment law concerns, practicing managers, individual providers, and employees should seek the input or representation of individuals or organizations that offer legal expertise in this area.

Responsibility for Compliance

Employment law applies to the rights and obligations that exist between employer and current employees, job applicants, and former employees. Because employment relationships can be complex, employment law covers issues as diverse as discrimination, wrongful termination, wages and taxation, and workplace safety. According to the *Equal Employment Opportunity Commission (EEOC)* (2008a) and the Department of Labor (DOL) (DOL, 2008a), employee rights include but are not limited to:

1. A workplace free of dangerous conditions, toxic substances, and other potential safety hazards

2. Fair wages for work performed
3. Freedom from discrimination and harassment of all types
4. Freedom from retaliation for filing a claim or complaint against an employer
5. Privacy

Employers have an obligation to follow federal and, where applicable, state and local employment and labor laws. The current social environment is focused on corporate responsibility. The ultimate responsibility for regulatory compliance rests with the senior leadership of the organization (Chapters 5 and 9). The Board has legal obligations to the:

• Corporation, stockholders, and its members (fiduciary duties)
• Government
• People or organizations with whom the corporation interacts

The Board can delegate their responsibility, but not the accountability, to meet these legal requirements to the Chief Executive Officer (CEO) and senior leadership. However, all managers and employees must be knowledgeable of compliance requirements, risks, and ways to avoid compliance violations. To protect themselves, health care businesses must take an organized approach to regulatory compliance.

It is in its value statements that an organization can best define its commitment to honest and ethical business practices. Value statements should be updated periodically to keep in sync with business and regulatory changes. Supported by organizational values that promote honest and ethical business practices and a strategic planning process that evaluates applicable regulatory requirements as an essential element of the internal environment, ongoing regulatory compliance can best be achieved though the establishment of a dynamic corporate compliance program (CCP). As discussed in Chapter 9, a CCP is designed to help mitigate risks of intentional or unintentional regulatory noncompliance. In 1991, the U.S. Sentencing Commission adopted sentencing policies and practices for organizations found guilty of a federal felony. These guidelines reflect the principle that organizations with effective compliance and ethics programs will receive lower **culpability scores** thus lessening the potential fines and penalties (Matyas and Valiant, 2006).

Culpability scores are a summation of points assigned for the grievousness of the offense minus points for mitigating factors like having an ethics program and additional points for the aggravating factors like failure to cooperate with investigators (McGreal, 2008). Like in golf, a high total score is undesirable.

Employment Regulation

Employment practices are regulated at all government levels: federal, state, and local. Regulation impacts all facets of employment practices including but not limited to:

• Recruitment, hire, and retention practices:
  Aliens authorized to work in the United States
  Applicant investigation
  Child labor
  Discriminatory practices
  Employee termination, rights and benefits
  Employment
  Equal employment opportunities
  Medical examinations
  Recruitment and recruitment advertising
  Retaliatory practices
• Compensation practices and levels requirements:
  Equal pay
  Minimum wage
  Overtime compensation
• Benefits plans:
  Continuation of employee health care insurance
  Retirement pension and welfare plans
• Occupational health and safety (Chapter 9)
• Compensation for employment injury or illness (Chapter 9)
• Family and medical leave of absence (Chapter 9)
• Military service leave of absence and reemployment (Chapter 9)

Federal Employment Regulations

The EEOC is responsible for the administration of several federal laws including:

• *Title VII of the Civil Rights Act* as amended in 1991 prohibits employment discrimination based on race, color, religion, sex, and national origin. It also provides for the recovery of compensatory and punitive damages in cases of intentional violations of Title VII, the Americans with Disabilities Act of 1990, and section 501 of the Rehabilitation Act of 1973 (EEOC, 2008a). Title VII applies to:

Employers with 15 or more employees
Employment agencies
Federal, state, and local governments
Labor organizations

Title VII also addresses sex-based discrimination related to *sexual harassment* and **pregnancy-based discrimination**. Sexual harassment covers practices ranging from workplace conditions that create a hostile environment for persons of either gender (including same sex harassment) to direct requests for sexual favors. Amended by the *Pregnancy Discrimination Act*, Title VII prohibits discrimination on the basis of pregnancy, childbirth, and related medical conditions (EEOC, 2008a). PT managers and practice owners are encouraged to pursue a deeper understanding of this act given that the majority of PT members are women (APTA, 2007).

- *Equal Pay Act of 1963*, a part of the Fair Labor Standards Act (FLSA), prohibits sex-based wage discrimination between men and women. To be subject to this equal pay provision jobs do not need to be identical. Job titles do not need to be the same. They must be substantially equal in job content. This applies to jobs that are "substantially equal in the same establishment who are performing under similar working conditions" (EEOC, 2008b). Employers may not retaliate against an individual for opposing employment practices that discriminate based on sex or for filing charges, testifying, or participating in an investigation, proceeding, or litigation related to sex discrimination charge. It is of interest to note that 2007 data on APTA members in all employment settings, women earned approximately 88% of what their male peers earned. However, a large part of this income difference was attributed to women private practice owners compared to male owners (APTA, 2008a).
- *Age Discrimination in Employment Act of 1967 (ADEA)* applies to

Employers with 20 or more employees
Employment agencies

Employees and job applicants with respect to any term, condition, or privilege of employment, including hiring, firing, promotion, layoff, compensation, benefits, job assignments, and training Federal, state, and local governments
Labor organizations

This act "prohibits employment discrimination against persons 40 years of age or older" (EEOC, 2008c). It also covers retaliation for opposing age discrimination employment practices including filing an ADEA related charge, testifying, or participating in any way in an investigation, proceeding, or litigation. ADEA protections extend to apprenticeship programs, job notices and advertisements, pre-employment inquiries, benefits through the *Older Workers Benefit Protection Act Of 1990 (OWBPA)*. It also addresses the requirements for an employee to voluntarily waive their ADEA rights (EEOC, 2008b). Analysis of recent APTA demographic data highlights the importance of PT managers and employers acting with due diligence regarding employment matters with experienced staff applicants and staff members. More than 58% of APTA members report being 40 or older (APTA, 2008b). However, with the progressive increases in full retirement age, more mature PTs can be expected to work for longer periods of time.

- *Rehabilitation Act of 1973* has two sections. Section 501 prohibits employment discrimination against individuals with disabilities in the federal sector. Section 505 contains provisions governing remedies and attorney's fees under Section 501 (EEOC, 2008d).
- *Titles I and V of the Americans with Disabilities Act of 1990 (ADA)* prohibits employment discrimination against qualified individuals with disabilities (Chapter 9). The ADA applies to:

Employers with 15 or more employees
Employment agencies
Federal (Section 501 of the Rehabilitation Act), state, and local governments
Labor organizations

Qualified employees and job applicants with respect to any terms, conditions, and privileges of employment including job application procedures, hiring, firing, advancement, compensation, and job training.

Retaliation for opposing age discrimination employment practices including filing an ADA related charge, testifying, or participating in any way in an investigation, proceeding, or litigation.

ADA protections extend to medical examinations, inquiries, and drug and alcohol abuse. An employer is required to make a reasonable accommodation to the known disability of a qualified applicant or employee if it would not impose an undue hardship on the operation of the employer's business. The EEOC (2008e) provides clear definitions of its key terms. For example:

An **individual with a** *disability* is a person who has, has had a record of, or is regarded to have a physical or mental impairment that substantially limits one or more major life activities.

A *qualified employee or applicant with a disability* is a person who, with or without reasonable accommodation, can perform the essential functions of the job in question.

Reasonable accommodation may include, but is not limited to making facilities accessible and usable, job restructuring, work schedule modification, reassignment, workplace modifications, training, accommodations for examination, and the provision of readers or interpreters.

Undue hardship is an action that would require significant difficulty or expense. When evaluating undue hardship, the employer's size, financial resources, and the nature and structure of its operation are considered. Employers are not required to make accommodations that would negatively impact their products or services nor are they required to provide personal items such as glasses or hearing aids.

- *Civil Rights Act of 1991* amended the laws enforced by the EEOC and established the *Glass Ceiling Act* (EEOC, 2007a). This act is particularly relevant for employers of women and minorities. The Glass Ceiling Act set up the Glass Ceiling Commission to study the existence of artificial barriers to the advancement of women and minorities in the workplace, and to make recommendations for overcoming such barriers (EEOC, 2007b). Clear written job descriptions, the

use of valid evaluation instruments reliably administered, consistency in scoring job-related criteria, and equal access to resources are organizational means of complying with this act. The private health care industry is one of the industries in which women are likely to attain managerial positions (EEOC, 2007c).

Noncompliance in any of the above areas can result in an employee filing charges with the EEOC. If found to be noncompliant, a business can be awarded significant monetary penalties. Table 17.1 provides EEOC, fiscal year 2006 statistics for numbers of charges made, the outcomes, and the costs to employers. While these EEOC statistics show that most of the filed claims are resolved with no cause being found, employers still bear the legal and administrative costs of defending their actions.

The DOL is responsible for the administration of several federal laws related to employment and employee compensation, benefits, safety, health and welfare. Many of the DOL administered laws may impact health care organizations and their employees (DOL, 2007a, 2008a). These laws include:

- The **Fair Labor Standards Act (FLSA)** sets standards for wages and overtime pay that affect most private and public employers. The Wage and Hour Division of the Employment Standards Administration administers FLSA (DOL, 2008b). The FLSA requires employers to pay covered employees who are not otherwise exempt at least the **federal minimum wage** and **overtime pay** of one-and-one-half-times the regular rate of pay. It also restricts the hours that children under the age of 16 can work and prohibits employment of persons under age 18 in certain nonagricultural operations jobs deemed too dangerous. While PTs are exempt from FLSA, physical therapist assistants (PTA) are not (APTA, 2008c).

The **Immigration and Nationality Act** enforces labor standards provisions that apply to aliens authorized to work in the United States under certain nonimmigrant visa programs. These standards could apply to the recruitment and employment of PTs or other professionals who may be foreign nationals (DOL, 2008c) (Chapter 1). See Additional Resources section for more specific information.

Table 17.1   EEOC 2006 Statistics Discrimination Charges, Resolutions, and Monetary Benefits Settlements

Category	Charges Received	Charges Resolved	Monetary Benefits Recovered[a]
Age	16,548	14,146	$ 51,500,000
Disability	15,575	15,045	$ 622,600,000
Equal pay	861	748	$ 36,100,000
National origin	8,327	8,181	$ 21,200,000
Pregnancy	4,901	4,629	$ 10,400,000
Race	27,238	25,992	$ 61,400,000
Religion	2,524	2,384	$ 5,700,000
Retaliation[b]	22,740	24,757	$ 90,000,000
Sex	23,247	23,364	$ 99,100,000
Sexual Harassment[c]	12,025	11,936	$ 48,800,000
Total	133,986	131,182	$ 1,046,800,000

[a] Not including monetary benefits recovered through litigation.
[b] 2004 data.
[c] 15% of charges received from males.
Source: EEOC, 2008b–f.

- The **Occupational Safety and Health Act (OSH Act)** regulates the safety and health conditions in most private industries and public sector employers. Employers have a general duty under the OSH Act to provide a workplace and work that is free from recognized, serious hazards (DOL, 2008d). Employers must comply with the regulations and the safety and health standards promulgated by the **Occupational Safety and Health Administration (OSHA)**. OSHA uses workplace inspection and investigation, compliance assistance, and cooperative programs as enforcement mechanisms. An example of how OSHA impacts health care workers is in the workplace requirements to prevent contact with blood born pathogens (DOL, 2007b) and support for workplace substance abuse programs (DOL, 2007c). There is a DOL website link for employers (DOL, 2008e) and one specifically for hospital physical therapy settings (DOL, 2007d). The latter site provides an online safety training module that covers blood born pathogens, electrical equipment, ergonomics, hazardous chemicals, slips and falls, and other potential workplace dangers.
- The **Federal Employees' Compensation Act (FECA)**, which is administered by the **Office of Workers' Compensation Programs (OWCP)**, establishes a comprehensive and exclusive workers' compensation program

that pays compensation for the disability or death of a federal employee resulting from personal injury sustained while in the performance of duty (DOL, 2008f). The FECA provides:

Benefits for wage loss compensation for total or partial disability

Schedule of awards for permanent loss or loss of use of specified members of the body, related medical costs, and vocational rehabilitation

This act pertains only to federal employees and agencies. Workers injured while employed by private companies, or by state and local government agencies, deal with their state workers' compensation board.

- The **Employee Retirement Income Security Act (ERISA)** as amended by the **Pension Protection Act of 2006** regulates employers who offer pension or welfare benefit plans for their employees. Title I of ERISA is administered by the **Pension and Welfare Benefits Administration (PWBA)**. ERISA deals with fiduciary matters, i.e., the duty of trustees to act primarily for another's benefit (Nolan and Nolan-Haley, 1990). It imposes a wide range of fiduciary, disclosure, and reporting requirements on fiduciaries of pension and welfare benefit plans and on others having dealings with these plans (DOL, 2008g).

- The **Comprehensive Omnibus Budget Reconciliation Act of 1985 (COBRA)** has several parts. Among the provisions, this law mandates that employers allow for the continuation of employee health care provisions (health care insurance) after termination of employment. The law does not address who pays the cost (DOL, 2008h). An example case where this act applies is when an employee retires prior to being eligible for Medicare. A common arrangement would be for the employee to continue in the employer's group health care plan if they pay the full cost of the plan out of pocket.
- The **Family and Medical Leave Act (FMLA)** is administered by the Wage and Hour Division of the Employment Standards Administration (DOL, 2008i). The FMLA applies to employers of 50 or more employees. It requires employers to allow up to 12 weeks of unpaid, job-protected leave to eligible employees for the birth or adoption of a child or for the serious illness of the employee or a spouse, child or parent. While this law is beneficial for employees, their absence can create a significant financial and operational hardship for employers who must often allow for the use of earned sick leave benefits or work shorthanded. In physical therapy organizations, it is common that the remaining staff members would absorb the work of the member or members on leave. This places everyone in the work setting under additional stress. For example, vacation days may have to be postponed, waiting lists can accrue when patient volume increases, continuing education leave may have to be postponed, and new programs are likely put on hold.
- The **Immigration and Nationality Act** is administered by the Wage and Hour Division of the Employment Standards Administration (DOL, 2008c). It requires employers who want to use foreign temporary workers (for less than a year) on H-2A visas to get a labor certificate from the **Employment and Training Administration** certifying that there are not sufficient, able, willing and qualified U.S. workers available to do the work. The provisions of this act must be met when recruiting foreign PTs or other health care professionals. There are also visas for those who want permanent residency to work in the United States. See

Chapter 1 and Additional Resources section for more information on this topic.
- The *Worker Adjustment and Retraining Notification Act (WARN)* requires that employees receive early warning of upcoming layoffs or facility closings. Employees must be provided with severance pay that covers the required notice period if notice is not given. WARN is enforced through the federal courts (DOL, 2008j).
- *Uniformed Services Employment and Reemployment Rights Act* is administered by the **Veterans' Employment and Training Service (VETS)** (DOL, 2008k). This act allows for certain persons who serve in the armed forces, such as those called up from the reserves or National Guard, to have a right to reemployment with the employer they were with when they entered service. As with FMLA, this law is designed to protect the employee but may cause a significant impact on the employer and/or coworkers, who may need to work shorthanded while the protected employee is away from the workplace. If someone is hired in place of the person on military duty they may be out of the job when that person returns.
- The **Americans with Disabilities Act (ADA)** (2007) has four parts:

1. Employment provisions
2. Communications provisions
3. Public accommodations
4. Transportation

These provisions are enforced by several federal agencies including the EEOC, Department of Justices' Civil Rights Division, Federal Communications Commission, and Department of Transportation. Of particular importance to employers are the employment provisions. These prohibit discrimination against a person with a qualified disability when the discrimination is attributable to the individual's disability. In addition, an employer is required to make reasonable accommodation to facilitate the employment or continued employment of a qualified applicant or employee, respectively (DOL, 2008l; Engel et al., 1996). Physical therapy managers should be well versed in the employment provisions of the ADA because health care industry workers have a high incidence of job-related injury and illness and the work is emotionally stressful (EEOC, 2008g). For more information, see the Additional Resources section.

- **Section 503 of the Rehabilitation Act of 1973** is enforced by the Employment Standards Administration's **Office of Federal Contract Compliance Programs (OFCCP)** within the Department of Labor (DOL, 2008m). This act prohibits businesses that contract or subcontract with the federal government for work exceeding $10,000 in payment from discriminating. This act is relevant to Medicare providers who receive this threshold amount. Contractors or subcontractors meeting this criterion must take affirmative action to hire, retain, and promote qualified individuals with disabilities. All covered contractors and subcontractors must include a specific equal opportunity clause in each of their nonexempt contracts and subcontracts.

  DOL's Office of Compliance Assistance Policy leads a variety of department-wide compliance assistance efforts. Its Web portal is designed to provide businesses, workers, and others with the knowledge and tools they need to comply with DOL's rules. See Additional Resources section for specific access information.

- **Health Insurance Portability and Accountability Act of 1996 (HIPAA)** is administered by the Centers for Medicare and Medicaid (CMS). The employment-related provisions of HIPAA are intended to "improve portability and continuity of health insurance coverage in the group and individual markets, to combat waste, fraud, and abuse in health insurance and health care delivery, to promote the use of medical savings accounts, to improve access to long-term care services and coverage, to simplify the administration of health insurance, and for other purposes" (Health and Human Service [HHS], 2007). Title I, Health Care Portability, and Renewability addressed the portability and continuity of health care insurance. It protects health insurance coverage for workers and their families when they change or lose their jobs. According to CMS (2007), this may help consumers:

  - Increase their ability to get health coverage when starting a new job
  - Lower the chance of losing existing health care coverage

- Maintain continuous health coverage when you change jobs
- Buy health insurance coverage on your own if coverage is lost

  HIPAA ensures these benefits by limiting the use of preexisting condition exclusions. It also prohibits group health plans from discriminating in coverage decisions based on past or present poor health. Importantly, it guarantees certain small employers and individuals the right to purchase health insurance. In most cases, employers or individuals who purchase health insurance can renew the coverage regardless of any health conditions of individuals covered under the insurance policy. In cases where someone has left a job or is between jobs, HIPAA and COBRA provide ways for them to continue health insurance coverage for themselves and their family. State laws may provide additional options. However, the cost sharing benefit from an employer is likely discontinued making the cost of continued health insurance being borne totally by the former employee (DOL, 2008n).

- **Title IV of P.L. 99-660, Health Care Quality Improvement Act of 1986** and the amendment of *Section 1921 of the Social Security Act (Section 5(b) of PL 100-93)*, the **Medicare and Medicaid Patient and Program Protection Act of 1987** deal with the *National Practitioner Data Bank (NPDB)*. The Department of Health and Human Services is the agency responsible for its administration. The NPDB was established to improve medical care by encouraging licensing boards, health care entities, and professional societies to identify and discipline individual providers who engage in "unprofessional behavior; and to restrict the ability of incompetent physicians, dentists, and other health care practitioners to move from state to state without disclosure or discovery of previous medical malpractice payment and adverse action history. Adverse actions can involve licensure, clinical privileges, professional society membership, and exclusions from Medicare and Medicaid" (NPDB, 2008a). The adverse action options used by NPDB are listed in Table 17.2. Certain employers may check on licensed applicants before they employ them. Licensing boards, health care organizations like hospitals, and profes-

Table 17.2 List of Adverse Actions: Individual Subjects and Health Care Plans

Related to Individual Clinical Privileges	Revisions to Clinical Actions
Revocation	Restored or Reinstated, Complete
Suspension	Restored or Reinstated, Conditional
Summary or Emergency Suspension	Restoration or Reinstatement Denied
Voluntary Limitation, Restriction, or Reduction while under, or to avoid, investigation	Reduction of Previous Action
Voluntary Surrender While Under, or to Avoid, Investigation	Extension of Previous Action
Summary or Emergency Limitation, Restriction, or Reduction	
Reduction Other Restriction/Limitation Denial	

Source: NPDB, 2008b.

sional organizations like the APTA, have a regulatory obligation to report to the NPDB. Other health care organizations that have a formal peer review process may also report (NPDB, 2008c). See Additional Resources section of this chapter.

State and Local Government Employment Law

State and local governments may also have employment laws and regulations. These may expand on federal law, such as extending anti-discrimination requirements to smaller employers, prohibit additional types of discrimination (e.g., sexual orientation, weight, or marital status), set minimum wage rates, or address other employment matters. For example, the Wisconsin "legislature finds that the practice of unfair discrimination in employment against properly qualified individuals by reason of their age, race, creed, color, disability, marital status, sex, national origin, ancestry, sexual orientation, arrest record, conviction record, membership in the national guard, state defense force or any other reserve component of the military forces of the United States or this state or use or nonuse of lawful products off the employer's premises during nonworking hours substantially and adversely affects the general welfare of the state" (Wisconsin Legislature, 2008). To learn about the antidiscrimination laws in your state, contact your state labor department or your state small business bureau. In addition, links to all 50 states, the District of Columbia and Puerto Rico employment laws and regulations can be found at http://www.law.cornell.edu/topics/Table_Labor.htm or DOL

Employment Standards Administration, Wage and Hour Division at http://www.dol.gov/esa/programs/whd/state/state.htm

Where an employment relationship is defined by a valid contractual agreement between employer and employee, state contract law safeguards the rights and duties of the parties (FindLaw for Small Business, 2008a).

Avoiding Trouble

Part of avoiding legal problems related to recruitment of employees is to have an organized advertisement, interview, hiring, and development process in place. An example process is shown in Figure 17.1.

Employers must be attentive to the requirements placed on them by federal, state, and local employment law and regulations. Employers are expected to follow federal, state, and local laws governing their relationships with their employees. According to FindLaw for Small Business (2008b), employers are expected to:

1. Follow proper hiring practices including:
   How to advertise
   How to conduct an interview
   How to investigate job applicants while protecting their privacy
2. Follow proper compensation practices such as:
   Minimum wage
   Overtime compensation
   Compensatory time
3. Avoid harassment and discrimination
4. Follow requirements for employee leave
5. Know how to conduct employee performance reviews and disciplinary actions

STEP 1

Define the work to be done.

STEP 2

Determine minimum requirements for any employee assigned the position.
- What physical abilities are required?
- What education is required and/or preferred?
- What knowledge and job skills does an entry-level employee require?
- What type of previous experience will an entry-level candidate require?
- What and how much previous experience will an entry-level candidate require?

STEP 3

Determine where the position fits in the organizational structure.
- Who will supervise the employee?
- Whom the employee will supervise?
- With which work teams will the employee work?

STEP 4

If this is a new position:
- Prepare a job description that reflects work to be done, minimum requirements, and organizational relationships. Include specific job competencies used to evaluate an employee's performance.
- Coordinate with human resources staff to get approval of the position description, determine the exemption status, assign a job code, set the compensation range, determine eligibility for other elements of the compensation and benefits plan, and obtain any needed approvals.

STEP 5

The department and human resources will collaborate to plan for candidate identification and the interview process. There are questions to be answered and responsibilities to be assigned to ensure that this part of the process goes smoothly. Interviewee training may be undertaken.
- How and when will qualified candidates be informed of the job opportunity?
- How and when will interested parties be instructed to respond?
- How and by whom will responses be screened?
- What criteria will be used to select candidates for interview?
- What interview expenses will be paid and out of what budget?
- Who will act as the point of communication with the interviewees?
- Who will schedule and coordinate the interview appointments?
- Who will participate in the interviews?
- What specific information will be shared with the interviewees and by whom?
- How will input be gathered and a candidate selected?
- Who will determine the specifics of the job offer?
- Who will make the job offer and negotiate with the selected candidate?
- Who will follow up with interested parties and interviewees when the interview process is completed?

STEP 6

Get new employees off to a good start.
- Develop a structured orientation plan.
- Prepare a work area with needed equipment, supplies, and reference materials.
- Assign a 'buddy' to help them through the first weeks of the new job.
- Keep the management door open so they can ask questions and get help.

Figure 17.1. A Six-step recruitment and hiring process.

6. Know how to terminate (voluntary, involuntary, or lay off) an employee without violating their legal rights
7. Know how to conduct workplace searches and employee monitoring

Job Advertisements

The American Bar Association (ABA) suggests that the goal should be to target qualified candidates without discriminating against any potential candidates. Words suggesting a race, age, sex, religious, or national origin preference should be avoided. For example, the use of the term "salesman" or "saleswomen" versus "salesperson" could be interpreted as sex discrimination. Reference to a "degree required" versus "recent graduate" would avoid the appearance of age discrimination. ABA also suggests that inclusion of the phrase "An Equal Opportunity Employer" in ads as it "implies that the employer will treat all applicants based solely on their qualification without regard to race, sex, religion, national origin, age or disability" (ABA, 2002).

Job Applicant Interviews

Job applicant interviews can be high risk for employers who are not prepared for employment law compliance. FindLaw for Small Business (2008c) suggests the following guiding principles that, when followed, will minimize risk and result in an acceptable interview process:

1. Employers should avoid any questions related to topics that the law prohibits them from considering in making an employment decision. Applicants can raise prohibited subjects but the employer cannot.
2. Respect the applicant's privacy. If federal law does not require the employer to do so, state or local laws may.
3. Don't exaggerate any facts or make promises you can't keep. Exaggerated reports about an organization's performance or future job security may lead to the risk of lawsuits for fraud or breach of contract.
4. Stay focused on the candidate's ability to perform the job.
5. Avoid making statements that might limit your right to make future personnel decisions. For example, a statement that "employees receive regular pay increases" may unintentionally obligate the business to provide that person, if hired, future increases even in the face of poor financial performance on the part of the company or poor performance on the part of the employee.
6. Use good taste in formulating interview questions. Avoid asking questions about things such as sexual preference, sex life, religious beliefs, political affiliations, family planning, or personal finances. This last item deserves more explanation. People with a history of having more debt then they can pay for might be tempted to defraud or steal. Employers, with written permission of an applicant, may check a job applicant's credit rating (Vault, 2008). This check is particularly common when an employee would have access to something of value to someone else (Weston, 2008). In the health care environment, things of value include patients' valuables, drugs, petty cash, records, and control of accounts. Judicious employers may check every applicant's credit, new graduates included. See Additional Resources section regarding the relevant law.

The use of an interview guide may help a prospective employer stay away from any prohibited questions or topics. There are ways to obtain information in a lawful way but doing so takes skill. There are several suggestions to prepare interviewers:

1. *Define the role of each interviewer.* Each interviewer should have a clear understanding of why he or she was selected to participate. For example, human resources may be involved to share information about compensation and benefits as well as to evaluate the character and fit of candidates.
2. *Prepare interviewers in advance.* Interviewers should be provided with information about each candidate and the selection criteria. They should also understand the type of feedback they will be expected to provide on each candidate interviewed.
3. *Interviewers should prepare and use standardized questions.* This will allow for a fair and accurate comparison of candidates.

A review of prohibited questions should be undertaken. In a group interview setting there should be a designated member who will intervene and rephrase any questions the others may broach that are inappropriate.

4. *Interviewers should prepare informational materials in advance.* If part of an interviewer's role is to provide candidates with specific information, then materials should be prepared and information shared in a consistent manner.

A well-planned interview will make the candidate selection process much easier as well as legally supportable. Candidates will have received the same information and responded to the same job-related questions.

Prevention Is Key

DelPo and Guerin (2005) suggest that employers can protect themselves from employment-related problems by treating employees well and handling employment problems as they arise. They provide employers with the following suggestions:

1. Treat employees with respect—employees who believe they have been treated poorly are more likely to seek recourse through the legal system. Moreover, if the evidence shows that they have been treated poorly, juries are more likely to treat their claims sympathetically.
2. Keep lines of communication open—employees will feel more valued and the employer is more likely to get an "early warning" when problems exist.
3. Be consistent—don't play favorites, treat everyone fairly and the same.
4. Evaluate employees regularly and honestly—it offers the opportunity to interact with employees on a regular basis and provides documentation of performance issues if action is taken.
5. Personnel decisions should be based solely on the job requirements—keep personal bias and/or personal considerations out of the equation.
6. Be careful not to punish an employee who brings a problem to your attention.

7. Adopt sound policies—share and follow them.
8. Keep good written records—in case you ever need to defend a personnel decision or action.
9. When problems arise, take action—fix a bad situation before it gets worse.
10. Protect employee privacy—give information regarding personnel matters to others on a need-to-know basis only.

Summary

This chapter focused on federal, state, and local laws that are most relevant to organizations that employ one or more persons. Many of the federal regulations apply to businesses that employ 15 or more employees. State and local laws often expand on federal legislation and can be more inclusive of employers with less than 15 employees. Employment laws apply to organizations of all types. A few regulations such as the establishment of the NPDB may apply specifically to the health care sector. In order to comply with regulatory requirements employers must become familiar with the sources and types of regulation impacting employment practices. There are many external and internal experts that can be of assistance. One of the keys to effective regulatory compliance is the adoption of an organized and consistent approach to regulatory compliance through a CCP. Failure to comply can result in civil and criminal prosecution. It is up to employers and managers to be knowledgeable about and comply with these laws and related regulations.

References

American Bar Association. Family Legal Guide. 2002. Available at http://www.abanet.org/publiced/practical/books/family_legal_guide/home.html. Accessed 2/14/08.

American Physical Therapy Association. Physical therapist member demographic profile 1999–2006. Available at http://www.apta.org/AM/Template.cfm?Section=Surveys_and_Stats1&Template=/MembersOnly.cfm&ContentID=46077. Accessed 12/27/07.

American Physical Therapy Association. 2007 median income of physical therapists summary report. Available at http://www.apta.org/AM/Template.cfm?Section=Surveys_and_Stats1&Template=/MembersOnly.cfm&ContentID=45849. Accessed 2/26/08a.

CASE STUDY 17.1

Worker Disciplined for Speaking Spanish

Background

Chez Ritz is a for-profit multistorey skilled nursing facility overlooking a large lake and well-tended gardens. Many residents pay for care from their own resources. The current census shows 100% of the residents are Caucasian. English is the preferred language of all residents. More than 50% of the patients have diagnosed cognitive deficits.

Inez, a rehabilitation aide/certified nursing assistant often spoke Spanish with a coworker during the workday as they passed each other in the halls. In the lunchroom at noon, Inez usually conversed in Spanish on the phone when she checked on her elderly non-English speaking mother. Both employees had satisfactory employment records.

The Issue

A recently hired nursing supervisor told the two Spanish-speaking employees that patients might become confused or agitated when they hear a language they do not understand. Patients might be distracted by the strange language and lose

their balance. Residents who are anxious may become more distracted because they do not understand what you are saying. She cited the organization's policy, which says that employees can speak any language that they choose privately outside of the workplace. She demanded that the coworkers stop speaking Spanish around patients. A reprimand was placed in both their personnel files.

The employees eventually quit. Inez filed a claim with a state and then a federal government agency.

Your Thoughts

1. List the possible legal issues you think this case reflects for the nursing supervisor and the organization.
2. Check your home state's agencies and federal regulations to support your choice.
3. What is the process for filing a claim with your state's agency?
4. What is the process for filing a claim with the appropriate federal agency?
5. What are the employees' rights?
6. What are the employer's rights?

CASE STUDY 17.2

Just a Little Thing

Here Is the Picture

Hooda Doneit is a contract therapist. She is filling in for a day in a private practice. She has never been to this facility before. Upon arrival, the office manager showed her the records for the day's patients. She also gave Hooda a very short explanation about documentation, coding for billing, and showed her commonly used pieces of exercise equipment and supplies.

Early in the day Hooda copied exercises for a patient's home exercise program.

While putting the handout together she sustained a staple puncture in her right (dominant hand) thumb. She squeezed the thumb to increase bleeding and blotted up the blood with tissue. She discarded the tissue in the copy room wastebasket. She carried the handout back to the patient with her dominant hand. On the back of the handout was a part of her thumbprint in blood. Hooda reviewed the home plan with the patient using both of her hands to correct the patient's performance. At the end

(Continued)

CASE STUDY 17.2

Just a Little Thing (continued)

of the treatment, they shook hands. Hooda washed her hands with a bar of soap and went to meet her next patient.

Review OSHA Regulations

1. Access and review the OSHA website regarding bloodborne pathogens.

2. Identify where Hooda's actions were below standards identified by OSHA.
3. Offer suggestions for the owner of the private practice regarding hiring contract therapists.

CASE STUDY 17.3

Think Before You Ask Questions

There are restrictions on questions that can be asked in the recruitment and hire process. Review three references to construct a list of 10 questions that might be interpreted as discriminatory under federal or state law. The categories you are to include are:

1. Sexual and marital discrimination, e.g., Do you have children?
2. Racial discrimination, e.g., Do you get darker in the summer?

3. Discrimination related to national origin, e.g., Is that a Middle Eastern name?
4. Religious discrimination, e.g., Are you a Christian?

Now, construct a list of 10 questions that are appropriate for an interview for a physical therapy position. You may choose any categories of questions related to a physical therapy inpatient position.

American Physical Therapy Association. Physical therapist member demographic profile 1999–2006. Available at http://www.apta.org/AM/Template.cfm?Section=Surveys_and_Stats1&Template=/MembersOnly.cfm&ContentID=46077. Accessed 2/26/08b.

American Physical Therapy Association. Summary of department of labor's final regulation under the fair labor standards act "fair pay rule." Available at http://www.apta.org/AM/Template.cfm?Section=Other_Issues&CONTENTID=18361&TEMPLATE=/CM/ContentDisplay.cfm. Accessed 2/26/08c.

Americans With Disabilities Act. A guide to disabilities rights laws, August, 2001. Available at http://ada.gov/cguide.htm. Accessed 8/15/07.

Centers for Medicare and Medicaid Services. Programs. Available from http://www.cms.hhs.gov. Accessed 8/10/07.

Conover CJ. Health care regulation, A $169 billion hidden tax. Policy Analysis, No.527, October 4, 2002.

Available at http://www.cato.org/pubs/pas/pa527.pdf. Accessed 8/10/07.

DelPo A, Guerin L. Everyday Employment Law: The Basics. Nolo, Berkley, CA. 2005. Available at http://www.nolo.com/article.cfm/objectId/9CDFC0B1-EDEA-4C78-A0F529405BEF37C4/111/259/CHK/. Accessed 2/22/08.

Department of Health and Human Services. Public Law 104-191. Available at http://aspe.hhs.gov/admnsimp/pl104191.htm. Accessed 8/15/07.

Department of Labor. Major laws. Available at http://www.dol.gov/opa/aboutdol/lawsprog.htm. Accessed 8/10/07a.

Department of Labor. Bloodborne pathogens and needle-stick prevention. Available at http://osha.gov/SLTC/bloodbornepathogens/index.html. Accessed 8/10/07b.

Department of Labor. Workplace substance abuse. Available at http://www.osha.gov/SLTC/substanceabuse/index.html. Accessed 8/10/07c.

Department of Labor. Hospital e-tool: Physical therapy

module. Available at http://www.osha.gov/SLTC/etools/hospital/clinical/pt/pt.html. Accessed 8/10/07d.

Department of Labor. Our mission. Available at http://www.dol.gov/opa/aboutdol/mission.htm. Accessed 2/25/08a.

Department of Labor. Fair Labor Standards Act (FLSA). Available at http://www.dol.gov/esa/whd/flsa/. Accessed 2/14/08b.

Department of Labor. Immigration and Nationality Act. Available at http://www.dol.gov/compliance/laws/comp-ina.htm. Accessed 2/14/08c.

Department of Labor. The Occupational Safety and Health Act of 1970 (OSH act). Available at http://www.dol.gov/compliance/guide/osha.htm. Accessed 2/26/08d.

Department of Labor. Find it! By audience-employers. Available at http://www.dol.gov/dol/audience/aud-employers.htm. Accessed 2/27/08e.

Department of Labor. Federal Employees' Compensation Act (FECA). Available at http://www.dol.gov/compliance/laws/comp-osha.htm. Accessed 2/14/08f.

Department of Labor. Employee Retirement Income Security Act (ERISA). Available at http://www.dol.gov/ebsa/compliance_assistance.html. Accessed 2/14/08g.

Department of Labor. Comprehensive Omnibus Budget Reconciliation Act of 1985 (COBRA). Available at http://www.dol.gov/opa/aboutdol/lawsprog.htm. Accessed 2/14/08h.

Department of Labor. Compliance assistance—Family and Medical Leave Act (FMLA). Available at http://www.dol.gov/esa/whd/fmla/. Accessed 2/14/08i.

Department of Labor. Worker Adjustment and Retr... Notification Act (WARN). Available at h... dol.gov/compliance/laws/comp-warn... 2/14/08j.

Department of Labor. Uniformed ... and Reemployment Rights Act... www.dol.gov/vets/programs/userr... pdf. Accessed 2/14/08k.

Department of Labor. Americans with ... (ADA). Available at http://www.dol.go... laws/comp-rehab.htm. Accessed 2/14/08...

Department of Labor. Section 503 of the Rehab... of 1973. Available at http://www.dol.gov/co... laws/comp-rehab.htm. Accessed 2/14/08m.

Department of Labor. Retirement and health care cov-erage: Q & A's for dislocated workers. Available at http://www.dol.gov/ebsa/publications/dislocated_workers_brochure.html. Accessed 2/29/08n.

Engel DA, Calderone BJ, Lederman BG, Wesolik CJ, War-nick MP. Human resources issues. In Health Insurance Portability and Accountability Act of 1996 Public Law 104-191 August 21, 1996. Available at http://aspe.dhhs.gov/admnsimp/pl104191.htm. Accessed 8/15/07.

Equal Employment Opportunity Commission. Civil Rights Act of 1991. Available at http://www.eeoc.gov/policy/cra91.html. Accessed 11/12/07a

Equal Employment Opportunity Commission. An act. Available at http://www.eeoc.gov/abouteeoc/35th/thelaw/cra_1991.html. Accessed 1/12/07b.

Equal Employment Opportunity Commission. Glass ceil-ings: The status of women as officials and managers in the private sector. Available at http://www.eeoc.gov/stats/reports/glassceiling/index.html. Accessed 1/12/07c.

Equal Employment Opportunity Commission. Title VII of the Civil Rights Act of 1964. Available at http://www.eeoc.gov/policy/vii.html. Accessed 2/14/08a.

Equal Employment Opportunity Commission. Equal pay and compensation discrimination. Available at http://www.eeoc.gov/types/epa.html. Accessed 2/14/08b.

Equal Employment Opportunity Commission. Age Dis-crimination in Employment Act of 1967 (ADEA). Available at http://www.eeoc.gov/policy/adea.html. Accessed 2/14/08c.

Equal Employment Opportunity Commission. Rehabili-tation Act of 1973, Sections 501 and 505. Available at http://www.eeoc.gov/policy/rehab.html. Accessed 2/14/08d.

Equal Employment Opportunity Commission. Titles I and V of the Americans with Disabilities Act of 1990 (ADA). Available at http://www.eeoc.gov/policy/ada.html. Accessed 2/14/08e.

Equal Employment Opportunity Commission. Enforce-ment statistics and litigation. Available at http://www.eeoc.gov/stats/enforcement.html. Accessed 3/02/08f.

Equal Employment Opportunity Commission. Questions and answers about health care workers and the Amer-icans with Disabilities Act. Available at http://www.eeoc.gov/facts/health_care_workers.html. Accessed 2/27/08g.

...aw for Small Business. Employment law and human ...urces. Available at http://smallbusiness.findlaw. ...mployment-employer/. Accessed 2/14/08a.

...r Small Business. Employer right's and responsi-...vailable at http://smallbusiness.findlaw.com/ ...nt-employer/employment-employer-over-...yment-employer-overview-responsibili-...ccessed 2/14/08b.

...Small Business. Conducting job inter-...Available at http://smallbusiness.findlaw.-.../employment-employer/employment-employer-hiring/employment-employer-hiring-interview-legal.html. Accessed 2/14/08c.

Longest BB Jr, Rakich JS, Darr K. Managing health serv-ices organizations and systems, 4th ed. Baltimore, MD: Health Professions. 2000.

Matyas DE, Valiant C. Legal issues in healthcare fraud and abuse: Navigating uncertainties, 3rd ed. Washington, DC: American Health Lawyers Association. 2006.

McGreal PE. Sentencing commission to study privi-lege waiver issue. Available at http://lawprofessors.typepad.com/compliance_prof/2005/08/sentencing_comm.html. Accessed 3/01/08.

National Practitioner Data Bank (NPDB). General infor-mation. Available at http://www.npdb-hipdb.hrsa.gov/npdb.html. Accessed 2/14/08a.

National Practitioner Data Bank. Adverse action clas-sification codes – Individual subjects. Available at http://www.npdb-hipdb.hrsa.gov/pubs/codes/Code_

List-Adverse_Action_Classification_Individual.pdf. Accessed 3/02/08b.

National Practitioner Data Bank. What is an eligible entity? Available at http://www.npdb-hipdb.hrsa.gov/pubs/gb/NPDB_Guidebook_Chapter_B.pdf. Accessed 2/29/08c.

Nolan JR, Nolan-Haley JM. Black's Law Dictionary, 6th ed. St. Paul, MN: West. 1990.

Vault. Can potential employers check your credit? Available at http://www.vault.com/nr/newsmain.jsp?nr_page=3&ch_id=420&article_id=14821453&cat_id=1691. Accessed 2/29/08.

Weston LP. The basics: How bad credit can cost you a job. Available at http://moneycentral.msn.com/content/Banking/Yourcreditrating/P87306.asp. Accessed 2/29/08/.

Wisconsin Legislature. Fair employment. Available at http://nxt.legis.state.wi.us/nxt/gateway.dll?f=templates&fn=default.htm&vid=WI:Default&d=stats&jd=111.31. Accessed 3/31/08.

ADDITIONAL RESOURCES

Current information about the various federal government Internet sites noted in this chapter may be found at the following sites: DOL http://www.dol.gov, DOL Employment Law Guide available at http://www.dol.gov/compliance/guide; HRSA http://www.hrsa.gov; and OSHA http://www.osha.gov. A candid analysis of the glass ceiling (women), the adobe ceiling (Hispanics), and the concrete wall (African-Americans) in the United States corporate environment can be accessed at http://www.dol.gov/esa/media/reports/ofccp/newgc.htm. EEOC's regulations are published annually in Title 29 of the Code of Federal Regulations (CFR). Internet links to EEOC's regulations can be found at http://www.eeoc.gov/policy/regs/index.html. A helpful book for managers who have challenging staff members is DelPo A, Guerin L. Dealing with Problem Employees: A Legal Guide, 4th ed. Berkeley, CA: Nolo. 2007. The EEOC has recently produced an ADA guide sheet specifically for the health care industry. PTs sustain injuries on and off the job as well as illnesses. For relevant guidance on continued employment there is a questions and answers sheet about health care workers and the Americans with Disabilities Act. It may be accessed at http://www.eeoc.gov/facts/health_care_workers.html. To review certification information for noncitizen health care workers see http://www.uscis.gov/portal/site/uscis/menuitem. There are several DOL sites that may provide problem specific information. These include the DOL's Office of Compliance at http://www.dol.gov/compliance and the DOL Employment Law Guide at http://www.dol.gov/compliance/guide. To check your own record or to learn more about the NPDB go to http://www.npdb-hipdb.hrsa.gov/npdb.html. For your own information, you should become familiar with the Fair Credit Reporting Act. A concise summary is available at http://www.yale.edu/hronline/careers/screening/documents/FairCreditReporting Act.pdf. Another comprehensive legal information site is the Cornell Law School Legal Information Institute. Laws by topic. Available at http://www.law.cornell.edu/topics/Table_Labor.htm.

CHAPTER 18

MARKETING BASICS

DEBORAH G. FRIBERG

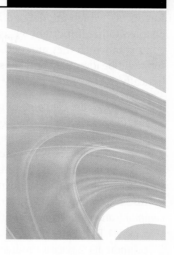

Learning Objectives

1. Become familiar with basic marketing concepts.
2. Understand the scope of activities that comprise the marketing process.
3. Describe the concept of product life cycle and how it applies to physical therapy.
4. Provide examples of a physical therapy target market, market segment, and niche market.
5. In your own words, define the 7P components in a service marketing mix.
6. Distinguish between a service marketing mix and the components of a communications mix.
7. Given physical therapy case studies, apply marketing concepts, utilize the 7Ps of service marketing mix, and develop a compatible communications mix.

Introduction

The concept of *marketing* is often approached from the viewpoint of the business and its need to sell its services and/or products. The process of finding *customers*, individuals, or groups who directly or indirectly may need or want to use a service or product is the foundation of a "selling" marketing philosophy (Kotler, 2000; Levitt, 1960). Drucker (1954) would encourage a different point of view. He advocates that the purpose of any business is to create customers because it is customers who are the "foundation of its business and

what keeps it in existence" (Drucker, 1954, p. 37). Because its purpose is to create customers, a business should have only two functions: marketing and innovation. "Marketing and innovation produce results, all the rest are costs" (Drucker, 1973, p. 61).

Health care businesses have many customers including patients, a patient's family and friends, physicians, other health care providers, private third party payers, government third party payers, **third party administrators (TPA)**, employers, and sometimes the communities they serve. These customers represent individuals who may want or need health care services. The purchase of health care services and/or products can involve complex transactions and include multiple customers. Consider the customers who may impact the purchase of a single dose of a pharmaceutical company's antibiotic. A pharmaceutical company advertises to the public in the hope that people will talk to their physicians about that company's product. Employers who provide health insurance select the prescription coverage plan for their employees. The **prescription coverage plan administrator** contracts with brick and mortar and online pharmacy providers. The physician or other licensed prescriber determines that an antibiotic is needed and writes a prescription for the antibiotic that best meets the customer's needs. The customer or their family, caregiver, and friends will select a place to purchase the antibiotic considering their insurance coverage, convenience, and more. The pharmacist may

Key Terms

Key terms, which are defined below, are bolded and italicized the first time they appear in the chapter. Other important terms are shown in boldface on first appearance and are defined by the context in which they are used. When either of these types of terms is used several times, its acronym will be identified and subsequently used in the chapter. Both types of terms are listed alphabetically in the online glossary with their definitions and (when applicable) their acronyms.

4 Ps: the four core elements of marketing (1) product, (2) price, (3) place, and (4) promotion). Also see communication/marketing mix.

7 Ps: the 4 Ps plus the 3 Ps of service marketing (5) physical evidence of effectiveness, (6) processes that instill customer confidence, and (7) people. Also see communication/marketing mix.

communication/marketing mix: the combination of ways (4 Ps/7 Ps) a business chooses to present/promote its services/ product(s) to potential and actual customers.

customer(s): those who buy services or products. In health care, this includes actual and potential patients, third party payers, and referrers.

market: a forum for transactions where buyers, influenced by their income and the price of goods and services will make purchases from sellers.

market development: one of Ansoff's intensive business growth strategies. Growing a business through expanded sales of existing products in new markets by expanding the qualified available market or the target market.

market diversification: development of new products for new markets.

market entry: offering a service or product to a new market.

market orientation: a customer centric organizational marketing philosophy that focuses on meeting customer needs by anticipating, identifying, and satisfying customer requirements efficiently and profitably.

market penetration: growing a business by expanding sales of its existing services/products in existing markets by capturing a larger market share from a competitor or encouraging its current customers to use more of its offerings.

market position(ing): the philosophical positions that an organization can pursue concerning how the organization wishes to be perceived by its qualified target markets: market leader (reputation for being the first to . . .), innovator (for quality and leadership), customer centric (humanistic and caring).

market retrenchment: dropping out of a market segment or the entire market by dropping an unprofitable service or product.

market segmentation: distinct groups of potential customers expected to buy certain services and products. Groups can be segmented by a number of variables like age, income, and gender.

marketing: the process that includes planning, design, and development of manufactured and service products. It also includes the pricing, promotion, and selling of products to customers and markets, and facilitate capital formation.

niche market: a small, narrowly defined group whose needs are not yet well served.

pricing: attaching a dollar value to a service or product. Options include adding a fixed percentage above cost, charging what the market will pay, charging what competitors do, building in a desired percentage higher than cost, adding enough to earn a certain amount by a chosen date.

product-market growth matrix: a comparison of ways management can consider to grow the business. Ansoff called these options market penetration, product development, market development, and market diversification.

product mix: all the services/products an organization offers to customers.

target market: a selected group of consumers who share specific characteristics that may affect their interest in a specific service or product. A specific group of consumers for whom services are products crafted to appeal to their senses.

recommend a generic alternative or another medication when filling the prescription. This example underscores why marketing health care services can be difficult. There are multiple customers.

The focus of this chapter is to explore the topic of marketing. According to the American Marketing Association (AMA), marketing "is the process of planning and executing the conception, pricing, promotion, and distribution of ideas, services and goods, to create exchanges [sales] that satisfy individual and organizational objectives" (AMA, 1985). If we accept Drucker's (1954) point of view on marketing, all business decisions should be tied to creating new customers while retaining current customers. For example, decisions about what products to offer, locations, and how much to charge should reflect only what customers need and want (Kotler, 2000).

Throughout this chapter, we explore the general principles of market-focused marketing and use examples to show how these principles interface with physical therapy (PT) practices. To facilitate the reader's understanding of the complexities of marketing health care, the terms "customer(s)" and "product(s)" will be used as generic terms. Customer(s) and product(s) are used when referring to a wide range of people and a variety of offerings, respectively. Customer(s) include(s) all purchasers of health care services and products. Product(s) include(s) goods, services, ideas, or a combination of these that are offered to the market for consumption. It is recognized that marketing products require the services of various types and service businesses can sell manufactured products. When additional clarity is needed, more individualized terms will be used.

So Much More Than Selling

One of the most important roles management plays is deciding what new products and interventions should be made available (MacStravic, 1977). Customers need and desire continuous change, and with change comes the need or desire for new products. For example, third party payers are continually looking for health care products that are more effective but cost less. At the same time, the customers want the latest technology, more convenience, and other amenities (Porter and Teisberg, 2006). What the customer wants is likely to cost more but will not necessarily improve the effectiveness of their care. Marketing is the process that includes the planning, design, and development of manufactured and service products. It also includes the pricing, promotion, and distribution of products to customers (Herzlinger, 1997; McCarthy, 1971). Distribution in health care relates to the act of **selling**, a

very specific part of the marketing process that deals with arranging the exchange and negotiating the details of that exchange (Chapter 19). In a marketing strategy that emphasizes selling above all else, the focus is on encouraging the potential buyer to purchase a specific available product. The needs of the customer are considered less important than selling what the seller has to offer (Kotler, 2000). It is clear that management of the marketing process involves much more than selling, however, if no exchange takes place, the marketing effort has failed (Chapter 19). The difference between a selling emphasis and a market emphasis is the difference between selling whatever is at hand and selling what the customer needs (Kotler et al., 2002). Meeting client needs requires management to identify, anticipate, and satisfy customer requirements efficiently and profitably (Cooper and Arcyris, 1998). Thus, products are developed to meet specific customer requirements This is called a **market orientation**.

Marketing Concepts

The term "*market*" refers to the collective of individual customers' or organizations' wants or needs for a product, who have the ability or authority to purchase that product, and who can obtain that product legally. Potentially, a market could include the total population, but for operational purposes markets are typically categorized more narrowly (NetMBA, 2007). Common market categories are

- **Potential market**: individual consumer or organization wants or needs a product
- **Available market**: those in the potential market who can afford to buy the product
- **Qualified available market**: those in the available market that can legally obtain the desired product
- **Target market**: those individuals in the qualified available market that the business wants to supply with its product
- **Penetrated market**: those who have purchased the product

Market Share

Market share is the percentage of the qualified available market that is served by a single organization (Cooper and Arcyris, 1998). Market share is demonstrated graphically in Figure 18.1.

If the entire pie represents the qualified available market for PT services (including PT products) in a particular geographic area, the various slices represent the relative size (share) of each seller's penetrated market. Our PT Company currently holds a 21% share of the qualified available market. Competitor A is the biggest competitor to our PT Company with 43% of qualified available market, followed by Competitor C with 29% of the qualified available market. The "Other" business has the smallest percentage of customers. Regarding market share, a business can do three things:

1. Grow market share
2. Maintain current market share
3. Drop out of the market altogether

Market Share Growth Strategies

Ansoff (1957) created the *product–market growth matrix* to help businesses consider different ways to expand. His *market penetration*, **product development**, *market development*, and *market diversification* model continues to offer businesses growth strategies.

1. Market penetration occurs when a business grows through expanded sales of its existing products in existing markets. This requires that the business either gain market share from a competitor or encourage its current customers to use more of its product. For example, a sale offering one shirt for $25.00 or two shirts for $35.00 may encourage current customers to buy more. For a PT practice, market penetration strategies might involve targeting a larger segment of the qualified available market. For example, promotional materials like flyers, billboards, radio advertisements, or personalized letters could be used to encourage potential customers to choose PT instead of chiropractic services for the treatment of spinal dysfunction.

2. Product development occurs when a business grows through the sale of new products in existing markets. For example, a health care provider might offer an alternative approach to the treatment of a chronic medical condition. For PT this could be PT targeting the market segment that has diabetes may be a new product. New products can be an important approach to growth and long-term business success.

3. Market development occurs when a business grows through expanded sales of existing products in new markets. This can be accomplished by expanding the qualified available market or the target market. The expansion of sales through the opening of an additional PT outpatient clinic in a neighboring community would be an example of expanding the qualified available market and the target market.

4. Market diversification occurs when a business grows through expanded sales of new products in new markets. The expansion of

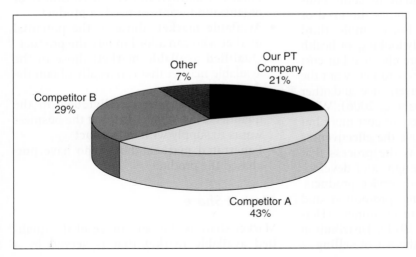

Figure 18.1. Market share.

sales by an adult PT provider through the opening of a new pediatric PT outpatient clinic near a cluster of schools would be an example of market diversification. Unlike the other growth options, **diversification** can have a greater impact on a business, as it typically requires new skills, techniques, equipment, and/or facilities. Diversification activities should be viewed in much the same way as a new product or service line or entry into a new market (Hiam and Schewe, 1992). There should be a systematic examination of the potential benefits and risks for each product or market decision.

Market Entry

Market development and diversification both involve meeting the needs of new markets. Both are *market entry* strategies. The environmental assessment performed as part of an annual strategic planning process (Chapters 3 and 13) may point out an opportunity for a new product to be offered. To bring this product to a new market at a price that customers will pay requires having the following information:

- How well competitors are doing in this market: if they are doing well, that may be good for new entrants if the market is underserved and/or market share can be captured
- How large the target market is: large is good for new entrants

- How many competitors there are: a large number is not good for new entrants
- How strong the potential competitors are: strong rivalries, brand recognition, and others with large marketing budgets make entry difficult
- How many other potential new entrants there are: too many competitors can negatively impact all sellers
- How quickly current sellers respond: slow is good for new entrants
- How sustainable is the product: the longer the better for new entrants

Obviously, some of the information needed by new entrants into a market is difficult to obtain. Some of it may not yet exist, and furthermore, predicting what others will and will not do is speculation. For all these reasons, gaining a share of the market through the market entry strategy can be challenging. Figure 18.2 depicts the integration of the overall market expansion strategy. A strategy is the conceptualization of the desired future and the actions to secure it (Macmillan and Tampoe, 2000).

Market Segmentation

Market segmentation is an alternative way of considering target markets. The concept of segmentation is illustrated in Tables 18.1 and 18.2. The tables demonstrate how the qualified available market can be divided into more

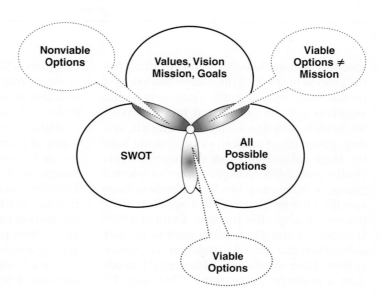

Figure 18.2. Integration of strategic and market planning.

Table 18.1   Examples of Market Segmentation and Target Markets

Business	Potential Market and Characteristics	Available Market	Qualified Available Market	Target Market	Service Differentiation
Pediatric PT Service Provider	Parents of children with developmental disabilities with: • High familial stress • Child care demands • Need for parental respite	Parents with private funding or coverage through a contracted third party payer	Patients with a physician referral or seeing a licensed physical therapy provider in a direct access state	Qualified available market within a 30-mile radius of the provider's clinic	Pediatric therapy provided in a day rehabilitation model with significant parental respite components
Adult PT Provider specializing in geriatric care	Elderly patients who: • Currently live alone • Are having difficulty with mobility • Are having difficulty with self-care	Patients with private funding or coverage through the Medicare or Medicaid programs	Patients with a physician referral	Adult children who are concerned about their elderly parents who currently live independently but who are beginning to have difficulty with independent mobility or self-care	Geriatric specialty care delivered in the patient's home. Service includes a patient evaluation, home safety evaluation, and cognitive assessment. Home checks, fall prevention training, lifeline service, and supervised outings are offered for an added fee
Adult PT Provider	All adults in need of physical therapy services offered in an outpatient setting	Patients with private funding or coverage through a contracted third party payer	Patients with a physician referral or seeing a licensed physical therapy provider in a direct access state	Clients under age 45 who have suffered a CVA	Services targeted at physical rehabilitation as well as vocational and social reintegration of the younger CVA survivor including a stroke survivor support group

specific target markets. Market segmentation is the process of splitting the known market for a product into separate parts. Customers within segments may be categorized in a variety of ways, such as by age, social class, lifestyle, setting, geography, vocation, or purchasing habits. These subcategories are the target markets (Kotler et al., 1983). A target market is a selected group, or submarket, in which members share specific characteristics that may affect their interest in a specific product. Demographics (Chapters 3 and 4) are often used to identify submarkets in a general population (i.e., senior citizens have significantly different PT needs than a pediatric population). Obviously, PT

programs will need to be customized for each of these groups. There are many possible ways to differentiate one selected target market or audience from others.

Rather than trying to satisfy the needs and wants of everyone, the astute manager directs his or her organization's efforts toward the unique needs and characteristics of the most favorable market segments. Organizations that use market segmentation strive to serve the market targets that they are able to satisfy rather than just "selling" to any group representing a sizeable market.

The advantages of market segmentation are substantial. Segmentation results in the creation

Table 18.2	Examples of Market Segments in Physical Therapy
Age	Pediatrics
	• Neurological
	• Developmental
	• Orthopaedic
	• Sports
	Adult
	• Sports
	• Orthopedics
	• Neurological
	• Work hardening
	• Pain
	Geriatric
	• Orthopedic
	• Pain
	• Mobility
	• Balance retraining
	• Wound care
Gender	Adult females
	• Seeking treatment for self
	Sports
	Orthopedic/Pain
	Pregnancy related
	Incontinence
	Other
	• Seeking treatment for family members
	Child
	Spouse
	Parents
	Adult males
	• Seeking treatment for self
	Sports
	Orthopaedic/Pain
	Incontinence
	Other
Occupation/ Avocation	Sports
	Wellness
	Dance
Special consider- ations, services, etc targeted at segments based on affiliations	Community groups
	Social groups
	Location or residence
	Employers/employment status
	Third party payment plans
	Socioeconomic factors
	Religious communities
Disease or disability	Risk for health problems
	Type of therapy needed
Personal require- ments	Shared vision/beliefs
	Self-ensured individuals
	Previous experience with PT
	Transportation method
	Location
	Operating hours
	Walk in service

of a specific way of communicating a product for each subgroup of potential customers that the company intends to satisfy (target) (Kotler et al., 1983). The goal is to produce goods that furnish substantial value to selected groups of potential buyers as efficiently as possible. Segmentation can lead to high customer loyalty, but it also has drawbacks. It can lead to a position where the marketing effort is focused on a portion of the population to the neglect of other portions. A second drawback is the potential for redundancy and increased costs. A business that pursues two or more market segments may have to invest in two or more product development processes, sets of promotional strategies, product distribution systems, price structures, locations and more. Depending on the specific circumstances, duplication may be costly. One example of segmentation that could impact a physical therapy department or clinic is when a hospital with a strong reputation for acute and post-acute cardiac care wishes to enter the pediatric market.

Market Retrenchment

When businesses have a small market share (see "Other" in Fig. 18.1) or flat growth in volumes, it is necessary for them to review their product marketing strategy. There are two major options to consider in this situation. The first is to accept the status quo. This option should be considered whenever the product is

- Profitable
- Contributes to a favorable market position or image
- A loss leader (something sold below cost) as an incentive to buy a product line that is profitable
- Helps sales of the company's other product lines

Option two is to drop the product or service. This is **market retrenchment**, or dropping out of a market segment or a full market. This option may potentially free resources to be reinvested in a company's more profitable products. The possible benefit can be an overall improvement in performance, possibly even total market share. When a physical therapy company changes from offering rehabilitation services (i.e., occupational, speech, and

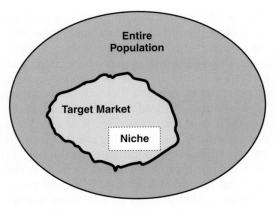

Figure 18.3. Target and niche markets.

physical therapies to a sports and orthopedic emphasis) it is leaving a market segment.

Niche Market

A *niche market* is a narrowly defined target market for a specific product (Fig. 18.3). Niche marketing can be very effective for small businesses that cannot afford the diversity of products to effectively serve a qualified available market or even a full target market. It may also be helpful for a business that simply chooses not to serve full markets. A good niche strategy can lead a company to profitability but may limit its growth potential. If a PT practice hopes to establish a strong niche in the market, it will need to differentiate its offering from those of competitors (MacStravic, 1977) (Chapters 4–6).

If, as many marketers believe, 20% of buyers consume 80% of product volume (Koch, 2000), then that key 20% and others like them could be reached much more efficiently with less effort and cost. Niche marketing involves targeting, communicating with, selling, and obtaining feedback about the heaviest users of your business's products. Picking the right segment of the market is the key to achieving the sales volumes that can make a niche strategy financially successful.

Market Positioning

Market positioning refers to the philosophical positions that an organization can pursue. Each involves decisions concerning how an organization wishes to be perceived by its qualified target markets. Three options for achieving a market position are to be a

1. **Market leader**: reputation will allow the organization to be perceived as a resource for the most advanced and effective treatment techniques.
2. **Innovator**: orientation will allow the organization to develop both a quality and leadership reputation in the community.
3. **Customer-centric**: focuses the efforts of the organization on the humanistic and caring aspects of products rather than arrogant self-serving pushing products on customers (Chapter 19). To promote a specific image, communication with potential and current customers has to take place. Promotion requires communication (Lewis, 1999).

Marketing Mix

Marketing mix refers to the variables that a business can actively manage to satisfy the needs of target markets. The mix is the combination of ways a business chooses to present itself to customers. The concept of the marketing mix originated with the work of Borden (1964) who introduced what became known as the traditional tools (**product**, **price**, **place**, **promotion**) or the core *4 Ps* of marketing (Kotler, 1976; McCarthy, 1971). For businesses whose products are primarily services, the "Ps" of marketing have been expanded to include **physical evidence**, **processes**, and **people** (Booms and Bitner, 1981; Kotler et al., 2002). The *7 Ps* in the marketing mix for service products is shown in Figure 18.4.

Product

Product (or service) is defined by the special characteristics of what is being offered for sale. Characteristics of a product can include its image (i.e., brand recognition, style, etc.), its features, and how it is presented or packaged to customers. Image could be recognition for a tradition of offering complementary and alternative health products. Packaging can include easy to read signage for parking, building locations, easily accessible internal phones, and multiple information kiosks. Electronic consultation services on all days in a week is a unique feature than

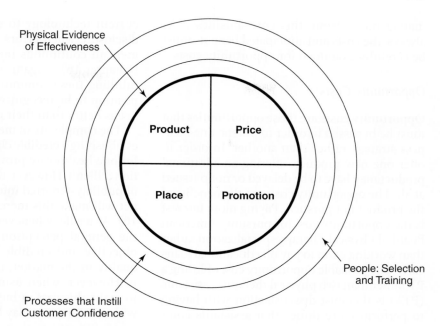

Figure 18.4. 7 Ps of service marketing.

might be available. The use of branded equipment like Balanced Body Pilates equipment is appropriate for a complementary and alternative health care product as is a delivery style involving an integrated team approach.

More on Product

Products have to be managed. **Product management** involves monitoring current products for market performance, changing strategy, and changing products (adding, deleting, or modifying) when performance fails to meet expectations. *Product mix* refers to all of the products an organization offers for consumption. Some organizations offering a variety of goods use a technique called **product portfolio analysis** to integrate goal achievement strategies for their entire product mix (Mintzberg et al., 1995). A portfolio analysis is possible only if the product line of the organization is diverse. A health personnel employment agency that provides full- and part-time occupational, speech, and physical therapies for hospitals, schools, and skilled nursing facilities in many locations across the states has a diverse product line.

Product Diversification

The **product diversification** approach to marketing is based on the principle that if man-

agement considers all product strategies in conjunction with one another, the company is more likely to benefit than if individual product decisions are made independently. This approach is analogous to the investment portfolio strategies (mixing growth and value stocks, bonds, and equities) used by various individual investors and companies (Chapter 23). PT providers can use this principle to produce a desirable and diversified portfolio of products. For example, a PT clinic may choose to add a variety of orthopedic-related durable medical products for customers and educational courses for professionals. An advantage of diversification for PT clinics is that a wide variety of services and products can establish the image of the clinic as a resource to the community instead of a niche provider. A bigger target market may also lead to more growth. The effect of new ventures on existing programs must always be considered. Synergy between new and existing products may be more attractive while conflicting programs can confuse a market. For example, a premier adult orthopedic practice that diversifies into care for pediatric customers may be perceived as being inexperienced in this new product area. They may also lose focus on their existing services as they dedicate more resources to the development of the new product. Product diversification can add cost and distract management from the core business. As always, the costs and anticipated benefits must be carefully examined for opportunity costs.

Opportunity Costs

Opportunity costs are those opportunities that must be bypassed in order to pursue one business strategy rather than another. In order to offer one new product, offering an additional product may have to be delayed or not pursued at all. The opportunity costs are the benefits of the product not pursued. Paying more interest is the opportunity cost for pursuing American Board of Physical Therapy specialization rather than working extra to pay off educational loans early. The probable opportunity cost of hiring a PT rather than two physical therapist assistants (PTA) is therapist dissatisfaction with having to perform more duties that assistants commonly perform.

Product Positioning

Product positioning involves establishing a unique image for the product in the minds of target market members. This image can be general, applying to the portfolio of products, or can specifically address one in particular. Management may position products according to target customers, product characteristics, or product benefits. In all of these cases, they attempt to create an image of value among target customers of what the product means and how it should be viewed.

All health care businesses should incorporate four product characteristics into their positioning strategy. These are

1. Quality
2. Safety
3. Technical leadership
4. Customer service

Quality is the most important qualification for success in a competitive health care environment. In today's era of transparency and public reporting of quality outcomes, a product positioning strategy based on quality is a commitment. It says to internal and external audiences that an organization is committed to providing products to customers based on accepted standards of practice, use of evidence-based care, provision of the most

current technology to support care delivery, disclosure when errors occur, and an investment in continuous improvement of quality (Chapter 16). Organizations that succeed in fulfilling these commitments will be in good position to be recognized by their target market as better than their competitors.

The complexity of measuring quality makes establishing a credible claim of superior quality for one health care provider over its competition difficult. However, the growing availability of publicly-reported information on the Internet will make this increasingly easy (Chapter 16). As a rule, whenever a provider has either the general perception of higher quality or objective and credible evidence of superior quality in the market, it should capitalize on it. However, when using public information to make this case, a business should proceed with caution, as it may become problematic if its quality ratings change in the future.

Product safety, an element of quality, is an essential ingredient in designing any health care product. Media coverage of health care-related errors has put safety at the forefront of customer consciousness. An internal commitment and plan for the prevention of medical errors must be part of every health care provider's product strategy. To "error-proof" their products, many health care businesses have begun incorporating industrial engineering principles into their process reengineering and new process design. Publicly-reported safety issues or noncompliance with safety regulations can shake the market's faith in an organization's product quality.

A PT practice might demonstrate quality or clinical effectiveness in several ways. Posting licenses, certifications, and certificates in a public areas demonstrates to the customer that certain basic requirements have been met for operating a PT business. Letters of commendation and statements of gratitude from past patients or referral sources might also add to the customer's perception of quality and safety. Mission, vision, and value statements along with a customer bill of rights posted in common areas show an organization's commitment to quality and safety. Any or all of these practices would help customers become aware that the business' commitment to quality and safety is indeed a priority. Also see the physical evidence section.

Marketing Related to Product Life Cycle

The **product life cycle** refers to the fairly predictable way that sales and profitability of products change over time (Fig. 18.5). While the cycle timeline may differ, few products escape the pattern of introduction, growth, maturity, and decline. Fad items such as clothing styles typically have very short life cycles, perhaps only months or weeks. At the inverse, market cycles for products like sheet steel and gasoline can span decades. An example applicable to PT is a set of therapeutic exercise techniques known as proprioceptive neuromuscular facilitation (PNF) (Knott and Voss, 1968). These techniques were introduced in the 1950s, reached maturity in the 1970s, and have since been in decline. In the late 1980s and mid-1990s, PNF was combined with other therapeutic techniques and became a new and viable continuing education product.

The product life cycle is helpful in anticipating the sales volumes and revenue from products over time. Although Figure 18.5 depicts a common growth path, it is not the only possible path. Some clinical products, such as aquatic therapy, may be obvious and immediately understood by customers and through constant evolution never reach a decline. Easily-understood products are more likely to progress rapidly into the growth stages. Products like constraint therapy take a significant

amount of time for customers to understand and utilize. Some products never make it past their introductory stage.

Digman's (1990) terminology for describing the product life cycle is useful for explaining this concept. The life cycle terminology is

- Introduction or embryonic stage
- Growth state
- Maturation stage
- Decline or aging stage

Analogous to the birth order of children in a family, successful business will have several product lines at various stages along the product life cycle. Each product, or "child," at different stages of their life cycle contributes different opportunities, challenges, and rewards to the "family," or business. For products, it is necessary to develop a balanced portfolio of products from each of the life cycle stages. When a product is doing well in terms of volume and revenue, its successor needs to be ready in the pipeline.

In the **introduction stage**, a new product is brought to a market. This stage is characterized by low sales, high expenses, and financial losses. Introduction usually requires a heavy financial investment in promotion activities as well as research, development, and production. During the introduction stage, the target market must be educated about product

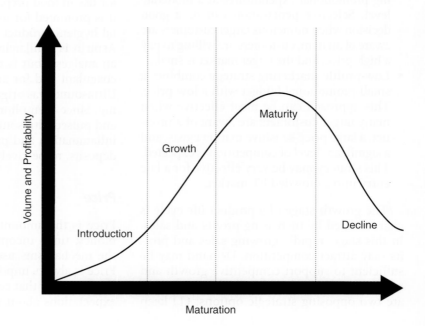

Figure 18.5. Model of the product life cycle.

benefits. Macmillan and Tampoe (2000) suggest that businesses can use the following strategies to speed up introduction:

- **High-profile marketing** strategy: introduces a product with a large investment in promotion. This strategy is most effective when a large portion of the target market is unaware of the item, price is relatively unimportant, and the organization wants to develop high preference for its brand because extensive competition is expected in the future. A health care example is a luxury woman's health pavilion attached to a community hospital that offers everything from skin care and stress reduction through exercise and nutrition programs.
- **Preemptive penetration** strategy also requires a heavy promotional expenditure accompanied by a low price. Used when the target market is largely unaware of their product's existence, price is relatively important to them, a large potential market exists with economies of scale possible from large sales volumes, and substantial competition is expected. Low margins (Chapter 21) and high costs tend to discourage competitors from entering a market, while scale economies (Chapter 20) are expected to help profitability.
- **Selective penetration** strategy consists of pricing a product relatively high while keeping promotional expenditures at a moderate level. Selective penetration can be a good decision when numerous target customers are aware of an item, customers are willing to pay a high price, and the target market is small.
- **Low-profile marketing** strategy combines a small promotional budget with a low price. This approach can be most effective when many target customers are aware of a product, a large price-sensitive market exists, and a significant level of competition is expected. This strategy may be very effective for a late entry into a crowded PT market.

The **growth stage** of a product life cycle is characterized by increasing profits and sales. In this stage, rapidly growing sales and profits may attract competition. Demand may be sufficient to support competitive growth and maintain prices and profits. At this stage there are two opposing strategic options: (1) keep prices stable, decrease spending, and maximize short-term profit, or (2) reinvest profits into substantial marketing efforts in order to build a strong market position for future profitability. At times, regulatory requirements, legal protections such as patents, or cost of market entry will inhibit or slow competitors' entry into a market.

The **maturation stage** is characterized by high volume and profit with little additional investment in promotion. Competing organizations may try to garner some of the market acceptance that the original service or product has earned with copycat products that will speed market saturation (Hannagan, 2002). Competitors may promote themselves as better or less expensive substitutes for the original product. For example, the National Athletic Trainers' Association (NATA, 2008) claims that its members provide cost effective services compared to PTs.

The **decline stage** is characterized by decreasing popularity and market share. The service or product is dated. Typically, unless there was no real utility in the original service or product (as is the case with fads), the market is being better satisfied by substitutes or replacement product. For a service or product in a true decline stage additional investment will not produce a revival unless the product fills a new demand. Baking soda is an excellent example of a customer product that was originally promoted for use in food preparation and baking. Today, it is promoted for use as fabric cleaning, dental hygiene product, and for odor absorption. Aspirin is similar in that it was first used as an analgesic but is now promoted as an anticoagulant and for arteriosclerosis prevention. Ultrasound was originally used for tissue heating. Since then phonophoresis, iontophoresis, and pulsed ultrasound have evolved to reduce inflammation and pain and break up calcium deposits, respectively (Belanger, 2002).

Price

Price is the amount a customer must pay in money, time, inconvenience, and so on and the mechanisms used to justify the amount. Price is always important to a customer. It is a characteristic that certain customers use to set expectations about how good the product is.

Price and expected benefits are related in most market segments.

More on Pricing

Setting the price of something or *pricing*, is mostly a managerial decision. There is a legal prohibition against price discrimination (i.e., when a seller sells the same item to competitive buyers, but charges it differently). However, if there is a difference in costs based on sales volume (i.e., fixed costs are less per item), different prices can be offered (Clarkson et al., 1995) (Chapter 20). As long as prices are not discriminatory, there are several approaches to pricing. These approaches support different marketing strategies and include:

- Cost-based pricing
- Competition-based pricing
- Demand-based pricing

Cost-based pricing are cost-driven strategies (Schoch and Yap, 1998). Prices are set relative to costs. Factors such as demand and competition have little influence. The four major cost-based strategies are

1. *Markup pricing* products are marked up by a fixed percentage over costs. Organizations that market many different items such as large retail outlets find standard markups to be the only feasible way to set prices.
2. *Cost-plus pricing* involves summing up the costs to develop, produce, market, and sell services and products, as well as an additional arbitrary margin of profit. Cost-plus pricing disregards competitors' prices and what potential customers are willing to pay. Difficulty in determining costs is a common problem for the following cost-focused pricing methods.
3. *Target return pricing* computes the price starting with a desired percentage of return on the investment. A target return percentage is then calculated and added to the sum of the costs to get the final price. Like the other cost-based pricing methods, customers and competitors are not given direct consideration.
4. *Payback period pricing* looks ahead to when the return on investment will be at a desirable level. Pricing this way can help assure cash flow (Wilson, 1999). Organiza-

tions that use this method of pricing do not look beyond their own profit needs when considering how to price their offerings.

Other pricing strategies include **competitor pricing**, where prices are set in relation to those of competitors. This method determines the typical price for services in a specific market. The greater the product differentiation, the more a firm is able to price independently from competitors. **Prestige pricing** is a form of demand-oriented pricing (Koschnick, 1995) and involves charging a premium price for a service or product. It is a strategy designed to capitalize on the perception that cost and quality are linked. Some customers strongly believe that "you get what you pay for." These customers perceive quality and prestige to be proportional to an item's price and they will pay more expecting that they will get the best.

While many exceptions exist, in an open market, as the price of a product rises, the demand typically falls. Price elasticity (Chapter 20) refers to the relationship between price and product demand (Kotler, 1982). Evidence suggests that the concept of price elasticity does not always apply to health care. A reason that health care can be insensitive to price is because in circumstances where the need for health care is emergent, people will seek services regardless of price. Another reason is the unique relationship between the providers and customers due to the traditional third party payment system (Chapters 2, 3, and 22). Under this system, the party or parties making purchase decisions are not the same as the parties that pay for the products. This "disconnect" between customers and price accounts for some of the price insensitivity. Efforts to "reconnect" customers with this transaction include increased deductibles, co-payments, and health care savings accounts. However, for the majority of patients with health insurance, price is a secondary concern in the selection of their health care provider. In an effort to correct price insensitivity on the part of the patient, the coverage strategies of third party payers have evolved to control access through provider purchasing agreements. These agreements can be very price sensitive, especially in a highly competitive market. Third party payment system and intense government regulation and oversight (Chapters 1 and 2) have had a profound effect on health care and PT pricing (Chapter 22). The stakes are high when making pricing decisions. A price set too high limits access for customers, while one set too low increases volume with insufficient reimbursement. As a result, pricing can be one of the most important marketing decisions made by management The nuances of health care reimbursement and finance will be covered in greater detail in Part V of this volume.

Place

Place includes the location(s) chosen to deliver a product to customers, the hours of operation, and other related information. As noted earlier in the discussion of product, "place" should match the expectations of targeted customers (Chapter 22). A sports-orthopedic practice in an indoor community soccer facility links the type of practice with an appropriate environment. Conversely, a general practice located on the second floor with only stair access is inappropriate for many patients who are older or have lower extremity or cardiorespiratory impairments. If an organization has a Website, information should be easily accessible and up-to-date.

More on Place

Place should match the tastes of the targeted customer groups as well as the mission of the organization. An attractive, tastefully-decorated, and well-maintained facility located in a safe, convenient area reinforces the perceived relationship between quality and high price (Chapter 4). Some key considerations for choosing a location for a health care service are accessibility and convenience for targeted customers, cost, distance from competitors' locations, space, and pricing strategy. The appropriate place to provide services is in line with customers' tastes, preferences, cost, competitors' locations, as well as the organizations goals. Some considerations to place include

- Accessible to persons with physical disabilities
- Parking
- Proximity to other health care providers
- Proximity to referral sources
- Rules about placing visible signs outside the location

- Safety: location, accommodations
- Site visibility and signage potential
- Target market density
- Traffic patterns and accessibility

Additional discussion on place was presented earlier in the product section.

Promotion

Promotion includes the various methods used to inform the public about the product and to sell the product. Promotion involves communicating to the general public and previous and current customers. Kotler et al. (2002) identify the communication options available to businesses as

Advertising (all the businesses paid for means of promoting itself and its products including websites)

Direct marketing (mail, phone, and electronic communications directed to a target market)

Personal selling (face-to-face communication with potential, current, past customers)

Public relations (all free information distributed by others about the business and its products)

Sales promotion (time-limited incentives associated with the purchase of product)

Based on the strategic marketing plan to promote the product(s), an integrated combination of these communication methods is selected. This combination of communication tools is known as the **communication mix** (Kotler et al., 2002). For example, a physical therapy practice could buy an advertisement on Google. Recognition is enhanced by an interview published in a local newspaper for work with a community service organization. For a minimal cost, diaper bags with the practice's logo and address could be handed out at a well baby screening clinic. Follow up e-mails could be sent to the parents who brought their child in for screening to inform them of the full range of products offered by the practice and third parties that have paid for services. Finally, in face-to-face meetings with potential and current customers, professional physical therapy offers meeting specific needs can be discussed and sold. The personal selling part of promotion is critical to the success of a physical therapy practice. It will be addressed in detail in a separate chapter (Chapter 19).

More on Promotion

According to Hannagan (2002), there are six overlapping steps in a successfully implemented promotional program. The progressive steps believed to lead to a sale are

1. Product awareness
2. Product knowledge
3. Product differentiation from alternative products
4. Support comparisons that favorably represent the promoted product
5. Form a product preference based on steps 1–4
6. Act on this preference by purchasing the preferred product

The objective of the communication mix discussed earlier (advertising, public relations, sales promotion, direct marketing, and personal selling) is to influence the customer to buy a specific product. Promotional campaigns for this purpose range from the simple message on a billboard to a national promotional campaign that includes media advertisements, contests, sweepstakes, and other promotional techniques that can help to position a product as a "must have" item. Lasting impact comes from delivering on promises and satisfying wants and/or needs. A very effective and cost-efficient method of promotion in health care is positive "word of mouth" endorsements from customers who have had positive personal experiences with individual therapists and the businesses they work for (Stone, 2001; Thompson, 2002) (Chapter 19).

Marketing Ethics

Ethical considerations are a priority for most health care managers. Goldman (1993) advises that to fall within ethical boundaries, health care marketing should

1. Put patient welfare first
2. Avoid unnecessary services
3. Maintain high standards of honesty and accuracy
4. Be accountable to the public

More specific information regarding promotional strategies, selling, and ethics is covered in Chapter 19.

Physical Evidence

The additional elements of the marketing mix specific to service products like physical therapy refer to indirect indicators often used by customers as proxies for the actual product. Quality and effectiveness of a service product is difficult to directly judge ahead of time because the service product is experienced at the same time that it is produced. Service products are not inherently "real" in the same sense as manufactured goods. The customer does not own them. Therefore, customers need other forms of physical evidence to help them judge if they are about to or have bought a high quality product and if it will be effective in meeting their needs. These "stand-ins" for quality and effectiveness have to be used to give some tangibility to an inherently intangible service product (Booms and Bitner, 1981) (Chapter 19).

Some ways customers infer quality and effectiveness are by observing what occurs at the business location and the clinic environment, the age and condition of equipment, the overall cleanliness of a facility, the decor, noise, and so forth. Customers also use the clarity and accuracy of pretreatment communications as an indicator of a practice's attention to detail and its quality on the whole. They listen to staff banter and watch their interactions to get an impression about what to expect when being treated. Every potential and actual customer has personal preferences and expectations. Meeting these through various forms of physical evidence can give them confidence that they will be treated appropriately.

Processes

Processes is another service product marketing tool. Processes refer to the way business activities flow and are coordinated. Customers recognize if there are consistencies in the operations or not. Smooth operations instill confidence that can be extended to the yet-to–be-experienced treatment. Specific operations of importance to customers include ease of setting appointments, timeliness of communications, and diligence in pursuing accurate information from third party payers. In a physical therapy clinic, processes include such things as waiting time, efficient use of treatment time, availability of appropriate treatment space and equipment, the amount of attention professional staff has to spend on them personally, and a customer-friendly cancellation policy.

People

The third marketing mix element related to service products is people. People includes all members of a business. All the members of a business a customer sees and hears can influence their perception of quality. Because clinical service products are provided by licensed professionals like PTs, such professionals are among the principle influencers of customers' perceptions (Forsyth, 2003). However, the behavior of everyone from the valet to the head of a department are observable indicators that contribute to customers' estimates of how well and how appropriately they will be treated relative to how well and how appropriately they expect to be treated. Customers often use customer service as a surrogate measure of quality.

Customer Service

Customer service starts at the first contact a potential or actual customer has with the business, be it a phone call, a stop at the reception desk, or visit to see a friend. Customer attention is on the basic observable and experiential elements like

Can they find someone to help them?
Is there excessive waiting time?
Do staff members look neat and organized?
Is the greeting appropriate?
Do staff show respect and common courtesy?
Is the staff knowledgeable?
Are directions, instructions, and written materials clear and comprehensive?
Are staff helpful, do they make it easy to access the product?

A negative response to any of these questions serves to diminish the confidence of the customer that the product is as good as they had hoped. It should be clear that each and every staff member could have tremendous impact on the customer's perception of the quality of the business. The manner in which all the staff members interact, hold themselves to the public, and even present themselves (i.e., dress and overall appearance) are critical factors to the image of the company. Therefore, it is important for all staff members to act in a professional manner and provide services that consistently meet or exceed customer expectations. This mandate applies to the professional clinical staff as well as to other staff members who encounter the public either in person, by phone, or via written communications.

Some less-personal indicators of quality are the way members of the organization are selected and trained. This can be made known to customers by printed material or Websites that highlight each staff member's background, accomplishments, and interests. A tasteful display of diplomas, continuing education certificates of completion, certifications, special internal and external organization training, publications, and internal and external awards and other recognitions is another way to positively inform customers about those who will care for them.

More on People

Technical leadership is one of the hardest characteristics to demonstrate to health care customers because it is hard for them to evaluate. Most patients do not know what the product should be and cannot easily assess if its quality. Technical leadership can be characterized by management's success in developing a high-performing staff, providing the best technical equipment, and appropriate settings. Offering customers a high-performing staff is the most difficult of these tasks. It starts with hiring those with superior credentials and a history of strong performance. Once hired, it means ongoing investment in their training and development. It also requires creating a working environment that fosters the best day-to-day performance (Chapters 11, 14, and 16). State-of-the-art technology and appropriate treatment facilities are dependent on a business' ability to stay current and access to adequate financial resources that come from sales.

The concept of a marketing mix reinforces the importance of selecting the elements to be used in the development of a market strategy. How a business defines these components determines its marketing mix. Because health care transactions usually involve multiple parties, it is imperative that health care business owners and managers understand their customers, their product characteristics that are important to each stakeholder in the transaction, and how those needs interrelate if they wish to do business with them (Mullin et al., 1993).

Summary

This chapter introduced the reader to the scope of activities that comprise the marketing process including planning, design, and development of products. Basic marketing concepts were reviewed to help create an understanding of the strategies that might be used to encourage potential customers to purchase an organization's products. The components of what is known as the traditional four core tools or the "4Ps" of product marketing were introduced. To these, three more tools for marketing products that are difficult for customers to experience beforehand like clinical services were added. These seven service marketing tools known as the "7Ps" were discussed at length and applied to physical therapy examples.

Special attention was given to marketing strategy and the selection and application of the 7P marketing tools. A marketing strategy utilizes marketing tools that are appropriate to its goals, product, and the target market. This selected group of tools is known as the marketing mix. A similar concept called the communication mix was also introduced. The communication mix is the combination of ways a business chooses to promote its product(s) to potential customers. The concept of a product's life cycle was introduced. The cycle relates to the income and volume of sales of products from their inception to the present. On average, newly introduced products, products that are gaining popularity, and long-standing products differ in the cost to market them, volume of sales, and revenue generated. Each stage of the cycle poses different marketing challenges. The marketing approaches appropriate for products at different stages of the life cycle were explored using physical therapy contexts to exemplify solutions at each of the stages.

The current chapter discussed several ways to enhance sales but left off addressing the specific knowledge and skills that facilitate the sale of products. Given that the final objective of marketing is to increase sales, how to do this deserves more attention. In the next chapter, the focus is on the sales process and the key contemporary concepts of personal selling of professional service products. The important sales related role of PTs and other health care organization personnel is analyzed and discussed.

CASE STUDY 18.1

Marketing to the Physical Therapy Customer

The Practice

Independent Physical Therapists, PC (IPT) is a privately owned company with six outpatient clinics located in cities along the border with a neighboring state. Until now, IPT has relied on physician, word of mouth, and payer referrals for its new business for its clinics. Because of the recent passage of the direct access legislation in their state, IPT's management believes that a marketing strategy is in order. Among the opportunities to consider is that the neighboring state's regulations do require practitioner referral for physical therapy. IPT's management believes that the strength of their orthopaedic and fitness related physical therapy products should be marketed directly to potential customers from both states. Since marketing has been an informal and occasional endeavor, it is felt that this is an ideal time to get serious about growing the business at all locations. At the

(Continued)

CASE STUDY 18.1

Marketing to the Physical Therapy Customer (continued)

request of management, the IPT board of directors has authorized the formation of a $25,000 marketing account.

Questions About a New Marketing Strategy

To begin formulating the marketing strategy you would like to see IPT answer the following questions:

1. What marketing resources will you consult?
2. Who is the target market or markets?
3. What is the physical therapy product or products?
4. What distinguishes IPT from similar providers?
5. What would the marketing mix include?
6. What would the communication mix consist of?
7. How would the product life cycle apply to products provided in IPT's state?
8. How would the product life cycle apply to products provided to customers from the neighboring state?

9. What are the desired results of the marketing effort(s)?

Sharing the Good News

Things will change for everyone with the decision to take a more active marketing approach. All members of IPT have a part in the marketing effort. Management must bring everyone up-to-date, answer questions, and provide training so everyone can be involved in growing the business. Based on your conceptualized marketing strategy, share your recommendations for:

1. Updating everyone on the marketing strategy and operational plans
2. Describing what the chosen marketing mix is and any changes the mix will have on what they do
3. Describing what the chosen communication mix is and any changes the mix will have on what they do
4. Answering questions the employees are likely to ask. The form below will help to organize this task.

Marketing and Communication Mix Work Sheet

Date: _____   Draft #: _____   **Market(s)**

Location(s): _____   Target/Segment: _____

Manager(s): _____   Niche: _____

YOUR MARKETING MIX

Product/Service characteristics:	Physical Evidence:
Price/Charge justification:	
	Processes
Place product delivered:	
Promotion/Communications mix:	People/Personnel Training:
Advertising:	
Public relations:	
Sales promotion:	
Direct marketing:	
Personnel selling:	
Comments:	

REFERENCES

American Marketing Association. Board approves new marketing definition. Marketing News. 1985; March 1:1.

Ansoff I. Strategies for diversification. Harvard Business Review. 1957;35(5[Sep–Oct]):113–124.

Belanger AY. Evidence-Based Guide to Therapeutic Physical Agents. Baltimore, MD: Lippincott Williams & Wilkins. 2002.

Booms BH, Bitner MJ. Marketing strategies and organizational structures for service firms. In Donnelly JH and George WR, eds. Marketing of Services. Chicago, IL: American Marketing Association. 1981:47–51.

Borden NH. The concept of the marketing mix. Journal of Advertising Research. June 1964;4:2–7.

Clarkson KW, Miller RL, Jentz GA, Cross FB. West's business law: Text cases legal, ethical, regulatory, and international environment, 6th ed. Minneapolis/St. Paul, MN: West. 1995.

Cooper CL, Arcyris C. The Concise Blackwell Encyclopedia of Management. Malden, MA: Blackwell. 1998.

Digman LA. Strategic management: Concepts, decisions, and cases, 2nd ed. Homewood, IL: BPI/Irwin. 1990.

Drucker PF. The practice of management. New York, NY: Harper and Brothers. 1954.

Drucker PF. Management: Tasks, responsibilities, practices. New York, NY: Harper Row. 1973.

Forsyth P. Marketing and selling professional services, 3rd ed. Sterling, VA: Kogan Page. 2003.

Goldman RL. Practical applications of healthcare marketing ethics. Healthcare Financial Management. 1993;47(March):46–48.

Hannagan T. Mastering strategic planning. New York, NY: Palgrave. 2002.

Herzlinger R. Market driven health care. Reading, MA: Addison Wesley. 1997.

Hiam A, Schewe CD. The Portable MBA in marketing. New York: John Wiley and Sons. 1992.

Knott M, Voss DE. Proprioceptive neuromuscular facilitation, 2nd ed. San Francisco, CA: Harper and Roe. 1968.

Koch R. The Financial Times guide to strategy: How to create and deliver a useful strategy, 2nd ed. New York, NY: Prentice Hall. 2000.

Koschnick WJ. Dictionary of marketing. Brookfield, CN: Grower. 1995.

Kotler P. Marketing management, 3rd ed. Englewood Cliffs, NJ: Prentice Hall. 1976.

Kotler P. Marketing for nonprofit organizations. Englewood Cliffs, NJ: Prentice-Hall. 1982.

Kotler P. Marketing management, The Millennium ed. Upper Saddle River, NJ: Prentice Hall. 2000.

Kotler P, Ferrell OC, Lamb C. Cases and readings for marketing for nonprofit organizations. Englewood Cliffs, NJ: Prentice-Hall. 1983.

Kotler P, Hayes T, Bloom PN. Marketing professional services, 2nd ed. Paramus, NJ: Prentice Hall. 2002.

Levitt T. Marketing myopia. Harvard Business Review. 1960;48(July–August):45–56.

Lewis B. Communication mix. In Lewis BR, Littler D, eds. The Blackwell Encyclopedic Dictionary of Marketing. Malden, MA: Blackwell Business. 1999:120–121.

Macmillan H, Tampoe M. Strategic management process, content, and implementation. New York, NY: Oxford University Press. 2000.

MacStravic RE. Marketing health care. Germantown, MD: Aspen. 1977.

McCarthy EJ. Basic marketing: A managerial approach, 4th ed. Homewood, IL: Richard D. Irwin. 1971.

Mintzberg H, Quinn JB, Voyer J. The Strategy Process, Collegiate ed. Englewood Cliffs, NJ: Prentice Hall. 1995.

Mullin BJ, Hardy S, Sutton WA. Sport marketing. Champaign, IL: Human Kinetics. 1993.

National Athletic Trainers' Association. The facts about athletic trainers and the National Athletic Trainers' Association. Available at http://www.iata-usa.org/docs/NATA_Fact_Sheet_About_Athletic_Trainers.doc. Accessed 3/27/08.

NetMBA. Market definition. 2002–2007. Available at http://www.netmba.com/marketing/market/definition/. Accessed 3/10/08.

Porter ME, Teisberg EO. Redefining health care: Creating value-based competition on results. Boston, MA: Harvard Business School. 2006.

Schoch HP, Yap TH. Cost-pricing relationship. In Abdel-Khalik AR, ed. The Blackwell Encyclopedic Dictionary of Accounting. Malden, MA: Blackwell. 1998:109–112.

Stone CE. Effective marketing of CAM services. In Faass N, ed. Integrating Complementary Medicine into Health Systems. Gaithersburg, MD: Aspen. 2001:135–140.

Thompson G. A niche master. Physical Therapy Products-The Magazine for Physical Therapy Professionals. 2002; July/August:14.

Wilson D. Pricing objectives. In Lewis BR, Littler D, eds. The Blackwell Encyclopedic Dictionary of Marketing. Malden, MA: Blackwell. 1999:160–162.

ADDITIONAL RESOURCES

A home study course on marketing is available for purchase from www.apta.org. Rehab Management is a free subscription publication with interdisciplinary interest that regularly has marketing articles. Contact http://www.rehabpub.com. Shi and Singh discuss the concepts of market justice and market forces (Shi L, Singh DA. Delivering Health Care in America—A Systems Approach, 3rd ed. Boston, MA: Jones and Bartlett. 2004). Marketing and organizational strategies including adaptive, market entry, and competitive strategies are discussed in Chapter 6 in Swayne LE, Duncan WJ, Ginter PM. Strategic Management of Health Care Organizations, 5th ed. Malden, MA: Blackwell. 2006. A book relating marketing and selling professional services that is very relevant to selling physical therapy services is: Forsyth P. Marketing and Selling Professional Services, 3rd ed. Sterling, VA: Kogan Page. 2003. A summary and access to the legal record regarding the term Pilates is available at http://www.pilates.com/BBAPP/V/about/pilates-trademark-lawsuit.html.

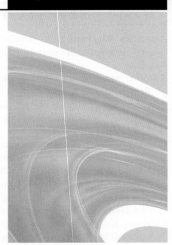

CHAPTER 19

The Selling Part of the Marketing Process

LARRY J. NOSSE

Learning Objectives

1. Discuss the relationship between marketing and sales.
2. Compare retail sales and professional service sales.
3. Identify the steps in a personal sales encounter.
4. Summarize the key concepts underlying a relational approach to professional service sales.
5. Identify parallels between professional service sales concepts and the practice of physical therapy.
6. Given practical physical therapy relevant scenarios, apply the selling model and application concepts presented in this chapter.

Introduction

After looking at the title of this chapter you might be saying to yourself, "Hey! I'm a therapist, not a sales person. Where's the connection between what I do in my clinical work and *selling*?" Such thinking is common among professional service "doers" like physicians, attorneys, accountants (Kotler et al., 2002), and physical therapists (PTs). A short response to such comments is that there is nothing incompatible between applying contemporary personal selling concepts and the ethical practice of one's profession. Furthermore, within or outside the workplace, selling skills are help-ful in influencing the decisions of those with whom we interact (Baron and Harris, 2003). In professional and personal interactions, we all engage in marketing and selling "something." We all have or can do something for someone in exchange for something others have or can do for us. "Something" is a broad term, but as Kotler (2000) noted, anything can be marketed and ultimately culminate in a satisfactory exchange. Table 19.1, a modification of Kotler's list of marketing opportunities with physical therapy examples, exemplifies this point.

The categories and examples in Table 19.1 show two general types of exchange between parties. Some examples reflect a monetary exchange (e.g., experiences, professional services, and property). In the other examples, the exchange is not necessarily monetary (e.g., attitudes, events, and organizations). This means across a broad range of interactions, whenever there are possibilities of mutually beneficial exchanges occurring, the exchange process can be facilitated by the application of contemporary selling concepts. This chapter presents selected concepts related to professionals selling their own knowledge and skills to clients. Physical therapy contexts are used in practical applications of the concepts. In Chapter 18, the general terms product and customer were used because the marketing principles were developed primarily for manufactured products and goods, which were sold to customers. Over the last twenty-five years, marketing literature has evolved specifically about professionals

Key Terms

Key terms, which are defined below, are bolded and italicized the first time they appear in the chapter. Other important terms are shown in boldface on first appearance and are defined by the context in which they are used. When either of these types of terms is used several times, its acronym will be identified and subsequently used in the chapter. Both types of terms are listed alphabetically in the online glossary with their definitions and (when applicable) their acronyms.

consumer driven: the theory behind consumer-driven health care is that by giving employees more financial control over their health care expenditures, they will become more conscious of the costs associated with their health care decisions and behaviors and they will make choices that are more cost-conscious thus slowing health care cost increases.

customer centric: the efforts of the organization are focused on the humanistic and caring aspects of services/products rather than arrogant self-serving pushing services/products on customers.

customer service: providing customers with the right information or service when they need it in ways that demonstrate to the customer that they are important to the organization.

personal selling: one of the ways of promoting services and products to potential, past, and current customers that requires sales agent–customer interaction.

professional service(s): in health care, services provided by licensed professionals like physicians, dentists, and physical therapists that meet customer needs and wants guided by the practitioner's professional association and state licensure regulations.

relational sales/selling: an approach to personal sales based on developing a longitudinal association with a customer. This entails learning about and meeting the customer's needs in a way that both the seller and the customer gain something important.

retail: businesses that sell manufactured products to the public as opposed to businesses that sell to other businesses for resale.

sale(s): a seller–customer/client exchange or transaction. The seller provides something that meets the buyer's needs or wants (therapy services) in exchange for something the seller wants (payment).

sales agent: a representative of an entity who interfaces with potential and actual customers. Agents are usually knowledgeable and skilled communicators who are able to facilitate converting a customer's needs and wants into a sale. When buying something he or she knows little about, a customer depends on accurate and relevant information from the sales agent. When professional services are involved in the transaction, the sales agent is often the provider of the service.

sales concepts: practical concepts a seller can apply to help clients understand how particular services and products meet their expressed needs and wants. Also see relational sales.

sales process: opening (to establish a working relationship), exploring and confirming client needs (by listening, questioning, and responding), presenting solutions (to match needs with appropriate services), responding to objections (to reduce concerns with accurate information), and closing (ask client if they are ready to buy [consent to treat]).

selling: facilitating a win-win exchange between a seller and a customer.

---

marketing and selling their own knowledge, skill, and expertise (Donnelly and George, 1981; Forsyth, 2003). This literature uses professional services to identify the product and client to identify the customer. Following this convention, *professional service*(s) and client(s) will be used in this chapter. These terms are appropriate for describing what a PT exchanges with others for payment.

Personal Selling Part of the Communication Mix

Personal selling, introduced in Chapter 18 as part of the communication mix, is a very important technique for promoting the sale of physical therapy services. When carried out appropriately, face-to-face promotion:

Table 19.1 Marketing Categories With Physical Therapy Examples

What Can Be Marketed	Physical Therapy Examples
Attitudes	"The culture of DIA Therapy fosters 'doing it all' for the client, for yourself, and for the organization"
Events	"Join us for a tour and refreshments as we celebrate the opening of our third Kind Care physical therapy location"
Experiences	"At our woman's health pavilion we pamper you in our plush surroundings, with our gourmet food, and an expert blending of traditional and complimentary and alternative medical offerings"
Ideas	"I am here to present to you (management, nursing, physicians, etc.) an exciting means of attracting new physical therapy referrals without a major expenditure"
Information	"This website describes the motor learning based physical therapy treatments we provide for adults with neurological conditions as well as a summary of the evidence underlying our approach"
Organizations	"The American Physical Therapy Association is a national professional organization representing over 71,000 PT, physical therapist assistant (PTA), and student members"
People	"All of our staff members are specialists certified by the American Board of Physical Therapist Specialties"
Places	"Our convenient location is handicapped accessible and we offer valet and transport services"
Products	"Improve your documentation and range of motion measurement accuracy with a digital inclinometer with wireless pc computer interface"
Professional Services	"We provide an integrated team approach involving occupational, physical, and speech therapies, along with medical, psychological, and social service consultants"
Properties	"Ideal for a physical therapy office. A ground level 1500 square foot office in a 5 year old building and available in 30 days. Utilities included. Near by parking. No lease. Option to buy."

Source: Modified from Kotler, 2000.

Allows the professional to begin building a relationship with the client

Provides the client an opportunity to meet and converse with the professional who will be providing the services they need

Allows timely responses to clients' concerns and misunderstandings

Is likely to influence a client's decision to buy once the relationship has evolved in part because saying no to a helpful person is psychologically uncomfortable.

Personal selling is very client/*customer centric*. For some, personal selling is the best way to convert a client's interest into a sale (Forsyth, 2003). It is an opportunity to learn about a client's needs, to inform them of the services available to meet their needs, and to sell them the relevant services. In a business context, this seller-client exchange or transaction is called a *sale*. In a typical sales transaction, the seller provides something that meets the buyer's needs or wants in exchange for something the seller wants. Usually, this is money. The revenue for a business to operate and grow comes from sales (Kotler, 2000; Miller and Sinkovitz, 2005). Increasing sales and revenue is the ultimate purpose of any marketing strategy (Chapter 18) (Forsyth, 2003). To facilitate the sale of physical therapy and like services, a marketing department chooses and implements means of

- Attracting new clients (new referrals and walk-ins where there is direct access)
- Fostering repeat business (a new course of treatment for previous clients)
- Retaining current clients (keeping those already being treated)
- Maximizing use of available treatments (offering current clients more or new services)

In a market-oriented organization (Chapter 18), there is a concerted effort to make a business "more effective than its competitors in creating, delivering, and communicating its value to its chosen target markets" (Kotler, 2000, p. 19). This view of marketing integrates sales into the marketing strategy. This is an advancement over earlier marketing approaches in which marketing focused on identifying the needs of the buyer and selling focused on fulfilling the needs of the seller (the *sales agent*) (Levitt, 1960). This often resulted in personal sales agents pushing their clients to buy whatever the agent had available to sell with little concern about the buyer's real needs (Kotler et al., 2002). The attitude many people had regarding sales people was understandably less than positive particularly when manufactured goods were involved in the exchange.

Retail/Product Sales

Many sales concepts have evolved to enhance the sale of manufactured products and goods. The types of businesses that sell manufactured products to the public are called *retail* businesses. Most of us have purchased goods from retail businesses. When shopping, our buying decisions have at times been influenced by helpful sellers or sales agents. Effective sales agents listen to the client's explanation of what they want, why they want it, and other information the client shares. Sales agents are usually knowledgeable and skilled communicators who are able to facilitate converting a client's needs into a sale. When buying something we know little about, we depend on accurate and relevant information from the sales agent. We weigh the information, determine if the goods meet our needs, and if so, purchase the item or items. At the end of the transaction we receive something tangible that we wanted or needed, in part, because of the sales agent's help. The result of the sale was a **win-win** experience. The buyer went home with a tangible product they liked, the sales agent earned their pay or commission, the business paid its bills, made a profit, and later paid taxes. Intuitively, we knew that the sales agent, as nice and helpful as they were, helped us so they could make a sale that in turn helped them keep their job and helped the owner keep their business open.

Professional Service Sales

Another type of business does not manufacture and sell tangible products. Rather, the exchange is a service for a fee. Selling encounters between clients and professional service providers like accounting, law, medicine (Kotler et al., 2002), and physical therapy differ from retail sales in several ways.

1. The properties of what is exchanged
2. How clients are involved in the exchange
3. Marketing challenges
4. Levels of consumer protection

First, professional knowledge and skill is what is offered for sale. Knowledge is not a tangible object like a pair of slacks, a computer, or a house. Professional services transactions involve providing the client with something that is intangible (Shostack, 1977). The professional offers service options to the client who has to digest the information and decide what to do next. For example, a consultant consults with the client and provides oral and written recommendations. The client can put the information on the shelf or implement some, many, or all of the recommendations. A certified public accountant provides figures and reports on paper. It is up to the client to pay the calculated taxes that are due, pay bonuses earned by employees, buy major equipment, or sell the business. A physician renders a diagnosis and presents the patient with next step options, which the client can follow or not. PTs also consult, offer treatment options, and recommendations. It is up to the client to return for treatment or to carry out all or some portion of a home exercise program. While the anticipated result of the physical therapy treatments is some type of improvement, the quantification of the progress or outcome is mostly subjective. It is the client who most accurately weights the costs and benefits (Bateson, 1977) of complying, keeping appointments, or continuing physical therapy.

The second difference between professional service and product sales is in how each is produced. For professional services to be developed and delivered requires client participation and services customized to meet the client's needs. The client also participates as the service is rendered. This makes the service and the service provider inseparable (Kotler et al., 2002). This in turn makes it difficult for a client to judge the merit of the treatment separate from the positive attributes of the service provider. This is sometimes difficult because, unlike a retail product, the client does not own the service so they cannot take the service home, try it out, reuse it, or enjoy it at their leisure. Typically a therapist gathers information in the interview, client goals are identified, and an individualized plan of care is developed and delivered. As these events occur, the client also observes the therapist's attributes including organization, appearance, sociability, and caring behaviors to judge if they expect the service will be "right" for them. In comparison, retail goods can be seen and judged before purchase. Most retail goods do not involve the client in their production because they are premade, usually by a distant producer. There is limited choice because retail goods come in limited variety. Finally, products can be objectively tested and retested because the client possesses them.

The third notable difference between professional services and retail selling is their respective marketing challenges. The major challenge in service marketing is giving a degree of tangibility to an intangible thing whose outcome has yet to be experienced. A service cannot be fully experienced beforehand. Its outcome can only be imagined. One way to provide a semblance of tangibility to a service is through the statements of those who have experienced the service. Word of mouth comments, testimonials, and positive results expressed in terms of the percentage of prior clients who achieved certain results are all plausible substitutes for experience.

However, such examples do not guarantee like results for future clients. To make a service more tangible to clients Baron and Harris (2003) recommend a triangulation of resources for giving reality to the construct service. They suggest

- Providing relevant videos, anatomical models, and written materials for client review
- Guiding potential/actual clients toward a variety of readily available information sources about the service
- Giving the potential/actual clients a sample of the service on a trial basis (when allowed by law)

- Pointing out the desirable change(s) the clients should look for from the sample service. In addition, Miller and Sinkovitz (2005) suggest:
- Arranging for the potential/actual clients to spend time observing the treatment or new treatment area (with appropriate consent of current clients)
- Facilitating interaction between current or past clients (with consent)

The marketing challenge for retail businesses is quite different as the products are tangible and they have observable physical properties. The task for retail business marketing is to draw attention to the key distinguishing characteristics of a specific product compared to many apparently similar products that are equally available elsewhere.

The last professional services-retail selling difference to be discussed is consumer protection. Professional services associations have codes of ethics (Direct Selling Association, 2007; Manufacturers Agents National Association, 2007) or other behavioral guidelines (American Institute of Certified Public Accountants, 2008) to protect members' rights as well as to protect clients from financial, physical, emotional, or other kinds of harm. Besides a code of ethics (American Physical Therapy Association [APTA], 2007a) and practice guidelines (APTA, 2007b) PTs and other health care professional services providers are also licensed by states to protect the public (Chapter 8). These professional cultures support following these guidelines and regulations throughout a professional's career. Requirements for continuing professional education as a criterion for relicensure is common. For example, PTs are required to earn continuing education credits in ethics and jurisprudence for relicensure in many states (Federated State Boards of Physical Therapy, 2008).

While retail and manufacturing associations have comparable guiding documents, the use of such documents in training retail sales agents, particularly in small businesses, is not well documented. Moreover, the effectiveness of larger corporate sales training programs with or without inclusion of guiding document information has been questioned (Eades and Kear, 2006). Finally, retail sales agents are not universally licensed by state agencies.

Personal Professional Service Sales Concepts

Principles of marketing and selling professional services sales have evolved from product marketing and sales methods. Selling methods consider the client's thought processes as they are making a decision to buy or not buy (Crissy and Kaplan, 1969; Miller and Sinkovitz, 2005). The utilization of selected sales concepts by the professionals who actually provide the service to clients is one of the most important tools for the personal selling of professional services (Forsyth, 2003; Kotler et al., 2002). In initial contacts, clients use what they have experienced pre-service and the current encounter as proxy indicators of how the provider organization and the professional service provider will perform in meeting their needs. Attire, decor, friendliness, professionalism, and knowledge are some of these observables. A positive impression about the professional is likely to result in a client buying the services offered, and in the future, buying additional recommended relevant services (Kotler et al., 2002).

Successful professional personal sales are a key means of retaining current clients and having them return for future services. How to be successful in creating client demand for current and future services has many answers. However, the promise of providing the reader with the keys to becoming competent in personal professional selling under all circumstances is one that no one can make has to be learned. At best, the reader's attention can be drawn to commonalities extracted from the writings of knowledgeable authors who have written about personal selling.

A Sales Sequence

To give a framework of the events that make up a sales process it is helpful to offer a general sales model and then embellish it with concepts that underlay successful personal professional service sales. Charney (2004) offers a seller's perspective on the general sequence of events in a sales encounter. The main steps in a personal selling interaction with a client are summarized in Table 19.2.

It starts with developing a long-term, partner-like business relationship. It involves greeting, introduction, explanation of who you are, what you do, etc. At this time, the client is watching, listening, judging the professional, and responding to questions. The purpose of exploring is to learn the client's perspective of their needs, problems, strengths, challenges, constraints, and the expectations they have of your service. It is the opportunity to develop trust, establish your expertise, and define the client's needs. Based on this information, the professional summarizes the basis for service, the goals, what will be done, and how it will be done in order to meet the client's particular needs. When a client shows concern about what has been discussed, the professional adds the information that the client needs to be able to see the match between their needs and the services offered. When the professional feels the client has enough information about the match between the services and the client's needs, they ask the client to buy. This is the closing.

Sales encounters may not always proceed as anticipated. The steps may be gone through in a less logical order because of the client's need

Table 19.2 Steps in Personal Selling Sales Encounter (Seller's Guide)	
Steps (2–4 order can vary)	*Tasks*
1. Opening	Establish a working relationship
2. Exploring and confirming client needs	Listen, question, and respond
3. Presenting solutions to meet client needs	Match needs with appropriate services
4. Responding to objections	Reduce concerns with accurate information
5. Closing	Ask client if they are ready to buy the service

to know certain things "now." For example, a client's first statement might be, "I don't need this therapy" (step 4—respond to objections). Eventually, all the steps are used. They may just be followed in a unique sequence. A way to facilitate moving through the selling steps is to apply the practical concepts associated with the *relational sales* approach to personal selling.

Relational Selling Concepts

The benefit of knowing about the general sales encounter progression is that it offers a framework for proceeding toward a sale. However, it lacks sufficient detail of how to get through the steps. There are eight literature-based *sales concepts* that add the detail needed to move from opening to closing. In Table 19.3 these *sales concepts* are intermingled with the author's perspectives on personal selling concepts and how they relate to early PT-client interactions.

Personal Selling Concept 1: Build a Relationship

Personal selling is a face-to-face encounter between sellers and their clients. What takes place early in the opening step influences client perceptions. We all know that introducing ourselves by name and profession, asking how the client wishes to be addressed, and other informational exchanges are part of establishing rapport before we begin gathering medical history and other pertinent pretreatment information. For the most part, the initial intent of gaining rapport reflects short-term thinking. Relationship building denotes long-term thinking. Relationship building requires investing time at the onset, during the course of care, and after the client's original needs have been met. This is the essence of *relational sales/selling*.

Client Expectations

Client expectations are a major consideration in contemporary sales concepts, which focus on relationship building (Gordon, 2000; Kotler et al., 2002; Swenson and Link, 1998). The initial meetings between the professional providing service and the client can be compared to a reciprocal research event (Shonka and Kosch, 2002). The professional wants to gather relevant business related data about the client's situation

Table 19.3   Parallels Between Relational Personal Selling Concepts and PT

Key Words	PT Parallels	Descriptions	Desired Outcomes
Build relation-ship	Rapport	Intend to develop and nurture a long-term professional relationship with the client	Build trust, foundation for continued and future sales
Collaborate	Patient autonomy	Commit to collaborating/partnering with the client	Win-win solutions
Listen	Patient goals	Focus on what the client says with the intent of learning the client's needs/wants, and how they think	Understand client's unique issues, constraints, expectations, and perspectives
Question	Clarify	Assist the client to add precision to their problem, need, goal, priority, and expectation statements	Better targeting of resources and solutions likely to meet the client's expectations
Educate	Educate	Provide resources and solutions for client to consider; encourage and respond to all questions	Reduce client's concerns; match service to client's needs
Confirm	Plan of care	Secure the client's confirmation that you have correctly stated their goals,and so on	Service specific to client's needs and special circumstances
Agreement	Informed consent	Obtain the client's agreement to buy service customized to their needs and expectations	Meet client's confirmed needs
Keep in touch	Satisfaction survey and others	Continually engage in actions that benefit the client	Sell new and additional services that can benefit the client

and the client wants to gather data to test the correlation between their expectations and their observations about this particular professional and the setting they operate in. In other words, when clients see that some of their expectations are being met they have reason to presume that when the service is actually provided, it too will meet many of their expectations. The most fundamental expectations clients have of a professional service provider are

- They will be safe in your care
- You will not waste their time
- Your services will be of value

Forsyth (2003) points out there are also behaviors that clients expect their professional service provider to demonstrate. These expectations are that the professional will

- Be nice, respectful, and treat them like they are important
- Be knowledgeable in technical areas
- Understand and be considerate of their needs and wishes
- Act on the understanding of their needs and wishes

These characteristics should look familiar. They were discussed in Chapter 18 under *customer service*. These behaviors are also comparable to the therapist behaviors described in the APTA core professional values (2007c).

From a relational sales point of view, the basis of a business relationship is doing things that are in the client's best interest (Eades and Kear, 2006). To do this requires investing time and effort to learn everything relevant about the client's circumstances (Chapter 12). According to Kotler (2000), the rewards for learning what a client's needs are and doing things that satisfy these needs include

Loyalty, for example, retention—they continue physical therapy treatment with you and may give less consideration to going to similar non-PT professionals
Sales of additional services, for example, they become members of the organization's wellness and fitness center
Repeat business, for example, they will return to have you meet their future needs
Positive recommendations, for example, they tell others of their satisfaction with you, your department, and your organization

A relational approach is good for all parties. When clients return for additional services, the professional service provider and their organization spend less time gathering background information. This allows services to be delivered quickly. A returning client is relieved from bother and some stress (Kotler et al., 2002). They do not have to go through the process of finding another physical therapy provider, and more importantly, another PT. When there is therapist continuity the client is relieved of the inconvenience of starting a new relationship (Gordon, 2000), worrying about the satisfaction the new therapist will deliver, and the boredom of rehashing history that the original therapist already knew.

For an organization, retaining current and former clients is eventually healthy for the organization. Relational personal professional sales is expensive because it is time consuming (Chapter 18). PTs are not paid for time spent in consultation (with Medicare beneficiaries). Relationship selling in physical therapy does not produce immediate income. However, according to several authors, eventually sales will increase and cover the early "expense" (Baron and Harris, 2003; Crissy and Kaplan, 1969; Kotler, 2000). In the long term, clients may see the merit of receiving more services, they may be more likely to want new services that become available, and when they have future needs, they are likely to return to where they have had a satisfactory business relationship. For a physical therapy business to sustain client volumes, clients who are discharged or leave for other reasons have to be replaced. Continual promotional marketing efforts can help bring in new clients and the return of past clients. Relational sales can help keep client volume up by focusing on the retention of existing clients who could choose to go elsewhere. After they are discharged, satisfied clients are likely to return when need arises. Satisfied clients are sources of new clients through their positive word-of-mouth recommendations (Kotler, 2000; Kotler et al., 2002).

Personal Selling Concept 2: Collaborate/Partner

Building relationships requires the parties to work together to solve problems of mutual interest. A willingness to work together constructively to achieve mutually agreed on goals is a short definition of collaboration. A seller seeks collaboration with a buyer to learn about their needs (in opening or during exploring) and in jointly resolving issues that are interfering with meeting the buyer's needs. A buyer's incentive for collaborating is to help formulate customized solutions to meet their needs. The parties agree to partner to develop and enact coordinated actions to meet the mutually defined goals (Morgan and Hunt, 1994). Collaboration also involves a willingness to give equal consideration to each other's ideas. There is respectful power sharing. In a collaborative relationship, the parties try to anticipate each other's needs and make adjustments for each other's benefit (Chapter 14). Drawing on product and service business research Chonko and Burnap (1998) and Liedtka (1996) have identified the core elements of a successful collaboration/partnership (Table 19.4).

The table makes clear that in professional service sales, planned collaboration assumes that the client is intellectually capable of cooperating, interpreting, analyzing, and challenging the professional service provider. This is not always possible in health care because some clients have temporary, progressive, or long-standing cognitive impairments. Respect for the individual is shown by making efforts to involve them in the planning and execution of their program. Substantive collaboration can also involve the client's caregivers or their advocates.

Personal Selling Concept 3: Listen

The fundamentals of listening and responding were reviewed in Chapter 12. Both are key skills for communicating and critical for exploring client needs. The professional must first listen in order to develop an enduring relationship and a collaborative partnership. Chapter 12 offered the logical suggestion that when gathering information, one should listen more than they talk. Several authors writing about sales also advocate for this perspective and they offer some quantitative suggestions. Super and Gold (2004) say that on average, the seller should adhere to a 75–25% listening to talking ratio. Shonka and Kosch (2002) offer a more stringent criterion. They suggest that learning as much as possible about a client's needs requires listening 95% of the time with the remaining 5% being used for asking clarifying questions. Clearly, successful interactions with clients can be developed when service providers have developed focused listening skills. Active, attentive listening is used to understand the client's unique circumstances and their needs and wants as completely as possible (Charney, 2004). Covey (1990) calls this empathic listening (Chapter 12). Listening requires an intention to fully understand the speaker's frame of reference. The seller needs to attend to all aspects of the communication: words, verbal changes, nonverbal signs, emotion, and so on, before responding. This level of aural listening includes hearing the client's voice modulations that may reflect emphasis, level of emotion, and pauses and silences which can indicate when the client is formulating their thoughts or waiting for the listener to give signs affirming that they have been heard or understood. Attention to the visual part of listening is equally important for the listener to determine the consistency between what the buyer is saying and how they are behaving. Visual messages are in speaker's eyes (eye contact and movement), facial expressions, mouth and head movements, hand gestures, and leg movements. Emotional stress can be seen as pupil dilation, perspiration, face/neck flushing,

Table 19.4 What Is Needed for a Successful Collaboration/Partnership	
Participant Mindset	**Participant Skills**
Belief that combining efforts provides an opportunity to achieve or exceed goals	Able to challenge one another
Willingness to trust each other	Able to negotiate and resolve disagreements
Commitment to working jointly toward goals	Able to create, negotiate for, and agree upon realistic expectations
Expectation that there will be reciprocal learning	Able to recognize that change is needed and make adjustment(s)

and dry mouth. Perspiration odor that becomes evident during discussion is another nonverbal sign of stress. For the seller, the combination of the words used by the client, the way they were expressed, and the observable concurrent physical signs that were seen suggest what questions need to be asked and how.

In professional sales, client stress can exist because of a great need to solve business problems, ambiguity of various solutions, penalty for making a choice that does not work out, and other reasons. In a physical therapy context, clients can show signs of stress because of their impairment(s), functional limitation(s), and disability. Stress can also be from unfamiliarity with the care environment, physical therapy, the therapist, costs associated with treatment, as well as other personal matters. The therapist is obligated to meet the client's need that includes lessening their stress. It is important to determine if stress from various sources has diminished the client's ability to assent to receiving services. This is acting in the best interest of the client.

Personal Selling Concept 4: Question

Intensive listening during the exploration step usually identifies voids in the information presented or understood, implied questions, inconsistencies, and concepts that were incompletely presented. To gain a clearer picture of what is important to the client, more exploring is needed for such things as specificity about the client's expectations, and additional information the professional needs to have clarified through questioning. There are four types of clarifying questions (Shonka and Kosch, 2002):

1. Open-ended questions intended to get a detailed response from the client. Questions beginning with: If, How, What, When, Where, Who, and Why often get the desired expanded response. Two examples are, "What would that entail?" and "Why did you do that?"
2. Assumptive questions that are open-ended and based on the assumption that what is asked or suggested is correct. A management example is "However it was that you calculated your client return rate it was below 30%, wasn't it?" Such questions can be used to segue to the topic of sales training

for staff to raise the rate. Assumptive questions also can be used as "feelers" to gauge the client's interest in a topic. "Am I right that the marketing department involves representatives from clinical departments when they are formulating their marketing strategies?" Assumptive questions could be answered with a few words, but they tend to elicit extended responses.

3. Impact questions are also open-ended. Impact means that the question makes the client pause to think before they respond. Impact questions are based on an understanding of the client's aspirations, expectations, needs, problems, and others. Inviting words like "Do you think that . . .?, What would happen if . . .?, and Can you tell me more about . . .?" This type of question can do two things. It can show the client how much you have learned already and it reflects your ability to examine, assess, and prioritize matters important to the client.
4. Close-ended questions that can be answered in one or a few words like correct, incorrect, no, yes, right, wrong, more important, and less important are close-ended. Close-ended questions can be used to quickly verify what was said or to add some information so a more precise open-ended question can be asked. Close-ended questions can also be answered nonverbally like a shoulder shrug, a head shake, a wink, or raising the arms in surrender.

From the Client's Perspective

An important clarification for professional service providers to have is what the client's expectations are about what will happen and what the result will be. In a professional relationship such questions have to be responded to clearly and as specifically as possible. Vagueness, shifting subjects, and giving an overly optimistic picture are detrimental to meaningful collaboration. PTs need to be prepared to handle a variety of client concerns about initiating or continuing therapy, like

High out-of-pocket costs (i.e., high deductibles and increasing co-insurance and premiums)
Time demands (i.e., travel time, waiting time, and duration of treatment sessions)
Perceived benefit of treatment (i.e., inconvenience and/or increased discomfort for small

or personally unimportant increments of improvement)

Amount of 1:1 contact, (i.e., the time a PT is actually involved in the delivery of treatment versus the client carrying out self-directed or nonprofessional supervised activities)

In response to a client who raises these kinds of concerns based on prior experience with other PT providers, the current therapist has an excellent opportunity to differentiate themselves, their setting, and their treatment program from others. Respect for the "experienced" client can also be shown by incorporating their terminology when answering questions and further questioning about their experience and preferences. "Inexperienced" clients may or may not have a template for their expectations. The therapist's behaviors, appearance, personality, and so on help the client refine or reframe their questions about what physical therapy is, the purpose of treatment, and how the professional provides it.

Clients also have concerns. They may express them as questions like, "this is really going to cost a lot won't it?" "What happens if I don't come 3 times a week?" Or, "are you experienced in treating what I have?" They can also make statements like, "my chiropractor can do that" or "I only want one PT to treat me—no assistant and no changing therapists." Once the client's concern is understood, the professional service provider and client can discuss ways to overcome the obstacles and deal with each other's objections to the possible solutions (Miller and Sinkovitz, 2005). A wise response to questions about outcomes is to under promise the level at the beginning and exceed that expectation at the end (Kotler et al., 2002).

Personal Selling Concept 5: Educate

Education is a deal maker for a professional service provider. It is part of formulating solutions to meet the client's needs. Educating a client helps establish the level of knowledge the professional service provider has and it is the foundation for the client's understanding of how a particular mix of services meets their expressed needs. Clients may or may not assume a professional has expert knowledge about the relevant services that are available

through their unit and organization, as well as services available through other sources. Professionals with expert knowledge can become a strategic resource for the client (Shonka and Kosch, 2002). In addition to technical competencies, PTs are usually knowledgeable about the assets of their unit and organization. Ideally, a PT is also versed on the benefits, risks, and cost of services and products available from local and regional competing professionals like chiropractors as well as similar therapy organizations and through Internet resources. The ability to explain services, deliver services according to contemporary standards, and share substantial knowledge about relevant variables and resources reflects a PT's broad expert knowledge. These variables make expert knowledge visible to the client. The reward for sharing knowledge and demonstrating competence in developing the service relationship is client trust. The likely short-term payoff is patient cooperation once treatment is begun. Educated clients can make informed choices that best serve to meet their perceived needs.

An educated client's main concerns about the professional service provider and the recommended services are reduced (objections have been dealt with) through new information and a confirmation of what they already assumed (Shonka and Kosch, 2002). The desired outcome is that the client has the appropriate information to make an informed decision to buy the services the professional is offering because they understand that the services meet their needs better than alternative services.

Sales Concept 6: Confirm Understandings

A pre-closing suggestion is for the professional service provider to summarize what they understand the client to have said about their needs and expectations. In response, the client confirms what they have said and, when necessary, clarifies what they said or mean. The parties continue the discussion until they have the same perspectives on matters they respectively believe are important. This may involve a mix of tactics such as additional education, making compromises, rephrasing, or clarifying terms.

A common physical therapy example of confirming understandings is the physical therapy goal. To a client, regaining independence may mean "walking like I was before the fall." To a PT, independence for this client may mean independent walking with a wheeled walker on all surfaces, in and out of doors, up to 200 feet at >2 mph within 3 weeks. The client's goal may or may not be realistic. The therapist's goal may or may not be a standard goal for like clients. To advance toward making the sale, i.e., buying into the treatment plan, one option is referred to as a change in the terms of delivery (Charney, 2004). In other words, if the care setting was a skilled nursing facility, the stated goal may be presented as the goal for discharge. Continued physical therapy services at an outpatient location could be arranged to continue the effort to achieve the client's vision. This goal clarification is in the best interest of both the client and the therapist. It is a win-win solution.

Concept 7: Agreement and Consent

In sales, getting a client's agreement to buy their service is known as closing the deal. It is the point where the client is asked to buy the service. The investment of time and effort the professional service provider has made on behalf of the client in the preceding six activities should allow the client to say "yes, I'll buy your services." The professional has to have worked thoughtfully and conscientiously throughout the sales encounter to have the privilege of asking the client to buy the service and expecting them to say yes (Charney, 2004). In the physical therapy context, closing the deal is asking for and receiving consent to treat. The consent is the client's agreement to participate in the physical therapy activities presented in the agreed upon plan of care. At this point, they (or their agent) understand(s) that the customized plan is appropriate for their circumstances and can lead to the consensus goal.

Sales Concept 8: Keep in Touch

Soon after the sales agreement, the professional often contacts the client. Some common reasons for a PT to follow up with a client are

Confirming the next appointment (starting and ending time and location)
Name and location of front desk person who will be expecting them

Updating them on any new matters that will be discussed
Reminding them of material they should bring
Letting them know if anyone else will be present and getting the client's agreement
Asking if they have any requests at this time
Offering additional contact information should the client need to contact them

During the service period sellers often discuss treatment and nontreatment matters in addition to providing the service. There are also reasons to contact clients between meetings. Examples include:

Informing the client of additional services the professional or their organization has that are appropriate for their needs (a new sales opportunity)
Letting the client know of any personnel, meeting time, or date changes that will occur

After services have been delivered, the professional or their marketing department makes periodic contact with the former client. Many of the reasons these contacts are made are relevant to physical therapy departments and to the individual PTs who provided services. For example:

Getting feedback on the sales experience, the professional, the organization, the service, the client's level of satisfaction, their current service needs, and other topics related to performance improvement
Announcing new services
Invitation to attend a promotional event
Introducing new staff members
Announcing staff and or organizational changes
Distributing annual and other reports
Announcing organizational awards, community service, publications, and other external recognition
Inviting clients to let others know of their satisfaction with the services provided
Asking them to share their service experiences with potential clients

A cost related aspect of recall business is of particular interest to PTs, managers, and practice owners. It has been estimated that sustaining positive client contact post-service costs one-fifth of what it does for marketing efforts to attract new clients (Kotler, 2000).

Help from the Marketing Department or a Consultant

Pre-, ongoing, and post-service promotion efforts are part of an integrated marketing strategy (Chapter 18). The strategic goal is to meet, even exceed, client expectations so they com-plete their course of treatment, return when they have future service needs, and they speak positively to others about their PT, the department, and the organization. Achievement of these goals requires collaboration between marketing and service providing departments like physical therapy. An important segment of such collaboration should be personal sales training for the professional service providers. The essence of such a program is outlined in Table 19.5.

Table 19.5   Example Program to Involve Clinical Professionals in the Sales Component of a Strategic Marketing Effort

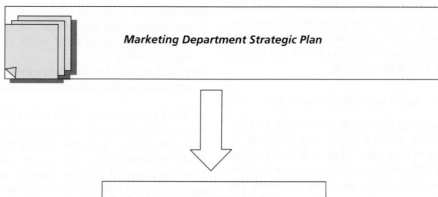

Marketing Department Strategic Plan

Professional Services Sales Training
Program For Clinical Dept. Managers

I. Organization marketing & sales plan
II. Department marketing & sales plan
III. Personnel training curriculum
A. Service sales model
B. 8 Personal service sales concepts
IV. Staff training time table
V. Follow-up reporting schedule

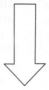

Training Modules for Professional
Services Sales: Physical Therapists

I. Service sales model, relationships,
    win-win partnering, collaboration
II. Communication = listen & question
III. Educate, confirm mutual under-
    standings
IV. Closing agreement, keeping in touch

Some Comments for PT Professionals

Delivering physical therapy services involves intense and frequent therapist-client contact. Time in front of clients is a valuable asset because it is a "value added" component of the service (Evans et al., 1998). This fosters mutual understanding and trust. This is a highly desirable position to be in for promoting sales. Clients buy services from those they trust, and not necessarily from those that they like (Swenson and Link, 1998). Being trusted is what is important in the relationship (Smith and Barclay, 1997). In a relational exchange process as advocated in this chapter, the initial sale is not the sole goal. Rather, the relationship and initial course of treatment are seen as the beginning of a long-term relationship involving future exchanges (Swenson and Link, 1998). Future exchanges are particularly important in an era of health care that is *consumer-driven* and competition for market share is keen (Chapters 4, 16, and 22). Potential and current clients seek information about their health care options, in part, because they have a financial interest in managing their own care (Gratzer, 2006; Porter and Teisberg, 2006). More than ever before, clients are demanding (Swenson and Link, 1998), better informed (Shonka and Kosch, 2002), and they want more say in the selection and delivery of their care services (Gratzer, 2006; Porter and Teisberg, 2006). Clients and their professional service providers need to converse. Therapists need to learn about their clients' needs so they can meet them efficiently and cost effectively in contrast to "selling" them something (Charney, 2004) just because the therapist likes a particular treatment or the equipment happens to be available. Therapists are obligated to learn about their clients' needs (goals) and respect their autonomy when they make choices. Informed choices require sharing appropriate information with clients about expected benefits, risks, costs, and other information believed to be helpful for the client to make appropriate choices about available services and products. The accuracy and timeliness of such information provided to clients enhances the likelihood of garnering the client's trust.

What's in It for Me?

Service volume has fiscal implications for the therapy unit and the organization. Under payment arrangements where providing more units of service or more products results in higher total payment (fee-for-service and discounted fee-for-service [Chapters 2 and 22]), providing the full spectrum of necessary services to satisfy clients' needs and wants has multiple benefits. Clients get what they should have or want, it helps therapists meet productivity expectations, the operational unit contributes more to the organization's revenue stream, and clients say good things about their therapist.

The Tough Situation

Clients insured under restrictive payer arrangements (fixed payment, limited number of visits) or without insurance, or who have no further physical therapy benefits can be informed that they have the option to pay out-of-pocket for continued or additional services. Many therapists are uncomfortable making this recommendation in such cases. Even answering inquiries about what Medicare's Advance Beneficiary Notice is all about may cause the therapist to take a deep breath before answering. These therapist reactions may be because the culture of the profession fosters benevolence over financial gain (APTA, 2007c; Nosse and Sagiv, 2005) (Chapter 7), or alternatively, they do not have sufficient sales skills, particularly in the area of closing the sale. There is evidence to infer that inadequate selling skills is at least part of the problem. Several documents have noted the importance of marketing knowledge and skill (which by definition includes sales precepts) for PTs (APTA, 2004, 2006; Schafer et al., 2007). The selling model and relational selling concepts provide means of strengthening practical selling skills. Regardless of the source of payment, professional guidelines support providing consumers with all the means available to help them satisfy their physical therapy related and other needs and wants, even those who have financial limitations (APTA, 2007a-c).

The opportunity to recommend physical therapy and other organizational services, and the obligation to meet clients' needs underscores the importance of having sufficient knowledge of the clients' financial constraints, professional guidelines, institutional policies, and payer requirements. When a client raises objections because of cost, a professional who believes in the value of their services, the strength of their expertise, and the potential benefits for the client, will go back to the sales steps, identify where the client is, and apply the appropriate selling concepts to deal with the objections. Not making this second effort is disingenuous. It is counter to the concepts of relational personal selling.

Selling Ideas to Others

The usefulness of understanding the progressive steps in a client's decision has applicability in most interactions where a win-win result is desired (Miller and Sinkovitz, 2005). For contrast purposes, Tables 19.6 and 19.7 present the sales steps and the application of the selected sales concepts for management and personal situations, respectively.

The five sales steps and the eight selling concepts can help to advance engaged parties toward making a decision that is good for both. Together they are a template for win-win encounters with clients, coworkers, and acquaintances. Being skilled in utilizing relational selling precepts helps broaden a therapist's scope of professional expertise.

Summary

This chapter expanded the discussion of the linkage between marketing and sales, discussed types of sales, defined sales in the context of professional services like physical therapy, introduced core information about the progression of events in a sales encounter, and presented contemporary service sales concepts believed to be useful in selling professional services like physical therapy. The chapter drew the readers attention to the potential advantages, practicality, and professionally compatible approach to personal selling based on relationship building. Marketing oversees organizational efforts to get clients in the door as well as to get them to return in the future. In health care, once a client is in the door, their needs, wants, and expectations have to be identified, discussed, clarified, and agreed upon before an individualized treatment plan can be delivered. This progression of interactions between a professional service provider such as a PT and their client is similar to those described in the personal selling approach utilized to enhance the sale of professional services through relationship building.

Relational selling is based on establishing trust with a client and building a collaborative, trust centered, relationship. The intent for a professional like a PT is to learn as much as they can from the client about what the client wants, needs, and expects and then show

Table19.6 General Application Selling Template: Staff Member and Their Manager	
Seller Progression	Selling Concept Applications
Opening	I have worked here x years. I have enjoyed it and I wish to do more to help the department grow.
Exploring and confirming	Let me know if I am paraphrasing you correctly. You have talked about the department's needs for expertise, for retention of staff, recruitment of new staff members, and growth in the area I work in.
Presenting solution(s)	Another senior staff member would help meet the needs you have voiced. I have the expertise, a willingness to teach, and an interest in expanding programs in my area.
Dealing with objections	Q: What will others think? A: Peers recognize my expertise. Q: Will they listen? A: They come to me now. Q: Will it raise labor cost? A: Over time it will bring in more, increase client satisfaction, and help staff retention and recruitment.
Closing	It is in the department's greater interest to have another senior staff member. Are you willing to recommend this new position be established?

Table 19.7	General Application Selling Template: Splitting Dating Expenses
Seller Progression	*Selling Concept Applications*
Opening	The price of gas just goes up and up.
Exploring and confirming	Is the tank full? Gas cost you $55 tonight, right?
Presenting solution	The tank is now full. It cost about what the tickets will cost. You bought the gas, so I would like to pay for the tickets.
Dealing with objections	Q: I invited you out didn't I? A: Yes, and you did the last two weekends. I can chip in. By sharing our resources we can enjoy more things we like more often.
Closing	So, I'll buy the tickets tonight, agreed?

how these criteria can be met by their professional abilities and by the resources of their department and their organization. The tools for accomplishing these personal selling tasks were a five-step progressive process of a selling encounter and eight integrated relational sales concepts. This provides the professional service provider with a template to follow that guides their progression and application of the relational sales concepts.

For a PT, no other form of promotion can provide the client with an experience as meaningful as personal selling. Personal selling allows the therapist to learn about the client's individual circumstances and expectations. With this knowledge, a collaborative treatment plan that is workable and expected to meet the client's needs can be formulated. Getting the client's agreement to commit to doing their part in carrying out the treatment plan is the "sale."

Clients buy expertise. Meeting their needs at the level they expect at every step in the service experience is a way for clients to confirm that they made the right choice of professional service provider. Satisfied clients usually stay with their provider to meet their current needs and often return when future services are needed or desired. Satisfied clients also speak well of their professional service provider, their department, and their organization to others who are in need of service. Ideally, successful personal selling results in an increase in sales volume. At a minimum, it can help sustain market share in a competitive environment. The importance of selling skills will be again brought up in the next chapter on physical therapy practice ownership. In this environment, staying in business is critically linked to the skill of all the professional members of the practice to promote the practice through personal selling.

CASE STUDY 19.1

What Have You Noticed?

Tasks

Based on your clinical experience, identify three physical therapy related selling opportunities that were used to enhance selling a service or idea and three that were not. Examples can come from your own actions or inactions with clients, department coworkers, managers, or interactions with members of other departments or organizations.

Applications

1. Think about the situations where selling did occur. List which of the eight relational selling concepts you think you observed in each case.
2. Think about the situations where selling opportunities were missed. Which of the eight relational selling concepts do you think were missed most often?
3. Outline a personal plan to improve your use of relational selling concepts in a variety of situations.

CASE STUDY 19.2

Selling Training

From your work on the previous case you could offer some suggestions to a marketing department representative who is interested in developing a workshop on promotion for therapists.

Develop an Outline of Suggestions

1. List things you would like to see covered regarding personal selling to clients.

2. List things you would like to see covered regarding personal selling to (choose one: peers, supervisors, physicians, other department members, family members, other).

3. Types of resources you would recommend be provided to the therapists.

REFERENCES

American Institute of Certified Public Accountants. Professional ethics/code of professional conduct. Available at http://www.aicpa.org/Professional+Resources/Professional+Ethics+Code+of+Professional+Conduct/. Accessed 4/05/08.

American Physical Therapy Association. Code of ethics. Available at http://www.apta.org/AM/Template. cfm?Section=Core_Documents1&Template=/CM/HTMLDisplay.cfm&ContentID=25854. Accessed 12/23/07a.

American Physical Therapy Association. Guide for professional conduct. Available at http://www.apta.org/AM/Template.cfm?Section=Core_Documents1&Template=/CM/HTMLDisplay.cfm&ContentID=24781. Accessed 12/05/07b.

American Physical Therapy Association. Professionalism in physical therapy: Core values. Available at http://www.apta.org/AM/Template.cfm?Section=Professionalism1&TEMPLATE=/CM/ContentDisplay.cfm&CONTENTID=39529. Accessed 7/14/07c.

American Physical Therapy Association. A normative model of physical therapist professional education. Alexandria, VA: Author. 2004.

American Physical Therapy Association. Education strategic plan (2006–2020). Available at http://www.apta.org/AM/Template.cfm?Section=Home&TEMPLATE=/CM/ContentDisplay.cfm&CONTENTFILEID=6170. Accessed 8/20/06.

Baron S, Harris K. Services marketing text and cases, 2nd ed. New York, NY: Palgrave. 2003.

Bateson J. Do we need service marketing? In Eiglier P, Langeard P, Lovelock CH, Bateson JEG, Young RF, eds. Marketing consumer services: New insights, Technical Report 77-115. Cambridge, MA: Marketing Service Institute. 1977:1–30.

Charney C. The instant sales pro. New York, NY: AMACOM. 2004.

Chonko LJ, Burnap HF. Strategic account strategies. In Bauer GJ, Baunchalk MS, Ingram TN, LaForge RW. Emerging trends in sales thought and practice. Westport, CN: Quorum Books. 1998:81-108.

Covey SR. The seven habits of highly effective people. New York, NY: Fireside. 1990.

Crissy WJE, Kaplan RM. Salesmanship: The personal force in marketing. New York, NY: John Wiley and Sons. 1969.

Direct Selling Association. Code of ethics. Available at http://retailindustry.about.com/gi/dynamic/offsite.htm?zi=1/XJ/Ya&sdn=retailindustry&cdn=money&tm=33&gps=87_228_963_767&f=10&tt=14&bt=0&bts=0&zu=http%3A//www.dsa.org/. Accessed 12/20/07.

Donnelly JH, George WR. Marketing of services. Chicago, IL: American Marketing Association. 1981.

Eades KM, Kear RE. The solution-centric organization. New York, NY: McGraw-Hill. 2006.

Evans KR, Good DJ, Hellman TW. Relationship selling: New challenges for today's sales manager. In Bauer GJ, Baunchalk MS, Ingram TN, LaForge RW. Emerging trends in sales thought and practice. Westport, CN: Quorum Books. 1998:31–48.

Federated State Boards of Physical Therapy. Examination information. Available at http://www.fsbpt.org/ForCandidatesAndLicensees/Jurisprudence/index.asp. Accessed 3/7/08.

Forsyth P. Marketing and selling professional services, 3rd ed. Sterling, VA: Kogan Page. 2003.

Gordon J. Selling 2.0. New York, NY: Berkley. 2000.

Gratzer D. The Cure: How capitalism can save American health care. New York, NY: Encounter. 2006.

Kotler P. Marketing management, The Millennium ed. Upper Saddle River, NJ: Prentice Hall. 2000.

Kotler P, Hayes T, Bloom PN. Marketing professional services, 2nd ed. Upper Saddle River, NJ: Prentice Hall. 2002.

Levitt T. Marketing myopia. Harvard Business Review. 1960;48(July-August):45–56.

Liedtka JM. Collaborating across lines of business for competitive advantage. The Academy of Management Executive. 1996;10(2):20–34.

Manufacturers Agents National Association. MANA code of ethics. Available at http://www.manaonline.org/?cat=6. Accessed 12/20/07.

Miller MS, Sinkovitz J. Selling is dead: Moving beyond traditional sales roles and practices to revitalize growth. Hoboken, NJ: John Wiley & Sons. 2005.

Morgan RM, Hunt SD. The commitment-trust theory of relationship marketing. Journal of Marketing 1994;58:20–38.

Nosse LJ, Sagiv L. Theory-based study of the basic values of 565 physical therapists. Physical Therapy. 2005;85:834–850.

Porter ME, Teisberg EO. Redefining health care: Creating value-based competition on results. Boston, MA: Harvard Business School. 2006.

Schafer DS, Lopopolo RB, Luedtke-Hoffman KA. Administration and management skills needed by physical therapists graduates in 2010: A national survey. Physical Therapy. 2007;87:261–281.

Shonka M, Kosch D. Beyond selling value: A proven way to avoid the vendor trap. Chicago, IL: Dearborn Trade Publishing. 2002.

Shostack GL. Breaking free from product marketing. Journal of Marketing. 1977;41:73–80.

Smith JB, Barclay DW. The effects of organizational differences and trust on the effectiveness of selling partner relationships. Journal of Marketing. 1997;61:3–21.

Super C, Gold RD. Selling (without selling) 4 1/2 steps to success. New York, NY: AMACON. 2004.

Swenson MJ, Link GD. Relationship selling: New challenges for today's salesperson. In Bauer GJ, Baunchalk MS, Ingram TN, LaForge RW. Emerging trends in sales thought and practice. Westport, CN: Quorum Books. 1998:11–30.

ADDITIONAL RESOURCES

An excellent, short, clearly written paperback on the marketing process and the communication mix is the Marketer's Toolkit: The 10 Strategies You Need to Succeed (Boston, Mass: Harvard Business School Press. 2006). The principles of customer-centric selling are reviewed in a short video clip available at http://www.allbusiness.com/3474087-1.html. The American Management Association provides audio summaries of its publications, podcasts, and seminars at http://podcast.amanet.org/edgewise/category/. To review information on the government's perspective on consumer driven health care, access Health and Human Services. Value-driven health care. Available at http://www.hhs.gov/valuedriven/index.html. General information about managers involved in marketing, advertising, and promotion is available at http://www.bls.gov/oco/ocos020.htm.

Business Acumen: Financial Awareness

CHAPTER 20

ECONOMIC PRINCIPLES

MARK DRNACH

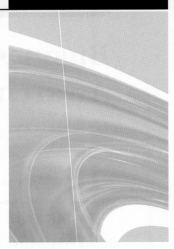

Learning Objectives

1. Understand the role of the government in a society and its role in the allocation of resources.
2. Describe basic economic principles.
3. Understand the role of competition in the market and the basic aspects of environmental scanning.
4. Identify the various costs and their behavior associated with the delivery of health care in the clinical setting.

Introduction

Health care has evolved over the past century into a multibillion-dollar industry. The need to remain financially solvent, make decisions that include the cost of services, and to maintain and prove effectiveness have come to the forefront of the health care industry. Health care providers can no longer have a narrow focus on the treatment of their patients. They must also have an awareness of the availability of resources, costs, and other economic factors associated with the delivery of services (Chapters 3, 4, 19, 21, and 22).

Economics is the study of economies. The term economy refers to the amount of services and goods that are produced and available, how services and goods are distributed, and how many and which types of services and goods are consumed (Gale, 2006). This chapter is intended to provide the reader with a fundamental understanding of commonly used economic terms and the principles that drive the U.S. economic system. Health care and physical therapy-specific examples are used to exemplify economic principles. In economic terms, physical therapy is a resource that is allocated among various health care markets (Chapter 18). On the supply side, there are an estimated 90,000 employed physical therapists (PT) with the unemployment rate for PTs of 0.2% (American Physical Therapy Association [APTA], 2005). Among the demand side components are the aging of the baby boomers (those born between 1946 and 1964) with higher utilization rates, increasing rate of chronic illness in the elderly such as heart disease and stroke, and an increasing awareness of the benefits of health in the maintenance of function and quality of life. PTs that have clinical doctoral degrees and a recognized area of specialization, for example, board certified specialist, completion of a residency program, or another professional degree or certification, are likely to have a competitive advantage over most substitutes. The pursuit of postgraduate education on a full-time basis does have what is called an **opportunity cost** (i.e., tuition, loss of income and possibly loss of direct clinical experience), but will provide valuable personal and economic rewards. Finally, in the workplace the concept of economy of scale may be recognized in the form of productivity expectations. If salaries are a fixed cost, by increasing the volume of work carried out by existing

Key Terms

Key terms, which are defined below, are bolded and italicized the first time they appear in the chapter. Other important terms are shown in boldface on first appearance and are defined by the context in which they are used. When either of these types of terms is used several times, its acronym will be identified and subsequently used in the chapter. Both types of terms are listed alphabetically in the online glossary with their definitions and (when applicable) their acronyms.

capitalism: an economic philosophy that espouses a market orientation that is a free-market economy and competition and an orientation favoring individualistic efforts to succeed.

command economy: an economic system where the resources are state owned and their allocation and use is determined by the centralized decisions of a planning authority.

competitive market: a market where there are ample like or similar services and products available to customers.

consumer price index (CPI): an economic indicator that measures the change in the cost of a fixed collection of services or goods. It is used as a measure of inflation.

demand: the ability and level of desire to buy a service or product. Marketing can help increase or meet demand.

economics: systematic study of the production, conservation and allocation of resources in conditions of scarcity, together with the interaction of consumers, producers, and government. Includes supply and demand in markets, employment/unemployment, growth and development, and income.

economy of scale: the savings in cost due to mass production.

elasticity: a measure of responsiveness. A health care example is looking at the demand for a service and changes in some other variable like price in the supply and demand equation.

inelastic: demand is insensitive to price changes such as when the service or product is essential to the consumer or when a consumer has sufficient income to buy the needed items when there is a substantial price change.

macroeconomic policy: monetary policy influencing the supply of money and the interest rate, and fiscal policy influencing taxes and government spending.

microeconomic principles: help predict how markets will respond to policy and other influences.

needs: according to Maslow, basic needs are hierarchically arranged. Fulfillment of the basics allows the higher needs to be pursued. Needs are physiological (most basic), safety, love, esteem, and self-actualization (highest level).

price elasticity: the sensitivity of demand to changing price.

public goods: services/products that benefit all of the people of a country and are available to all regardless of ability to pay.

resource allocation: distributing limited resources to people/departments/organizations who have unlimited wants.

scarcity: the market condition when wants exceeds the availability of supply.

supply: supply refers to the amount of services or goods available at a given price at any time.

supply and demand curve: demand is how many consumers desire the services or goods that are in supply. A curve of the supply and demand relationship shows that the variables are inversely related. As selling price or supply goes up, consumer demand goes down.

utility: a measure of the satisfaction or benefit a consumer receives from a service or good.

want: something a person desires or would like to have.

staff, the fixed cost is distributed over a larger number of **units of service** (UOS), lowering the labor cost per unit and thereby increasing financial productivity and ultimately profits. A deeper understanding of general economic concepts is useful for PTs in planning their personal and professional endeavors, for clearly,

no one operates in an economic vacuum (Stossel, 2005).

Economics

The systematic interactions between producing, distributing, and consuming wealth can be applied to a country or segment of business. Economists investigate how people use their limited resources to fulfill their wants and needs under conditions of scarcity, together with the interaction of consumers, producers, and government. How an economic system or economy functions is one of life's important domains. The national economy influences quality of life through *macroeconomic policies* (e.g., monetary policy influencing the supply of money and the interest rate, and fiscal policy influencing taxes and government spending). Principles known as *microeconomic principles* help predict how markets will respond to policy and other influences. Examples include the supply and demand of a specific service or good in a given market, inflation and unemployment status, and in turn, the standard of living (Hajiran, 2007). Economics is often presented in terms of the production of a good or service and is commonly understood in relation to the buying and selling of consumer goods, like food or other tangible items (Chapter 19). The application of basic economic principles to the behavior of the health care industry is not straightforward, given the complex nature of health care as a product and service (Scott et al., 2001). Folland et al. (2007) suggest that what makes health care a distinctive economic system is the following:

1. The presence of uncertainty inherent in a person's health, making demand irregular for the individual. Consumers of health care are uncertain of their needs for any specific period in the future, which makes demand for health care irregular from the individual's or individual practice's perspective.

2. The presence of health insurance that guards against uncertainty but also reduces the costs of health care at any one point in time. The demand for a costly health service (e.g., heart bypass surgery) may rise in the presence of health insurance, since that insurance costs less (e.g., $350.00/month in premiums) than the costly intervention ($8,000.00/surgery). This affects demand for health care by those consumers who may be candidates for the intervention, and depending on the insurance, may affect the incentives of the health care provider. For example, diagnosis-related groups, **pro-**spective payment systems, and resource utilization groups (Chapter 22).

3. The lack of information on what constitutes good or needed health care is a problem. Consumers do not know the details of what they need to stay or become healthly without the advice of health care professionals like physicians or PTs. The professional also does not know with 100% certainty the outcome of any specific intervention or episode of care, and may perform several diagnostic tests or evaluations to guide him in the diagnostic process and subsequent provision of care.

4. The restriction on competition through state legislation, licensure laws, Certificate of Need programs, professional education requirements and educational costs, as well as other imposed regulations. This can impact the supply of health care by restricting the number of people who can become health care providers (Chapter 8).

5. The lack of health care in another individual often evokes feelings of sadness or concern, leading people to believe that something should be done to provide health care, although exactly how that should be accomplished in the United States is under debate (Chapter 1).

6. Government subsidies and programs which are present in most developed nations provide structured means of service delivery at a certain level and are primarily funded by mandatory taxes on the citizens (Chapter 1). With government-sponsored programs comes the basic economic problem of the type and level of health care to provide (e.g., vaccinations, preventative services, comprehensive or limited rehabilitation), how to provide it (e.g., through government or private clinics/facilities), and who is eligible for the government program (e.g., the poor, people without current access, people with disabilities, etc.).

7. The fact that health itself is not bought with money; health care is bought and the factors or influences that produce health, or a return to a healthy state, are sought by the consumer. Health is desired because it makes people feel better and allows them to work, thereby increasing their income and tax revenue for the government (Folland et al., 1993).

Similar to providing for financial health (e.g., Social Security), providing for a citizen's physical health may also be viewed as the responsibility of the government. Given the distinctive features of health care, the rising demand and cost of coverage, some government intervention may be warranted.

The Role of Government

What is the role of government and why do people organize themselves with a central governing body? This is a fundamental question that is the basis of understanding why people form governments and what is expected of them. Intervention by a government comes mainly through the activities of provision, distribution, and regulation of health care (Folland et al., 2007). First, a government has the duty to protect the people from violence, both within its borders and from external attacks. This is done in part by the establishment of a national defense system, a legal system, and a police force that are responsible for protection and the maintenance of order. Second, a government has the duty to establish certain social practices that protect its citizens from oppression and injustice, which in turn promotes internal order and general satisfaction among the people. This is addressed in part by the establishment of rules and regulations and a justice system, which includes a system of incarceration and rehabilitation for individuals who break the law. Third, a government has the duty to establish and maintain a system of *public goods*. Public goods are services and products for the benefit of the people. No one is excluded from accessing them regardless of who paid for them. Public goods include such things as the building and maintenance of public highways, harbors, airports, and railways for the public use. These systems support and promote trade among people and factor into the economic growth of a society (Lipford and Slice, 2007).

Prior to the 1900s, the role of the government in the United States and other developing countries was minor, with relatively low taxation and few regulations (Lipford and Slice, 2007). However, governments started to change; instituting more social programs such as public education, workers' compensation

for work-related injuries, old-age pension, and the funding of health care. This broadening of the role of government has brought about profound changes, not only in the programs that the government has to offer but the amount of funds needed to financially support and maintain the various social programs that have developed. The availability of funds is influenced by many factors including the economic system that is adopted by a government or country, the system and level of service provision, and the utilization of the services by the people (Chapter 1).

Capitalism

Capitalism can be defined as an economic system based on private ownership of capital in which the production and distribution of goods is done in a relatively free (limited government influence) for-profit market (Fig. 20.1). It is the main economic system in North America. Capitalism is based on four main pillars: a

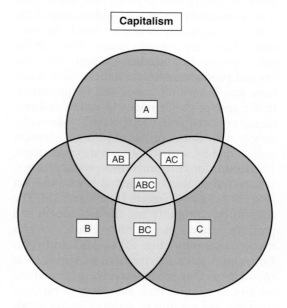

Figure 20.1. Capitalism. The controlling powers in a society: (A) Individuals with private control; (B) Governments with state control; (C) Natural resource constraints or property control. (If A>B then AB = Democracy. If B>A then AB = Dictatorship). The four pillars of capitalism: (AB) Democracy; (AC) Free markets; (BC) Governmental regulations; (ABC) Private property rights (Hajiran, 2007).

democratic or freely elected government; free markets for economic competition and the pursuit of an improved quality of life; private property rights which empower profit motives by owners/entrepreneurs; and governmental regulations regarding enforcement of commerce related contracts both nationally and internationally (Hajiran, 2007).

The U.S. government, which is part of the world's largest and most successful capitalistic society, is faced with the same problem of most industrialized nations: how to provide basic health care to all of its citizens (Chapter 1). Through a system of taxation and governmental programs (i.e., Medicare and Medicaid) the U.S. government has made some attempt to provide health care for some of its citizens, the elderly and the poor, but continues to debate the questions of who should receive health care, who should pay for it, and what level of care should be provided while maintaining a balance between government regulations, free markets, and private rights in a capitalist society. When a central authority such as a government answers these questions based on a master plan it is a *command economy*. A modification of the command economy is one in which the consumer has some limited choices. Through the price systems in a **market economy** consumers and producers interact to determine what, how, and for whom goods will be produced. In the case of public goods (e.g., law enforcement, military, and transportation services), they may be better provided by a government rather than by individual (private) producers. The forum for consumer and producer interactions/transactions is referred to as a **market** (Fig. 20.1, AC) (Chapters 18, 19, and 22). The right to own property and the consumer's and producer's freedom of choice characterizes a market economy (Fig. 20.1, ABC and AC). Consumers have the freedom to spend their resources as they see fit. Producers (providers) are free to allocate their resources to produce the type and amount of services and/or products they desire. The role of government (Fig. 20.1 B) in a market economy is to:

1. Provide goods or services that would not otherwise be produced, such as public safety.
2. Accommodate for weaknesses in the market economy that may result in misallocation of resources, such as health care.

3. Establish restrictions to the free market that are in the interest of the public good or health.

In support of a market economy there is a core set of economic principles and related concepts. The following sections discuss these principles and concepts.

Basic Economic Principles

Needs and Wants

A basic discussion on economics can begin with an understanding of human beings' needs and wants (Chapter 23). Maslow (1943) presented a human-centered theory on motivation that categorized a human's basic needs in a hierarchical fashion, where the appearance of one need rests on the prior satisfaction of another. Every drive or motivation is related to the state of satisfaction or dissatisfaction of other needs or desires. These basic needs are categorized as

1. Physiological needs such as food, clothing, and shelter
2. Safety needs such as safety from harm, tyranny, or extreme temperatures
3. Love needs, both giving and receiving such things as affection, belonging, or the need for a life partner
4. Esteem needs such as personal achievement, independence, or prestige
5. Self-actualization needs such as the feeling of self-fulfillment, living a life that one was meant to live, the actualization of one's full potential

The emergence of these needs rest on the satisfaction of the preceding or more fundamental need.

A "want," on the other hand, is something that a person desires or would like to have (Chapter 23). These wants can motivate a person, especially if the person has the financial means to obtain them. Understanding the difference between what a person needs and what he wants is important in both the delivery of health care services and in running a business, as well as in personal life.

Scarcity

Scarcity is an economic condition when human wants and needs exceed the available supply. A society cannot fulfill all of the wants or needs of the people at one time; there has to be a point where the supply of one item is sufficient given the total amount of all the various wants and needs that can be identified. Whenever resources are limited in the presence of unlimited wants it can be said that there is a scarcity of the resource. Goods and services are scarce because of limited availability (natural resource constraints) along with the limits in technology and of trained people relative to the total amount of the item desired (Wikipedia Free Encyclopedia, 2008).

The concept of opportunity cost is related to scarcity of resources. Consumers have finite resources. When expending limited resources consumers strive to gain maximum value (best outcome for low cost) (Chapter 4). They cannot afford all of the goods and services they might desire. As a result, they must choose between all of the possible goods and services available to them. The goal is to make the choice that results in the greatest added value. To do this, the consumer must compare the relative value of alternative purchases under consideration. The opportunity cost of an acquisition is the value of the alternative opportunity that was foregone (Finkler and Ward, 1999).

In the United States, many Americans may not believe that health care resources are scarce. A general hypothesis is that everyone is entitled to live as long as possible and as healthy as possible, and that this is attainable given enough health care. When combined with the opinion that health care resources and the money to buy them are readily available, it may become clearer why some individuals resist restrictions on health care, even when they might agree that health care resources are not being used efficiently. Few people will tolerate limits on health care when the limit is viewed not because of scarcity but as someone else's refusal to spend money on available care (Mariner, 1995).

But is health care really scarce, or are the shortages of health care personnel and technology due to limited government funding or other market barriers in accessing health care services, such as the price of the professional education, or practice costs? A problem with the current health care system may not be associated with scarcity but rather *resource allocation*; how to allocate limited resources

to people who have unlimited wants. This is based on opportunity cost more than financial cost, the main concerns being the efficiency, choice, and distribution of health care (Scott et al., 2001). If the allocation is efficient then the quantity and type of health care that the consumer wants would be available and produced at the lowest possible cost. The value that is placed on a service or good will be reflected in the allocation of funds to produce an adequate supply of those services or goods. How money is allocated towards resources is a reflection on the importance placed on those resources. In the United States, only a portion of the available monies is allocated to health care. How we allocate resources reflects how we value different resources such as national defense, health care programs, and public education.

Value and Utility

Value is the importance that an individual good or service attains for a person because he or she is dependent on it to satisfy a want or need (Menger, 2007). Value may be **tangible** (quantifiable), **intangible** (not quantifiable) or both. Consider the process of deciding on a summer vacation. Assume that the decision has been narrowed down to either a ski trip or a tropical cruise. If the ski trip and cruise are the same price then both trips will result in the same decline in the vacationer's resources. His final choice will be based on his assessment of intangible value. Intangible value might be measured in prestige or expected enjoyment. If the cruise were twice as expensive as the ski trip, then the vacationer would have both tangible and intangible value to consider. Intangible value may weigh the decision in favor of the more costly alternative. The concept of intangible and tangible value also applies to organizational decisions. When an organization has the opportunity to invest in one of two alternative business ventures, management will use financial information to identify the resource requirements (cost) and projected value to the organization. Often they want to determine which venture will yield the greatest projected financial return. However, under some circumstances the venture with the lower financial return may be selected based on intangible value. For example, a community hospital may select a venture that does the most to further its mission of community service or has a lower short-term return but positions it for greater return to the community in the long run.

Marginal analysis is used to solve microeconomic problems by looking at the cost and benefit associated with the next, or marginal, unit that is either bought or sold. In order to maximize profits, producers must produce at a level where marginal cost is equal to marginal revenue. If marginal revenue is greater than marginal cost then there is a potential to make more profit, so the producer will produce more. If marginal cost is greater than marginal revenue then the producer is over producing and losing profit on each unit. The **marginal value** of a good or service is the value of the last increment of the good or service sold or purchased.

Utility is a measure of satisfaction or benefit one receives from a product or service. People will attempt to maximize their utility (satisfaction) given their unique constraints like available funds. This helps to determine how much a person would be willing to pay for a good or service (Finkler et al., 2007). **Marginal utility** is defined as the extra utility achieved by consuming one more unit of a good. For example, utility will increase to a certain point for bottled water before it increases at a decreasing rate as the addition of one more bottle of water decreases the satisfaction or benefit of having bottled water. This concept is formally known as the law of diminishing marginal utility. As a person increases his consumption of a service or product there is a diminishing of satisfaction or benefit with each additional unit consumed. How consumers go about choosing the mix of services and goods that maximize their utility is based on their needs, wants, and preferences, the amount of money they have to spend, and the price of the goods or services available to them in the market. By collecting relevant data on the individual consumer's choices based on various determinants of demand such as price, income, and price of alternatives, a market demand can be estimated (Chapter 18).

Supply and Demand

According to the Department of Labor, the *demand* for PTs is expected to grow 27% from 2006 to 2016 (Bureau of Labor Statistics, 2008). This increase is facilitated by the growing elderly population, the aging of the baby boomers, and the advancements in technology that save the lives of infants born too soon or with life-threatening disabilities. The *supply* of PTs in the United States is roughly 50/100,000 (New York Center for Health Workforce Studies, 2008) A basic concept in economics is the relationship between the quantity supplied of an item, such as a PT's services, and its relationship to the quantity demanded for such an item in a market. This is commonly represented in a *supply and demand curve* (Fig. 20.2).

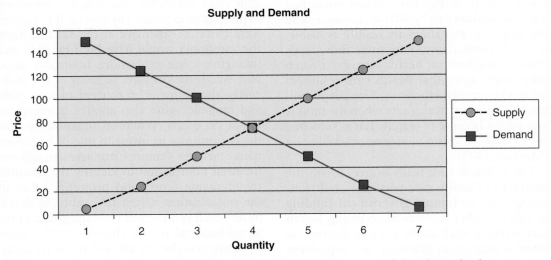

Figure 20.2. Supply and demand diagram. A basic economic representation of the relationship between the quantity supplied of a good or service to the quantity demand and its relationship to price. As demand increases the price decreases. As the price increases the supply increases.

In economics, this is one of the simplest ways to explain the price behavior resulting from the willingness of consumers to buy and the willingness of producers to produce. At a given level of demand, as the supply of an item or service increases the price that a consumer is willing to pay for that item decreases. This explanation of a consumer's behavior assumes that all other factors in the market are held constant, such as an individual's income, perceptions, and the price of other items in the market at that time.

An example of a supply and demand relationship could be applied to the demand for physical therapy services in a local community or market. If the services are available and provided for free, the quantity demanded would be expected to be at its maximum with other factors held constant. If the price for a physical therapy service was increased to $75, the quantity demanded would be expected to drop as the consumer makes a decision that the service is not valued at $75, or living on a finite amount of dollars, he chooses to spend his $75 on something else that is of value to him in the market. If the price of a physical therapy service increases to $150, the demand will continue to drop. That is why the demand curve slopes downward. The law of demand states that the quantity demanded would decrease as the price increases.

Supply can be looked at similarly. As the price (payment) that is paid to the physical therapy provider increases, the supply (number of PTs providing services) will also increase. For example, if PTs were not paid to perform a service, the supply of PTs would be expected to be very limited given that other factors remain constant. If the price paid to a PT was increased to $75 per service, the supply of PT would be expected to increase. If the price paid for a service increases to $150, the supply would continue to rise. That is why the supply curve slopes upward. The law of supply is that the quantity supplied would increase as the price increases.

Under ideal conditions, the point at which the supply and demand curves meet is the point of **equilibrium** in the market. This is the point where the supply of PTs meets the demand for physical therapy services. If the quantity of physical therapy services supplied exceeds the quantity demanded, theoretically, the price for a physical therapy service

is forced to decline, leading to a decrease in the quantity supplied. Conversely, if the quantity of physical therapy services falls short of the quantity demanded, the price for physical therapy services would rise, leading to an increase in the quantity of PTs willing to supply their services to the market. Theoretically, in a free market without government control, supply and demand vacillate until an equilibrium point is reached.

Elasticity of Demand

A basic economic question is, as the price of a health care service rises will the quantity demanded be affected? This question reflects the economic concept called *elasticity*. Elasticity is a term used to describe the responsiveness of any variable. Relating this to health care services is to look at the demand for a health care service, and changes in some other variable like price in the supply and demand equation. The sensitivity of demand to changing price is called *price elasticity*. Price elasticity of demand (PED) is calculated by dividing the percentage of change in the quantity demanded by the percentage change in the price.

$$PED = \frac{\text{Percentage change in quantity demanded}}{\text{Percentage change in price of the product}}$$

The absolute value of the price elasticity reflects the relationship between price and the quantity demanded, and is not expressed in any particular units. Demand is price *inelastic* when the percentage of change in price results in a smaller percentage of change in quantity, resulting in a PED less than 1 in absolute value (i.e., ignore the negative sign). Demand is price elastic when the percentage of change in price results in a larger percentage change in demand, resulting in a PED greater than 1. As an example, suppose that a physical therapy practice offers evaluations for fall risks to the elderly population in the community. The practice charges $50 for the evaluation and currently provides ten evaluations per month. What if they increase their charge to $55 dollars (+10%) and only get requests for seven evaluations per month (−30%).

Then:

PED = −30% ÷ +10%
PED = −3

The PED indicates that the price for the evaluation is very sensitive to the change in price.

The price elasticity of a service or product will dictate the shape of the demand curve for any specific service or product. Demand may be inelastic or insensitive to price changes when the service or product is essential to the consumer. Compared to luxury products, basic necessities are price inelastic. Demand may also be inelastic because the consumers have sufficient resources (income) to buy the needed items when there is a substantial price change. This is seen when the cost of luxury products such as designer clothing increases but demand stays high. When the quantity demanded changes significantly in response to a price increase, demand is said to be highly elastic. Under conditions of high elasticity, price increases may result in an overall decrease in the quantity demanded or, in a competitive market, the consumer may switch to a competitor's service or product or an alternative service or product. When consumers turn to an alternative source or product, it is called a **substitution**. The closer the alternative service or product to the original, the more likely it is that the consumer will turn to a substitution when prices increase. For some consumers, chiropractice physicians, athletic trainers, occupational therapists, and massage therapists are substitutes for PTs.

Income will also have an impact on demand by causing a shift in the demand curve to the right. This might happen if income growth provides consumers with more disposable income to spend on desirable services or products. For example, as income rises, the overall demand for high-end day spa services might increase. Conversely, if disposable income declines, the demand for high-end day spa services may decline while the demand for less expensive personal care services may increase.

The impact of price on profit is of great interest to producers. Producers desire to maximize their profit. Their goal is to charge a price that gives the greatest net income or profit.

Total Revenue =
Price per unit × Quantity of units sold
Total Expense =
Cost per unit × Quantity of units produced
Net Income (profit) =
Total revenue − Total expense

Producers attempt to maximize their net income (profit) by:

1. Identifying and charging the highest price that consumers are willing to pay.
2. Producing goods or services at the lowest per unit cost of production.

As price rises, producers are motivated to increase the amount of service or product they provide to consumers. However, price elasticity may result in diminishing demand as prices rise. As price increases, demand will decrease. At some point, total revenue (units of service/product multiplied by price) will reach a maximum and then began to decline. Producers must determine how much of which products to produce based on their available resources and price.

At market equilibrium, demand for a product equals its supply. The interaction between price, supply, and demand work in concert to maintain a demand–supply balance. For example, holding supply constant, when demand increases some consumers are willing to pay more which drives the price upward. A new equilibrium between quantity supplied and quantity demanded will be achieved. The increase in price will also act as an incentive for producers to increase the quantity supplied. As long as there is a positive impact on total revenue and net income, producers will be motivated to increase the quantity supplied (Chapter 22).

In health care the utilization of services is different from supply of health care providers and the demand from the consumer who does not know if he will need health care during a certain period of time (Folland et al., 2007). The consumer does not necessarily know what makes a good PT or what constitutes appropriate physical therapy services. A PT provider provides both the information and the service, which affects the concept of supply by influencing the consumer's perception of the value and expected benefits of the service (Chapter 19). In addition, other factors can influence supply and demand such as the availability of physical therapy services in a local market, the cost associated with becoming and practicing as a PT, the consumer's health care insurance, or lack thereof, the consumer's personal income, and other prices in the market (Chapter 18). The supply and demand model, as it applies to health care, does provide a basic understanding of the forces of supply and demand in a free market, and allows the PT to better understand the behavior of the consumer.

Role of Competition in the Market

A *competitive market* is characterized by multiple producers each having a minority share of the market. In a competitive market consumers have a choice of services/providers and products/producers from which to choose. If one provider or producer raises his price or decreases production, the consumer has the ability to substitute another or similar provider or producer. The result is price increases are constrained. When one provider or producer dominates a market, it is called a **monopoly**. In a monopoly market, the consumer is unable to substitute. As a result, demand is price inelastic.

At times, a free market economy may find a monopoly (i.e., natural monopoly) desirable because of the lower cost per unit of producing essential services or products due to the *economy of scale*. For example, a community may have only one source for utilities, phone, cable TV, or hospital care because the cost of supporting multiple service providers of the same service or products prohibitive. When a monopoly for an essential service is present in a market, the government may impose regulations on the monopoly to control production, the price, and to ensure equitable distribution of the services.

A practical example of economic modeling applied to PT data was the Vector report (Anonymous, 1997; Vector, 1997), which was commissioned by the American Physical Therapy Association (APTA). The issues of supply, demand, and competition were addressed along with the potential effects on employment, salaries, and use of substitutes. One of the predictions from the economic models was

that there would be a progressively increasing oversupply of PTs and physical therapist assistants (PTA) starting in 1998 and a leveling of salaries and an assessment of the impact of potential substitutes for PTs. There was also the implication that enrollment in physical therapy and PTA educational programs would likely decline. While subsequent employment surveys conducted between 1998 and 2005 by the APTA Department of Research (APTA, 2005) had some potential to verify a number of the Vector predictions, verification was complicated by the implementation of the Balanced Budget Act of 1997 and the emergence of conflicting reports on the future of the physical therapy job market (Bureau of Labor Statistics, 2008). According to the most recent study by the APTA, the employment problems created by the Balanced Budget Act of 1997 have ceased and the employment environment for PTs has greatly improved (APTA, 2005).

Understanding the Market

As the practice of physical therapy continues to expand in the area of private practice, PTs, as individual practice owners as well as managers of physical therapy departments, will need to continue to develop their skills in leadership, professionalism, administration and management, including skills with economic relevance (Schafer et al., 2007). Focusing on specific aspects of the market, the PT can make decisions about his practice based on what is happening in the market, both nationally and locally. **Environmental scanning** (Chapters 4 and 13) is a behavior of collecting information about the current status or changes in the market and prices in order to make decisions about the direction of a particular practice or program. It includes both searching for information and viewing information and can range from information gained from casual conversations to formal marketing research (Choo, 2001). Environmental scanning can cover several environmental sectors, such as attributes or needs of the customer, advances in technology, pending or possible regulatory issues, socio-cultural, political or demographical trends, competitors' statistics, and economic indicators. It is a behavior (environmental assessment) that a new PT should have a basic understanding as he begins his clinical practice (Schafer, 1991; Schafer et al., 2007). Full details of environmental scanning are in Chapters 3–6, and 13.

A basic way to gain information about the health care market is to follow aggregate data provided by government agencies concerning costs and demographics. See Additional Resources section for some example sources. On an individual and local market, information from patients, durable medical equipment suppliers, referral sources or other PTs, is also valuable. During one-on-one conversations, the PT can pick up on common themes or concerns such as the price of health care in the community, the access to services on the weekend, or the outcomes of certain health care clinicians. Local information about the number and type of health care facilities in an area, the local unemployment rate, the average household income, and the population demographics and trends can aid in strategic planning and decision making regarding the type of services to develop or expand (Chapter 22). See Additional Resources section for example sources. At the national level, there are many economic indicators that are monitored and periodically reported. Some of the more common indicators are

- **Consumer Price Index (CPI):** An economic indicator that measures the change in the cost of a fixed collection of goods or services. Typically includes housing, electricity, food, and transportation. It is a widely used measure of inflation.
- **Gross Domestic Product (GDP):** The total money value of all goods and services produced in a country in a given year. It is one indicator of a country's economic size and health. Typically the U.S. economy grows at around 2.5–3% per year. If growth varies from this expected range, the federal government typically steps in to try to influence the economy.
- **Unemployment Rate:** Defined unemployment as a percentage of the labor force. Monitoring the monthly unemployment rate is a good guide to economic development (The Economist, 2007). For every 1% rise in the unemployment rate, more than 1 million beneficiaries are added to the Medicaid program (Holahan and Garret,

2008). The cost of this program is shared by the federal and state governments and the additional cost can have an affect on the federal and state budgets for health care and other social programs.
- **Population Demographics/Trends:** The aging population with its higher utilization rates and increasing rates of coronary heart disease point to increasing demand for health care services. In addition, the changing ethnic and cultural diversity of Americans requires services and service deliveries that are responsive to the needs of this population (Catholic Health East, 2003). The GDP must grow at least as fast as the population if the standard of living is to be maintained (The Economist, 2007).

Cost

Cost is defined as a measure of economic sacrifice (Morse, 1984). It is what is given up in order to obtain something else. The issue of the cost of health care has been in the forefront of the public debate on universal health care coverage and the cost of employee benefits in businesses as the cost continues to rise. Since the late 1990s, health care spending has increased at a faster rate of growth than has the GDP, inflation, and the population (Office of the Assistant Secretary for Planning and Evaluation [ASPE], 2008). Workers with employer-sponsored health insurance often experience a reduction in wages in response to increasing health care costs. Increased cost are also offset by direct wage reductions, increased employee cost sharing, or in cases where wages are fixed (i.e., contractual obligations), by increasing the number of hours worked (ASPE, 2008). Increasing cost means a shifting of resources towards health care and away from other goods and services, which impact the economy at a local, national, and international level. In 2005, the share of federal revenues going to fund health care was approximately 30% with state and local governments contributing approximately 30% of their expenditures for health care (Centers for Medicare and Medicaid Services [CMS], 2008a). In 2006, health care spending was approximately two trillion dollars in the United States, or $7,026 per person (16% of the GDP; CMS 2008b). Out of pocket spending accounted for 12% of this cost. Health care spending is expected to continue to increase over the next decade reaching 4.3 trillion dollars and accounting for approximately 19.5% of the GDP by the year 2017 (CMS, 2008c). Out of the 2.1 trillion dollars spent in 2006, 58.9 billion was spent on professional services that includes therapists, chiropractors, optometrists, and podiatrists (CMS, 2008b).

Cost as a factor in the price of a service is an important component in the decision-making process of both the consumer and producer. An understanding of the cost associated with the service or goods must be identified and understood by the provider in order to set a price that is acceptable to the consumer and is conducive to the financial viability of the business. Identification of the most commonly treated conditions in a physical therapy practice is the first step in the cost identification process. Once the common conditions are identified, the cost associated with the interventions and treatment of the people with these conditions can follow and a general picture of how much it costs to provide services to a person with a specific condition can become clearer.

Cost can be divided into various categories. **Implicit costs** are those costs that are more intangible and related to things like time and effort put into the maintenance of a company by the owner, or the use of assets for which no payment is made or value reduced. The most common implicit cost is opportunity cost, the cost of the next best alternative. Although not recorded in financial statements, opportunity cost should be considered when discussing or evaluating alternative courses of action in a business. For example, if a practice owner is considering what to do with the additional space in the clinic, he may consider expanding his current outpatient services, which will allow him to provide services to an additional three patients per hour. Another alternative would be to make the space a pediatric treatment gym that would allow the practice to expand its current services into the area of pediatrics and to provide additional programs to the community. One factor in the decision on what to do would be to estimate the opportunity cost associated with each decision.

The other category of cost is **explicit costs**. These are tangible costs that can easily be accounted for, such as wages and supply costs. There are two types of explicit costs: direct and indirect costs. **Direct costs** are those costs directly associated with the production of goods or services. In a physical therapy clinic, these would include such things as the salary and benefits given to the PT, the supplies and equipment that are used in the delivery of physical therapy services, and the tools that are used in the evaluation process. These are directly related to the production of the physical therapy service. **Indirect costs** are those costs that are indirectly associated with the production of goods or services, often referred to as overhead costs. Indirect costs may not be so readily identified. These costs include such things as administrative salaries, utility bills, building and grounds maintenance, or laundry services (Fig. 20.3) (Chapter 21). In larger organizations, indirect costs are generally allocated to departments within the organization based on the size of the department, the number of employees in the department, the revenues the department generates, or some other formula derived by the organization's management. Indirect cost allocations can vary depending on the type and size of the organization.

Explicit costs can also be classified as either fixed, variable, or semi-variable. **Fixed costs**, such as salary and wages, rent, interest expenses on loans, and depreciation of equipment, are set and do not change over an extended period of time or with service volume. Fixed costs are more easily budgeted and managed because they are not affected by service volume. **Variable costs** are the costs, which vary depending on volume. A PT exerts the most control over these costs. Variable cost items could include supplies such as ultrasound gel, home exercise program forms, office supplies, printing costs for brochures and pamphlets, and the costs for small equipment or any item that is "used up" in the process of service provision. Because variable costs are the easiest to control they are generally the first to be affected in order to meet short-term financial goals. A business owner's request to turn off lights when not in use, keeping the thermostat set at a specific temperature, and copying on both sides of a piece of paper may sound insignificant to an

Cost Worksheet

DIRECT COST:

1.	Salary			
		a.	base	$ 66,000[a]
		b.	overtime	0
		c.	**Total salary =**	$ 66,000
2.	Fringes (approx. 30% of lc.)			
		a.	FICA (7.65% of lc.)	$ 5,049
		b.	Workman's comp. (4% of lc.)	$ 2,640
		c.	State unemployment (av. $250/yr)	$ 250
		d.	Fed. unemployment ($56/yr)	$ 56
		e.	Pension Plan (av. 3–4% of lc.)	$ 2,640
		f.	Professional Liability (1% of lc.)	$ 660
		g.	Insurance (health, life, disability) (12% of lc.)	$ 7,920
		h.	**Total fringes =**	$ 19,215
3.	Other			
		a.	mileage	$ 150
		b.	continuing education	$ 500
		c.	tuition reimbursement	$ 0
		d.	license/dues/subscriptions	$ 500
		e.	**Total other =**	$ 1,150
4.	**Direct Total** (1c + 2h + 3e) =			$ 86,365
5.	INDIRECT COST (allocation)[b]:			
	Private clinic or home health agency (add 50%–60% of direct total)			
	Hospital based (add 30%–40% of direct total)			$ 43,182

TOTAL COST (4 + 5) = $129,547

TOTAL COST of 129,547/2080 **HOURS PAID TO WORK PER YEAR =
COST PER HOUR** of $62.28

Typically 2080 hours per year for a 40-hour workweek. 1950 for a 37.5-hour workweek.
For a 10-month school year, 7 hours per day: 1400 hours.

[a] Median annual earnings for a physical therapist. Bureau of Labor Statistics, U.S. Department of Labor,
    Occupational Handbook, 2008–09 Edition.

[b] Includes nonrevenue-generating staff and overhead costs.

Figure 20.3. Cost worksheet (Drnach, 2008).

employee, but it is one way to control costs. Decreasing salaries or limiting benefits would be a more drastic measure. **Semi-variable costs**, sometimes referred to as mixed costs, fall between fixed and variable costs. Semi-variable cost items have a fixed cost compo-

nent and a variable cost component, which is affected by volume. Examples of these items include cellular phone service that has a fixed monthly rate for a specific amount of minutes. If the user exceeds those minutes an additional cost is incurred. The PT has limited control over variable cost items. The **total cost** can be determined with the following formula:

Total costs = total fixed costs + total variable costs

Identifying the total costs associated with the provision of services provides necessary information in the calculation of needed revenue to sustain a business. Generating revenue in excess of total costs (a profit) is important in maintaining the business, updating equipment, increasing salaries, or to expand into new markets (Chapters 2 and 22).

In health care, cost is usually associated with a unit of service (UOS) which can mean different things to different organizations (Table 20.1). A UOS may be defined as a patient encounter, a 15-minute increment of physical therapy service, a specific treatment intervention, or the length of the episode of care. Understanding how an organization defines a UOS is an important aspect of understanding and calculating costs.

Marginal cost (or incremental cost) is the additional cost required to provide one more UOS. This is an important piece of information when deciding to see one more patient, or providing services for one more day (or UOS). How much money will be spent? How much additional revenue will be realized? The difference in total cost before a change is made and after the change has been made represents the marginal cost of that change. In addition, many managers or owners of a practice may want information on the cost per diagnostic group or cost per intervention or treatment modality. This represents average cost and is calculated using the total volume of the UOS provided for the target segment. **Average total cost** can be determined with the following formula:

Average total cost = Total cost/Total volume of UOS

Table 20.1	Examples of UOS
Service	*1 Unit Equals*
Inpatient	15 minutes
Outpatient	Intervention CPT code
Skilled nursing facility	8 minutes
School-based therapy	30 minutes
Home care	One patient visit

For example, if the total cost associated with providing physical therapy services for one year was 95,000.00 and the total UOS delivered in that year was 1560, then the average total cost for the provision of services would be $60.90 per UOS. Similarly, marginal cost (MC) is:

MC = change in total cost / change in UOS output

If it cost $50 to provide one more UOS then the MC would be:

MC = $50.00/1
MC = $50.00

The MC to produce one more UOS is less than the average cost in this example

Break-Even Analysis

Identifying and categorizing the costs of doing business can lead to a better understanding of the behavior of a UOS in making money, losing money, or breaking even. This is not simply looking at the average cost and the revenue generated, but also looking at the volume of patients or UOS that are provided with the fixed costs for the program or service. Fixed costs are not influenced by volume, but as the volume increases the fixed costs per UOS decreases because of the sharing of the fixed cost with an increasing number of patients. This is referred to as economy of scale; the reduction in the cost of providing services with increased volume because fixed costs are used more, thereby decreasing the average cost per UOS (Table 20.2).

The **break-even analysis** is a technique to find the specific volume at which a business neither makes nor loses money (Finkler et al., 2007). It is based on the following formula:

Break-even quantity = Fixed costs / Price – variable cost per UOS

Using the information in Table 20.2, a manager would want to know how many UOS it would take to break even given a program that has a fixed cost of $200 and a variable cost of $100. The price for one UOS is $150. Using the formula:

Table 20.2   Costs in Dollars

Volume	Fixed Cost	Variable Cost	Total Cost	Average Cost	Marginal Cost
1	200	100	300	300	
10	200	1,000	1,200	120	100
15	200	1,500	1,700	113	100
20	200	2,000	2,200	110	100

Note as volume increases the average cost decreases (economy of scale).
Marginal cost = change in total cost / change in UOS
When the volume goes from 1 to 10: MC = 900/9 = 100

Break-even quantity = $200 / 150 – 100
Break-even quantity = $200 / 50
Break-even quantity = 4 units

Therefore, until 4 UOS are provided the business will be operating at a loss. Once 4 UOS are provided the business will be making neither a profit nor loss, but will break even. After 4 UOS, the business will be operating at a profit. Note that Figure 20.4 can be used to estimate the break-even point.

When trying to achieve the break-even point a manager has several options. One is to lower the fixed cost associated with the UOS. As stated previously this may be difficult to do given the nature of fixed costs and those items associated with them, such as salary and benefits. The appropriate utilization of a less costly employee, such as a PTA instead of a PT, is one way to lower fixed costs. Lowering variable cost, or the price for the service are other options, although lowering the price in an insurance-driven industry is not always prudent. The easiest way to achieve the break-even point and beyond is to increase volume, recruiting more patients (Chapters 18, 19, and 22).

Operating at break-even may sustain a business for a short period. Unfortunately, a business must have some level of profit to maintain its current financial position over time. Additional resources will be required for nonroutine expenses such as equipment replacement or routine building maintenance. Overtime, reserves will be depleted and the break-even business will be unable to sustain operations. The bottom line, to exist into the future, a business must bring in more money than it spends (Chapters 2, 19, and 22).

Cost-Effectiveness Analysis

All players in the health care system, employers, insurers, providers and consumers, as well

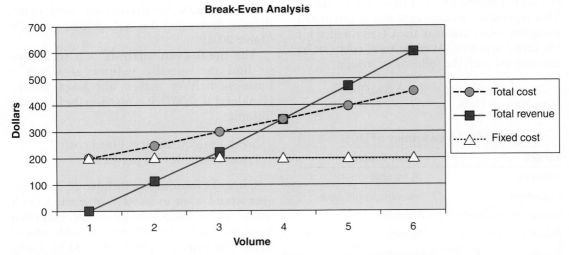

Figure 20.4. Graphic representation of a break-even analysis.

as federal and state policy makers, need objective, scientifically based information to help them make decisions about the allocation of the scarce health care resource (Agency for Healthcare Research and Quality [AHRQ], 2002). PTs have to make decisions every day regarding the allocation of resources and the effectiveness of the services they provide (Finch et al., 2005). AHRQ is the federal government's agency charged with supporting research designed to improve the quality of health care, reduce its cost, address patient safety and medical errors, and broaden access to essential services (Chapter 16).

Once a PT understands costs, it can be factored into clinical decision making regarding the most cost-effective method to produce an outcome in a given patient population or program. Articles are just now appearing in the literature that address or include the concept of cost effectiveness in the study of the effectiveness of certain physical therapy interventions (Critchley et al., 2007; Korthals-de Bos et al., 2003; Struijs et al., 2006).

A **cost-effectiveness analysis (CEA)** is done to promote an efficient use of finite resources. It is the measurement of the relative costs and outcomes associated with a particular activity or program in comparison to another similar program, which produces the same outcome. It is important that the outcome measurement tool is consistent between the two programs under consideration to assure that the patient/client achieves the same result. When performing a CEA, the costs (both direct and indirect) for each program are identified, categorized, and monitored along with other quantitative and qualitative data. After the provision of services for the duration of the program are complete, patient outcomes are obtained and decisions made regarding the efficient use of resources to produce the optimal outcome for the patients. A problem that may arise in the clinic is the inclusion of less costly services or the exclusion of more costly services in an attempt to control cost, without looking at the effects such substitutions have on the outcomes of the services provided. If a new approach produces the exact same outcome for less money, then it can be concluded that the new approach is cost effective. Being less costly is not the sole goal of physical therapy intervention. Being cost effective and produc-

ing the same outcome for the patient over alternative interventions is the ultimate goal.

Summary

Economics studies how people use their limited resources to fulfill their wants and needs. In a free market economy consumers interact with producers to determine what, how, and for whom services and goods will be produced. Some goods and services (i.e., public goods) are produced by governments. It has only been during the recent century that governments have expanded their role into more social programs such as health care, in addition to public education and national defense. This expansion has created opportunities as well as challenges as capitalistic economies balance the influence of government with individual and private control.

The need for providers (such as PTs) to have a basic understanding of economic principles such as scarcity, resource allocation, value, utility, and demand has become more important in clinical-decision making as health care cost continues to rise and cost containment measures are discussed and implemented in the health care industry. Such measures often introduce the concept of opportunity cost and the value associated with the foregone alternative action. Consumers have finite resources. When expending limited resources consumers strive to gain maximum value. Value is often associated with price, which has an interesting elastic component and is important in determining the effect a change in price would have on the quantity demanded by the consumer. Supply of a resource affects quantity demanded as well as the price. Assuming all other factors are constant, as the price of a product or service increases, the quantity demanded by the consumer is likely to decrease and vice versa. Less expensive substitutes become more attractive to buyers.

When there are alternative providers of services and products there is competition in the market. A competitive market is characterized by multiple producers each having a minority share of the market. In a competitive market, consumers have a choice of products/producers from which to choose. Having a basic understanding of how to scan the market or environment provides information about the current status or changes in the market and aids in strategic planning for a business.

The cost associated with the provision of health care is an important component in the decision-making process of both the consumer and producer. An understanding of the various cost associated with the service or goods (i.e., fixed costs, variable costs, and mixed costs) must be identified and understood by the provider in order to set a price that is acceptable to the consumer and is conducive to the financial viability of the business.

Activities such as a break-even analysis and a cost-effectiveness analysis can aid the PT in maximizing his economic potential while maintaining quality care made evident through his clinical outcomes.

To know what costs and expenses are and if there is a profit requires keeping financial records. The next chapter deals with such accounting. One benefit of having accurate and up-to-date financial records is being able to compare what has occurred to what was expected. This is the basis of budgeting, which is a major component of Chapter 21.

CASE STUDY 20.1

From a Consumer's Perspective

Review the section on value. Take a consumer of physical therapy services perspective and form three possible tangible and three intangible values a customer might have regarding the following physical therapy services:

1. Hospital-based services
2. Home health services

3. Early intervention services provided under the Individuals with Disabilities Education Act (IDEA)

Be prepared to participate in a class discussion on this case.

CASE STUDY 20.2

There is No Business Like Your Business

Situation

You are a PT making $60,000 per year (fixed cost). The price for a patient visit is $75. The variable cost of a UOS is $3.50. Given this information calculate the break-even quantity. The following assumptions will help you solve this problem:

a. The PT can complete eight patient visits per day. How many days will it take to reach the break-even quantity?

b. What would be the percentage change in the break-even quantity if the PT were given a 4% salary raise?
c. How many more working days would it take to reach the new break-even quantity?

REFERENCES

Agency for Healthcare Research and Quality. Health care cost. September 2002. AHRQ Pub. No. 02-P033. Available at http://www.ahrq.gov/news/costsfact.htm. Accessed 2/27/08.

American Physical Therapy Association. APTA employment survey. Alexandria, VA: Department of Research Services. 2005.

Anonymous. APTA workforce study looks at supply and demand of PTs. PT Bulletin. 1997;12(20):1, 10.

Bureau of Labor Statistics. Occupational outlook handbook, 2008-09 edition, physical therapists. Available at http://www.bls.gov/oco/ocos080.htm. Accessed 2/24/08.

Catholic Health East. Healthcare strategic environmental scan 2003. 2003. Available at http://www.che.org/publications/pdf/Environmental-Scan-2003.pdf. Accessed 2/29/08.

Centers for Medicare and Medicaid Services. Sponsors of health care costs: Businesses, households, and governments, 1987–2005. Available at http://www.cms.hhs.gov/NationalHealthExpendData/downloads/bhg07.pdf. Accessed 2/27/08a.

Centers for Medicare and Medicaid Services. National health expenditure accounts 2006 highlights. Available at http://www.cms.hhs.gov/NationalHealthExpendData/downloads/highlights.pdf. Accessed 2/27/08b.

Centers for Medicare and Medicaid Services. National health expenditure projections 2007–2017. Available at http://www.cms.hhs.gov/apps/media/press_releases.asp. Accessed 2/27/08c.

Choo CW. Environmental scanning as information seeking and organizational learning. Information Research. 2001;7(1). Available at http://www.InformationR.net/ir/7-1/paper112.html. Accessed 3/08/08.

Critchley D, Ratcliffe J, Noonan S, et al. Effectiveness and cost-effectiveness of three types of physiotherapy used to reduce chronic low back pain disability: A pragmatic randomized trial with economic evaluation. Spine. 2007;32:1474–1481.

Drnach M. The basics of billing. In Drnach M. ed. The clinical practice of pediatric physical therapy: From the NICU to independent living. Baltimore, MD: Lippincott Williams and Wilkins. 2008 of pp. 339–349.

Finch E, Geddes E, Larin H. Ethically-based clinical decision making in physical therapy: Process and issues. Physiotherapy Theory and Practice. 2005;21:147–162.

Finkler S, Kovner C, Jones C. Financial management for nurse managers and executives, 3rd ed. St. Louis, MO: Saunders Elsevier. 2007.

Finkler SA, Ward DM. Essentials of cost accounting for health care organizations, 2nd ed. Gaithersburg, MD: Aspen. 1999.

Folland S, Goodman A, Stano M. The economics of health and health care. New York, NY: Macmillan Publishing Company. 1993.

Folland S, Goodman A, Stano M. The economics of health and health care, 5th ed. Upper Saddle River, NJ: Pearson Prentice Hall. 2007.

Gale. Encyclopedia of business information sources. Detroit, MI: Gale Research. 2006.

Hajiran H. Interdisciplinary teaching tools for economics 101. Available at http://ssrn.com/abstract=643384. Accessed 9/25/07.

Holahan J, Garret B. Rising unemployment and Medicaid. Available at http://www.urban.org/UploadedPDF/410306_HPOnline_1.pdf. Accessed 3/08/08.

Korthals-de Bos I, Hoving J, van Tulder M, et al. Cost effectiveness of physiotherapy, manual therapy, and general practitioner care for neck pain: Economic evaluation alongside a randomised controlled trial. BMJ. 2003;326:911–916.

Lipford JW, Slice J. Adam Smith's roles for government and contemporary US government roles. The Independent Review. 2007;11:485–501.

Mariner W. Rationing healthcare and the need for credible scarcity: Why Americans can't say no. American Journal of Public Health. 1995;85:1439–1445.

Maslow A. A theory of human motivation. Psychological Review. 1943;50:370–396. Available at http://psychclassics.yorku.ca/Maslow/motivation.htm. Accessed 2/27/08.

Menger C. Principles of Economics. Auburn AL: Ludwig von Mises Institute. 2007.

Morse W, Roth H. Cost accounting, 3rd ed. Reading, MA: Addison-Wesley. 1984.

New York Center for Health Workforce Studies. The United States workforce profile. Available at http://chws.albany.edu. Accessed 2/24/08.

Office of the Assistant Secretary for Planning and Evaluation. (ASPE) Effects of health care spending on the US economy. Executive summary. Available at http://aspe.hhs.gov/health/costgrowth/index.htm. Accessed 2/27/08.

Schafer D. Environmental-scanning behavior among private practice physical therapy firms. Physical Therapy. 1991;71:482–490.

Schafer D, Lopopolo R, Luedtke-Hoffman R. Administration and management skills needed by physical therapist graduates in 2010: A national survey. Physical Therapy. 2007;87:261–273.

Scott R, Solomon S, McGowan J. Applying economic principles to health care. Emerging Infectious Diseases. 2001;7:282–285.

Stossel T. Regulating academic-industrial research relationships—solving problems or stifling progress? New England Journal of Medicine. 2005;353:1060–1065.

Struijs P, Korthals-de Bos I, van Tulder M, et al. Cost effectiveness of brace, physiotherapy, or both for treatment of tennis elbow. British Journal of Sports Medicine. 2006;40:637–643.

The Economist. Guide to Economic Indicators: Making Sense of Economics, 6th ed. New York, NY: Bloomberg Press. 2007.

Vector. Physical therapy workforce study executive summary. Ann Arbor, MI: Vector Research. 1997.

Wikipedia Free Encyclopedia. Scarcity. Available at http://en.wikipedia.org/wiki/Economic_scarcity. Accessed 2/27/08.

ADDITIONAL RESOURCES

Information on the local market can also be obtain through the local government or business organizations such as the Chamber of Commerce (www.chamberofcommerce.com) or through the Census Bureau (www.census.gov). Some basic ways to gain information about the health care market is to follow aggregate data provided by the government concerning costs and demographics. For example, the U.S. Department of Labor Bureau of Statistics (Available at http://www.bls.gov) provides on line information on the current CPI and unemployment statistics to name a few. It also has access to the Occupational Outlook Handbook which provides regional information on employment, earnings, and projection data for physical therapy. An excellent site for current information on inflation and what PTs are earning.

The American Physical Therapy Association practice link available at http://www.apta.org, provides information on the supervision of support staff, documentation guidelines, and employment surveys. This is a valuable site for PTs especially if they are managers in a business, owners of a private practice, or independent contractors.

Cleverley W, Cameron A. Essential of Health Care Financing. 5th ed. Aspen Publication. Gaithersburg MD. 2002

offers in-depth information on the concept of cost and the costing process. It would be helpful to a PT who is involved in the budgeting or strategic planning process.

There are a number of reports indicating that high school and college students as well as the general adult population have a poor understanding of economic principles. For areas in need of improvement see http://www.ncee.net/cel/WhatAmericans KnowAboutEconomics_051105-ExecSummary.pdf; http://www.jumpstart.org/national_standers.html. Free e-books on economics may be obtained at http://www.asiaing.com/index.php. Free summaries on cost benefit analysis and other topics covered in this chapter are available from the Concise Encyclopedia of Economics at http://www.econlib.org/library/CEECategory.html#M. Personal finance education information is available from the Federal Reserve at http://www.federalreserveeducation.org/pfed/indextext.cfm#Economics. Common terms used in federal government reports are defined at http://www.federalreserveeducation.org/teachers/FedChallenge/FedChallenge_Research.htm and http://www.federalreserveeducation.org/Teachers/glossary/glossary.cfm.

CHAPTER 21

ACCOUNTING AND FINANCING

MARK DRNACH

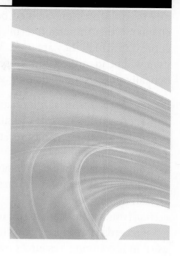

Learning Objectives

1. Describe basic processes in accounting.
2. Demonstrate an understanding of the application of standard accounting practices.
3. Explain and construct the four basic financial statements.
4. Describe the process of budgeting.
5. Demonstrate the ability to perform basic financial analysis of financial information.
6. Understand management's role in revenue and expense management.
7. Given essential information, apply selected accounting and financing concepts presented in this chapter.

Introduction

"No money, no mission" was a point made in other chapters (Chapters 2, 5, and 22) to underscore the balancing that has to take place between business decisions and fulfilling service needs. The money part of the comment means that the need of any business is to remain financially solvent to serve its customers or fulfill its mission. The constant need to achieve and maintain a positive bottom line (making a profit) in the health care industry has expanded the role and responsibilities of health care providers in the delivery of services. This includes physical therapists (PTs). Whether it is a sole proprietor practice or part of a larger group or organization, such as a hospital, the need to organize, manage, and understand finan-

cial information is now an important aspect of health care. Understanding the established rules and regulations for identifying, recording, and reporting financial information allows PTs to participate in the business of health care, program evaluation, cost-effectiveness analysis, and in the development of plans for the future, which contribute to long-term organizational sustainability. Having a basic understanding of the terms and processes used in accounting is one of the first steps in this process, and necessary in order to participate in the conversations about health care finances. Basic accounting practices are used to develop four *fundamental financial statements*:

1. *Balance sheet*
2. *Income statement*
3. *Cash flow statement*
4. *Retained earnings statement*

An understanding of the information in these statements will allow a physical therapist (PT) to see the relationship between the delivery of patient care services to the **revenues** and *expenses* of operating a health care business. Decisions about new or expanded programs, staffing, and purchases that would otherwise be based on a "best guess" will become clearer and more objective. Application of objective information about the performance of an organization, as compared to what was planned (the budgeting process) and/or what competitors are doing, will help the organization stay on target with performance objectives.

In addition, every PT should have a basic understanding of how to maximize revenues.

Key Terms

Key terms, which are defined below, are bolded and italicized the first time they appear in the chapter. Other important terms are shown in boldface on first appearance and are defined by the context in which they are used. When either of these types of terms is used several times, its acronym will be identified and subsequently used in the chapter. Both types of terms are listed alphabetically in the online glossary with their definitions and (when applicable) their acronyms.

account: a way financial information is accumulated (recorded) for its sub classifications of assets, liabilities, owners' equity, revenue, and expenses. Also see chart of accounts.

accounting: a systematic way of keeping track of financial activities and their results to guide decision making.

accrual basis: in accounting, this relates to the timing of recording financial transactions.

asset: in accounting, resources owned by an organization that can be used to benefit future operations. Something owned that has value.

balance sheet: a date-specific fundamental financial statement that provides information about an organization's assets, liabilities, and owner's equity. It shows what assets the firm owns, and how those assets are financed in the form of liabilities and owner equity.

cash basis: in accounting, revenue is recorded when cash is received and expenses are recorded when bills are paid. It is an alternative to the accrual method often used in small businesses with cash flow concerns.

cash flow: the changes in cash, cash inflow–cash outflow, resulting from normal operating activities.

chart of accounts: a listing of the account titles and account numbers used by a business to track money spent and money earned.

debit: a debt to be paid. In accounting, this is an entry made on the left side of an account.

equity: a claim to the assets by the owner. Owner's equity for example.

expenses: the resources used to generate revenue.

fund accounting: in accounting, this means that there is a separation and tracking of financial transactions to meet restrictions and reporting requirements imposed by funding sources. A common accounting procedure in not-for-profit entities.

fundamental financial statements: in accounting, these are a balance sheet, income statement, cash flow statement, and retained earnings statement.

gross: the amount left after deducting the cost of a service or product from net sales.

income statement: in accounting, this is a fundamental financial statement that shows the results of an organization's operations over a specific time period. It includes revenue, expenses, and net income for the period.

liabilities: in accounting, this is the current and noncurrent financial debts.

liquid assets: anything that can be quickly turned into cash.

net: in accounting, the result of subtracting two relevant amounts. For example, the net profit is the result of subtracting the cost to provide a service from the amount received for administering the service.

operating margin: a profitability ratio. The ratio of net income to total revenue.

retained earnings statement: also referred to as an owner's equity statement. The statement explains the differences in an owner's equity on the balance sheet and provides information on how profits are used in a business, either distributed to the owners or reinvested into the business.

It is necessary to understand the payment options available for services rendered, either by the first party (the patient/client), the second party (the provider), or a third party (an insurance company, state or federal government program, philanthropy), and how to balance **productivity** between providing quality care and maximizing revenues. Once the principles of health care accounting and financial planning are understood, financial management skills can be applied to health care operations to maximize an organization's productivity and financial performance.

This chapter will cover the basic accounting practices and financial issues that can help a PT understand these fundamental aspects of an organization. In doing so, he or she will be better equipped to participate effectively in this important aspect of health care. The accounting concepts have direct application to personal financial management as well.

Accounting

Accounting is a system of record keeping that allows an organization to keep an account of its financial activity. It is a process of identifying, recording, summarizing, and reporting in monetary terms information about an organization during a specific period of time. Accounting is not a science, but rather a set of rules and conventions that apply to the way an organization identifies, records, summarizes, and reports financial information. In the United States, these rules and reporting requirements are established by the Financial Accounting Standards Board (FASB) and are called the Generally Accepted Accounting Principles (GAAP). The GAAP provides some consistency to the accounting process, which allows an individual or investor to analyze or compare companies' financial statements. An example of some of the more common accounting principles include the *identification of the entity*, which is the business unit, the person, or business that is the focus of attention and for which the financial statements are being prepared; and the *expectation of going concern*, which is the belief that the business is going to continue into the future. If the entity is planning on going out of business, then disclosing that information is required. The *matching principle* states that a business must record the expenses that are associated with the revenues generated for a given period. Matching is the only way an organization can determine if a specific product and/or service is contributing to the organization's financial performance. The *identification of the cost* of any quantifiable resource, which typically is the amount the organization paid for that resource (historical or acquisition cost), measured in the United States in U.S. dollars. This may significantly underestimate the current value of a resource (compared to its replacement cost or market value). Nonetheless, it is the easiest and most objective way to capture a resource's value. The *availability of objective evidence* means that the information in the financial statement is based on objective and verifiable evidence (e.g., receipts); and the *acceptance of materiality* or tolerance of the inherent errors or omissions (e.g., the small stuff; the useful life of a paper clip or push pin) in the financial statement. Some error is unavoidable. Financial statements are not expected to be error-free, but the error or intentional omission should not be sufficient (or material) to cause the reviewer of the financial statement to change his or her decision based on the information provided. The inclusion of the *application of consistency* in the accounting methods used in the business from year to year, and the *trust in full disclosure* of the financial position and results of operations of a business in accordance with GAAP are mandatory (Finkler et al., 2007) (Chapter 5). Because these common principles are expected to be followed by all organizations, reporting transactions and the results of such activity will allow a potential investor or external reviewer to understand the financial aspects of an organization.

Many organizations hire a **certified public accountant (CPA)** once a year to examine their financial statements because of their importance to the organization as well as to assure compliance with the various U.S. taxation requirements. The credentials of CPA is a designation given by the American Institute of Certified Public Accountants to those individuals who successfully pass the Uniform Certified Public Accountant Examination and meet the state's requirements for licensure, indicating a level of expertise in accounting, financial planning, and auditing (a process of examining the accuracy and completeness of a financial statement). CPAs are required to report whether the financial statements have been prepared in accordance with GAAP.

In certain circumstances the GAAP are modified by specific accounting conventions. The accounting conventions common to health care are allowances for contractual deductions and fund accounting. The convention of **allowances for contractual deductions** addresses the difference between the price charged for a service and the price paid by third party payers. This approach is taken because the utilization of a variety of contractual third party payers in health care may cause prices to be set much higher than the average payment (in order to maximize revenues). The amount of payment varies significantly between payers and is seldom under the control of the health care provider. To capture and account for the difference between the amount charged and the amount paid, an account called *allowances for contractual deductions* is used. Contractual allowances are accepted in order to increase patient volume by providing services to the people in the area who carry a specific health insurance (i.e., Medicare). In this agreement, the business agrees to accept the payment of the insurance company as payment in full for the services rendered. *Fund accounting* is often found in not-for-profit hospitals and health care organizations (HCO) (as one form of oversight in the absence of stockholders). An HCO may need to separate into a specified category or fund the financial information of one or more sections from that of the total entity, especially when funds are provided for a specific purpose. For example, if a HCO received a philanthropic gift to be used only for the support of a pediatric program or building project, a separate fund would be set up to account for this donor-restricted gift. This separation prevents the comingling of restricted funds with general funds. Types of accounting funds that may be seen in health care are endowment funds, plant replacement and expansion funds, and specific-purpose funds (Cleverley and Cameron, 2002). Each fund is considered an independent entity with its own set of accounts, but is part of the larger financial entity; therefore, the performance and condition of the fund accounts are included in the financial reports of the total entity.

Accounting involves the creation of an internal system of record keeping and reporting which ultimately results in the creation of financial statements for the business. These systems include such aspects as the creation of a chart of accounts, adherence to a double entry system of accounting, and the classification of financial activities such as debits, credits, assets, and liabilities.

Chart of Accounts

The process of accounting begins with the identification of the entity for which the financial information will be gathered and then the identification of the entity's accounts. An *account* is a category of assets, liabilities, owner's equity, revenues, and expenses. A chart of accounts is the foundation for accounting information systems within an organization and serves as the nucleus for the development of standard financial statements (Gans et al., 2007). It is simply a listing of an organization's

accounts by title and corresponding numerical code. The chart of accounts is often arranged in the order that the accounts appear on the balance sheet (assets, liabilities, then owner's equity) and income statement (revenues then expenses) (Gans et al., 2007). A numerical code is used to classify and differentiate between accounts. The number and types of accounts will depend on the size, type, and complexity of the business. Management information needs will influence the number and degree of specificity of the chart of accounts. For example, management may wish to have one general account to record revenue from equipment sold. If it is important to know the sales revenue for each type of equipment sold, management may choose to have one account for each type or category of equipment. The total of these equipment revenue accounts would then be combined to determine total revenue from equipment sold. Table 21.1 provides an example of a chart of accounts at the primary classification level. Each of the major account types from the balance sheet and income statement is assigned a series of numbers that define the characteristics of the account (e.g., revenue or expense). Within each numerical series, the major accounts are further defined by sub-groupings of funds or sub-groupings of accounts (e.g., revenue from patient services; expenses for support services).

Table 21.2 contains a more detailed example of numeric coding for the expense category of salaries and benefits. The logic that has been used to assign a numeric code to each of the sub-classes, such as employee type, is provided. The chart of accounts is specific to a business. Once the logic of the numeric coding is provided, it should be easily understood and used as the reference for the accounts included in budgets and other financial statements.

The development and utilization of the chart of accounts is a significant aspect in the generation of uniform financial statements, which in turn are vital in the analysis of outcomes, cost effectiveness, and comparative studies (Gans et al., 2007).

Double Entry

When a financial event occurs, it is recorded (posted) in a book of accounts, also referred to as a ledger. This event, considered a transac-

Code	Type	Subcode	Fund
Table 21.1 Physical Therapy Practice Chart of Accounts Primary Classification September 30, 2009			
100–199	Assets	110	Operating fund
		120	Capital equipment fund
		130	Other funds
200–299	Liabilities	210	Operating fund
		220	Capital equipment fund
		230	Other fund
300–399	Capital accounts	310	Operating fund
		320	Capital equipment fund
		330	Other fund
400–499	Revenue accounts	410	Patient service revenue
		420	Deductions from revenue
		430	Other revenue
500–599	Expense accounts	510	Patient services
		520	Support services
		530	Management services
		540	Purchased services
		550	Other expenses

tion, has two aspects, the change in the entity's assets and the change in the entity's liabilities. For example, if a patient owes a practice $75 and pays that amount after 30 days, the account for cash on hand will go up, while the account for **accounts receivable** (what is owed the business) will go down. Both aspects of a transaction should be recorded. The accountant debits the transaction to one account and credits it to another.

Debits and Credits

Debits and credits, from the Latin words *debere*, which means to owe, and *credere* to entrust, preceded the concept of positive and negative numbers (Wikipedia, 2008). Historically the posting of debits is placed on the left hand side of the ledger and the posting of credits is placed on the right hand side. Debits and credits are not assigned negative values, nor is the sum of the debits or credits assigned a negative value. They are terms used to describe the basic accounts in a double entry accounting system in which one account is debited while another is credited. Whether or not this has a positive or negative effect on the organization's financial statements depends on what type of account is involved (e.g., revenue accounts increase with credit postings, and expense accounts increase with debit postings).

Asset, Liability, and Equity

Assets are economic resources that are owned by a business and are expected to benefit future operations (Weltman, 1997). Assets include such things as

• Prepaid expenses
• Inventories
• Accounts receivables
• Capital assets
• Intangibles
• Cash
• Investments

Prepaid expenses include such things as salary advanced or insurance payments made for a future period. Inventories represent the value of supplies or products that will be used or sold during future periods. Accounts receivable are a type of asset in which the patient or client has an obligation to pay the organization for a product or service rendered on credit. (Some transactions are done "on account." This means that payment was not made when the service or product was delivered; instead an account was opened and is tracked until payment is made in full.) **Capital assets** include land, buildings, and equipment. Sometimes assets are called intangible, meaning the asset has no physical substance.

Table 21.2   Chart of Accounts Logic

500–599	Expense
	Salaries
531.10	Management
511.10	Therapist
511.12	Technical
521.10	Billing
521.12	Clerical
	Benefits
532.10	Management
512.10	Therapist
512.12	Technical
522.10	Billing
522.12	Clerical
	FICA
533.10	Management
513.10	Therapist
513.12	Technical
523.10	Billing
523.12	Clerical

Summary-Coding Logic

Digit	Meaning	Code	Technical Salaries
1st	Type of account	5	Expense
2nd	Subgroup/fund	1	Patient services
3rd	Account class	1	Salaries
4th and 5th	Subclass/department	.10/.12	Technical/billing

Patents, trademarks, copyrights, and goodwill (e.g., reputation for excellence, good relationships with community partners) are examples of intangible assets (Weltman, 1997).

Assets are important in determining the financial health of the organization. For the purposes of reporting, the value of an asset represents its current value to the organization and its ability to continue the operation of its business. Potential creditors view assets as resources available to cover the organization's debt, including the creditor's investment. For the creditor, more assets mean a better chance of repayment if the operation of the organization does not produce enough income to cover expenses. Creditors value assets based on the value and the speed with which the asset can be converted to cash. Cash and assets that can be readily converted to cash are referred to as *liquid assets* (e.g., checks, cash in savings accounts, easily converted securities). Assets that require a long conversion period are referred to as **fixed assets** (e.g., real estate, equipment, furniture).

Liabilities are debts of the organization. Total liabilities are the amount of the organization's assets that are owned by its creditors. Liabilities that are repayable within 1 year are considered to be short term. Liabilities not due or payable for greater than 1 year are considered to be long-term liabilities. Liabilities include such things as

- Accounts payable
- Accrued expenses
- Notes payable

Accounts payable are debts payable to individuals who have provided products or services to the organization on credit. Outstanding bills for supplies, professional and cleaning services, are examples of debts that would fall under accounts payable.

Accrued expenses represent the value of debts that are held for payment in the future (Berman et al., 1994). The time or need for payment may not be known. Vacation time or paid time off (PTO) is a good example of an accrued expense. The organization owes to its employees the value of their accrued time off. Often, employees are able to bank or use accrued time off at their discretion. Should they terminate their employment, they may or may not be able to claim the value of their banked time. If accrued PTO is paid at prevailing wages instead of the wage at the time of accrual, the value to the employee and size of this accrued debt can grow over time. As long as the employer has the potential to pay for this accrued debt, it is listed as a liability.

Notes payable are promises (notes) to pay a certain amount of money at a certain time in the future. Generally, these are loans evidenced by loan agreements indicating the loan amount, repayment schedule, and the interest due at future dates. Amounts owed for lines of credit, start-up capital, and mortgages are examples of debts that would fall under the category of notes payable.

Equity or ownership is often associated with a publicly traded stock, but is also the value of an organization beyond its liabilities or what it owes (*net* worth = what is left after debts were paid). The owner's equity is the difference between the organization's total assets and its total liabilities. It is the portion of the assets that the owner owns as opposed to what he or she borrowed. The net worth of the owner can increase in two ways. First, the owner can invest additional resources into the organization or the net worth can increase as a result of profitable operations (an increase in income greater than an increase in expenses).

Accrual and Cash

The concept of accrual refers to the practice of recording financial transactions within an appropriate period of time. The *accrual basis* of accounting requires that revenue be recorded within the period it is earned. Likewise, expenses must be recorded in the period when the resources are consumed for the production of related revenue. For example, an organization using the accrual method would record the cost of PTO earned by employees as a liability in the period it is earned. This liability is then carried until the employee takes the PTO benefit. When the PTO is used, the liability is reduced. In this way, the expense of the PTO is recorded in the time period it was earned, not when it is paid out. If it was not recorded (accrued) in this manner, the expenses for the period when PTO was earned would be understated, the expenses for the period when PTO was actually paid to the employee would be over stated, and the organization's real liabilities would be understated by the total amount of PTO pay owed to employees. For example, one employee who is paid $25 per hour, a bank of 20 PTO days (160 hours) would represent a liability of $4,000 to the organization. Consistent recording procedures prevent the manipulation of financial performance during any specific period of time. The rules for transaction recording are

1. Revenue and expenses should be recorded when services and/or products are sold or costs are incurred.
2. Expenses should be recorded during the time period in which the item purchased is used in the production of the entity's goods or services.

The *cash basis* of accounting is used as an alternative to the accrual method. Under the cash basis for accounting, revenue is recorded when cash is received and expenses are recorded when bills are paid. This approach fails to match revenue and expenses. It will not support management efforts to determine the costs of individual products and services and is used on a limited basis in health care, most commonly in small private practices and partnerships (Weltman, 1997).

Revenues and Expenses

Revenue is gross income (*gross* = before anything is taken out or paid). A HCO has several potential sources of revenue.

- Income from the sale or delivery of a service or product
- Seminars or continuing educational programs provided
- Income from grants or philanthropic gifts
- Income from investments (Chapter 2)

Under the accrual basis of accounting, revenue is recorded in the period the revenue is earned. Under a cash basis, revenue is recorded when the money is received. Revenue from the sale of a service or product is calculated by multiplying the price of the service or product times the number sold. The revenue recorded for items sold at discounted or a third party payer's established and agreed upon price should be adjusted by recording a deduction to revenue. For example, a $150 evaluation provided under a contract with a third party payer requiring a 10% discount would be recorded with two entries. The first entry would record revenue of $150. A second entry would record a $15 deduction from revenue. The net amount would equal $135, the discounted price. Revenue is also classified by its origin. Revenue for the sale of a service or product provided by the company is referred to as revenue from operations or, simply, operating revenue. Revenue from all other sources is referred to as nonoperating revenue.

An expense is money spent to produce or purchase a service or product that is sold. Under the accrual basis of accounting, expense is recorded in the time period the service or item is produced. Under a cash basis, expense is recorded when the bill is paid.

A HCO has several potential expenses related to the provision of services.

- Salary
- Benefits
- Equipment
- Supplies
- Utilities

When an organization's revenues exceed expenses for a scheduled period of time, the excess is classified as a **profit**. When expenses exceed revenue, the difference is classified as a loss. Making a profit allows the organization to increase salaries to keep up with inflation, purchase new or updated equipment, or to expand the practice if so desired. Having excess cash or a profit is beneficial to the livelihood of any organization. Understanding the financial aspect of health care is necessary in order to generate sufficient revenue to sustain a business (Chapter 22). Understanding the basic financial statements that capture the financial aspect of an organization is vital to this process.

Financial Statements

Financial statements are a set of financial reports that generally include

A balance sheet
An income statement
A cash flow statement
A retained earnings statement

Each statement is interrelated and is collectively used to view the financial health, stability, and growth potential of an organization. Financial statements can also be used to compare past to current performance revealing trends that can be used to evaluate current performance or to predict future performance. These statements can be as simple or complex as the business and should be prepared with the aid of a professional such as a CPA.

Projected financial performance is reflected in financial plans or budgets, which are referred to as "pro forma" (for the sake of form) statements. Pro forma statements present financial information in advance, or in the future. An annual financial business plan or budget represents management's best estimate of what will happen in the future (Chapter 22). It is the internal benchmark against which day-to-day performance can be assessed.

The FASB sets the standards for accounting and financial reporting. The FASB defines the objectives of financial reporting which include the provision of information:

1. That is useful to present and potential investors, creditors, and other users in making a rational investment, extending credit, and similar decisions.
2. That lists the economic resources of an organization, the claims to those resources, and the effects of transactions, events, and circumstances that change resources.
3. That describes an organization's financial performance during a stated period.

4. That identifies ways in which an organization obtains and expends cash, about its borrowing and repaying of borrowed funds, about its capital transactions, and about other factors that may affect its liquidity or solvency.
5. That states how management has discharged its stewardship responsibility for the use of the organization's resources.
6. That is useful to managers and directors in making decisions in the interest of owners.

Financial statements are typically prepared to represent the financial activity for a specific period of time. The specific date of the statement is the last date for which information was included. The time frame may vary based on the needs of the organization. Common time frames are yearly, quarterly, monthly, or every 2 weeks. Detailed activity tracking reports may be produced weekly or even daily. Financial reporting does not always follow the chronological year, depending on the nature of the business, but follows a **fiscal year** (FY). A FY follows any established 12-month cycle, ending historically when the organization experiences a decrease in the volume of activity (e.g., the lowest time in a 12-month cycle). This allows additional time to be spent on closing the books and preparing the financial statements. Once an organization has established its FY, it will continue to operate and report performance on that FY cycle. The FYs of related organizations are often the same, which allows for the comparison and cumulative reporting of financial results among related businesses.

Some additional basic accounting practices that are used in creating financial statements include the justification or alignment of all numerical information. All of the decimal places for the numbers in the statement must be vertically aligned. In addition, if the statement includes specific information on the cents for one account, it is assumed that all of the accounts are correct to the cent. This is typically done with personal checking account balances. However, by contrast, most financial statements round off to the nearest dollar amount. The dollar sign ($) is generally used only with the top and bottom figures in a financial statement; at the bottom indicating the total figure for a group of accounts. Double lines indicate the final figure in the statement (Table 21.3). Financial statements also use parentheses to indicate a negative number as opposed to the dashed line. Understanding these basic accounting practices can lead to a better understanding of the fundamental financial statements, which include the balance sheet, the income statement, the cash flow statement, and the retained earnings statement.

Balance Sheet

The first statement in the set of financial statements is the balance sheet, a statement of an organization's *financial condition*. A balance sheet is a listing of assets, liabilities, and owner's equity. At all times the total assets will equal the total liabilities plus the owner's equity, which is called the balance sheet equation.

Table 21.3   Balance Sheet for Physical Therapy Practice September 30, 2009

Assets		*Liabilities and Owner's Equity*	
Cash	$45,000	Liabilities:	
Investments	60,000		
Prepaid expenses	2,000	Accounts payable	$50,000
Inventories	10,000	Accrued expenses	5,000
Accounts receivable	60,000	Notes payable	225,000
		Total liabilities	$280,000
Land	$40,000		
Buildings	90,000		
Equipment	200,000	Owner's equity	$227,000
		Total liabilities and	
Total	$507,000	owner's equity	$507,000

Total assets = Total liabilities + owner's equity

The balance sheet is for a past period of time, prepared to reflect the organization at a certain point in time, giving a picture of an organization's pluses (assets and owner's equity) and minuses (liabilities) at a glance. Table 21.3 depicts a balance sheet for a physical therapy practice ending September 30, 2009. The clinic runs from October 1 to September 30. This balance sheet represents an end of the year status, but includes all activity of the organization prior to that date.

Income Statement

The income statement is a report on the *financial performance* of an organization over a specific period of time. It provides a comparison of monies earned (revenues) to monies spent (expenses). The difference between revenues and expenses is the net income or loss from operations during the reporting period. In an income statement, revenues are listed first, followed by allowance for contractual deductions to revenue, then expenses. Revenues in physical therapy practices are typically vol-

ume driven so that an increase in the number of patients treated increases the revenue the business generates (Drnach, 2008). Revenues can also be contractually based, meaning that for a stated service a negotiated amount of revenue will be paid to the organization.

Expenses follow revenue on the income statement. Some expenses are volume driven while others are fixed (Chapter 20). The income statement is a summary of revenues generated minus the expenses incurred resulting in net income. Income statements are also known as *Profit and Loss Statements* or a *Statement of Operations* because net income shows how much of a profit or how big a loss has been generated for a specific period of time, typically in the past not the future. The income statement is represented by the equation

Revenue – Expenses = Net income

Table 21.4 is an example of the income statement for a physical therapy practice for the FY ending September 30, 2009. This is an example of an annual income statement. Income statements can be prepared to cover any increment of time, but should be prepared at a minimum of once per year. Net income (profit or loss) from the income statement will affect the

Table 21.4   Physical Therapy Practice Income Statement Year Ending September 30, 2009

Revenue:		
Gross Revenue		
Services	$832,818	
Equipment	60,000	
Total operating revenue		$892,818
Less:		
Allowance for deductions		203,563
Gross revenue net deductions		689,255
Nonoperating revenue		23,000
Total revenue		$712,255
Expenses:		
Salaries	$361,421	
Benefits	65,056	
FICA	28,191	
Education	6,300	
Recruitment	5,000	
Professional services	11,000	
Purchased services	600	
Supplies	51,095	
Travel	4,000	
Dues	2,000	
Equipment	1,200	

(Continued)

Table 21.4 continued		
Rent/Lease	20,000	
Utilities	9,000	
Communication	3,375	
Environmental services	5,300	
Accrued expenses	40,083	
Insurance	6,100	
Total expenses		$619,721
Net income (loss)		92,534
Taxes		30,536
Net income after taxes		$61,998

owner's equity on the balance sheet. Accrued expenses on the income statement will affect accounts payable on the balance sheet.

Cash Flow Statement

The cash flow statement is a mandatory part of an organization's financial statements. It reports on the cash that flows through the business from core operations, financing, or investing. It reports on the actual cash and not any future incoming or outgoing cash on account. The availability of cash to cover short-term liabilities, such as payroll, is of critical importance especially for small business who cannot borrow against future profits like a large business (Ransom, 2008). This financial statement will show how an organization's cash position changes over time and provides a basic report on the financial health of an organization. Table 21.5 is the cash flow statement for a physical therapy practice for the period October 1, 2008 through September 30, 2009. Cash flow statements can be prepared for past, present, and future time periods. Cash flow statements that look to the future (called a pro forma statement) can help management identify potential problems in available cash before they happen. The cash flow statement is represented by the equation

Table 21.5 Physical Therapy Practice Cash Flow Statement Year Ending September 30, 2009

Cash Balance, October 1, 2008		
Cash in bank	$39,517	
Petty cash	500	
Cash balance		$40,017
Sources of cash		
Cash from operations	$51,613	
Accounts receivable	751,910	
Owner investment		
Total sources of cash		$803,523
Uses of cash		
Accounts payable	$213,110	
Payroll	495,568	
Owner withdrawal	25,000	
Capital purchase	4,862	
Cash Flow Statement		
Land and building	60,000	
Total uses of cash		$798,540
Increase (decrease) in cash		$4,983
Cash balance, September 30, 2009		$45,000

Current cash balance = Beginning cash balance + Cash received – Cash spent

The cash flow statement is useful in financial planning and is usually required when seeking financial support from a bank or other financial institutions (Chapter 22). It is prepared from the information on the balance sheet and income statement and captures the changes in cash over a period of time. For example, if the cash balance on the balance sheet has increased over the year, the cash flow statement can indicate the reason. It may show that the accounts receivable balance was reduced or that payments are being stretched out over a longer period of time, reflected as a growth in the accounts payable.

Note that the cash balance on the cash flow statement always equals the cash asset on the balance sheet.

Retained Earnings Statement

A retained earnings statement is also referred to as an owner's equity statement. Retained earnings are commonly influenced by the organization's net income and the payment of dividends to stockholders or owners of the company. The retained earnings statement explains the differences in an owner's equity on the balance sheet and provides information on how profits are used in a business, either distributed to the owners or reinvested into the business. Table 21.6 is the retained earnings statement for a physical therapy practice for the period October 1, 2008 through September 30, 2009. In the early years of a business, the owners may reinvest more of the profits into the business for growth and development. As the business matures, the owners may take out a larger portion of the profits for their personal income. Net income on the income statement will affect the retained earnings on the retained earnings statement.

Table 21.6 Physical Therapy Practice Statement of Retained Earnings Year Ending September 30, 2009	
Beginning balance	$190,002
Net income	61,998
Dividends paid	(25,000)
Current balance	$227,000

The retained earnings statement is represented by the equation:

Current retained earnings = Beginning retained earnings balance + (Revenues – Expenses) – Dividends paid

Budgeting

Financial planning often includes the creation of a **budget**. A budget is a financial statement of the estimated income and expenditures for an organization or an aspect of the organization, covering a specified future period of time. The format of a budget follows the income statement format, but reflects the anticipated performance of the organization, a discrete department or program, or a major capital undertaking. There can be several types of budgets such as an operating budget, a strategic budget, a capital budget (e.g., for buildings or equipment), a cash budget, or a special purpose budget (e.g., pediatric services only), to name a few (Finkler et al., 2007). The focus of this section is the operating budget that plans for the operating revenues and expenses of an organization within a period of 1 year. (Strategic budgeting is done for a long-range plan, typically 3–5 years). All of the budgets of an organization make up the budget for the whole organization or practice.

Budgeting requires the manager to plan ahead, forecast, and anticipate what will happen in the next year from a financial point of view. It is a dynamic process that requires monitoring and making revisions as the revenues and expenses fluctuate for any given month (Chapter 22). Budgeting is an important process that establishes an organization's financial or activity goals along with benchmarks to measure progress throughout the year.

There are a variety of ways to prepare a budget for the upcoming year, depending on the size of the organization and the program for which the budget is being prepared. Typically the budgeting process would include

- Environmental scanning (Chapters 2–6, 13, 14, and 22): In preparing a budget a manager should be aware of what is happening in the local and national markets of health care in order to anticipate any significant changes that may occur within the next year, to identify opportunities for growth, or make adjustments for anticipated changes in reimbursement or revenue levels. This would also include the identification of any anticipated changes such as the need to acquire new equipment, the need for additional personnel, the need to increase salaries, or to cover the expected increase in the cost of a provided benefit, such as health care insurance.

- Identification of goals and objectives (Chapter 3): Clear financial goals and objectives should be determined and understood by all parties in the budget-making process so that all participating parties are working towards the same goal and have a clear understanding of what that entails. If the organization wishes to increase its profits in the upcoming year so it can expand its services by opening up a new clinic, or create a library for staff and patients, or to cover the rising cost of benefits, the amount of funds needed and the rationale for the objective should be clear and appropriate (Chapter 22).
- Identify the relationship between the established goals and objectives with the organization's mission, structure, strategic plan, and current policies and procedures (Chapters 2, 13, and 14): The goals and objectives identified in the previous step should clearly relate to the mission of the organization. The relevant polices and procedures and the positions in the organization (organizational chart [Chapters 11 and 14]) responsible for the functions that will be affected by the goals and objectives related to the proposed budget (both revenues and expenses) should make sense to the organization as a whole and to the employees individually (e.g., spending money to update equipment which is in line with the mission to provide current and up-to-date interventions). The financial information contained in a budget should reflect the mission and strategic growth of the organization.
- Gather data on estimated costs and revenues: A manager or team should develop specific measurable operating objectives (Chapters 3 and 13). How much revenue would be needed to support the expenses of the department or program? What **profit margin** would be necessary in order to make the budgeted program viable and add to the overall financial success of the organization? What would be the break-even point? How

much time will it take to reach the break-even point? Is there enough cash to start up a new program? What is the expected fee for the program or service? What are other organizations currently charging for this service? These are just a few questions that would facilitate the investigation and acquisition of information in the development of a budget.

- Develop a proposed budget: The next step is to develop a budget which will then be used in the overall decision-making process for the development of the program or service. The accounts in the budget should be from the established chart of accounts of the organization. The expenses should be accounts (or sub-accounts) that are also listed on the income statement. The source of the proposed revenues should be identified. How will the anticipated revenues be generated? Are they coming from an established source or will the organization need to take out a loan? Note that revenues provided to an aspect of an organization may not reflect the total revenues generated from that aspect or department. Physical therapy departments or programs often bring in more revenues than their expenses, contributing a significant profit to the overall organization. They are referred to as **profit centers**, or loss centers depending on their net income. Therefore the program or department may only get a portion of the total revenue that is generated from the programs or services provided, with the additional revenue going to offset the costs of another aspect of the organization. This is not necessarily negative. There are many aspects of a business that may not generate revenue but are necessary for the delivery of services, such as building maintenance, administrative personnel, or housekeeping. The amount of operating revenues provided to such a department or program is considered the allocated operating revenue for a specific period of time (Table 21.7).

Once a budget has been developed and approved, it has to be implemented and monitored. Basic accounting practices are applied to the budget as with other financial statements. Capturing the variances in what was budgeted versus what is actually happening is an important aspect in financial management.

Table 21.7 Annual Operating Budget Physical Therapy Practice Year Ending September 30, 2009			
REVENUE		YTD	Variance
Operating revenue		$619,721	
EXPENSES			
Salaries	$361,421	$361,421	0
Benefits	65,056	65,056	0
FICA	28,191	28,191	0
Education	6,300	7,000	(700)
Recruitment	5,000	5,000	0
Professional services	11,000	11,000	0
Purchased services	10,600	10,600	0
Supplies	51,095	50,000	1,095
Travel	4,000	5,250	(1,250)
Dues	2,000	2,000	0
Equipment	21,283	21,083	200
Rent/lease	30,000	30,000	0
Utilities	9,000	9,300	(300)
Communication	3,375	4,125	(150)
Environmental services	5,300	5,300	0
Insurance	6,100	6,100	0
Total expenses	$619,721	$621,426	$(1705)

YTD, Year to date.

Note: Variance is the difference between what was budgeted and what was spent. This practice is over budget by $1,705. Why do you think this happened?

Financial Analysis

A key to effective financial management is the ability to analyze projected to actual performance. This is referred to as **variance analysis**. Variance analysis compares the actual entry to the projected or budgeted amount. The difference between the two is considered a variance which is listed as a positive number if the variance is less than expected or a negative (noted by parentheses instead of a negative sign) when the variance is over what is expected (Table 21.7). Variance analysis identifies the difference between the actual and the projected amounts for a specific period of time. More detailed information is often necessary to determine causal factors.

Information in financial statements can also be subjected to a variety of analytic techniques to assess a company's performance, financial position, and relative financial viability. These techniques include **common size, comparative**, and **ratio analysis** (Berman et al., 1994). More often than not, financial statements are used for comparative analysis. Comparison can be made between the elements of one financial statement for one period of time, between

two or more time periods, or between planned (budgeted) and actual performance. To aid in the comparison of financial statement entries, numbers are expressed as a percentage of a total category. For example, in Table 21.8 salary expense for FY 2009 could be expressed as an amount, $361,421 or 58.3% of the total expenses. When comparative percentages are used to define elements of a financial statement it is referred to as a **common-size statement** (Dillon and LaMont, 1983). Information on a financial statement can also be expressed for more than one date or period of time and are called **comparative statements**. Table 21.8 is an example of both a common-size and comparative financial statement.

Comparative analysis allows for the identification of trends and financial patterns. It is up to management to determine the value of the information relative to the performance of the business. In the case of the example in Table 21.8, the statement shows an improved financial performance between FY 2008 and 2009. Note that although **gross revenues** from services increased $166,564 (a 25% increase) it still continued to make up 93% of the total operating revenue due to the increase

Table 21.8 Comparative Common-Size Income Statement, Physical Therapy Practice, Year Ending September 30, 2009 and September 30, 2008

	FY 2009	FY 2008	Common-Size Percentages FY 2009 (%)	FY 2008 (%)
REVENUE:				
Gross revenue				
Services	$832,818	$666,254	93	93.3
Equipment	60,000	48,000	6.7	6.7
Total operating revenue	892,818	714,254	100.0	100.0
Less:				
Allowance for deductions	203,563	162,850	22.8	22.8
Gross revenue net deductions	689,255	551,404	96.8	96.8
Nonoperating revenue	23,000	18,400	3.2	3.2
Total revenue	$712,255	$569,804	100.0	100.0
EXPENSES:				
Salaries	361,421	335,124	58.3	55.6
Benefits	65,056	60,322	10.5	10.0
FICA	28,191	25,805	4.5	4.3
Education	6,300	4,500	1.0	0.7
Recruitment	5,000	5,000	0.8	0.8
Professional services	11,000	15,000	1.8	2.5
Purchased services	10,600	8,480	1.7	1.4
Supplies	51,095	40,876	8.2	6.8
Travel	4,000	2,500	0.6	0.4
Dues	2,000	1,500	0.3	0.2
Equipment	21,283	15,500	3.4	2.6
Rent/Lease	30,000	63,300	4.8	10.5
Utilities	9,000	9,000	1.5	1.5
Communication	3,375	3,375	0.5	0.6
Environmental services	5,300	5,300	0.9	0.9
Insurance	6,100	7,100	1.0	1.2
Total expenses	$619,721	$602,682	100.0	100.0
Net income (loss)	92,534	(32,878)	10.4	−4.6
Taxes	$30,536	0	33.0	0.0
Net income after taxes	$61,998	($32,878)	6.9	−4.6

in gross revenues from equipment (which also increased 25%). Using common size percentages also allows a comparison *between* organizations based not on absolute numbers in dollar amounts, but by percentages of totals, which eliminates the size of the organizations being compared. This allows an investor to compare such attributes of an organization such as the percentage of gross revenues from services as a percentage of total operating revenue or the percentage of total expenses paid to salaries.

Financial Ratios

Another technique that can be used to compare financial performance over time, between elements or between similar organizations is the use of **financial ratios**. The purpose of ratio analysis is to find two ratios, that when compared provide some beneficial insight into the financial health of the organization. Financial ratio analysis refers to the use of the relationships between two mathematical quantities that have management significance. The idea

behind the use of financial ratios is to summarize key financial data in a format that is easy
to understand and evaluate (Berman et al.,
1994). Common size, liquidity, efficiency, and
profitability ratios are examples of ratios used
to evaluate an organization's performance.

Common size ratios allow comparison
of one account to the total account (e.g.,
accounts receivable to total assets). They also
allow the comparison of an organization to
other organizations of different sizes as discussed previously (e.g., common-sized financial statements). Common size ratios answer
the question: what percentage of account X is
made up of the sub-account Y? Several financial accounts can be common sized including

- Cash to total assets = cash / total assets
- Current liabilities to total equity = current
  liabilities / total equity
- **Operating income** to total revenues = operating income / total revenues

Common size ratios put absolute dollar
amounts into perspective by eliminating the
factor of the size and are helpful in the analysis
of historical information or trends.

Liquidity ratios are used to assess an organization's ability to meet its short-term financial
obligations (liabilities). Does the organization
have available cash to pay off current liabilities
when they come due? Two of the more common liquidity ratios are

Current ratio is the ratio of current assets to
  current liabilities. It is a common index of
  liquidity. The higher the ratio, the better a
  business is positioned to meet its current
  obligations (Berman et al., 1994). Generally
  this ratio is considered healthy at approximately 2:1 (Wallace, 1990).

  Current Ratio = current assets / current
  liabilities

The **acid test ratio** is the most rigorous test
  of liquidity. It takes into consideration only
  cash or those assets that can be immediately
  liquidated for cash. The higher the ratio, the
  better the organization's potential to meet
  its current obligations (Berman et al., 1994).
  Generally this ratio is considered healthy at
  approximately 1:1 (Wallace, 1990).

  Acid test ratio = (cash + marketable
  securities) / current liabilities

Efficiency ratios can provide some information on how efficiently the organization
is run. A common efficiency ratio is the **days
receivable** that is a measurement of the average time it takes to collect the cash from the
accounts receivable. Days receivable is calculated by first finding the net patient revenue
per day (net patient revenue for the year / 365
days per year), then dividing that number into
net accounts receivable.

Days receivable = accounts receivable /
patient revenue per day

Days receivable will have a direct affect on the
cash flow statement and the amount of available
cash to meet expenses, such as payroll.

Another common efficiency ratio is **revenue
to assets**, which provides information on how
many dollars of revenue have been generated by each dollar invested in assets (Finkler
et al., 2007). It is calculated by the following
formula:

Revenue to assets = total revenues / total
assets

If Business A generates $1 of revenue for
each dollar invested in assets, compared to
Business B that generates $2 of revenue for
each dollar invested in assets, Business B
would appear to be more efficient in its use of
assets than Business A.

Profitability ratios are other ratios used
in both for-profit and not-for-profit organizations. The need to make a profit is vital in both
types of organizations in order to keep up with
inflation, the cost of living expenses, and to
sustain growth. The *operating margin* is the
ratio of net income to total revenue. Operating margin can be calculated for all or discrete
parts of an organization. Good financial performance results in a high operating margin.
This ratio provides a basis for comparison of
the economic performance of one organization
to industry standards, previous performance,
and other investment opportunities. Operating margin can also help an organization
assess the relative contribution of one operating unit to another.

Operating margin = (total revenues – total
expenses) / total revenues

Return on assets is the relationship of total
income to the total investment (assets) of the

organization. Return on assets can be calculated for all or discrete parts of an organization. A higher return on assets indicates good performance. This ratio also provides a basis for comparison of the economic performance of one organization to industry standards, previous performance, and other investment opportunities. Return on assets may be used as a criterion for selecting between alternative business strategies.

> Return on assets = (income + interest expense) / total assets

It should be noted that a variety of ratios can be developed or used other than those described earlier.

Performance Indicators

Financial ratios offer a set of standardized assessment tools that allow for the comparison of current financial performance to past performance, current expectations as well as the performance of similar organizations on an individual or industry wide basis. Some additional financial performance indicators that may be of particular value for assessing the performance of a physical therapy practice are the following (Skula and Psetian, 1997).

Volume
Number of referrals
Number of scheduled treatments or units of service (UOS)
Number of completed (billed) treatments or UOS
Number of visits
Case mix
Revenues
Net revenue per referral
Net revenue per visit
Net revenue as a percentage of charge
Costs
Labor cost per volume measure
Nonlabor cost per volume measure
Employee benefits as a percentage of salary
Efficiency
Productive hours paid per billed UOS
Nonproductive hours paid per billed UOS
Number of visits per referral
Number of visits per referral by diagnosis, age, or other defining factor
Number of billed UOS per patient visit

Performance indicators can be used to create a report card for organizational performance. Management should use performance indicators that are meaningful to its success. Through careful selection, clear performance expectations, sometimes called performance benchmarks can be established and communicated to members of the organization. Organizational performance indicators should be tracked, trended, and the outcome should be shared with everyone who has a role in meeting performance targets (Case, 1995).

There is an increasing trend in health care toward the use of industry performance standards to evaluate the performance of individual HCOs (Chapter 16). Industry performance standards can help management assess performance in a rapidly changing environment when historical performance has less relevance, set reasonable improvement targets and for competitive positioning. However, the use of external performance standards should be done only with a complete understanding about the source and applicability of the standard. Care should be taken to be sure that selected industry standards are clearly applicable, represent comparable data, and that regional and organizational differences have been identified. A common performance indicator is the measurement of an employee's productivity.

Productivity

Productivity refers to the amount of a resource consumed in the production of an increment of output. As with any other aspect of organizational performance, an objective performance target will help direct management and staff efforts in the right direction. Productivity standards are performance targets. To be of maximum benefit, productivity standards should be

- Based on a measurable unit of output
- Objectively measured
- Readily available
- Understandable
- Achievable

Management is responsible for setting productivity standards (performance expectations) for resources consumed. Where productivity standards do not exist or are out of date, new standards should be set using internal data and external benchmarks or standards. Internal data will demonstrate how well the organization is performing in comparison to historical performance. Comparison of external benchmarks to internal performance measurements will show how the organization is performing in comparison to other similar organizations (Chapters 6, 13, and 16). External benchmarks may be available through professional organizations, business associations, consultants, proprietary databases, or directly from similar business. In 2006, the American Physical Therapy Association (APTA) published a report on productivity expectations of PTs (APTA, 2006). More than half of the respondents (57.9%) reported that the facility where they work have productivity standards but that there was considerable variability of a standard within similar types of practice settings. Even if the organization exceeds external benchmarks, management may still find opportunities to improve performance.

Productivity standards are generally based on financial activity or billable time (Table 21.9). A PT could be productive in the true sense of the word, but not financially productive. For example, researching the latest evidence of the effectiveness of an intervention commonly used in the practice, learning to use a new database system, learning to use new technology to supervise support personnel, or a piece of assistive technology may be productive in the sense that these activities promote the knowledge and skills of a PT, or promote the efficient delivery of services, but they may not be billable to a third party payer.

Financial productivity will become more clear and understandable if the PT understands the importance of providing cost effective services in a productive manner. If the activity is associated with increasing referrals (by providing a more cost effective and efficient intervention thereby improving outcomes), decreasing nonlabor cost (by decreasing the need for support staff for certain activities), or maximizing the amount of billable time available (by the use of technology to complete a supervisory visit of a support personnel) for example, the relationship of these activities to financial productivity will become more clear and understandable to all persons involved. Productivity, or the amount of billable hours available, is also influenced by several other factors, which include

Table 21.9   Calculating Financial Productivity

Time	PT	PTA
Hours paid/yr[a]	2080	2080
Nonproductive hours:		
PTO: 15 days	120	120
Continuing education: 3 days	24	24
Required meetings: hrs/year	40	40
Total nonproductive/yr[b]	184	184
Available productive hours/yr	1896	1896
Billable hours		
6 hrs billable / 8 hrs worked[c]		
75% productivity expectation	1422	1422
UOS (=15 min)/yr[d]	5688	5688
UOS/day	24	24
Cost[e]		
Salary	47008	37918
Benefits	8461	6825
FICA	3596	2901
Education	500	300
Human resources	200	100
Total cost	59765	48044
Total cost/hours paid	28.73	23.1
Total cost/productive hour	42.03	33.79
Total cost/UOS	10.51	8.45

[a]A full-time employee gets paid for 40 hours per week for 52 weeks per year or 2,080 hours. This is considered a full-time equivalent (FTE).
[b]In-home care time should be allocated for travel, which is nonbillable and would significantly affect the available productive hours per year.
[c]Six hours per day takes into consideration 1 hour for a paid lunch and 30 minutes at the beginning and end of the day for documentation and other patient management activities. 6/8 = 0.75 Seventy-five percent of the available productive hours 1,896 = 1,422
[d]1 UOS = 15 minutes. Four 15 minutes units = 1 hour. 1,422 hours × 4 units per hour = 5,688 UOS
[e]Cost accounts may vary. See Figure 20.3, Cost Worksheet.

- Patient cancellation rate
- Utilization of appropriate personnel and resources
- Physical plant design and layout
- Documentation requirem   ents and access procedures
- Supervisory requirements of paraprofessionals
- Use of technology

To become more productive does not automatically mean to "see more patients" and should begin with an examination of current practices and making them more efficient.

Revenue Management

For most HCOs revenue management is the management of accounts receivable. It is the actions taken to increase total revenue and improve the collection of accounts receivable. Revenue management is a lengthy process that involves several activities including

1. Measuring services and products for sale
2. Setting prices (fees)
3. Identifying the payer(s) for each service or product
4. Establishing policies and procedures that address the provision of the service, recording the delivery of the service, and collecting reimbursement
5. Estimating expected payment
6. Following procedures for payment receipt, account reconciliation, and cash management
7. Financial reporting

The goal of revenue management is to maximize income from operations and investments. This can be done by increasing the volume of patients seen or maximizing the payer mix to optimize reimbursement (i.e., have more patients with better paying insurance; requires marketing) (Chapters 18 and 19), decreasing the cost of services provided (Chapter 20), raising the fees charged for services rendered, or improving the collection of accounts receivable.

Fees

Under the current U.S. health care reimbursement system, the majority of health care payments come from private health insurance and governmental health payment plans. A minor but growing percentage of payment is self-payment (patients paying out of pocket). Commercial (private) health care insurance plans typically use standardized payment schedules that determine the amount that they will pay for a specific health care service. This is called the **usual and customary rate** (UCR) which is consistent with the average rate or fee for similar services in a particular geographic area. Often, commercial health care insurance will pay the provider charges up to the UCR. The patient is sometimes required to pay the difference. Governmental payers, such as Medicare,

use a variety of payment methods that range from paying some percentage of the provider cost (expenses) to paying a fixed amount per service regardless of the health care provider's cost. Who and how payment is provided will influence the organization's fee schedule.

The **fee schedule** is a listing of the services provided and the charge for each of those services. The established fee can be based on an amount of time, on the type of service, on a per session or per visit basis, a per day basis (per diem), or for a set number of sessions. A fee based on time is more common in physical therapy.

Typically each listing on a fee schedule is defined by

1. Numeric charge code
2. Description
3. Unit of measure for the product or service
4. Price

An organization's fee schedule will vary based on the size and complexity of its business. It will also vary based on management and customer information needs. The more specific the information needs of management, the more specific the charges on the fee schedule.

The actual dollar amount of the fees can be calculated using several different methods. Two of the more common methods are the going-rate pricing and the markup pricing. The **going-rate pricing** is what others in the marketplace are charging for the same or similar service. This method is easily established, but runs the risk of not covering all the cost of the business. The cost associated with the delivery of a service for one organization may be significantly different from those of other organizations in the marketplace. A more common method is the markup pricing method. The **markup pricing** is similar in most industries whereby a fee or price is estimated based on several factors such as cost, time, location, and type of service provided, and then a markup or an additional percentage of the fee is added on so that the organization can make a profit on the specific product or service (Drnach, 2008). Decisions about fee setting need to balance the desire to maximize net income against market sensitivity to the price for the service. All organizations must also be mindful of laws that govern pricing.

The Robinson–Patman Act of 1936 prohibits organizations from charging similar customers different prices unless the differences are based on differences in production cost, transportation, sale, or quantities in which commodities are sold (Garrison, 1979). Differential pricing must be based on real cost differences. As a result, the organization must set charges to maximize the potential payment from all sources while using one level charge for all patients. All of these factors can be accommodated if the fee is set somewhere above the highest payment rate.

Billing

Establishing a fee schedule is one step; obtaining payment is another. An important aspect in billing for services rendered is clear communication with the third party payer on what exactly is being billed. Current Procedural Terminology codes or CPT codes were established by the American Medical Association (AMA) to aid in this process (AMA, 2003). CPT codes are five-digit codes used by health care providers to designate the type of service provided. PTs generally use codes in the Physical Medicine and Rehabilitation section, or 97000 codes. Examples of several common CPT codes used in physical therapy are

97000	Physical therapy evaluation
97002	Physical therapy re-evaluation
97110	Therapeutic exercise
97112	Neuromuscular re-education
97116	Gait training

The Centers for Medicare and Medicaid Services (CMS) is responsible for setting the reimbursement rates at which the government pays health care providers. To assure that claims are processed efficiently, CMS uses the **Healthcare Common Procedure Coding System (HCPCS)**, commonly referred to as "hick picks." Level I HCPCS use the CPT codes, which are used primarily to identify medical services and procedures furnished by physicians and other health care professionals such as PTs. Level II of the HCPCS are used primarily to identify products, supplies, and services not included in the CPT codes. Because Medicare and other insurers cover a variety of services, supplies, and equipment that are not identified by CPT codes, the Level II HCPCS

codes were established for submitting claims for these items. Level II codes are also referred to as alpha-numeric codes because they consist of a single alphabetical letter followed by four numeric digits. An example of some HCPCS codes include the following:

2008 HCPCS Alpha Numeric Index (CMS, 2007)

A4565	Sling
L0100-L0200	Cervical spinal orthosis
L3040-L3100	Orthopedic shoe arch support
E0305-E0310	Bed rail
E0992	Wheelchair seat insert

When billing by CPT code it is important that the ICD-9 code is also indicated, especially when billing Medicare/Medicaid and third party insurers. The ICD-9 code is the **International Classification of Diseases**, Ninth Revision, developed by the World Health Organization (The National Center for Health Statistics, 2007). This code identifies the patient's disease (or diagnosis) for which he or she is being treated which should complement the diagnosis made by the PT. Currently an updated version of the ICD-9 codes is available (ICD-10). The ICD-10 update includes expanded detail for many conditions and moves from using numeric codes to using alphanumeric codes. Example IDC-9 codes include

331.3	Communicating hydrocephalus
717	Internal derangement of the knee
726.31	Medial epicondylitis
756.51	Osteogenesis imperfecta
781.2	Abnormality of gait

In addition to coding, several payment factors have been developed over the years to assist health care providers in defining their revenues. Two of the more common payment factors are the **Resource Based Relative Value Scale (RBRVS)** and **Diagnosis-Related Groups (DRGs)**, which are two ways of including similar or related services into one payment (Drnach, 2008). **Relative Value Units (RVUs)**, developed by Medicare, assign a value to a particular service or procedure identified by a CPT code. There are basically three types of RVUs: work (wRVU), malpractice (mpRVU), and practice expense (peRVU). These three factors are associated with the reasonable price or reimbursement that Medicare will pay for a unit of service. They are contained in the formula

Reasonable amount = [(wRVU × wGP-CI)] + [(peRVU × peGPCI)] + [mpRVU × mpGPCI)] × a conversion factor

In addition to the values associated with the RVUs, the Medicare payment is adjusted to reflect variations in practice expenses among various geographic regions by using a specific geographic practice cost index (GPCI). There is also a GPCI for each RVU. A conversion factor (CF) is determined annually by Congress and the CMS. Medicare also distinguishes between a facility and nonfacility practice expense RVU, based on where a service is provided. Facility locations, under the resource-based system for calculating payments, include inpatient and outpatient hospital settings, emergency rooms, skilled nursing facilities, or ambulatory surgical centers. Outpatient rehabilitation services are usually reimbursed at the nonfacility per RVU. Although the formula is complex it is a good way to estimate appropriate revenues from services provided and does attempt to provide a fair and equitable distribution of payment based on several factors other than the organization's fee.

Collections

A high percentage of health care services are provided on credit, an aspect of accrual accounting. Credit purchasing occurs when the customer is billed through the use of an invoice for money owed after the service or product is provided. Organizations that provide services on account should have clear policies and procedures regarding the extension of credit. Policies on the provision of services *pro bono publico* (Latin "for the public good"), providing services at a discount, self-pay obligations, coordination of third party benefits, billing procedures, and cash receipts management should be clear and communicated to the patient and provider prior to the delivery of services. Effective management of accounts receivable starts before admission or at the point of patient registration (Berman et al., 1994).

The APTA encourages PTs to provide pro bono physical therapy services when appropriate by

- Providing professional services at no fee or reduced fee to persons of limited financial means.

- Donating professional expertise and service to charitable organizations.
- Engaging in activities to improve access to physical therapy.
- Offering financial support to organizations that deliver physical therapy services to persons of limited financial means (APTA, 2008).

The benefits of engaging in these types of activities can include an enhanced public image and an increase in both personal and collective work satisfaction; both intangible assets of an organization (Scott, 1993).

When a third party payer is involved, services should not be provided until the payer authorizes them. This is called **pre-authorization**. Pre-authorization does not guarantee payment, but it may limit loss of payment due to technical or contractual issues. Usually, it is the responsibility of the enrollee (patient or person who bought the insurance plan) to understand and comply with the terms of his or her health care insurance. In practice, it is in the provider's best interest to assist the patient with benefit verification and pre-authorization compliance. Not only is it good customer service (another intangible asset), pre-authorization of service coverage has the potential to increase the speed and rate of payment.

Key factors that can improve the collection of payments for services rendered include

- Clear understanding by both the patient and provider on how payment will be made prior to the delivery of services.
- Appropriate understanding of the benefits and limits of an individual's health care insurance prior to the delivery of services.
- Clear and appropriate documentation of services rendered and the patient's response to the intervention.
- Timely submission of invoices.
- Timely provision of documentation needs of the third party payer or medical claims reviewer.
- Adherence to an established plan of care.
- Clear communication with both the patient and the third party payer on the benefits and limitations of physical therapy interventions.

Expense Management

Expense management is controlling operating and capital expenses. Operating expenses are associated with the cost of resources used in the production of goods and services in a limited (typically 1 year) period of time (i.e., expenses in the income statement). Capital expenses are associated with the purchase of equipment, facilities, and other high priced items that contribute to the delivery of the service or product over an extended period of time (typically more than 1 year). An organization will often use a dollar threshold, such as $500, to differentiate between operating and capital expenses. Equipment with an extended life and a value greater than the threshold will be classified as a capital expense. Controlling operating or capital expenses requires close attention to the variances that may occur in budgets for operations (operation budget) or capital ventures (capital budget). Management may also attempt to control operating expenses by influencing the utilization of mixed or variable cost items such as utilities, supplies, or recruitment (Chapter 20).

The goal of expense management is to maximize net income. To reach that goal, the spread between gross revenue and total expenses must become wider. Armed with a working knowledge of cost characteristics, managers should be able to predict the impacts of their decisions regarding the purchase and use of resources on net income. The importance of efficiently managing resources has increased as payment cuts reduce the net income of most HCOs. As health care costs continue to rise, the need and payment for services will continue to be scrutinized. HCOs will need to continuously improve revenue and/or decrease cost. To manage expenses effectively requires knowledge of the types of expenses, what expenses can be controlled, how expenses are controlled and how expenses behave in relation to the volume of service and/or goods produced. Some basic activities associated with expense management include

- Monitoring budgets and investigating variances.
- Implementing policies and procedures and monitoring the utilization of mixed or variable cost items (including overtime pay to nonexempt employees).
- Monitoring the market (environmental scanning) in anticipation of increases in benefits, salaries, or other expense items.
- Engage in cost-effectiveness analysis of services rendered.

Summary

This chapter provided a financial and accounting background for physical therapists to enhance their ability to participate in business financial discussions and decision making. The discussion stressed the importance of accounting and financial information to support organizational decisions. The application of standard accounting practices ensures that financial reports have a consistent meaning between time periods and organizations. Reliable financial information is essential to management efforts to maximize financial performance. To assure consistency, an understanding of GAAP and the basic accounting concepts of a chart of accounts, double entry, debits and credits, assets, liabilities and owner's equity, accrual versus cash method of accounting, and revenues and expenses were defined. The accounting conventions of fund accounting and allowances for contractual deductions were also introduced as they are commonly seen in HCO's financial documents. The standard financial reports (i.e., balance sheet, income statement, cash-flow statement, and retained earnings statement) were introduced and used to present the financial status of an entity for the FY ending September 30, 2009. In assessing financial reports common-sizing, comparing, and using financial ratios were discussed that help in understanding the variances seen within and between financial reports and budgets as well as to understand better the financial health of an organization. The monitoring and investigation of variances from what was expected or budgeted is an important duty in financial management. Revenue management, including the setting of fees and coding for services rendered is vital to the communication process with payers of health care services. Likewise expense management is important in maximizing net income. This financial information is a necessary prerequisite for what comes next: entrepreneurship-starting, and owning a physical therapy practice.

CASE STUDY 21.1

Individual Case

Introduction

Table 21.10 presents demographic, patient, payer, treatment, and reimbursement information from a hypothetical physical therapy practice. This information is the basis for dealing with the questions that follow the table, so review the information. You will have to do some calculations.

Questions

1. Determine the annual number of visits per year. Assume 50 weeks in 1 year.
2. Determine the number of visits per week in each program. Assume 5 days per week.
3. Determine the number of patients, by patient mix, that are seen each day.
4. Determine the annual number of patients seen for each payment group.

5. Determine the annual amount that you charge each year. This is based on the fee and the number of patients seen annually.
6. Determine the annual amount of revenue that is brought in based on the reimbursement schedules.
7. Choose option a or b.

Option a: Summarize your findings as if you were describing this business to a PT who potentially could become your assistant manager in a small hospital department where everyone treats patients.

Option b: Summarize your findings as if you were describing this business to a PT who potentially could become a partner in your private practice. You both treat patients and deal with management matters.

Table 21.10 Information for the Individual Case Study on Accounting

Type	Private physical therapy clinic
Location	Columbus, OH
Programs	(75%) outpatient, (15%) contract services to schools, (10%) home care
Patient mix	(40%) geriatric, (50%) adults <65 yrs, (10%) pediatric
Diagnostic mix	Musculoskeletal 60%
	Neuromuscular 20%
	Cardiopulmonary 19%
	Integumentary 1%
Payer mix	(60%) Medicare, (0%) Medicaid, (20%) private insurance
(20%) HMO, (0%) self pay	
#Visits/week	250
Fee	$100 per visit
Reimbursement schedule	
Medicare	$80/visit
Medicaid	$67/visit
Private insurance	$90/visit
HMO	$80/visit

CASE STUDY 21.2

Group Case

Instructions

Get together with one or more peers who chose the same option as you did. Discuss and answer the question, "what types of skills the assistant manager or potential partner would need to meet the anticipated needs of the patient mix." List the types of therapy services that would be provided (i.e., evaluation, therapeutic exercises, gait training, etc). Develop a fee schedule for the services. Finally, determine how much more money would be brought in if all patients paid cash.

REFERENCES

American Medical Association. Current Procedural Terminology. CPT 2004 Professional Edition, Chicago, IL: American Medical Association Press of the American Medical Association. 2003.

American Physical Therapy Association. Practice profile survey. Reported productivity expectations of PTs 1999–2005. Alexandria, VA: The American Physical Therapy Association. 2006.

American Physical Therapy Association. Guidelines: Pro bono physical therapy services. HOD G06-93-21-39. Alexandria, VA: American Physical Therapy Association. 2008.

Berman H, Kukla S, Weeks L. The Financial Management of Hospitals, 8th ed. Ann Arbor, MI: Health Administration Press. 1994.

Case J. Open book management: The coming business revolution. New York, NY: Harper Business. 1995:19–36.

Center for Medicaid and Medicare Services. 2008 HCPCS Alpha Numeric Index. Available at http://www.cms.hhs.gov/HCPCSReleaseCodeSets/downloads/INDEX2008.pdf. Accessed 5/01/07.

Cleverley W, Cameron A. Essentials of health care finance, 5th ed. Gaithersburg, MD: Aspen. 2002.

Dillon R, LaMont R. Financial statement analysis. A key to practice diagnosis and prognosis. Clinical Management. 1983;35:36–39.

Drnach M. The basics of billing. In Drnach M ed. The clinical practice of pediatric physical therapy: From the NICU to Independent Living. Baltimore, MD: Lippincott Williams & Wilkins. 2008:339–349.

Finkler S, Kovner C, Jones C. Financial management for nurse managers and executives, 3rd ed. St. Louis, MO: Saunders Elsevier. 2007.

Gans D, Piland N, Honore P. Developing a chart of accounts: Historical perspective of the Medical Group Management Association. Journal of Public Health Management Practice. 2007;13:130–132.

Garrison R. Managerial accounting: Concepts for planning, control, decision-making, Revised ed. Dallas, TX: Business Publications. 1979.

National Center for Health Statistics. Classification of diseases and functioning and disability. ICD-9-CM. US Department of Health and Human Services. Available at www.cdc.gov/nchs/about/otheract/icd9/abticd9.htm. Accessed 12/01/07.

Ransom D. Small business woes. Available at http://www.allbusiness.com/energy-utilities/oil-gas-industry-oil-processing/10063332-3.html. Accessed 5/14/08.

Scott R. For the public good. PTMagazine. American Physical Therapy Association. 1993:82:82–85.

Skula R, Psetian J. A comparative analysis of revenues and cost-management strategies for not-for-profit and for-profit hospitals. Hospital and Health Service Administration. 1997;42:117–134.

Wallace W. Financial Accounting. Cincinnati, OH: South-Western Publishing. 1990.

Weltman B. The Big Idea Book for New Business Owners. New York, NY: Macmillian Spectrum. 1997.

Wikipedia. Debits and Credits. Available at http://en.wikipedia.org/wiki/Debits_andcredits. Accessed 5/01/08.

ADDITIONAL RESOURCES

Financial Accounting Standards Board can be accessed at http://www.fasb.org/.

Ittelson T. Financial Statements. A Step-by-Step Guide to Understanding and Creating Financial Reports. Career Press, Franklin Lakes NJ. 1998.

Private Practice Section of the APTA. Private Practice Physical Therapy: The How-To Manual.

Glinn J and McMenamin P, eds. Private Practice Section, American Physical Therapy Association. Alexandria, VA. 2002.

Pam Pohly's netguide offers free reviews of hundreds of health care accounting and related books 1999 through the most current editions. The list of available texts are found at http://www.pohly.com/books_healthcare_finance_accounting.html.

The APTA website has several links that would assist a PT entering into private practice or as a manager of a department. These include Practice and Reimbursement links which include access to information on coding, working with insurers, use of personnel, and other resources for owners or managers of a practice. See American Physical Therapy Association at www.apta.org.

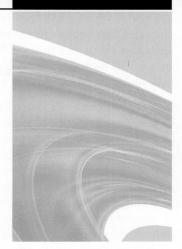

CHAPTER 22

ENTREPRENEURSHIP: PHYSICAL THERAPIST PRACTICE OWNERSHIP

DON OLSEN AND LARRY J. NOSSE

Learning Objectives

1. Compare and contrast the opportunities and threats of self-employment and working for someone else (another person or an organization).
2. Define entrepreneur.
3. List and discuss key characteristics attributed to entrepreneurs.
4. Locate and utilize relevant information to assess the current physical therapist owned practice environment.
5. Compare and contrast the application of business principles as typically applied in small physical therapist owned practices and hospital physical therapy departments.
6. Utilize the information in this book to develop a general plan to become a physical therapist entrepreneur.
7. Construct reasonable, reference supported solutions to scenarios related to planning, and managing physical therapist owned private practices.

Introduction

Much service business management material has been covered in the preceding chapters of this text. However, large business concepts have prevailed. This emphasis was chosen because large business is most written about and several of the authors' management experiences have been in large not-for-profit health care organizations. The current chapter applies many of the principles presented in earlier chapters to small, private, physical therapist (PT) owned practices. This is the kind the authors are engaged in. We, and others (Black and Glinn, 2002; Fiebert et al., 1990), have found that many physical therapists (PTs) who want to start their own practice find that they have not been prepared by their basic education or experience to face the complexities of planning and operating their own business. The intent of this chapter is to contribute to PTs' understanding of the benefits and challenges of ownership and to provide a planning **process** to guide the formation of a private physical therapy practice. Our approach has three main focuses:

1. Describe the characteristics of **entrepreneurs** and the opportunities and threats associated with ownership of a small physical therapy practice.
2. Emphasize the practical application of selected business principles and procedures to the *entrepreneurial* physical therapy business environment.
3. Offer experience-based guidance for becoming a small private physical therapy practice owner.

We direct this chapter to PTs who may consider becoming practice owners at some point in their career. As small private practice owners ourselves, we offer our perspectives on the benefits of ownership along with the inherent challenges and risks associated with pursuing an entrepreneurial career path.

Key terms, which are defined below, are bolded and italicized the first time they appear in the chapter. Other important terms are shown in boldface on first appearance and are defined by the context in which they are used. When either of these types of terms is used several times, its acronym will be identified and subsequently used in the chapter. Both types of terms are listed alphabetically in the online glossary with their definitions and (when applicable) their acronyms.

budgeting: the process of forming budgets. A budget provides a prediction of income and expenses so financial decisions can be made.

business plan: a comprehensive planning document that clearly describes the developmental objective of a proposed or existing business. The plan is a written guide for starting and running a business successfully.

direct access: patients have access to physical therapists without a written referral from a licensed prescriber. State practice acts vary as to the conditions under which direct access can occur.

entrepreneur/entrepreneurial: a person who is willing to start a business under the assumption that their talents are sufficient to avoid losses and will lead to autonomy and prosperity. A bent to start and conduct an enterprise or business, assuming full control and financial risk with the intent of making a profit rather than work as an employee.

overutilization: providing unnecessary but reimbursable physical therapy or other health care services.

physician-owned physical therapy service(s) (POPTS): financial arrangements based on the referral of physical therapist services for the financial benefit of the referrer.

professional autonomy: in physical therapy, this is practice characterized by independent, self-determined professional judgment and action.

referralfor-profit: when state statutes allow for various practitioners to refer patients to physical therapists, and various referrers have an ownership interest in physical therapy businesses, and these referrers send their patients to their own physical therapy settings, these conditions are called referral-for-profit. This term is more inclusive than the older term, POPTS, which did not clearly include other referrers.

self-employed: working for oneself rather than being an employee working for someone else. A business owner is self-employed. According to the IRS, the self-employed are owners of unincorporated businesses who rely on profit from their businesses for their primary source of income. Owners of incorporated businesses, whose primary form of compensation is a regular wage or salary from their business are not considered by the Bureau of Labor Statistics as self-employed, but rather they are counted as owners.

small business: to participate in federal government programs the Small Business Administration sets small business criteria based on the average annual receipts or number of employees. These numbers differ by business and relate to for-profit organizations. For a hospital the maximum annual receipts is $31.5 million. For physical and occupational therapists, and speech therapists and audiologists the maximum is $6.5 million.

small practice: for physical therapy practices an arbitrary number is less than 20 employees. The number of employees is important for insurance purposes and the size of a small business varies by state.

Stark I, II, III: statues regarding the regulation of physician self-referral. Named after its chief congressional sponsor, Pete Stark in the Omnibus Budget Reconciliation Act of 1989 (Stark I), and 1993 (Stark II and III).

start-up: a new business.

What Is a Small Business?

Small is a relative term. A *small business* is defined differently depending on who you ask and why you are asking. The Small Business Administration (SBA, 2007a) says to do business with the Federal government, a small physical therapy business is one that generates a yearly average of $6.5 million in receipts. The same agency adds that a small business is one that is independently owned and operated and is not dominant in its field. For industry analysis, to distinguish small from large businesses, 500 employees is the dividing point. The Wisconsin Office of the Commissioner of Insurance (State of Wisconsin, 2007) says for health insurance policy purposes, a small business is one with 2–50 employees. Finally, the National Association for the Self-Employed (NASE; 2008) uses ten or fewer employees in their literature. Our practical definition of a *small practice* is a practice with 1–20 employees.

Contributions of Small Businesses

Historically, small businesses have contributed more than 50% to the U.S. gross domestic product. In the health care sector, more than half the businesses meet industry definition of a small business (Small Business Notes, 2007). Small businesses contribute to their local communities in several ways. Small businesses

1. Account for most of the new jobs created in this country.
2. Are more likely to try new methods of doing business in order to get a foothold in a market and continue to grow.
3. Are more likely to develop new ideas, test new services and products before larger businesses.
4. Are more likely to provide services and products larger businesses choose not to pursue.

Regardless of size, to be profitable and successful over time, a business must provide something customers value and deliver it efficiently (Chapter 2). The benefits attributed to small businesses are easily translatable to the private physical therapy practice environment.

Small businesses offer opportunities for innovations in management (Chapter 11), service delivery, service and product development, and other areas. The more people who are free to innovate and profit from their efforts, the more likely innovations will occur. Successful innovations are those that will improve the performance and profitability of a business by increasing or retaining its **market share**. Kuratko and Hodgetts (2007) suggest that innovations stem from:

Demographic changes
Incongruities between what is and what could or should be
Market and industry changes
New knowledge/new concepts

Innovations have the potential for improving the physical therapy service delivery process and increasing the value a private practice offers to its customers. Examples of physical therapy related innovation include establishing a specialized program for people with diabetes, a program to assist in weight loss, or to improve balance and prevent falls, or establish ongoing exercise programs for clients to continue at their facility after discontinuing treatment. Innovation may also involve complementary alternative medicine services, for example, acupuncture, hypnosis, personal training, Pilates, ti chi ch'uan, yoga, and various types of massage. These alternative services provide opportunities for cross referrals and may attract a larger client base. A larger client base can lead to referring more patients to or back to physicians and other referrers. In order to continue to thrive in an environment that includes increased competition and declining reimbursement, innovation is necessary. See Additional Resources for more innovation ideas.

Entrepreneur Characteristics

"Entrepreneurs are the aggressive catalysts for change in today's world of business" (Bangs, 1995, p. v). Entrepreneurs are often independent thinkers who dare to be different and assume the risks of creating new products and services. Their quests include responsibility and desired results achieved through their own efforts (Timmons and Spinelli, 2006).

Given the changing environment of health care such as declining payment rates from federal and state agencies and managed-care organizations, PT entrepreneurs/owners and operators/employees of private practices are challenged to alter service delivery models to meet the needs of the clients while remaining viable financially (Beckley, 2005; Percy, 2006). Private practice owners of small-size practices often have the opportunity to lead the way to new delivery models because (1) they are the primary decision maker(s), (2) they can quickly respond to changing needs (Chapter 5), and (3) succeeding in business is a very personal goal.

While meeting the needs of patients is the core element of any PT's practice, developing and managing an environment within which quality care is provided and sufficient revenue is received requires significant organization of efforts, knowledge, and skill (Lopopolo et al., 2004; Private Practice Section [PPS], 2007; Schafer et al., 2007). In a small practice, this is in addition to maintaining **direct care** skills. This duality of business and clinical competence extends to the salaried personnel who work in a private practice. Ideally, private practice physical therapy owners and their employees should be:

- Able to manage multiple life roles
- Committed to adhering to professional ethical precepts and laws
- Confident in their clinical practice skills
- Familiar with, and able and willing to apply basic business principles in their practice
- Flexible so they are able to adapt rapidly to the ever changing health care delivery issues
- Interested in management
- Motivated to deliver quality care efficiently
- Technically skilled and capable clinicians

Nominally, the private practice owner also requires: knowledge of strategic planning (Chapters 2–6, and 13), marketing (Chapters 18 and 19), hiring (Chapter 17), managing people (Chapter 11), and **fiscal** management (Chapters 20 and 21). Personal qualities that complement good clinical and business skills include creativity, vision, wisdom, responsibility, enthusiasm, perseverance, and physical endurance.

Who Is in Private Practice?

The statement, "I'm in private practice," sometimes is not a true statement. In physical therapy, there are several groups encompassed in the terms private practice. Included are PT practice owners, PTs, and PTAs employed in PT-owned practices, and PTs and PTAs employed in physician-owned practices (American Physical Therapy Association [APTA], 1994). However, only owners are "in private practice" (Wojciechowski, 2005).

A Perspective on Physical Therapists and Business

PTs have been described as bright and dedicated professionals who have endured the rigors of an intense formal academic and clinical education (Kastantin, 1994; Newsweek, 2008). In addition, PTs have been found to be highly motivated to work toward improving the status of those they work closely with (Nosse and Sagiv, 2005). Honorable intentions notwithstanding, like other revenue generating health related services, physical therapy practice is a business. For practitioners with an entrepreneurial spirit, it is necessary to recognize this fact if they hope to survive financially. For those who choose to be employees of large organizations, the force of the financial viability message may be less inspiring. This may be because the message is filtered through management levels and "reworked" for their consumption. This could contribute to some employees feeling that the organization's financial problems are the leadership's problems rather than their own. This attitude is the opposite of that of an entrepreneur.

Private Practice Employees

Because there are fewer staff members, and less access to specialized management services (Chapter 11) like marketing or human resources departments (Chapter 18), therapists employed in private practice settings are usually expected to be involved in nonpatient care activities such as marketing, budgeting, developing new services, and participating in the hiring process. Such experiences can increase staff members' breadth of knowledge and experience with a range of business activities. These experiences may lead them to management positions or practice ownership. PTs with the characteristics and skills noted earlier who are not yet ready for ownership are needed as employees in private physical therapy practices for the model to remain viable. Without such capable employees growth of private practice physical therapy will be difficult.

Private Practice: The Good and the Bad News

Many PTs at some time have thought about practicing on their own (Ramsey, 2007). With or without the aspiration of becoming a business owner, having knowledge of principles of business management (Chapter 11), marketing (Chapter 18), and finance (Chapters 20 and 21) is useful in many employment settings (Schafer et al., 2007) as well as in personal life. Management principles have general applicability in the many roles therapists play as small practice owners, family members, and community leaders.

In addition to business and management knowledge, an entrepreneurial PT must be willing to take financial risks, have stamina to work long hours, and be committed to being self-employed. In return for a willingness to take financial risks and hard work, there are tangible and intangible rewards.

Opportunities

Among the possibilities that can be achieved through practice ownership are

- Financial reward
- Self-expression/creativity
- Autonomy
- Leadership skill development
- Contribution to the profession and community

Financial Reward

In return for investing their money at the risk of losing it, if there is a profit from operations, it belongs to the owner(s). This profit may be taken in addition to a salary for his or her efforts. For more than a decade, gross earned income (Chapter 21) comparisons have shown PTs who are self-employed on a full-time basis earn approximately twice as much as their full-time salaried colleagues (APTA, 1994; Phoenix Strategic Surveys, 2003; PPS, 2004).

Self-Expression

A private practice owner has the opportunity of choosing the type of clinical practice, location, organizational configuration (Chapter 14), and legal structure. Figure 22.1 depicts common legal structures.

An owner may choose to do home care as a solo practitioner. They may operate a clinic with a partner or operate several clinics under one of several forms of incorporation and with any number of shareholders (Wojciechowski, 2005) (Chapter 6).

Self-expression can also be reflected in the innovative ways client concerns are dealt with. The small private practice model must recognize, and in unique ways, minimize the impact of key deterrents to clients decisions' to seek or continue physical therapy services (Chapter 19). Deterrents include

High out-of-pocket costs, i.e., high deductibles and increasing co-insurance and premiums

Demands on client's time, i.e., travel time, waiting time, and duration of treatment

Perceived benefit of treatment, i.e., increased discomfort and small increments of improvement

Amount of time a PT was actually involved in the delivery of treatment

PT practice owners typically seek to self-define their practice, control the business decisions relevant to their practice, and maintain *professional autonomy* (Wojciechowski, 2005).

Autonomy

At the end of 2007, 88% of state statutes and the District of Columbia allowed patients to see PTs without a written or verbal referral from a medical practitioner (APTA, 2007a). This is a very large step toward professional autonomy for PTs.

There has been stimulating discussions as to what professional autonomy or autonomous practice means. The operational definition for the term as used in the APTA 2020 vision statement is a "physical therapist practice characterized by independent, self-determined, professional judgment and action" (APTA, 2007b). There is also an ethical obligation noted in the APTA Code of Ethics, Principle 4 that deals with exerting professional responsibility in managing the care of patients (APTA, 2007c).

Sinnott (2004) and Sandstrom (2007) have called attention to differences between practice or technical autonomy and business or socioeconomic autonomy, respectively. While all PTs are ethically required to "own" their technical practice, they are not ethically

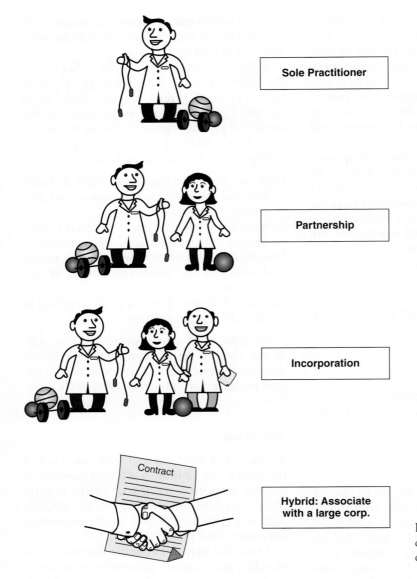

Figure 22.1. General schema of private practice ownership opportunities.

required to "own" the business where they utilize their technical skills in an autonomous manner (Advance for Physical Therapists and PT Assistants, 2007; Sinnott, 2004). Sandstrom (2007) noted that the attainment of complete autonomy is not possible. An example of technical autonomy limitation is being required to provide different postoperative care according to various surgeon mandated standard protocols. A socioeconomic limitation is the restriction of a patient's choice of providers when a patient is encouraged, even directed, by their physician to seek treatment at a *physician-owned physical therapy service (POPTS)* (Chapter 9).

In contrast to an employer perspective of autonomy there is an entrepreneurial view of autonomy. This view suggests that professional autonomy should include control of the financial aspects associated with providing services in addition to control of the direct-care aspects (McMenamin, 2004). This perspective melds business ownership with the concept of autonomy. We agree with Sandstrom (2007) that no one in health care can be totally autonomous. We also believe that practice ownership plus autonomy in clinical matters is as close as a PT can get to fulfill the spirit of autonomy.

Opportunity to Lead

Leadership is driven by a manager's leadership style, the situation, and the characteristics of the personnel involved. Ownership of a private practice offers the owner the opportunity to develop a leadership style appropriate to their unique mix of personality, circumstances, peers, and staff members. As a leader, the owner must facilitate interrelationships between people, identify opportunities and threats that will impact the practice, and make decisions regarding these situations so the practice continues to grow and prosper (Schneller, 1997; Senske, 2003). The owner-leader is in a position to develop and enhance their leadership skills, their ability to apply business principles, and their clinical skills in a unique way to promote the delivery of quality PT services that are distinguishable from their competitors.

Community Contribution

A successful PT practice owner supports activities that increase the influence of their organization within the local community. Such involvement has also been called civic engagement and social entrepreneurship (Johnson, 2008). The goal for engagement in community activities is to garner a positive community view of the organization (Black and Glinn, 2002; Schneller, 1997). Accordingly, the PT owner has the opportunity to be involved in efforts that address community health problems. This may be accomplished through involvement with service organizations or working with local leaders to provide needed services. Some examples of this type of community involvement are posture and balance screening clinics, providing pro bono care at and following Special Olympics events, participating in volunteer wheelchair ramp building projects or Habitat for Humanity, providing observation opportunities for local students, speaking to local nonprofit and government agencies associated with health care and business groups. These activities enhance the community while promoting PT as a profession in general and the PT practice in particular.

Money-Related Skills

An entrepreneur is in business to make a profit from his or her own efforts. These efforts are diverse so private practice owners have to wear many hats. Often, one of the hats is to serve as the chief financial officer responsible for maintaining profitability and growth. However, most practice owners we know are like us. They have had little formal training in the areas of accounting (Chapter 20) and finance (Chapter 21). One of the most common finance-related tasks for practice owners is *budgeting* income and expenses.

Budgeting

Budgeting is necessary as the outcome of the process is a budget that provides a prediction of income and expenses so financial decisions can be made (Chapter 21). To determine income, an owner will need to find common reimbursement rates for third party payers they expect to deal with and estimate how many treatments they will provide for the budget time span.

Consultation with a certified public accountant can facilitate developing a budget, which will help keep expenses within the estimated revenues for the practice. This budget should include a projected salary for the owner to pay their nonbusiness expenses (Anderson, 2002).

Chapter 21 has already introduced basic budgeting concepts. The following suggestions apply budgeting concepts to a small private practice. A budget should consider

- Labor—plan for expenses including an income for yourself and staff.
- Taxes—estimate taxes, benefits, insurances, and for yourself and staff.
- Operational expenses—estimate other expenses such as rent, phone, utilities, cleaning, supplies, transcription, billing, advertising, and consultant services.
- Income—estimate the charges to be billed and the number of patient visits needed to meet projected expenses.
- Allocation—distribute the resources to meet expenses using the estimated income.
  Control of expenses and income require following the budget plans for operations.

Control in turn requires regularly evaluating performance and incentives compared to actual expenses and income.

It has been suggested that budget projections and actual performance be discussed with staff and owners so that everyone understands the goals and expectations of the practice as well as potential consequences. Following the preceding list and keeping stakeholders informed should keep financial performance within 10% of estimates (Anderson, 2002).

Billing and Cash Flow

PT services, like other medical services, are among the few areas of business where the provider is unable to confidently set the price for their services with expectation that their price is what third party payers will pay. With the exception of an occasional cash customer, the service provider may not know what the actual reimbursement will be until payment is received from a third party payer.

Transactions in health care are seldom clear-cut when it comes to billing and payment. Billing often has little relationship to the payment. Payments vary by health insurance plan. Some plans may limit the number of PT treatments. Different plans require beneficiaries to pay different deductible and co-payment amounts. These payments are income for the practice. Payment rates also vary by the contracts a provider has entered into with managed-care organizations, the government, and other third party payers. Insurance carriers may deny payment for certain current procedural terminology (CPT) codes. To get paid all or some of the amount billed, an appeal may have to be made to the payer by the provider. Thus, at the time treatment is given, and possibly for an extended time, neither the patient nor the service provider knows with certainty what will be paid by one, and at times, more than one third party. The actual amount received for services rendered may be considerably less than the amount billed as the usual and customary fee.

To keep a steady cash flow, frequent billing is necessary. This will likely require appropriate computer software to facilitate electronic billing. A **billing service** can be used or an employee can be hired. A billing service can add a practice expense of 6% or more of the amount collected by the biller. The issue then becomes one of determining if it is as efficient and less costly to hire/train an in-house person to do the billing rather than contracting for the service.

A clear billing strategy has to be implemented including a step-by-step process for the billing cycle. This strategy includes verbally explaining to patients their benefits and their personal financial obligations before treatment begins. The patient should be provided the same information in writing. The customer's signature on a document affirms that their benefits and potential costs have been discussed and are understood (Anderson, 2002). Depictions of the billing process of two different private practices are presented in Figures 22.2 and 22.3. Adhering to the elements in either example is likely to facilitate sufficient cash flow and reduce the frequency of payer challenges.

Regular comparisons between income and budget estimates need to occur. Where there are variations, they need to be addressed by making necessary adjustments for the near future.

If costs increase more than expected, options for controlling increases include:

Downsizing the clinic and office space to reduce rent
Employing staff part-time rather than full time
Laying off staff
Offering incentives to employees for increased productivity and bringing in new clients
Paying staff an hourly rate rather than a salary
Reducing benefits
Relocating to a more moderate rent area
Sharing office space

Financial Stress

A private practice owner has autonomy in his or her business. Owners are relatively free to make clinical decisions based on their professional judgment and business decisions based on current circumstances. Since the business is theirs, the pressure to sustain their financial viability is very personal. The owner and their employees are dependent on the success of the business for their incomes.

It is common for a small private practice owner to take out a home equity loan to pay employees or to meet personal expenses because reimbursement payments have been

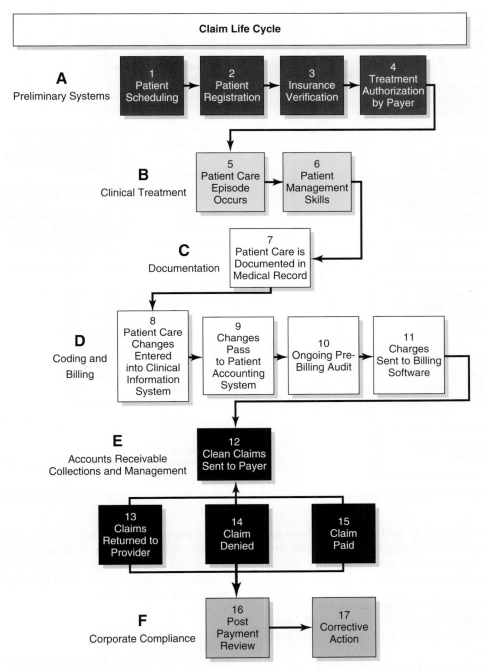

Figure 22.2. Example billing process from marketing through turning account over to a collection agency. Permission to reprint granted by Peter R. Kovacek.

delayed or there have been fewer customers than usual for a time. The pressure to make the right business decision is again personal. Making the right decision may keep the business viable. Making a wrong decision may lead to multiple problems and lead to a loss of business or even lead to closing the business.

Challenges to the Private Practice Model of Physical Therapy

As opportunities for small PT owned practices continue to evolve, so do challenges and threats to this model of providing services.

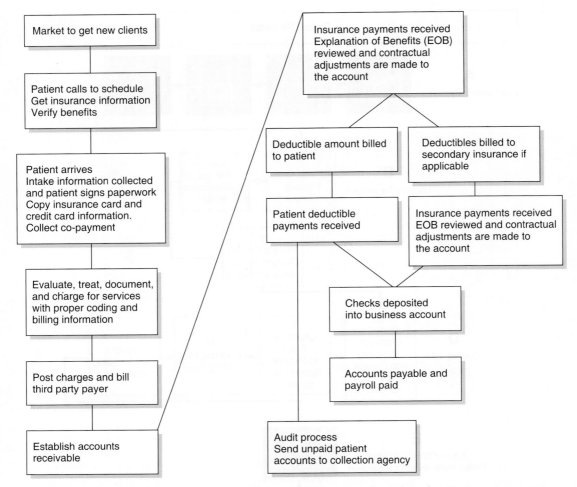

Figure 22.3. Example billing process from making initial appointment through quality improvement measures.

We have chosen to address several personnel and business challenges we perceive as limiters to the growth of private practice physical therapy. These issues are

- Number of **private practitioners**
- Employee characteristics and availability
- Selected aspects of competition and payment
- Balancing work and personal life

When the Majority Is a Minority

A potential threat to the private practice of PT is limited numbers of people contributing their talents to the development of innovative ways to deliver services in an entrepreneurial environment. In a changing health care environment, the more talented people involved in private practice, the more likely challenges will be met successfully. This is necessary for this model of delivering PT to grow alongside traditional hospital and medical clinic environments that employ PTs.

The Numbers

Most PTs are women. Most practice owners are men. Therefore, there is a large pool of talented PTs who could become practice owners. The most comprehensive demographic information on this topic comes from APTA surveys. Since 1978, APTA has monitored the employment status of its members (APTA, 1994). Of particular interest to our discussion is the percentage of APTA members who work in private practices (Tables 22.1 and 22.2), the percentage of members who are *self-employed* on a full-time

Table 22.1   Changes (%) in Selected Employment Settings Reported by APTA Members

Selected Settings	Year				
	1999	2000	2002	2004	2005
Private outpatient office or group practice[a]	27.5[b]	30.4	22.4	31.8	32.9
Health system or hospital outpatient facility	19.6	21.2	21.8	19.1	20.2
Acute care hospital	13.6	13.1	14.2	11.8	12.0
Patient's home/Home care	10.0	8.8	6.1	7.4	6.8
SNF/ECF/ICF	7.2	5.9	5.1	4.8	4.9
School System	5.0	5.2	3.2	4.6	4.1
Subacute rehab hospital	5.1	3.8	4.7	2.6	2.5

[a]Includes physical therapist practice owners, employees of physical therapist–owned practices, and physical therapists employed in physician-owned practices.
[b]Percentiles.
Reprinted from Physical Therapist Member Demographic Profile 1999-2005 p.4, with permission of the American Physical Therapy Association. This material is copyrighted, and any further reproduction of distribution is prohibited.

basis (some individuals in private practice would be in this category), and estimates that parse data on women practice owners.

Data from 1999 to 2005 show the employment arrangements for PTs (Table 22.1). Throughout this time span, the largest percentage of APTA members have reported working in privately owned outpatient settings (APTA, 2007d). However, this figure includes practice owners as well as PTs employed in these settings (Wallace, 2008). Further confounding the effort to identify practice owners is that some individuals worked in more than one setting. For example, owners can take a salary as employees do. Moreover, someone can be an owner who also works for someone else full or part-time. This makes the 32.9% figure less informative than one would prefer. A better estimate of practice ownership can be found in the full time self-employed category in Table 22.2. Since 1999, somewhere between 8% and 14% of APTA members had some level of practice ownership. Three earlier surveys found that women made up nearly one-third of respondents who were self-employed full time (APTA, 1994). Corollary information comes from PPS membership data. In 2004, 35.7% of the PPS members were women (PPS, 2004). This percentage corresponds to other survey findings. However, the PPS has the highest dues of all sections, which may be a disincentive to join. An owner just starting out may defer APTA and PPS members hip because of limited income or poor cash flow (Chapter 21).

Table 22.2   Remuneration and Employment Status Reported by APTA Members

Remuneration	Employment	Year				
		1999	2000	2002	2004	2005
Salaried	Full-time	61.4[a]	65.0	76.2	69.1	59.6
	Part-time	13.1	13.0	9.8	10.9	4.6
Self-Employed	Full-time	11.6	10.8	8.3	13.9	11.9
	Part-time	6.4	5.2	3.6	4.7	2.8
Hourly	Full-time	—	—	—	—	12.0[b]
	Part-time	—	—	—	—	7.2[b]

[a]Percentiles
[b]Initial year data were collected.
Reprinted from Physical Therapist Member Demographic Profile 1999-2005 p. 4, with permission of the American Physical Therapy Association. This material is opyrighted, and any further reproduction or distribution is prohibited.

Another gross estimate of private practice ownership is to divide the number of PT members of the PPS (N = 20, 105) (personal communication, Monica Baroody, 3/14/07) by the estimated number of PTs in the U.S (155,000) (Bureau of Labor Statistics [BLS], 2007). This calculation yields approximately 13%. Since APTA and section memberships are voluntary, and PPS membership is the most costly of all sections, this figure may also underestimate the number of PTs who are small practice owners, particularly those who are self-employed part-time. Another caveat about these figures is that about 30% (47,174 [APTA, 2007e]/155,000 [BLS, 2007]) of U.S. PTs are APTA members.

The near future does not promise much change. A recent report on a large sample of first year entry-level student PTs reported a gender difference in interest in private practice ownership. Survey respondents were mostly females (74%). The pertinent question students responded to was, "do you plan to own a PT practice"? Of 899 respondents, a smaller percentage of women (40.3%) than men (57.7%) agreed with the statement. However, more than one-third of the women and a quarter of the men chose the "do not know" answer option. The author pointed out a need for faculty to expose students, particularly women, to the full spectrum of PT career opportunities (Johnson, 2007).

Some Start-up Challenges

Anyone trying to start a business will experience similar challenges. These include limited liquid assets, difficulty obtaining loans, and miscues because of lack of business experience.

Ownership challenges expressed by women expand this list and add insight about why there are fewer women than men in private practice. Sanders (2006) and Wynn (1997) summarized the business related and personal difficulties several women PTs had in developing their private practices. These were

- Becoming part of local business organizations
- Family commitments
- Limited mentoring opportunities/few role models
- Limited networking opportunities
- Little business knowledge

- Making contacts with referral sources
- Securing financing

The general experience of the women who identified these issues was that it was difficult for women to start a private practice because they may be treated more cautiously by business and banking communities than are men. This translates to lesser acceptance within some business organizations and greater difficulty in obtaining loans.

Differences in value priorities have also been associated with the lower percentage of women in private practice. Rozier et al. (1998) studied the relationship between gender and perceptions of employment success. The group surveyed a random sample of APTA members and obtained responses from more than 1,900 individuals of whom 83% were women. In defining career success, the women respondents placed greater importance on balancing their family and work roles and less importance on working full time than men. Other survey data indicate nearly 40% of APTA women member respondents have experienced career interruptions (APTA, 1993). This poses difficulties for anyone starting, developing, and growing a private practice.

Some Solutions

Steps are being taken to facilitate entering into private practice. As more women enter private practice, more role models become available. This may bolster APTA (2007f) and PPS (2007) mentoring services to aid those seeking to enter private practice. APTA (2007g), PPS (2007), and the Section on Administration (Kovacek et al, 1999) and its successor, the Section on Health Policy and Administration (Sinnott, 2006), have taken active roles in this area by fostering entrepreneurship, private practice, and business-related education, respectively. There is also a need for professional education programs to include more intense and expanded instruction in principles of entrepreneurship and business by developing clinical internships and mentoring experiences in private practice for students, fellows, and residents who have such interests. The combined efforts of professional groups and educational programs can help achieve the essence of Vision 2020

(APTA, 2008a). See Additional Resources section for more suggestions.

Competition—Large Versus Small Private Practice

Large national and regional corporations often offer benefits that a small local practice owner may not be able to afford to purchase or offer their employees (Small Business Administration, 2007b). Benefits can include easy access to financial resources and a variety of support services such as legal staff, training and development personnel, marketing, and technical expertise in many areas from computer networking to acquisition specialists. Acquisition specialists are individuals who identify other businesses worth purchasing. Large corporations can also offer employees competitive salaries, continuing education resources, low cost health insurance (U.S. Physical Therapy [USPT], 2007a), concierge or personal legal services, mortgage assistance, and other unique benefits.

There are national organizations that assist PTs to get into private practice. These organizations offer financing, leasing assistance, business systems, consultation, and other services to PTs, who join the organization as partners or associates (USPT, 2007b). Arrangements vary, but for a minority share of the profit, a partner can be in business and have health care and other benefits with little up-front investment. Clearly, legal advice is needed to go over the agreement conditions before taking such a step.

A goal of national publicly traded corporations is to increase the value of their stock for shareholders. Strategies to accomplish this include striving for market dominance and high profit levels. Strategies can include buying independently owned practices.

Referral-for-Profit: Practices Not Owned by PTs

The number of small, independently owned physical therapy practices fluctuates. Reasons for this include retirements, closures, consolidations, acquisitions by large national and regional corporations (Percy, 2006), and the expansion of the number of medical doctor (physician) associated practices (Chapter 9). There are also chiropractor-owned physical

therapy services (Coshocton Tribune, 2008; Kane County Chronicle, 2008). Because by statute various practitioners can refer patients to PTs, and various referrers have an ownership interest in physical therapy businesses, the more inclusive term referral-for-profit is more appropriate than POPTS (PT Bulletin on Line, 2008). However, morel physicians have employed physical therapists than others with referral rights so the literature has focused on medical physicians.

Several health care professions have been successful in restricting ownership of their practices to licensed members of the same profession (APTA, 2005). Some example professions are: medicine (Medical Board of California, 2008), veterinary medicine, dentistry (State of New York, 2008), and chiropractic (Office of the Professions, 2008). These groups have prospered with licensure and business ownership restricted to like licensed professionals. There have been exhortations for this to become the norm for PTs also. From a PT owner's perspective, "Ownership means control and is a key to independence. Without dominant ownership in our practices, we will fail to have full professional autonomy and will be at the mercy of non-PT owners" (Gauvin and McMenamin, 2002, p. 42). The APTAs (2007h) position is similar, it opposes physician ownership of physical therapy services and advocates for "exclusive PT ownership and operation of physical therapy services" (APTA, 2005, 2007i). However, there are financial incentives for referrers to make this goal tough to realize.

Referral-for-Profit Practices

Currently, individual physicians, physician groups, and hospital systems are striving to retain or increase their market share of patients. Many groups are entering new markets to increase the numbers of patients they serve (Gabel et al., 2008). A physician or medical group has at least three strong incentives to offer physical therapy services in which they have an ownership interest. First, it is convenient for the patient and the referring physician. Second, physicians can have control over all aspects of patients' pre- and post-surgery care (Maryland Orthopaedic Association, 2008; Wichita Eagle, 2008). And third, referrals to physical therapy can be a means of increasing revenue. Who knows the true reason or reasons? The opportunity to limit patient choice, to overuse services, and to diminish therapist technical autonomy are inherent in such situations.

Some examples of referral-for-profit practices that we have recognized are worth discussing because they are not necessarily obvious to most people. Many physicians are associates in large medical groups or are employees of a hospital system. When physical therapy is a service offered by the group or hospital, the associated or employed physicians may be strongly encouraged to refer their patients to their organization's physical therapy service. This is a subtle form of referral-for-profit. Other ways this occurs include

- Non-PTs employing PTs and/or PTAs
- Making referrals in exchange for some form of gain
- Owning or having a financial interest in physical therapy clinics
- Utilizing unlicensed or staff trained on the job to provide care in the physician's office

Referral-for-profit creates a potential conflict of interest pitting physician financial benefit against what is in the best interest of stakeholders (Mason, 2009). History has shown that significant percentages of physician owned health service businesses including physical therapy and rehabilitation businesses are more costly for payers than nonphysician owned businesses of the same type (Mitchell and Scott, 1992; Swedlow et al., 1992; Thornton, 1999). A Department of Health and Human Services (2006) report pointed out that between 2002 and 2004 there was a doubling of the number of physicians submitting claims for physical therapy services exceeding $1,000,000. The report also noted that longstanding concerns about service quality and Medicare regulatory compliance remain problems.

APTA (2007h,i; Mason, 2009) has long been in opposition to arrangements where professional autonomy may be limited and *overutilization* of services may be encouraged. These are ethical and core value issues (Matoushek, 2005) as well as financial issues. Referral-for-profit situations can limit the consumers' right to choose their PT and overutilization increases co-payment costs to the consumer

and costs to third party payers. Overutilization could occur if a physician orders, and a PT administers, unnecessary but reimbursable PT. For patients in federally subsidized programs such as Medicare and Medicaid, the federal government has passed protective legislation (*Stark I, II, III*) (Chapter 9) to limit physicians profiting from services provided to Medicare beneficiaries at locations where the physician has some means of profiting. The negative impact of such referral-for-profit arrangements on private practice PTs is the loss of access to the market share controlled by referrers. While *direct access* to PTs is nearly universal, third party payers require physician referrals to assure the medical necessity of physical therapy. Therefore, the adage here is "he or she who controls the referral wins." In these situations, direct access or not, the winner is not the local PT private practitioner. Referral-for-profit is one issue that private practice PTs need to be politically aware of, and active in and supportive of advocacy efforts (Chapter 1) to remedy unfair business practices like the plan of care authorization by a physician to get paid for treating Medicare beneficiaries.

A Critical Assessment of Small Private Practice Finances

When any business is bringing in only a little more money than it takes to keep the business operating, the owners or board has to confront the need to change how the business operates as well as the possibility of closing the business. A commercial website reported that more than three-quarters of their 3,000 webinar private practice participants (predominantly PTs) said they were at or near this breaking-even point (Survivalstrategies, 2008; personal communication, Harry Schmiedeke, 2/06/08). We are aware of owners who have not drawn a salary for months. Two easily identifiable contributors to this financially undesirable position are staff therapist salaries increasing more than 27% between 1999 and 2005 (APTA, 2007d) and concurrent outpatient payments decreasing up to 8% (Wallace, 2008). The reality is there is a need for more economical models of private practice service delivery and employee payment methods for small practices to remain financially viable.

Balancing Life Demands

Any new business owner is under stress for a variety of reasons. The pursuit of professional goals may lead to the exclusion of wider interests and other responsibilities to health, family, community, and professional associations. The number of hours full time self-employed PTs work in a week is typically greater than the average number of hours worked by salaried PTs (APTA, 1994). Eighteen-hour days are common in the life of a private practice owner, particularly an owner starting out (Wynn, 1997). As pointed out in Chapter 2, personal values need to be understood because they are expressed in professional life. Values guide the many decisions that confront health care practitioners whether owner or employee. With the additional responsibility of managing a practice that one depends on for their livelihood, consideration of morality, professional ethics, and personal values is all the more important (Chapter 7). It is important to balance pursuit of all life goals and to do so in ways that reflect respect for ethical principles.

With the background of the opportunities and challenges associated with private practice ownership having been dealt with we address the practical information on how to start your own practice.

Getting Your Practice Started

Two attributes are necessary to start a private practice. The first is self-determination manifested as a strong desire to be in control of your future, i.e., an entrepreneurial spirit. The second is a clear vision of this future. Many direct and indirect learning experiences may stimulate these attributes.

Direct Experience

An invaluable source of stimulation is direct experience. Working in a private PT practice gives a first hand picture of all aspects of the business and clinical aspects of self-employment. Being mentored by someone in this environment provides an additional opportunity from which to grow.

Other Experiences

Many additional experiences may stimulate a desire for self-direction and help formulate a personal vision of the future. Some of these learning experiences are

- Discussing private practice with owners of private practices and consultants
- Reading professional journals and books from many fields, materials of the APTA and the PPS
- Consulting community business organizations such as the Chamber of Commerce and the Better Business Bureau
- Attending meetings of national associations including the APTA, PPS and other local, state, and national organizations
- Seeking advice from governmental sources like the Small Business Administration (http://www.sba.gov) and Service Corps of Retired Executives (http://www.score.org)
- Acquiring further education through continuing education courses or for credit courses offered by educational institutions
- Exploring Internet business resources

In general, the above experiences provide a foundation to assess personal strengths and weaknesses, set reasonable expectations, identify when and what assistance is needed, and help develop an organized planning process for decisions and actions (Chapters 5, 6, and 13).

Planning Is a Must

Planning is an important aspect in many life roles. We do planning for vacations and social events, meeting personal financial goals, purchasing or building a home, changing jobs, running a marathon, or moving. To reduce the risk of complications in business *start-up* and operation stages, and eventually disposing of the business, an aspiring PT entrepreneur needs to plan.

In today's rapidly changing health care environment, all health care providers are faced with high levels of uncertainty and strong competition for market share (Chapters 1 and 6). Under such conditions, informal planning is insufficient to lead to business success. Formal planning fosters strategic thinking (Chapters 3–6) while synthesizing intuition and creativity into the future vision of the business

(Bangs, 1995). A good plan enhances the odds for success. A plan serves as a sign of visionary management. While the development of a business plan is advisable (Berry, 2008), not every business has a written business plan (Spors, 2008). For example, a survey of sports medicine centers, for which 44% PT had some form of ownership, found just two-thirds had written business plans (Olsen, 1996).

Historical records make it clear that planning is a necessity for a business to survive (Ellis and Pekar, 1980). Yet, as thorough as a planning process may be, it is often difficult to control the environment and actions of others. As noted in Chapters 3–6 and 18, markets and competitors are constantly changing. For this reason, plans need to be dynamic with flexible estimates of what is to be done initially. Continual research and innovation are required to accommodate the demands of a changing business environment. Realizing that the most diligently constructed plans are imperfect (McDaniel, 1997) encourages the adaptation of a continuous planning process (Chapter 13). Doing so rewards planners with minimal surprises in market conditions and competitors' strategies.

Know Yourself: Self-Assessment

A person's education, personal traits, and experience interact to give them an individualized perspective or frame of reference when encountering life's personal and professional tasks. Self-assessment is useful to anyone considering starting any major project. The key purpose of self-assessment is to gain insight into personal strengths and weaknesses relative to the project under consideration. Self-assessment will help the entrepreneur identify personal assets and deficits that can impact on goal achievement.

Self-understanding can be gained by completion of selected self-assessment instruments. One self-assessment method is a checklist. Table 22.3 contains an example checklist of questions that potential entrepreneurs should ask themselves early in their exploration period.

The information gained from this checklist includes identification of essential strengths, weaknesses, tendencies, preferences, and values. The overall picture allows exploration of feelings of comfort and discomfort when moving forward to start a business. Weaknesses should be of particular interest. Are there personality characteristics that may interfere with the ability to make certain decisions like firing an employee? By learning of these potential limitations, consideration can be given to alternative solutions. Four options to consider to augment your personality, strengths, and experience:

1. Pursuing further relevant education
2. Hiring an employee with personal characteristics or skills that supplement your own
3. Acquiring a compatible partner with supplemental skills and experience
4. Hiring a consultant

Values and Philosophy

Each individual should understand and be comfortable with their personal and professional philosophy and values. This is saying that personal and professional values and philosophy should be indistinguishable. The private practice owner is challenged daily by ethical situations. As suggested in Chapter 7, harmony between values and behaviors facilitates psychological comfort.

Goals

A useful conceptualization of goals is a necessity as goals are the destinations and objectives are the tactical action plans that serve as the roadmaps to get to the destination (Chapters 2, 3, 5, 6, and 13). Goals are needed for direction and balance between life roles. This however, fewer than 3% of Americans have reported having written long-range goals (Smith, 1994).

An acronym for a process for developing and assessing goals is SMARTER (Dolgoff, 2005). This suggests that goals should be

1. *Specific* so they can be understood
2. *Measurable* to be able to tell if desired progress is being made
3. *Acceptable* to those who have to take action to bring about the desired end
4. *Realistic* enough to try to achieve
5. *Time* bound so a completion date can be approximated

Table 22.3   Example of Prospective Entrepreneur Self-Assessment Checklist

Questions	Yes	No	Notes to Yourself
BEFORE YOU START:			
• Have you thought about why you want to own your own business?			
• Do you think you are the kind of person who can get a business started and make it go?			
• Do you want to start a business enough to keep you working long hours with little assurance of how much you will end up with?			
• Have you worked in a business like this before?			
• Have you worked for someone as a manager?			
• Do you have any business training?			
• Do you know how much money you will need to start the business?			
• Do you know how much money you have to invest initially and where you will obtain more if you need it?			
• What net income do you expect annually from the business?			
• Do other businesses like the one you have in mind do well in your community?			
• Is another business like yours needed in the area you intend to locate in?			
PERSONAL TRAITS			
• Are you a self-starter?			
• Do you enjoy interacting with others?			
• Can you lead others?			
• Can you take responsibility?			
• Are you a good organizer?			
• Are you a hard worker?			
• Can you make decisions under pressure?			
• Do people find you trustworthy?			
• Can you stick with a project when things get difficult?			
• Does your health allow you to work long hours?			
DIFFICULTIES			
• Have you had any difficulties in areas that you believe can negatively impact on your starting a business?			
• Have you had any difficulties in areas that you believe can negatively impact on the operation of your business once it opens?			
• Have you thought about how you will deal with anticipated difficulties?			
• Have you thought about other possible difficulties?			
• Do you have a support system for dealing with business or personal difficulties?			

6. Evaluated at intervals for gauging progress toward desired end
7. Reviewed at the end with a focus on improving future goal setting processes

Goals and action plans need to be periodically reviewed and updated. Setting goals in all facets of life will help achieve a balance in use of energy and time. Waitley (1987) and Smith (1994) identify six groups of major life goals to plan for

1. Personal well-being goals: these include physical and mental health, which is a reasonable prerequisite to achieving other goals
2. Affiliation goals: families, partners, personal friends
3. Work group goals: professional associations, networks, community groups, and work related friends
4. Community goals: contributions, relationships with fellow community members
5. Environmental goals: preservation of natural resources, green areas, and recreational areas
6. Spiritual goals: setting goals with an awareness of a higher power than oneself

The preceding discussion on goals has presented a frame of reference for dealing with the next important topic, the *business plan*.

Strategic Plan Compared to Business Plan

In the context of larger health care businesses, a strategic plan was described as a business's roadmap for success in qualitative terms (Chapters 3 and 21). It addresses in broad terms why the business should focus its attention on specific markets, products, services, technologies, processes, or other opportunities. Strategic plans are the responsibility of upper management who use input from others within the organization. In contrast, a business plan builds on the strategic plan. A business plan is more specific and contains highly detailed information about a specific element of the operational plan (Harris, 2008).

When starting out, a small business owner is likely to have a business plan that they use as their strategic plan. Key elements of a business plan include

- Market plan
- Operations plan (including management, staffing)
- Financial plan

The basic elements of these plans are summarized here as they were covered in depth earlier (Chapters 2, 3, 14, 18, 19, and 21). A market plan starts with a clear definition of the opportunity under consideration. The market plan includes analysis of such things as market size, market characteristics, growth trends and projections, customer preferences, service locations, partnering opportunities, the competitive environment, and so on. It will also include strategies to product/service positioning within the market, and communication and promotional strategies (Chapter 18).

An operations plan addresses issues related to management/governance, business structure, relationship of new services/products to other components of the business, human resource/staffing requirements, business capacity, technology requirements, infrastructure requirements, building and equipment requirements, the proposed implementation strategy, and post implementation methodology for tracking performance and measuring success (Chapters 11, 13, 14, 16, 17, 19, and 21).

A financial plan includes a detailed analysis of capital expenses, operating budgets inclusive of revenues, expenses, profit/loss projections, and return on investment (Chapters 20 and 21). The financial plan should also address the opportunity cost of the project under consideration. Opportunity costs are those opportunities that must be bypassed in order to pursue one strategy rather than another (Nosse et al., 1999). For example, a business may not have the resources or capacity to pursue two attractive expansion opportunities. One opportunity must be chosen. The other opportunity must be delayed or not pursued at all.

The length of the preceding discussion underscores the importance of doing thorough background work as the initial exploratory step in the process of going into business for yourself. Once there is self-understanding, knowledge of the local business environment, a realistic assessment of opportunities and challenges, and a commitment to the goal of ownership, then, a sound business plan is likely to evolve.

A Business Plan Format

Planning for a trip is a useful analogy for describing a business plan. The trip plan should include the destination, method of travel, lodging, cost, and source of the funds for the trip. One is likely to be disappointed if they showed up at the airport without identification, a reservation, or at the destination, without having made arrangements for accommodations. Unfortunately, many individuals spend more time researching a trip than researching the environment for a business venture. Information relating to a trip is often found in the itinerary. A business plan should accomplish the same goal as a trip plan. The business planning process creates a game plan for a specific purpose, to enhance the likelihood that the business will progress as anticipated.

A business plan is a method for potential lenders and investors to assess the owner's background, and business preparedness as well as to analyze the owner's business strategy. Business plans also serve as a reality check and a means to hone ideas (Zacharakis, 2004).

Business plans need to be constructed by the originator of the idea because the planning process can be a form of self-education in all aspects of the business. A plan assists in realistically and objectively putting pieces of the business puzzle together.

Business Planning Process

A process is a set of coordinated actions that when carried out are likely to produce the desired outcome. The process presented entails thinking about the future, seeking advice, doing homework, and crafting a plan that will lead to the desired future. It starts with a dream.

Dream Your Vision of the Future

Be excited and enthusiastic about the idea of planning for your future as a PT in private practice. Envision your future practice as if it was already operational and successful. Your vision should include the environment, types of patients, staff, referral sources, marketing, image, owner's roles, and how the practice will impact your life on a professional and personal level.

Talk and Listen, but More of the Latter

As part of the planning process, discuss the plans and financial needs with bankers, investors, advisors, partners, other PTs, physicians, family, and friends. Explain the scope of practice for PTs based on the state practice act, education, and experience you bring to the project. Once the plan is written, those who have an interest in the business may review it. Writing the plan and presenting it to numerous individuals for feedback will help refine your thinking and enhance the viability of the final product. Their insights, questions, and advice will assist in forming your practice model. Future support in the project by these individuals may also be assessed. For example, if your spouse is planning on a remodeling project in the near future, and you intend to use the funds to finance the practice, this creates a potential problem that needs to be recognized and addressed early in the planning process.

Do Your Homework

Research the current and potential market for the type of physical therapy services you intend to provide. Chapter 18 contains a contemporary overview of marketing principles applicable to health care businesses. A review of the sections on market orientation, pricing, market segmentation, and niche markets, will provide information on how and what to research for the envisioned future physical therapy business.

Write and Rewrite

Transform informal ideas and notes into a logical, organized document. Steps that can be taken to move from ideas to coherent written statements are

1. Write down whatever information you have at the moment. A partial written plan is an advancement.
2. Use plain English in writing. Avoid technical terms that may confuse readers who are not health care professionals. Use references when possible and cite these in the plan.

3. Tackle the fun parts first. Write your values and mission statements (Chapters 2–7). Perhaps your vision is clearest regarding where your practice will be. Pick a location and draw a plan for your office.
4. When the writing is not progressing, use software, a good book, or consultants to help translate your ideas into words others will understand and interpret as you do. A business owner must do the work of planning. Software programs such as those by Microsoft (2008) for small businesses are available and may assist in compiling the information you gather. Libraries, bookstores, or the Internet all provide resource materials to serve as a guide for your project. See Additional Resources section for more sources.
5. Be your own devil's advocate—Ask questions that need to be answered before seeking support. Try to include answers to questions that others will ask when reading the plan. Including information that answers questions raised by reviewers is a way to know if this plan will work. For example, what are the costs to establish and operate this practice? And, where will resources for the project come from?
6. Form a marketing plan (Chapters 2, 3, and 18) for the initial start-up period of the practice through the first year of operation. Estimate the cost of marketing efforts for the first year.
7. Project start-up expenses. These include consultants, renovation costs, equipment, supplies, marketing, and salaries.
8. Project cash flow for 3 years on a monthly basis (Chapter 21). Remember to include a salary for the owner(s) and employees while considering the lag in time between providing service, billing, and collections. Remember, that there will be ongoing personal living expenses to meet in addition to the expenses of the business.
9. Do a break-even analysis (Chapter 21) to determine on average, how many customers or how many treatments are needed to cover costs. Cut to the chase. Determine fees based on your research on reimbursement rates, estimate the numbers of patient visits, and collections to show the potential for the business to succeed.

When the resources are available, implement and follow the plan, continue to refine the plan as new information becomes available, regularly evaluate your plan by matching the estimates in your plan with your accomplishments (Stern, 1995).

A Seven-Part Business Plan Package

The discussion of the business plan relates to both the formation of a new business as well as an enhancement to an existing business. The example business plan format to be discussed in depth has seven major headings. A tabbed and numbered binder helps everyone follow and participate in the discussion of the plan. The major headings of the business plan are

    I. Transmittal letter
   II. Cover page
  III. Executive summary
  IV. Table of contents
   V. Business description
  VI. Financial information
 VII. Supporting documents

Table 22.4 is an expanded outline of the seven parts of a business plan. The outline and related discussion integrates the thoughts of several writers (Bangs, 1995; Kastantin, 1994; Nosse et al., 1999; Singer, 1995; SBA, 2008), and the practical experiences of the authors. The outline and accompanying discussion guide the reader through the process of developing a concise and substantive business plan.

Part I: The Transmittal Letter

A transmittal letter is a cover letter written on your business stationery that formally and concisely tells the reader what your goal is, i.e., explaining to a financial organization loan officer that you want a loan. While it is not part of the business plan per se, it introduces your plan to a busy loan officer or possibly a non-PT investor. The letter explains why the plan is being sent and what the recipient is expected to do with the plan. The transmittal letter usually includes the content listed in Table 22.4.

Table 22.4   Example Outline for a Business Plan Package

I. Transmittal Letter
   A. Purpose of the business
   B. Identity of the person requesting funds
   C. Amount and type of financing requested
   D. Amount of equity the owners will apply to the business
   E. Use of the funds
   F. When the funds will be needed
   G. Goals and market potential that can be achieved with the new funds
   H. Collateral available to secure financing

II. Cover Page
   A. Name of company
   B. Address
   C. Phone, fax, email
   D. Principal(s) (the major person or people with a financial interest in the business)
   E. Logo
   F. Submitted to (use only if plan is for financing)

III. Executive Summary
   A. Describe the business, location, legal status
   B. Mission
   C. Stage of development
   D. Services offered
   E. Target market(s)
   F. Marketing strategy
   G. Competitor(s)
   H. Operational location(s)
   I. Management and organization
   J. Financial information
   K. Long-term goals
   L. Funds sought, uses, and estimated return on investment

IV. Table of Contents
V. Business Description
   A. Mission (state what you do best, to whom, where)
   B. Industry analysis (describe industry, current trends and opportunities, economic cycles, supply and demand data)
   C. Market analysis and target market(s) (demographics, describe all customers)
   D. Competitor analysis (who and where, market distribution, position of competitors, barriers to entry and opportunities for growth)
   E. Marketing plan and strategy (how will services be made known? What is unique to the proposed business?)
   F. Synopsis of operations and location(s) (how will the business be run? capacity, productivity, quality control, map, photos, construction plans for location(s))
   G. Organizational structure (lines of authority, board, advisors, principles, management experience, consultants, key employees, management style)
   H. Long-term goals and exit plan (vision, what will happen to the business in the future?)

VI. Financial Information
   A. Personal capital being applied (personal financial information—how much you have, how much money is needed, when, for what purposes?)
   B. Equipment list (priorities, vendors and costs)
   C. Break-even analysis
   D. Balance sheets (personal and business if it already exists)
   E. Pro-forma cash-flow analysis (estimate of first year month by month and annually for years 1–3)
   F. For existing business, current audited tax returns, and other significant financial data

(Continued)

Table 22.4   continued

VII. Supporting Documents
    A. Resume(s) of principle(s), managers, key personnel
    B. Letters of intent
    C. Letters of recommendation
    D. Current contract(s)
    E. Job description(s)
    F. Special awards, achievements, relevant recognition
    G. Portfolio (newspaper clippings, magazine and journal articles, on principles or type of business)
    H. Equipment photos
    I. Appendices (optional)

Part II: The Cover Page

The cover page on your business stationary should be neat, short, and clear. The cover page includes the items noted under heading II of Table 22.4. If the plan is submitted to different entities, there should be an individualized cover page for each.

Part III: Executive Summary

After the cover page comes the executive summary. This summary provides an overview of the total business plan. After reading the executive summary, the reader should be sufficiently informed to ask in-depth clarifying questions. The executive summary

- Identifies the purpose of the business
- Describes the business and its uniqueness
- States the legal business structure
- States goals
- Establishes a timeline for plan implementation
- Identifies the target market(s) and major competitor(s)
- Provides a marketing strategy
- Notes key manager(s) and their skills, experience, and education
- Describes financial needs and how funds will be used
- Describes the financing payback timeline supported by earnings projections

Part IV: Table of Contents

The table of contents lists the major areas of the plan with the page number(s) where the information is in the plan. It is organized in standard outline format including various heading levels.

Part V: The Business Description

This very important part of the business plan has the purpose of clearly describing the business in detail. Because of the need for details, this section has eight main components. These components are the description (mission), industry analysis, market analysis, competition analysis, marketing plan, operations and location synopsis, structure, goals, and exit (termination) plan. Each component is summarized below. Pertinent questions are asked to highlight the kind of information that needs to be provided in each part of the business section of plan.

- Philosophy and mission—state the philosophy and mission of the practice. Describe what objectives will be accomplished through the business.
- Business description—define the situation of the practice. Is it a start-up practice, an acquisition, or an expansion?
- Ownership—identify the owners. If there are multiple owners, explain how much of the business each will own, what each person will invest, and how and when they will be paid. Identify the role of the various owners. Determine valuation of stock and buyout terms. Include employment agreements with pay and benefits. Include methods of handling buyouts due to illness, incompetence, or other reasons.
- Legal structure—describe the legal form of business structure, for example, incorporated and type, sole proprietorship, or partnership and type.
- Payment sources—identify provider payment agreements that will be pursued or exist (e.g., Medicare, Medicaid, and private

insurance plans). Explain if the practice will be arranging to contract with hospitals, nursing homes, home health agencies, medical clinics, or physician offices. Describe any types of contractual arrangements that are in existence or anticipated. Identify any cash-based programs the practice plans to offer.

- Services, programs, and benefits—explain the benefits of services provided by the practice and why people will buy the services. List services or products the practice will offer with an explanation of how these services are unique.
- PT industry—describe the industry of physical therapy and where it fits in the medical services industry, current trends, and strategic opportunities that are present within the industry. PT is primarily a service industry and has enjoyed remarkable growth. Is the future growth pattern of PT conducive to supporting new practices? Describe the educational level including the Doctor of Physical Therapy (DPT) and how this may impact the future of the profession. Does regulation and certification impact the industry? Medicare (i.e., $1810 2008 private practice cap per beneficiary), and private insurance limitations need to be addressed. Typical referral sources for similar businesses should be identified. Include industry standards or benchmarks, for example, Phoenix Strategic Surveys (2003) for billings, markups, salaries, profit margins, and other information that may be used for comparison. Identify common barriers for entry into the industry. Do you have to be a licensed PT to own a physical therapy practice? If not, what impact does this have on the industry? Do you want partners or investors who are not PTs?
- Customers—market analysis focuses on customers. Who are the customers? Remember the broad concept of customers includes referral sources, patients, patients' family and friends, healthy individuals, employers, insurance companies, managed-care organizations, local industry, health maintenance organizations, as well as sales and contracting groups. An explanation of how your state's licensure act allows you to access patients is helpful to nonmedical readers.

Identify physicians by medical specialties and other licensed referrers that are expected to refer patients to the clinic. Describe the size of the market population and your expected market share. Demographic data of the target population(s) is useful. Identify the population base, ages, income levels, large employers, transportation options, housing values, and employment rates (Chapters 3 and 4). Often, demographic information is available through local libraries, Internet sources, and Chambers of Commerce. For example, a market description might say the practice will target individuals ages 14–65 years who have health insurance coverage for physical therapy services, and live within a 5-mile radius of the proposed office site. See Chapter 18 for more specific information on market analysis and targeting segments of the market.

- Competition—list all of the competitors in the local market. Identify competitors' locations on a map and the distance from the proposed clinic location. What similar services do they offer? Identify the relevant competing local PT practices. These may include national and regional corporate chain practices, hospitals, satellite clinics, chiropractors, massage therapists, occupational therapists, other private physical therapy practices, and physician owned clinics that offer PT services. Learn from meetings with competitors, their websites and their literature, and your own networks. Examine competitors' strengths and weaknesses (Chapters 3–6) to support your claims of uniqueness and need for the type of proposed services compared to the competitors.
- Operations—the operations and location segment of the business plan describes how the business will be operated and what is essential to succeed. This section also includes the description of the proposed clinic's location and physical layout. Several important questions need to be considered. Among the key questions are

What leadership style will management use?
How will policies and procedures be developed and implemented?

Will you be a Medicare provider as a certified rehabilitation agency, or a PT in independent practice?

Will your policies and procedures meet Medicare and other payer guidelines?

Will you need a site survey by Medicare prior to being able to bill Medicare for your services? How much time will be allocated for managerial responsibilities in addition to patient care responsibilities?

There are also operational questions that need to be considered relating to the business' capacity to generate revenue. These important questions include

What type of billing and collections system will be used?

What type of computer and software and related peripherals are needed?

What kind of training will be done and by whom?

Who will handle billing, collections, and do follow-up work?

What will the productivity standards be for patient care employees?

What are the benchmarks for the industry?

Will you use care extenders in the practice such as PTAs, certified athletic trainers, and aides?

Are there statutory limitations and insurance carrier limitations in use of care extenders (Chapter 8)?

In the plan, relate this information to the expected numbers of patients to be treated or units of service to be delivered and expected revenues.

- Quality assurance needs to be discussed (Chapter 16). Questions to answer that relate to defining and measuring the quality of the services to be delivered include:

What internal and external quality assurance measures will be used?

How often will assessments be carried out and by whom?

How will the information be used?

What kind of follow up will be done to improve quality?

For external assessments, who will be contacted to assess quality and at what cost?

Do third party payers in your area already have an outcomes measure in place?

Do local networks have outcomes tools in place for members?

- Is Pay-for-Performance a factor with the current third party payers in your area? If so, what is their method of determining "quality" performance and what are the ramifications to your practice (Chapter 16)?

- The location and **physical plant** synopsis identifies why the location was chosen and provides comparative information regarding competitors' locations. Physical plant refers to the building and grounds. The content of this section includes:

Description of the neighborhood, building, and the office

Pictures of the building and office plans

Location of major pieces of equipment

A comparison of the desired facilities to those of local competitors

- Management structure is very important. It is likely to receive scrutiny due to the belief that many small business failures are attributable to management weaknesses (Bangs, 1995).

Content in this section should provide the reader with:

Your organization's structure including how decisions will be made

How company policies will be established and implemented

Your organizational chart

If there is a board of directors, who will be on the board and what will be the role of the board

Indicating if there will be a separate advisory board

Description of the management style that will be employed within the practice. As evidence of a positive track record in managing a business the organizational structure discussion should include a short personal history of all principles (the owner's). These histories should include:

Related management experience including duties and responsibilities with emphasis on those related to the proposed business

Education

Skills

Salaries and benefits

Resources the principal will make available to the business as equity investments or loans.

If loans are involved, what are the payback terms?

Additional management related resources that will be utilized should also be noted. Include names and credentials of these persons or organizations. Examples of such resources are advisors, financial and legal consultants, community associations, organizations, and educational programs.

- Future—the final element of Section V deals with the future of the business. Included in the discussion are the long-term aspirations of the owner(s) and what will happen if the owner(s) go(es) out of business or one owner wishes to exit the business. Long-term goals may include:

Expansion of space

Adding partners, locations, specialty programs

Changing role of the owner, including retirement or sale of the practice

The vision (Chapters 2, 3, and 7) may express where the owner would like to see the practice in 5 or 10 years.

The inclusion of considerations for terminating a business that may not yet exist is not out of context (Quatre, 2007). Thinking about the disposition of a business is similar to what PTs do in clinical practice. They think about, and begin planning for, the patient's discharge early in the course of treatment. In business planning there are several reasons to consider the termination of the business. An owner may retire or die. In a partnership or corporation a partner or shareholder may wish to leave the business or there may be a disagreement among the owners that would lead to a buyout or termination. The business may also be sold. Sale options include outright sale to another practitioner or corporation, selling to employees or partners, merging with another practice while maintaining ownership, or **liquidating** (selling the equipment, fixtures, and furniture).

An important consideration in the termination of a business is its value. The value of a practice is partially based on referral sources and the ongoing relationship with these sources and contracts with insurance companies, home health agencies, or other entities. Consultants should be used to evaluate and set a practices' market value (Quatre, 2007; Rhoades, 2003). This is a necessary procedure for determining a price in a buy–sell agreement between partners and for establishing corporate stock value. Identifying who will fix the market value should the practice ownership change is a foresightful inclusion in a business plan.

Part VI: Financial Information

If a business plan is being used for raising capital, there will be a financial information section that presents personal and business related income and expenses. The basic purpose of providing such information is to describe how money, if loaned, will be applied and its effect on starting or expanding the business. An explanation of the use of funds includes how much will be spent on various start-up expenses as well as initial operating costs. If money is loaned, it is important to explain the effect these borrowed funds will have on making the practice successful.

- Owner's personal financial information—a personal financial report includes a personal balance statement (Chapter 21). This statement shows how much capital owners will invest and how the capital will be used. Capital can come from many sources. In addition to personal resources, Stern (1995) suggests the following potential sources of funds for small businesses:

Arrange to delay payment to others for 60–90 days

Basic bank loan

Borrow from friends and relatives

Credit cards

Home equity loan

Invite partners or shareholders

Lease equipment to others

Prepaid consulting fees (contracts)

Public stock offering

Retirement funds

Sell uncollected accounts receivable (a business in existence)

Small Business Administration guaranteed bank loan

Small Business Administration micro loan

Venture capitalist

- Business financial information—if the practice is already in operation, a current balance sheet for the practice will be needed. For a new business, an estimated revenue projection has to be developed. This is called a **pro-forma** cash-flow analysis. Pro-forma means before formation. The purpose of this analysis is to present the anticipated long-term financial picture of the practice. This involves estimating anticipated revenues and expenses (Chapter 21). Accompanying this analysis should be a short narrative description providing supplementary information about the projected income statement.

Another required analysis is a break-even analysis (Chapter 21). The break-even point refers to the volume point where total revenue equal total cost. This analysis allows identifying when the business is expected to generate enough revenue to cover expenses. Such an analysis can help identify the sum needed to cover expenses until the break-even point is reached.

Part VII: Supporting Documents

This final section of a business plan includes anything that will make the plan more likely to be supported. Items in this section that may be considered include:

- Complete resumes of management personnel
- Drawings of the proposed facility
- Key contracts
- Letters of intent
- Letters of reference
- Marketing materials
- Market research data
- Newspaper or trade publication articles relevant to this type of business
- Photos of equipment
- Other materials the planner believes will support the purpose of the plan

Additional Considerations Related to Becoming a Private Practice Owner

Planning a private physical therapy practice requires some insight into the options that are available to provide such services. Figure 22.1 introduced the options in general, but more needs to be said.

Among the options to consider are providing services on a contractual basis, serving Medicare eligible patients, forming an agency, participating in a **joint venture**, and membership in a network of PTs. The following discussion focuses on these options in the context of small PT practices.

Contracting to Provide Services

Contracting may involve arranging with hospitals, skilled nursing facilities, outpatient clinics, or other types of facilities to provide PT as an independent contractor. To do this successfully, an individual PT or a practice owner, must be able to accomplish two things. First, meet the setting's staffing and service needs. And second, do so at a reimbursement level that covers the cost of personnel, contract administration, other overhead expenses plus a reasonable margin of profit.

Contracting allows a PT to enter private practice with a minimal investment. Arranging a contract with an organization that allows flexibility in scheduling allows an employed PT to work as a contractor on a part-time basis. Contracts may be developed for time periods ranging from a few hours a day or for several years. Payment rates for contracted services are usually higher than a typical salary and often taxes are not withheld. However, a common risk a contractor takes is that enough work may not always be available and there may be considerable travel time involved that limits income.

A PT contractor has different legal and tax obligations than a salaried PT. These obligations underscore the need to use qualified legal and accounting consultants. The worker classification impacts responsibility for income tax, withholding social security and Medicare taxes, unemployment compensation and worker's compensation premiums. State and federal employment laws, pension benefits, and liability are also impacted by classification as contractor or employee. The employer is responsible for paying the abovementioned costs for employees. Independent contractors are responsible for paying these costs themselves. In terms of professional liability, a contractor assumes the liability risk and is usually responsible for purchasing liability insurance. In an employment situation, employees are typically provided some professional liability coverage through an employer paid policy. There are a variety of tests the government applies to determine worker classification (Internal Revenue Service, 2008a, b). These tests are applied case by case. For this reason, it is important to consult an attorney regarding employment status as well as to review any contract to provide services prior to signing the contract.

Participation in the Medicare Program

In order for a private practice to bill for Medicare services the PT and the practice must obtain a Medicare billing number and decide how the practice will be classified for Medicare purposes. Each classification has certain advantages and disadvantages. For Medicare reimbursement, the **PT in independent practice** classification is the simplest form. However, there is currently a $1810 (for 2008) per year maximum limit for combined PT and speech therapy services per Medicare patient. There are limitation exceptions for certain cases and certain diagnoses being exempt from these caps (APTA 2008b).

Form an Agency

Another option available to a private practice PT is to form a **rehabilitation agency** or a **certified outpatient rehabilitation facility** (CORF). Currently, rehabilitation agencies and CORFs are reimbursed on a fee-for-service basis (Centers for Medicare and Medicaid Services [CMS], 2008). A rehabilitation agency under Medicare guidelines is a business that provides an integrated multidisciplinary program designed to upgrade the physical function of people who are handicapped or disabled through the efforts of a team of specialized rehabilitation professionals. At a minimum, this team includes PT, speech pathology services, and social or vocational services (APTA, 2008c; CMS, 2008).

A CORF under Medicare guidelines is a nonresidential facility that provides at least medical, PT, and psychological or social services. In addition to the above requirements, PTs in independent practice, rehabilitation agencies, and certified outpatient rehabilitation facilities must meet specific requirements relating to clinical records, policies governing services, state and local licensure, plans of care, adequate facilities, equipment, personnel qualifications, budget plan, and utilization review.

To gain status as a rehabilitation agency or CORF, a comprehensive application for accreditation must be completed and a site survey scheduled. Prior to a site survey, a facility must be operational, financially solvent, and have patient records for the site surveyor to review. This certification process may take several months to complete before a practice is accredited and able to bill and collect for services provided to Medicare enrollees.

In-Home Services

In-home physical therapy involves providing services in a person's residence. Medicare allows individual and groups of PTs who are Medicare approved to treat beneficiaries and bill as they would if treatments were provided in a clinic (e.g., CPT code—fee-for-service). Doing this part time is a way to begin ownership of one's own practice. Referrals may be obtained through contracts with physicians, hospitals, or local home health agencies. Home health agencies such as visiting nurse associations have specific accreditation requirements and are usually nursing focused. These agencies do contract with therapists and the therapist or contracting practice is often paid a fee per visit and, at times, additional payment for mileage. In home and home health practice allows flexibility for the therapist, however there may be a significant amount of traveling. This may result in a small number of patients that can be served per day. Home health practice usually provides a wide variety of patients. However, documentation requirements may differ with each contract source.

Joint Ventures

A joint venture between individuals and organizations involves creating a relationship wherein both groups share risks and benefits. Insurance carriers are seldom interested in negotiating with individual providers for services. Therefore, to survive, private practice PTs need to establish linkages with hospitals and other provider groups who contract with managed-care organizations (Sullivan, 1995). The key element in a joint venture for a private practice PT is finding a willing partner who can benefit from the therapist's experience and who will allow the therapist to maintain managerial control over the practice. One form of a joint venture is between groups of PTs and physicians. Such a venture provides the PTs with a flow of referrals. However, these arrangements may be interpreted as referral-for-profit or kickback situations (APTA, 2005). This kind of joint venture needs to be carefully reviewed by an attorney (Mitchell and Scott, 1992) in addition to consideration of the ethical issues associated with the arrangement (APTA, 2008d).

Network Participation

Private practice PTs as well as other health care providers may join forces, i.e., form a network, to negotiate with insurance companies and managed-care organizations to provide services. Groups of therapists can also combine administrative functions to increase efficiency. This consolidation can reduce the costs and improve network member competitiveness on a price basis. Prior to opening a practice, investigation of network options and membership criteria may be beneficial (Advance for Physical Therapists and PT Assistants, 2007).

Many local and national physical therapy networks exist (e.g., Midwest Rehabilitation Network, 2008 and Physical Therapy Provider Network, 2008, respectively). As individual small local PT practice owners find it increasingly more difficult to become preferred pro-

viders in managed-care plans, the need to join a network becomes more apparent. The expected benefit of membership in a network of PTs is that there will be a regular flow of patients to treat who have insurance that pays for PT services. This becomes possible for two reasons. First, one contract, covering all members of a network, can be developed. By not having to negotiate contracts with individual PT providers, a managed-care organization saves time, money, and it increases the options available to their members. The members of the managed-care organization have an increase in choices of PT providers. These are the members of the network. The second benefit for PT providers from membership in a network is the ability to develop and share outcome data. The network members can pool their data to get large numbers of cases to provide satisfactory evidence of efficacy and cost effectiveness.

Investigating membership in existing local networks could be beneficial for a new or existing practice. For comparative purposes it is important to know the:

- Contracts each network holds
- Expenses involved in joining the network
- Process and costs (if any) for terminating membership
- Reimbursement method
- Restrictions on members
- Value of network participation versus non-participation

Under network arrangements, reimbursement rates may be based on a discounted fee for service, limited fee per visit, **case rate**, or **capitated rate** (Chapter 21). In addition, a fee may have to be paid to the network for membership and ongoing administrative and marketing services. Certain networks may have exclusive arrangements with insurers to send patients to network member clinics. Other networks may be nonexclusive and open to other PT practitioners. Networks may restrict members from joining competing networks. Networks may be local, regional, or national in the scope of their contracts. As with any contract, there should be an escape clause that identifies the means, timeline, and possible financial penalties associated with terminating membership.

Final Thoughts

One result of a dynamic health care environment is that clinicians and nonclinicians, often with conflicting agendas, are becoming more involved in the design of patient care processes including service determination and outcomes analysis. Employers and insurance companies negotiate for a package of health care services and empower those who authorize services to make decisions regarding the services covered and the administration of these services to patients. Health care providers are having less say regarding the types and duration of treatments they provide to clients.

Changing ownership and management concepts include diversification and development of interorganizational arrangements and governance structures. In an environment of complex interrelationships between federal government agencies, insurance companies, health care providers, and employers offering health care benefits, the traditional, small, privately owned PT practice will face greater challenges in the near future. Entrepreneurial PTs, who studiously plan, innovate, maintain clinical competence, network, and continue learning will meet these challenges by developing new practice models to deliver quality care profitably.

Among the skills that are increasingly important to do this are: competency in case management, understanding insurance plans, risk management, outcomes analysis, as well as maintaining clinical expertise. Because managerial and clinical work increasingly overlap, health care managers and patient care staff need to master a broader range of knowledge than has been included in traditional educational programs.

To varying degrees, every PT is a manager. However, every manager is not an owner. Those choosing to be employees need to keep in mind that their efforts directly affect the business success of their employer.

Summary

This chapter is unique in that it is the only chapter dedicated to the application of business principles to a small business setting. The reader was introduced to entrepreneurship, the benefits and challenges of small business ownership, and a process to plan a business. Several perceived opportunities available to become private practice PTs were discussed. The opportunities were tempered with candid discussions of the challenges particular to becoming a successful private practice owner. Options for dealing with challenges were noted.

To gain more experience in thinking about private practice issues, the reader is encouraged to complete the case studies at the end of this chapter and the private practice scenarios on the web site. These engagement activities will challenge the reader to integrate many of the business and management concepts presented in the preceding and current chapters.

Regardless of employment status, salaried or owner, financial planning for personal financial security is a necessity. A successful practice makes money. Salaries increase. To prepare for the future, money needs to grow. It is appropriate that the final finance related chapter deals with personal financial planning. To help the reader become informed about this important aspect of life, principles of personal financial management for PTs are addressed next by a licensed financial planner.

CASE STUDY 22.1

Financing Your Dream Practice

Your dream is to open a practice in a specialty area.

1. Identify the specialty area that most appeals to you

2. Develop a summary statement about your practice
3. Project your financial needs
4. Identify your financial sources including amounts available from each source

CASE STUDY 22.2

At Home with Home Care

Introduction

You have had experience doing some home care through your current employer. You have seen that patients and their families are very engaged in the treatments you provide. This type of practice appeals to you. It is time for you to take an entrepreneurial approach to your professional life and do home health on a contractual basis with a local **home health agency**. They ask for a proposal for providing services.

Tasks

1. Develop a short proposal that includes the services you will offer and payment for services.
2. How many patients do you estimate you will be able to treat in a day?
3. Analyze the effect you expect this venture to have on your financial situation. Specifically, how does what you expect to earn compare to the salaried position you have or what you would expect to earn if you were employed?

CASE STUDY 22.3

A Hard Look at What You Are Worth

The Situation

A local private practice would like to have you join the practice. You would have to develop a caseload to support your pay level and benefits. What type of incentive-based program would you propose that would be fair to both parties?

To-Do List

1. Get three estimates of the payment and benefit costs for someone with your experience and credentials.
2. Analyze the criteria used for payment.
3. Determine what method you expect would be satisfactory to the practice owner(s) as well as meet your financial needs.

CASE STUDY 22.4

Should You or Shouldn't You?

Background

You have an existing office practice. Another local physical therapist group practice would like to contract with you to use your space to treat their patients who live near your office.

Questions to Answer

1. What financial arrangement would you propose if they provide the therapists and do their own billing?
2. What if you provided the services and they do the billing?

CASE STUDY 22.5

Safety Net or Snare?

The Scenario

You are an in-network provider. The network provides you with a listing with the insurance companies in their provider book and on their website. Your costs to provide services are $70/visit. One of your largest network third party payers is only willing to pay you $65 per visit. If you were to leave the network:

You are likely to receive $128 per visit

Clients will have higher deductibles and co-payments

You would no longer be listed as an in-network provider in the provider book or on their website

It may be difficult to get back into the network once you leave it

What Would You Do?

Do you take any action? If so, what action, and why? If not, explain why not.

REFERENCES

Advance for Physical Therapists & PT Assistants. Rehab roundtable: Is joining a physical therapy partnership network a good choice? 2007;18(8):130.

American Physical Therapy Association. 1993 Active membership profile report. Alexandria, VA: Author. 1994.

American Physical Therapy Association. Position on physician-owned physical therapy services (POPTS). An American Physical Therapy Association white paper. 2005.

American Physical Therapy Association. Direct access to physical therapy services. Available at http://www.apta.org/AM/Template.cfm?Section=Top_Issues2&TEMPLATE=/CM/ContentDisplay.cfm&CONTENTID=42072. Accessed 12/02/07a.

American Physical Therapy Association. Working operational definitions of elements of 2020 vision. Available at http://www.apta.org/AM/Template.cfm?Section=Vision_20201&CONTENTID=39951&TEMPLATE=/CM/ContentDisplay.cfm. Accessed 11/02/07b.

American Physical Therapy Association. Code of ethics. Available at http://www.apta.org/AM/Template.cfm?Section=Core_Documents1&Template=/CM/HTMLDisplay.cfm&ContentID=25854. Accessed 11/02/07c.

American Physical Therapy Association. Physical therapist member demographic profile 1999–2005. Available at http://www.apta.org/TEMPLATE=/CM/ContentDisplay cfm&CONTENTID=41544. Accessed 10/26/07d.

American Physical Therapy Association. PT demographics: Employment status. Available at http://www.apta.org/AM/Template.cfm?Section=Demographics&CONTENTID=41544&TEMPLATE=/CM/ContentDisplay.cfm. Accessed 11/03/07e.

American Physical Therapy Association. Members mentoring members. Available at http://www.apta.org/AM/Template.cfm?Section=Mentoring_2&Template=/TaggedPage/TaggedPageDisplay.Cfm &TPLID=52& ContentID=19791. Accessed 11/09/07f.

American Physical Therapy Association. Women in business. Available at http://www.apta.org/AM/Template.cfm?Section=Women_in_Business1&Template=/TaggedPage/TaggedPageDisplay.cfm&TPLID=124& ContentID=15770. Accessed 11/09/07g.

American Physical Therapy Association. Opposition to physician ownership of physical therapy services. HOD P06-03-27-25. Available at http://www.apta.org/AM/Template.cfm?Section=About_APTA&CONTENTID=42264&TEMPLATE=/CM/ContentDisplay.cfm. Accessed 11/09/07h.

American Physical Therapy Association. Physical therapist ownership and operation of physical therapy services HOD P06-02-24-48. Available at http://www.apta.org/AM/Template.cfm?Section=Policies_and_Bylaws1&TEMPLATE=/CM/ContentDisplay.cfm&CONTENTID=25679. Accessed 12/02/07i.

American Physical Therapy Association. Vision 2020. Available at http://www.apta.org/AM/Template.cfm?Section=Vision_20201&Template=/TaggedPage/TaggedPageDisplay.cfm&TPLID=285&ContentID=32061. Accessed 1/31/08a.

American Physical Therapy Association. CMS instructions related to the implementation of the therapy cap. Available at http://www.apta.org/AM/Template.cfm?Section=Medicare1&TEMPLATE=/CM/ContentDisplay.cfm&CONTENTID=30309. Accessed 2/04/08b.

American Physical Therapy Association. MED-MANUAL, §250–§253.2 Outpatient Physical Therapy, Comprehensive Outpatient Rehabilitation Facility and Community Mental Health Center Manual (HCFA—Pub. 9). Available at http://www.apta.org/AM/

Template.cfm?Section=CORFs1&CONTENTID =18879&TEMPLATE=/CM/ContentDisplay.cfm. Accessed 2/04/08c.

American Physical Therapy Association. Frequently asked questions about POPTS and referral for profit. Available at http://www.apta.org/AM/Template.cfm? Section=Ethics_and_Legal_Issues1&TEMPLATE=/ CM/ContentDisplay.cfm&CONTENTID=43091. Accessed 2/04/08d.

Anderson S. Budgeting: Plan for your business. In McMenamin PJ, Glinn JE Sr. Private practice physical therapy: The how-to manual. Alexandria, VA: PPS Publications. 2002:77–85.

Bangs DH Jr. The business planning guide, 7th ed. Chicago, IL: Upstart. 1995.

Berry T. Business plans: No plan, no problem? Available at http://www.entrepreneur.com/startingabusiness/ businessplans/businessplancoachtimberry/arti-cle175792.html. Accessed 1/31/08.

Beckley NJ. Get the buzz. Rehab Management. 2005;18(7):38–39.

Black J, Glinn JE Sr. Marketing your practice. In McMenamin PJ, Glinn JE Sr. Private practice physi-cal therapy: The how-to manual. Alexandria, VA: PPS Publications. 2002:117–130.

Bureau of Labor Statistics. Occupation search. Available at http://data.bls.gov/oep/servlet/oep.noeted.servlet. ActionServlet?Action=emprprt&Occ=291123040 6&Number=10&Sort=nchg&Base=2004&Proj= 2014&EdLevel=&Search=List&Type=Occupation &Phrase=&StartItem=0. Accessed 2/01/07.

Centers for Medicare and Medicaid Services. Medicare claims processing manual. Chapter 5-part B outpa-tient rehabilitation and CORF/OPT services. Available at http://www.cms.hhs.gov/manuals/downloads/clm-104c05TXT.pdf. Accessed 2/04/08.

Connell M. Focus on private practice: Should you start a practice from scratch or purchase one? Avail-able at http://www.apta.org/AM/Template.cfm? Section=Archives3&TEMPLATE=/CM/HTMLDis-play.cfm&CONTENTID=8598. Accessed 11/10/07.

Coshocton Tribune. Brief: Advance adds physical therapy department. Available at http://www.coshoctontribune. com/apps/pbcs.dll/article?AID=/20080127/NEWS01/ 801270313/1002/NEWS01. Accessed 1/28/08.

Department of Health and Human Services. Semiannual report to Congress. Available at http://oig.hhs.gov/ publications/docs/semiannual/2006/Semiannual%20 Final%20FY%202006.pdf. Accessed 1/29/08.

Dogoff R. An introduction to supervisory practice in human services. Boston, MA: Pearson. 2005.

Ellis DJ, Pekar PP Jr. Planning for nonplanners. New York, NY: AMACOM. 1980.

Fiebert IM, Zane LJ, Hamby EF. Private practice manage-ment in physical therapy. New York, NY: Churchill Livingstone. 1990.

Gable JR, Fahiman C, Kang R, et al. Where do I send thee? Does physician-ownership affect referral patterns to ambulatory surgery centers. Health Affairs. Avail-able at http://content.healthaffairs.org/cig/content/ abstract/hlthaff.27.3.w165v1. Accessed 3/18/08.

Gauvin J, McMenamin PJ. Establishing your practice: Basic considerations. In McMenamin PJ, Glinn JE Sr. Private practice physical therapy: The how-to manual. Alexandria, VA: PPS Publications. 2002:39–61.

Harris HM. Business plan or strategic plan: What's the difference. Available at http://www.planning.org/con-sultant/businessplan.html. Accessed 1/31/08.

Internal Revenue Service. IRS talk today focuses on worker classification. Available at http://www.irs.gov/ newsroom/article/0,,id=175309,00.html. Accessed 2/04/08a.

Internal Revenue Service. Employment taxes and classify-ing workers. Available at http://www.irs.gov/newsroom/ article/0,,id=177092,00.html. Accessed 2/04/08b.

Johnson MA. Sex differences in career expectations of physical therapist students. Physical Therapy. 2007;87:1199–1211.

Johnson M. Entrepreneurs & civic engagement 'social entrepreneurship'. Tapping the 'E' spirit. Presented at the 2008 APTA Combined Sections Meeting, Nashville, TN. February 8, 2008.

Kane County Chronicle. Chiropractor's new approach includes physical therapy. Available at http://www. kcchronicle.com/articles/2006/08/31/business/ archive-329448162589.txt. Accessed 1/31/08.

Kastantin JT. Phycial therapy practice planning. Physi-cal Therapy Today. 1994:17–27.

Kovacek P, Powers D, Iglarsh ZA, et al. Task force on leadership, administration, and management prepara-tion (LAMP). The Resource. 1999;29(1): 8–13.

Kuratko DF, Hodgetts RM. Entrepreneurship: Theory, process, practice, 7th ed. Mason, OH: Thomson South-Western. 2007.

Lopopolo RB, Schaefer DS, Nosse LJ. Leadership, admin-istration, management, and professionalism (LAMP) in physical therapy: A Delphi study. Physical Therapy. 2004; 84(2):137-150.

Maryland Orthopaedic Association. Current practice issues in orthopaedic surgery: Physician owned physical therapy services. Available at http:// www.mdortho.org/Current%20practice%20issues %20in%20orthopaedic%20surgery.doc. Accessed 1/28/08.

Mason D. Government Affairs. Comprehensively address-ing referral for profit. Available at http://www.apta.org/ AM/Template.cfm?Section=Home&TEMPLATE=/CM/ HTMLDisplay.cfm&CONTENTID=30255. Accessed 1/25/09.

Matoushek NB. In pursuit of (clinical) excellence. Rehab Management. 2005;18(9):40–47.

McDaniel RR Jr. Strategic leadership: A view from quan-tum and chaos theories. Health Care Management Review. 1997;22:5–9, 21–37.

McMenamin P. What does autonomous practice mean from an intellectual and business perspective? Presentation at LAMP Summit V. Philadelphia, PA. July 21, 2004.

Medical Board of California. Corporate practice of medi-cine. Available at http://www.medbd.ca.gov/licensee/ corporate_practice.html. Accessed 1/28/08.

Microsoft Office Online. Business plan. Available at http://office.microsoft.com/en-gb/results.aspx?qu= business+plan. Accessed 1/31/08.

Midwest Rehabilitation Network. About us. Available at http://www.mrninetwork.com/aboutus.aspx. Accessed 2/04/08.

Mitchell JM, Scott E. Physician ownership of physical therapy services. Effects on charges, utilization, profits, and service characteristics. Journal of the American Medical Association. 1992;268(15): 2055–2059.

National Association for the Self-Employed. Frequently asked questions. Available at http://news.nase.org/ nase_about/FAQ.asp. Accessed 1/28/08.

Newsweek. Today's physical therapist-Do you have what it takes? Available at http://www.newsweekshowcase. com/physical-therapy/. Accessed 4/30/08.

Nosse LJ, Friberg DG, Kovacek PR. Managerial and Supervisory Principles for Physical Therapists. Baltimore, MD: Lippincott Williams and Wilkins. 1999.

Nosse LJ, Sagiv L. Theory-based study of the basic values of 565 physical therapists. Physical Therapy. 2005;85:834–850.

Office of the Professions. Practice alerts: Multidisciplinary practice. Available at http://www.op.nysed.gov/ chiroalertmulti.htm. Accessed 1/28/08.

Olsen DL. A descriptive survey of management and operations at selected sports medicine centers in the United States. Journal of Orthopedic Sports Physical Therapy. 1996:315–322.

Olsen D. Entrepreneurship: Ownership and private practice physical therapy. In Nosse LJ, Friberg DG, Kovacek PR. Managerial and supervisory principles for physical therapists. Baltimore, MD: Lippincott Williams and Wilkins. 1999:278–298.

Percy S. The dawn of a new era. Rehab Management. 2006;19(1):46–49.

Phoenix Strategic Surveys. Outpatient rehabilitation industry best practices guide. Alexandria, VA: Private Practice Section. 2003.

Private Practice Section. Member demographics. 2004.

Private Practice Section. Overview of 20 step plan for opening up a private practice. Available at http://www. ppsapta.org/links/. Accessed 11/02/07.

PT Bulletin On Line. Referral for profit is preferred over POPTS: Communication strategies needed. Available at http://www.apta.org/AM/Template.cfm?Secti on=Archives2&Template=/Customsource/Tagged-Page/PTIssue.cfm&Issue=11/15/2005#article26969. Accessed 1/28/08.

Physical Therapy Provider Network. Markets. Available at http://www.ptpn.com/markets_1_8.htm. Accessed 2/04/08.

Quatre T. It's never too soon: Starting early on a successful exit plan. PT Magazine. 2007;15(10):30–33.

Ramsey E. A fresh start in the dream of practice ownership still alive? Advance for Directors in Rehabilitation. 2007;16(3):18–20.

Rhoades PW. The valuation of a physical therapy practice, 2nd ed. Alexandria, VA: Private Practice Section. 2003.

Rozier CK, Hamilton BL, Hersh-Cochran MS. Why students choose physical therapy as a career. Physical Therapy. 1998;78:43–51.

Sanders K. Lucy Buckley: Private practice history made by a woman. Impact. 2006;3(8):34, 36.

Sandstrom RW. The meanings of autonomy for physical therapy. Physical Therapy. 2007;87:98–110.

Schafer DS, Lopopolo RB, Luedtke-Hoffmann K. Administration and management skills needed by physical therapist graduates in 2010: A national survey. Physical Therapy. 2007;87:261–281.

Schneller ES. Accountability for health care: A white paper on leadership and management for the U.S. health care system. Health Care Management Review 1997;22:38–48.

Senske K. Executive values a Christian approach to organizational leadership. Minneapolis, MN: Augsburg Books. 2003.

Singer DW. Diversifying your practice. Rehab Management. 1995(June/July):145–146.

Sinnott M. Practice ownership and autonomy—A matter of perspective. HPA Resource. 2004;4(2):5.

Sinnott M C. LAMP: Lighting the way to vision 2020. HPA Resource. 2006;6(1):1, 3.

Small Business Administration. Table of small business size standards matched to North American industry Classification System codes. Available at http://www.sba.gov/idc/groups/public/documents/ sba_homepage/serv_sstd_tablepdf.pdf. Accessed 12/02/07a.

Small Business Administration. Small business research summary. Available at http://www.sba.gov/advo/ research/rs262.pdf. Accessed 11/10/07b.

Small Business Administration. Write a business plan. Available at http://sba.gov/smallbusinessplanner/plan/ writeabusinessplan/SERV_WRRITINGBUSPLAN. html. Accessed 2/02/08.

Small Business Notes. The small business share of GDP, 1998–2004. Available at http://www.smallbusiness-notes.com/aboutsb/rs299.html. Accessed 12/02/07.

Smith HW. The Ten Natural Laws of Successful Time and Life Management. New York, NY: Warner Books. 1994.

Spors KK. The 100-page plan-Don't bother. Milwaukee Journal Sentinel. 2008;Feb:50.

State of New York. Corporate practice of the professions. Available at http://www.op.nysed.gov/corporate_ practice.pdf. Accessed 1/28/08.

State of Wisconsin. Office of the Commissioner of Insurance. Available at http://oci.wi.gov/sm_emp/health. htm. Accessed 12/02/07.

Stern L. Conquer business plan phobia. Home Office Computing. 1995;Feb:26–28.

Sullivan T. Managed care and the survival of private practice. Rehab Management. 1995;(Oct/Nov): 22–29.

Survivalstrategies. Tip of the week. Available at http:// www.survivalstrategies.com. Accessed 1/16/08.

Swedlow A, Johnson G, Smithline N, et al. Increased costs and rates of use in the California Workers' Compensation System as a result of self referral by physicians.

New England Journal of Medicine. 1992;327:1502–1506.

Thornton, DM. Testimony before the Subcommittee on Health of the House Committee on Ways and Means Hearing on Medicare "Self-Referral" Law. Available at http://waysandmeans.house.gov/legacy/health/106cong/5-13-99/5-13thor.htm. Accessed 1/29/08.

Timmons JA, Spinelli S. New Venture Creation Entrepreneurship for the 21st Century, 7th ed. New York, NY: McGraw-Hill. 2006.

U.S. Physical Therapy. Benefits overview. Available at http://usph.hrmdirect.com/employment/custom.php?page=usph_benefits&. Accessed 11/07/07a.

U.S. Physical Therapy. Partnership benefits. Available at http://www.usph.com/oyoc/benefits.aspx. Accessed 11/07/07b.

Wallace J. Your patients, your practice, your business. PTmagazine. 2008;16(1):46–47.

Waitley DE. The psychology of winning, audio tape 4. Chicago, IL: Nightengale-Conant. 1978.

Wichita Eagle. Health News: Major reshuffling, remodeling. Available at http://www.kansas.com/business/healthcare/story/292420.html. Accessed 1/28/08.

Wojciechowski M. Group ownership and autonomous practice. PTmagazine. 2005;13(9):48–53.

Wynn KE. Breaking through the barriers. PT Magazine. 1997;10(5):44–46, 48–50, 52–56.

Zacharakis A. Writing a business plan. In Bygrave WD, Zacharakis A, eds. The Portable MBA in Entrepreneurship, 3rd ed. Hoboken, NJ: John Wiley. 2004:107–140.

ADDITIONAL RESOURCES

The evolution of the concept of autonomous practice in Vision 2020 is available at http://www.apta.org/AM/Template.cfm?Section=Professional_Resources&CONTENTID=32604&TEMPLATE=/CM/HTMLDisplay.cfmy. Several viewpoints on practice autonomy can be found in *Physical Therapy Magazine*. 2007;15(3):68–71. A retrospective by Pete Stark on the Stark Laws (related to referral for profit) is at http://blogs. forbes.com:80/sciencebizblog/2007/11/stark-regrets-i.html. The Small Business Administration's business planning resources can be found at http://www.sba.gov/index.html. SCORE's questionnaire to stimulate thinking about starting a business is at https://secure.e-myth. com/cs/scoreassessment/create/ba_results. IRS information related to starting a business is located at http://www.irs.gov/businesses/small/article/0,,id=99336,00.html. Free tax related educational materials for the small business owner is available at http://www.irs.gov/businesses/small/index.html. Goal setting is often difficult. A site with over 100 questions to help formulate goals is available at http://www.hr-guide.com/data/G336.htm. Free on line entrepreneur self-assessment questionnaires are available at http://theacorncentre.com/entrepreneur-questionnaire.pdf, http://www.bdc.ca/en/business_tools/entrepreneurial_self-Assessment/Entrepreneurial_self_assessment.htm?cookie%5Ftest=1. A business resource guide to help develop a business is provided by the Boston Department of Neighborhood Development at http://www.cityofboston.gov/dnd/obd/BRG/A_intro.asp. Free on line business courses can be accessed at http://www.sba.gov/services/training/onlinecourses/ index.html. Free consultation and low cost courses for small business entrepreneurs are available through America's Small Business Development Center Network at http://www.asbdc-us.org/About_Us/aboutus.html. The National Association of Women Business Owners can be found at http://www.nawbo.org/. For an article on the pros and cons of cash only practice see http://www. apta.org/AM/Template.cfm?Section=Archives3&TEMPLATE=/CM/HTMLDisplay.Cfm&CONTENTID=8646. APTA resources include private practice as part of a professional development plan (http://www.apta.org/AM/Template.cfm?Section=Professional_PT&Template=/MembersOnly.cfm&NavMenuID=1254&ContentID=38666&DirectListComboInd=D). The APTA also tracks emerging PT practice trends. See http://www.apta.org/AM/Template.cfm?Section=Emerging_PT_Practice&Template=/TaggedPage/Tagged Page Display.cfm&TPLID=202&ContentID=19869, http://www.apta.org/AM/Template.cfm? Section=Demographics&TEMPLATE=/CM/HTMLDisplay.cfm&CONTENTID=8471, and http://www.apta.org/AM/Template.cfm?Section=Home&Template=/CM/ContentDisplay.cfm&ContentID=43038. Weinper provided a look at future private practice opportunities in Rehab Management. Private practice premonitions, the sequel. 2004;17(1):48–50, 57. PTmagazine has a resource called the Small Practice Advisor at http://www.apta.org/AM/Template.cfm?Section=Current_Issue1&TEMPLATE=/CM/HTMLDisplay.cfm&CONTENTID=35844 or contact TygielPT@aol.com.

CHAPTER 23

MAKING STRUCTURED PERSONAL FINANCIAL DECISIONS

JOHN (JACK) NELSON

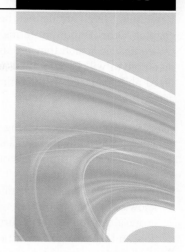

Learning Objectives

1. Identify the components of a properly designed personal financial foundation that can lead to economic stability and consistency of income.
2. Acquire a working knowledge of a personal financial decision-making process that is sufficiently dynamic and robust to meet your needs over time and under varying conditions.
3. When you are ready, be able to apply the personal financial decision-making process to plan your financial future.

Introduction

Being financially stable is the goal of many professionals. Unfortunately, this goal eludes many people. This is partly because financial security means different things to different people and partly because each individual has a unique set of circumstances that contributes to or takes away from the individual's financial security. This unrealized goal of financial security has led to an entire industry of self-help, quick-fix, and overgeneralized solutions.

Financial security or *fiscal health* is very similar to physical health. Both are the result of the following factors:

1. Family history
2. The external environment
3. Dedication to prudent behaviors
4. Well thought out courses of action to respond to new experiences and exposures

5. The use of trained professionals to guide us along the way

In other words, achieving fiscal health is the result of a lifelong process of making sound financial decisions that are centered on a core set of *financial values*. Since each individual's goals and values hierarchy will differ (Chapter 7), this chapter will concentrate its efforts toward establishing the process rather than providing tips and techniques. Once established, a sound process will support you in making decisions that will lead you towards your goals and will be consistent with your prized values. The process will also provide you with a very practical tool to cut through the marketing hype surrounding financial services and products and an understanding of the pros and cons of various strategies as they relate to you specifically. This is important because financial service and product marketing often casts a wide net to capture a large general target market. Therefore, the purpose of this chapter is twofold (1) identify an individualized financial decision-making process that is sufficiently dynamic and robust to work over time and under varying conditions and (2) to discuss the components of a properly designed personal financial foundation.

Note: Detailed explanations of various financial strategies would exceed the constraints of this book due to the level of detail needed to describe these strategies and the inability to provide any guidance without specific knowledge of a particular person's position and goals.

Key Terms

Key terms, which are defined below, are bolded and italicized the first time they appear in the chapter. Other important terms are shown in boldface on first appearance and are defined by the context in which they are used. When either of these types of terms is used several times, its acronym will be identified and subsequently used in the chapter. Both types of terms are listed alphabetically in the online glossary with their definitions and (when applicable) their acronyms.

consistency: in financial planning, this refers to the ability to regularly make financial decisions that are cohesive and supportive of achieving prioritized future financial goals.

current position: in financial planning this is (1) your knowledge, feelings or biases, (2) your personal financial timeline, (3) your current financial position, and (4) your goal priorities.

financial advisors: trained professionals who guide you through the process of planning your financial future. Some specialize in particular areas of finance (i.e., investing, insurance, retirement planning, etc.). Others focus on the creation of planning documents to help you through the process of financial planning.

financial product: general name for stocks, bonds, and other market related investment opportunities.

financial stability: in financial planning, this is a desired state that is realized when there are sufficient resources to meet challenges/opportunities in a cost efficient manner.

financial values: prioritized financial goals to meet anticipated needs and wants. These values must be identified for an appropriate financial plan to be formulated.

fiscal health: this is attained by consistently engaging in prudent financial behaviors, well thought out courses of action to respond to new experiences and exposures, and guidance from one or more trained professional advisors.

needs: according to Maslow, basic needs are hierarchically arranged. Fulfillment of the basics allows the higher needs to be pursued. Needs are: physiological (most basic), safety, love, esteem, self-actualization (highest level).

prudent behaviors: in financial planning means regularly putting money away (savings, investing, insurance, employee benefits, etc.), so it grows to meet financial goals, monitoring growth, and reassessing goals. A dedication to pursuing planned financial behaviors.

SMART: a format for stating a strategic goal that is (S)pecific, (M)easurable, (A)cceptable, (R)esults orientated, and (T)ime bound.

wants: things that a person desires or would like to have.

Growing Money to Meet Goals

Financial stability and *consistency* are likely to be achieved if there is a process and a structure to foster these goals. Financial stability and consistency have been established when:

There are sufficient resources that can be used to meet challenges/opportunities in a cost-efficient manner.
This process can be repeated in a structured fashion.
The outcome fits within an established financial structure.

In other words, if you follow some rules consistently, you are likely to have sufficient resources to use judiciously to have the wealth sufficient to meet your needs and priority wants (Chapter 21).

Things That Get in the Way

The challenges that impede the establishment of a process and structure are dynamic environment, misconceptions, stale data, generalized advice, lack of access to information, intimidation, and confusion. Advisors can aid in advancing the process by obtaining a base level of understanding about you, your financial circumstances, and the life goals you wish to achieve (Chapters 7 and 22). These variables will eventually have a greater impact on your financial well-being than any specific *financial product* or strategy. Like physical health, the ultimate responsibility for fiscal health lies with the individual.

More on Fiscal Health Factors

Let us further explore the five factors mentioned earlier that govern fiscal health.

1. Family history—Each individual comes to their fiscal maturity with the exposures and training they had when they were growing up (Kiyosaki et al., 1998). Individuals who grew up in a fiscally stable environment and were exposed to adults making good decisions have an advantage as they mature. Individuals who were encouraged to research and analyze situations prior to making decisions will be better prepared to establish good decision-making processes as they grow up. Unfortunately, the opposite is also likely. Poor decisionmaking and lack of intellectual curiosity will make establishing fiscal stability more difficult. It is good to note however, that family history is but one influencing factor in fiscal health.

2. External environment—The fiscal environment is composed of many factors. This environment is constantly changing due to demographic trends, government policy, scarcity of resources,and so on. Some of the external factors that make up the financial environment are

   Economy
   Employee benefits (or lack of benefits)
   Financial services and products
   Taxes
   World events

   The effect of this ever-changing external environment is that decisions that made good sense historically may not be appropriate today. The dedication to ongoing education and awareness of the economic changes that are occurring around us will help to modify our financial process to be current with the existing environment.

3. Prudence—A commitment to prudent financial behaviors means regularly putting money away so it grows. Fiscal health is a direct result of making consistently sound decisions and having an understanding of the relationships between the various elements of fiscal health such as

Employment benefits
Financial goals
Insurance
Investing
Saving

The ability to use your financial resources to support your personal goals is established by saving on a regular basis and by having access to your money so that you can take advantage of opportunities as they are presented to you. A helpful learning tool to remember this concept is the acronym LUCKY:

L = liquidity—the ability to have access to your financial resources (Chapter 21)
U = use—the right to use your resources as you need to
C = control—the ability to manage your resources to maximize the benefits for you and your family
K = knowledge—the understanding of how your resources work together to meet your goals.
Y = you—the individual must be able to take action given the available resources, the opportunity presented, and the knowledge gained as a result of ongoing financial education.

In other words, being LUCKY is not having luck per se, but the result of being dedicated to engaging in prudent planned financial behaviors.

4. Having a set methodology for making financial decisions prior to making the decision allows the individual to analyze the situation without regard to marketing hype and generalities. Well thought out courses of action facilitate responding to new experiences and opportunities.

5. The use of trained professionals is one way to explore financial growth options by sorting fact from fiction. The complexities of the financial landscape as well as the many pressures of daily living (job, family, community commitments, etc.), makes using a trained professional almost a requirement at some time during your life. More discussion on this topic will be presented later.

Of the five fiscal health components, only family history and the external environment are outside the direct control of the individual. Therefore, the last three factors, prudence, planned actions, and professional guidance are the primary focus of this chapter. Focusing on these factors at any age regardless of the first two factors can result in improved fiscal health.

Prudent Behaviors

Just as there are prudent professional behaviors (Chapter 8), there are certain prudent behaviors that will provide a solid foundation from which to build a sound financial platform. There is little disagreement among trained *financial advisors* that these behaviors are the initial starting point for fiscal health. These behaviors, when initiated and sufficiently repeated, will have two positive outcomes:

1. Sound financial habits will be formed. Good habits will be lifelong guideposts for financial stability.
2. Fiscal noise (money-related confusion) will be eliminated.

Often, it is difficult to take action towards improving your financial situation. This difficulty stems from random, ad hoc decisions that have been made in the past. Confronting such fiscal noise can appear to be a daunting task. However, sorting through this quagmire can be done by developing a direct, consistent, and disciplined path toward achieving your goals. This advice should sound familiar, it is the essence of strategic planning (Chapters 2–6, 13) applied on an individual basis.

Behaviors for Reaching Your Financial Goals

The following list contains the top ten behaviors (in deference to David Letterman) that will allow you to establish a stable base from which actions can take place that can impact your financial goals.

1. Check your emotions at the entryway to this exercise. Building a sound financial structure that will enable you to focus on the important things in life is a thoughtful, analytical process. The only emotions that should be a part of the exercise should be your personal dedication to your individual values (Chapter 7). What other people think, have, or desire should not influence you. You are not entitled to anything more than that which you can earn.

2. Take some time—Initially; spend two half-hour sessions per week that are dedicated to getting your financial house in order. This time should be scheduled as if it were a significant appointment or meeting. The time should be scheduled when you are relaxed and clearheaded. As you progress through the process this time can be reduced to allow you to focus on those things that have higher value to you (family, faith, work, self-improvement, community, etc. [Chapters 7, 22]).

3. Write it down × 2—Write down what is happening now: your expenses, debts, and sources of income? This data is historical. This information will be needed in the next stage of your financial process. At this stage you are just gathering data. As the process evolves, you will begin to organize the data and make judgments about what you are doing with your money. There are many tools on the Internet that can help you with this process (see Additional Resources).

   The second writing exercise is to state your desired outcomes. Some authors recommend that you use this exercise as a fantasy motivator, i.e., "I want $1,000,000" or "I want a Mercedes Benz." My professional experiences have not shown this to be useful. A goal is more easily dismissed if it is not readily achievable. But the goal should not be too immediate either. At this initial stage, a 3–5 year projection is sufficient (Chapter 13).

4. Pay yourself first—The act of saving is contagious. Once begun, it will last a lifetime. It is important that saving should not be done *for* you. Payroll savings plans do not count. After you made the decision to enroll you have "removed" yourself from the act of being a habitual saver. You must take the initiative to put away some money for you and your family. It does not have to be much. There are countless stories about significant sums of money being saved by people of modest means just because they had the habit of saving. How the money is invested is also not as important as the fact that you have taken the action to save.

5. Individuals and pundits only brag about their success. So do not listen to them or be influenced by them. Your situation is unique. The process and structure that you will implement with the help of your advisor will be a better predictor of financial stability and goal realization than the random implementation of strategies recommended by outsiders who are not fully aware of your situation.

6. If you read about or hear about once-in-a-lifetime opportunities, forget about them. The financial markets are very efficient. If there was a golden opportunity, it has already happened and you would be getting in at the back end of the opportunity, not the front end. The more people jump on an opportunity; the prices can be driven up by the demand generated by these individuals. If the opportunity was that good, why would someone take the time to write about it or talk about it rather than just doing it? Chasing opportunities without knowing how they fit into your personal financial structure can be a costly mistake.

7. Buy low and sell high—This is intuitively obvious, but few people do it because most individuals are motivated to take action by their stomachs not their brains. Wealth has been created historically when someone has saved money, and had the brains to use that money when other people were having their stomachs or their greed tell them to take a different course of action.

8. Protect yourself and your family—Most individuals cannot cover the cost of a loss (health, death, accident, etc.) just using their own resources. Insurance providers provide protection for your family. Do not ignore this area as a part of the financial growth process. As you start to accumulate financial resources, insurances become increasingly important. Rarely does anyone complain when they get a check from an insurance company after a claim has been paid. Insurance is every bit as individual as your personal financial situation. There should be no knee jerk financial decisions. Seek professional advice.

9. Select your advisory team carefully—This team is made up of your accountant, attorney, insurance agent(s), investment specialist, and financial planner. At times these professionals can wear multiple hats. This is appropriate as long as full disclosure is made as to the details of the relationship. Developing expertise in these areas is not a simple matter. People who have not dedicated themselves to continuing professional development in their area of professional specialization have not earned the right to be on your team.

10. Stay true to your process.

The next section of this chapter deals with setting up your individual financial decision-making process. The process that you develop will be specific to you and will help you make decisions that will be in line with your personal goals.

Well Thought-Out Actions

Sound financial decisions can be facilitated following a dynamic process based on six phases: documentation, analysis, decision-making rules, implementation of strategies, review, and finally re-definition (Chapters 13–15, and 21). The primary outcome of this process is a methodology for making decisions that, when put in place, will allow the individual to respond to life events that have a financial component (virtually all do).

Phase 1: Documentation

Documenting your *current position* is essential before any decisions can be made. Your current position is made up of four components, your

1. Knowledge, feelings, or biases
2. Personal financial timeline
3. Current assets and liabilities
4. Goal Prioritization

Knowledge, Feelings, and Biases

A set of questions that facilitate gaining an understanding of these psychological variables are presented in Table 23.1.

After working through this discovery process it is common to find that some of your previous knowledge base is inconsistent with newfound information. This growth is normal

Table 23.1   Questions About Your Knowledge, Feelings, and Biases About Financial Planning

1. What do you know about your current financial position?
2. Do you understand how debt works and are you comfortable with your understanding?
3. How have you made financial decisions in the past?
4. Are you happy or unhappy with the results of these decisions?
5. How do you feel about the process of decision making?
6. Have you gone to anyone for financial advice, and if so, were they a qualified professional?
7. Were you happy with their service?
8. What would you like to see improved in your overall strategy?
9. Do you have specific beliefs or values that would impact your goals and decisions?
10. What is your level of understanding of financial products/services?
11. Do you understand how debt works and are you comfortable with it?
12. Have you taken risk?
13. How did it make you feel?
14. What are the influences in your life that have an impact on your financial decisions?
15. What general goal do you hope to accomplish from your financial plan?
16. How would you respond if what you thought was true, turned out not to be true?

and desirable. In fact, as you grow financially many things that seemed appropriate based on your financial situation at that time might not be the best course of action later on.

Personal Financial Timeline

A personal financial timeline is a sketch of what you know, what you hope, what you need, what you want, and what you assume will happen in the future. This timeline will be essential in identifying what opportunities (+ or −) might be presented to you in the future. This timeline will provide a starting point for discussion. It is not intended to predict the future. Table 23.2 provides a format for creating this timeline.

By creating a financial timeline, a practical element is introduced into the process. In your financial life there are times when there are things of such a pressing nature that a decision must be made immediately. In other words, sometimes a process is not what is needed. Action must be taken. These must be accommodated. It is also true that some events that occur in the short and mid range might take

Table 23.2   Developing a Personal Financial Timeline Worksheet

What life events will impact your financial goals and plans?
What is your projected time frame for them?

Goal	Time Frame
Attending college/completing higher education	
Marriage	
Purchase a home	
Pay off educational debt	
Parenthood	
Paying for children's education	
Retirement	
Providing for long-term care	

preference over larger but longer range events. This need not change the prioritization of the goals; just accept that at times an element of pragmatism must be introduced into the process. For example, retirement and accumulating sufficient resources for that period is arguably on of the largest financial challenges we will face. Before retirement many other life events will occur that will need to be addressed, i.e., education, purchase of a car, job changes, and others. The creation of this timeline will allow you to identify early on that financial decision making is rarely sequential and in most instances there are simultaneous financial events. Coordinated decisions are best because they force prioritizing the use of resources.

Current Assets and Liabilities

Documentation of your assets and liabilities (Chapter 21) is essential for determining where to begin in the development of your financial decision-making process. It is part of your internal environmental scanning process. Table 23.3 offers a form for capturing the critical elements of your current position.

It is better to be inclusive and detailed at this stage of the process. Seemingly unrelated facts can often prove to be related upon analysis. Documenting your current financial position allows you to identify areas of redundancy, inefficiency, and incompatibility. It also allows you to determine if any resources are being spent unknowingly or unnecessarily. The next part of the process will guide you through eliminating these inefficiencies and potentially recapturing lost resources.

Goal Prioritization

The first three components of documentation deal with what is currently known to you. The final component deals with what you want. It is important to distinguish between **needs** and **wants** at this juncture. Needs dictate short-term resource utilization. Wants are a driving force behind how we use our financial resources. The only time at which needs and wants are the same is when the ultimate goal is status quo.

In order to prioritize your goals both needs and wants must be identified. Short-term goals are more needs based. Long-term goals are more closely identified with wants. When

---

Table 23.3   Financial Planning Worksheet

Occupation/Income
Yourself: Salary _____
Spouse: Salary _____
Combined Income: _____

Real Estate/Mortgages	Monthly Payment	Current Market Value	Unpaid Balance
Your residence			
Other home			
Vacation home			
Other			

Savings	Institution	Joint	Yourself	Spouse	Child
Savings/Checking Account					
Savings Bonds					
Annuities					
IRA:					
☐ SEP					
☐ Simple					
☐ Roth					
☐ Rollover					
☐ Other					
Section 529 Plan					
401(k) Annual Contribution					
Company Match					
Defined Benefit Plan					
Profit Sharing					
How much are you saving on a monthly basis?					

(Continued)

Table 23.3   continued

Investments	Joint	Yourself	Spouse	Child
Stocks/Bonds				
Stocks/Bonds				
Stocks/Bonds				
Stocks/Bonds				
Mutual Funds				
Mutual Funds				
Mutual Funds				
Mutual Funds				
Mutual Funds				

Other Assets	Joint	Yourself	Spouse	Child
Item *(auto, boat, additional investments, etc.)*				

Debts	Monthly Payment	Months Remaining	Unpaid Balance
Credit Card			
Credit Card			
Credit Card			
Credit Card			
Credit Card			
Credit Card			
Credit Card			
Personal Loan			
Home Equity Loan			
College Loan			
Car Loan			
Car Loan			
Other			

Insurance	Company	Insured	Premium	Cash Value	Loans	Amount Coverage

Accountant _____

Attorney _____

Investment Broker/Advisor _____

Insurance Agent _____

Banker _____

Other Professional Advisor _____

identifying goals, beginning with the end in mind is critical. To achieve this, goals must have five common characteristics that make up the mnemonic *SMART* (Chapter 13):

1. Specific
2. Measurable
3. Achievable
4. Results orientated
5. Timely

As with the other parts of this section on documentation, it is important to capture your prioritized goals in writing so that they can be used in later stages of the process. Table 23.4 will be helpful in capturing your important goals.

The four current position components: (1) knowledge, feelings, and biases, (2) financial timeline, (3) assets and liabilities, and (4) goals; document the environment within which your financial decisions must be made. Without these highly personal identifiers, the ability to make financial decisions that will work for you would be corrupted. One of the keys to making sound decisions is establishing the unique outcomes that fit your financial situation. Most financial theories work when the theorist gets to set the parameters and the assumptions. My task here is to help you make decisions that will work for you given your unique fact pattern. Financial decisions are rarely made in an isolated environment. Decisions have reper-

cussions throughout your financial position. Several very common examples are (1) having a very low deductible on your car insurance and paying for any minor car claims out of your emergency cash account or worse, paying on a credit card, (2) maximizing your qualified savings plan (e.g., 401[k]) at work and not having sufficient ready assets to meet current financial demand.

Phase 2: Analysis

The current position information needs to be examined and interpreted. This is the analysis portion of the process. It is the most technical. Working with an advisor is recommended at this step. Keep in mind that an advisor who specializes in the product specific area of financial planning (i.e., investment and/or insurance planning) might not be best suited

---

Table 23.4   Financial Life Goals

Part I

In any order, list your most important financial goals.
- _____
- _____
- _____
- _____
- _____
- _____
- _____
- _____
- _____
- _____

Examples:
- Asset protection/debt reduction
- Business growth
- Business start-up
- College funding

- Estate planning
- Financial security for retirement
- Financial security for survivors
- Wealth accumulation/management

Make sure your goals are SMART

Part II

Now prioritize your financial goals. Listing the most important first and least important last, then fill in the remaining values according to their personal importance.
1. _____
2. _____
3. _____
4. _____
5. _____
6. _____
7. _____
8. _____
9. _____
10. _____

for this type of engagement. Since most people have not gone through a detailed analysis of their financial position, and most people make many financial decisions during the course of each year, it makes sense that the longer an individual waits prior to performing this analysis the more time consuming the process will become. Each financial position you are currently in must be judged relative to the goals and objectives identified in the documentation process. Each position must also be reviewed in light of the other position to ensure proper coordination, as well as reduction of redundancies and inefficiencies. The objective criteria established in Phase 1 are the guiding light of this process. The objectivity of these guidelines allows the individual to judge the relative effectiveness of any financial position or strategy. Without the documentation obtained in Phase 1, no true objective analysis could be done on your financial position. The result of this analysis is to formulate the strategies and positions that are consistent with your goals and identifying those positions that need to be brought into alignment. Table 23.5 is a tool that brings together much of the information that was gathered separately in one place.

Phase 3: Decision-Making Rules

Once you have identified those positions and strategies that do not appear to be aligned with our goals, we must determine if these positions and strategies were the result of faulty analysis, change in environment, or lack of full consideration (Chapters 13, 15). Knowing why you are in a position that is not properly aligned will allow you to make changes in how you make decisions going forward. If for example, proper consideration was not given the proper control of your money, or the eventual cost of the position was too high. This knowledge will help you fine-tune the process in making future financial decisions.

The following is a generic listing of factors that can be considered when making financial decisions. The determination if any of these factors should be considered as well as what weighting they should be given will be driven by your specific situation. Considerations include

- Adequate compensation for committing resources

Table 23.5   Opportunities, Problems, Wealth Transfer, Resources Worksheet

Part I: Opportunities

1.
2.
3.
4.
5.
6.
7.
8.

Part II: Problem Identification

1.
2.
3.
4.
5.
6.
7.
8.

Part III: Wealth Transfer

1.
2.
3.
4.
5.
6.
7.
8.

Part IV: Resources

1.
2.
3.
4.
5.
6.
7.
8.

- Additional benefits of taking action
- Affect on existing relationships
- Alignment with goals
- Availability of resources
- Cost of taking action
- Liquidity and use and control of resources
- Risk tolerance
- Tax ramifications
- Time frame or holding period

Phase 4: Implementation of Strategies

Especially after the initial analysis, it is quite possible that a number of new strategies will be considered. Some of these strategies might be competing for the same resource dollar. If that is the case, then a review of the goal priorities (Table 23.4) is needed in order to reset the implementation priorities. Additionally, your personal timeline should be reconsidered to determine if implementation could affect other elements of your timeline. These three elements: priority of goals, availability of resource, and personal timeline will determine the implementation action plan.

Phase 5: Review

As in any strategic planning process, a review of results is necessary (Chapter 13). This step is taken at a reasonable interval after the implementation action plan has been executed to determine if the desired outcomes have been realized thus far and to determine if any additional or corrective action is needed. The review should use the same criteria as the action plan to determine viability. If there are any unintended consequences or unanticipated outcomes, they should be passed forward into the next step (Chapters 15, 16).

Phase 6: Re-definition

If there are any issues flagged by the review, then it must be determined if a goal was not a SMART goal (Chapter 13) or if there was incomplete analysis of the factors involved. Any new information can be used to modify the data contained in the initial documentation. This step is also used to re-visit the initial goals and timelines and to initiate any addition action plans to keep on track with existing goals as well as to initiate any additional analysis needed to review environmental changes that have occurred.

Using Trained Financial Advisors

The complexity of the financial environment, the frequency at which the environment changes combined with your unique fact pattern makes developing a financial decision process difficult. Having a financial advisor guide you through the process can be helpful if not necessary. There are many types of advisors available to help you through the process. Like physical therapists there are generalists and specialists. Some financial advisors specialize in particular areas of finance (i.e., investing, insurance, retirement planning, etc.). Others focus on the creation of planning documents to help you through the process of financial planning. Over the course of your financial life, each of these advisors may have something to offer you. At the initial stage, the advisor's ability to act as a guide/mentor is more crucial than the area of specialization. In fact, introducing specific focus areas at this stage of the process could prove to be detrimental to a successful outcome. Make sure that the communication between you and the advisor is bidirectional and that your unique situation is driving the process. Professional referrals and references are a good place to start when seeking an advisor. Just as in other professions, credentials are important, but ultimately it is the ability to communicate and connect with each other that will result in successful outcomes (Chapter 19). Credentials that focus on a planning process are ultimately more desirable in helping you establishing a sound financial structure. Like physical therapists, there are numerous educational/professional designations. However, in the financial planning arena there are several dozen different designations (Vohwinkle, 2008). Of the major credentials listed in Table 23.6, the three that currently focus on process and require a comprehensive understanding of the multiple disciplines within a financial process are CFP®, ChFC/CLU, and PFS.

Individuals who have completed these courses of study have not only completed the work necessary to pass thorough examinations but are required to maintain ongoing competency by taking continuous education courses. These individuals typically maintain relationships with allied specialists that might be needed for the ongoing operation of your financial process. In most instances, the allied professionals understand that underlying the success of the positions and strategies is the robust process of analysis that drives the mechanisms used to achieve desired outcomes.

The following are the anticipated benefits of initially using an advisor and a structured financial planning process:

Table 23.6   Major Financial Planner Designations

Title	Initials	Description
Certified Financial Planner	CFP	A highly respected designation that is earned by completing 3 years experience in the field, and passing a series of examinations on a broad range of financial topics.
Chartered Financial Consultant	ChFC	Often insurance professionals specializing in some aspects of financial planning. Requires meeting advanced education in economics and investments.
Chartered Life Underwriter	CLU	This credential indicates expertise regarding insurance products. It requires completion of seven American College courses and passing an exam.
Certified Public Accountant	CPA	An experienced accountant who has met stringent educational requirements and licensing requirements. Knowledgeable about accounting and tax matters.
Chartered Retirement Planning Counselor	CRPC	A credential issued by the College of Financial Planning after passing an exam. The credential signifies that a planner has specialized in retirement planning.
Personal Financial Specialist	PFS	This is a designation for CPAs who have additional financial planning education and who have passed an exam.

- Professional guidance—Not all financial decisions require the input of a professional. It is recommended that setting up the initial structure, decision-making process (as discussed earlier in this chapter), and strategy analysis should be reviewed with the help of a trained, experienced, financial advisor.
- Efficient use of resources—Financial opportunities occurs in each individual's life. These opportunities can present themselves as either a positive (promotions, raises, business opportunity, inheritance, fellowships, etc.) or negative (termination, disability, business failure, higher taxes, etc.). Financial security is determined by how well you utilize the financial resources you have at your disposal to meet these opportunities
- Outside influences—The effect of outside influences cannot be overstated in the development of a sound financial structure. Taxes, government entitlements, macro economies, political forces all are changeable and can and will have an effect on your financial process.
- Consistency—All of us make a stream of financial decisions each and every day. Our ability to make these decisions in a consistent manner that is cohesive to our long-term goal is a significant determinant of our future financial success.

- Expansion of our knowledge base—Most knowledge on which we make financial decisions is historic in nature. Most financial decisions we make are forward looking. This presents a dilemma. How can good decisions be made if the decision will be made on stale data? A commitment to a dynamic and robust process of reevaluation should be a lifelong commitment. If what you previously thought to be true is no longer true, adjustment to your financial process is required.
- Stability—Financially successful individuals often have been ready to take action toward their goals and ambitions. Most times what the layman has seen is the bold action that resulted in the financial success. What is not so readily seen is the work done behind the scenes to establish a stable financial structure that allows the individual to take action. Sometimes this foundation is built by previous generations (wealth transfer), other times the individual themselves have spent enormous amounts of time establishing a stable base. One way or another, stability is a strong determinant of financial success.

Summary

The purpose of this chapter was to establish the core guidelines for a stable financial growth process. The guidelines incorporated many of the concepts of strategic planning applied on an individual basis. The key components of a stable financial process identified included

Five important determinants of fiscal health

A tool for analyzing prudent fiscal actions (LUCKY)

Key prudent behaviors that contribute to fiscal stability

A six-phase process for stabilizing current positions and strategies that includes adjusting and modifying the process as needed.

Ten key suitability factors in analyzing strategies and financial services

Selection criteria for financial advisors including credentials

Worksheets to aid in the process of attaining financial stability

With this core process in place, individual strategies (stocks, bonds, insurance, retirement planning, debt management, etc.) can be analyzed and decisions made regarding their suitability in a person's specific long-term financial goals.

It was understood that each individual would have a greater (or lesser) desire to delve into the details of establishing a personalized financial process. Because most individuals have not been exposed to the tools and techniques described in this chapter it was anticipated that a novice to this process would be well served by utilizing the services of a financial advisor to guide them through the process.

In developing the material for this chapter, I relied most heavily on my own experience. This includes more than 30 years in the financial services industry and more than 20 years as a practicing financial planner. Other practitioner's opinions may differ from mine due to their different experiences and areas of specialization. The profession of financial planning is relatively new as compared with other professions, i.e., law medicine, accounting. The profession is evolving. Any definitive comments may change in the future due to new information as well as external environmental constraints. In other words, financial stability requires a dedication to a process not dogma and a certain commitment to being forever curious.

CASE STUDY 23.1

Smile, There Is No Case Study

Case studies or rules of thumb that could guide an individual in taking certain financial actions or making financial decisions has been a staple in financial writings. What I have said in this chapter makes such an approach counter productive to sound financial planning. Decisions made as a result of specific data and environments are unique to that set of facts. Hopefully this chapter has given you a process to look at your own situation (either by yourself or with a trained professional financial advisor) and to make decisions that will work for you. Any specific guidance other than process that you derive from this chapter will have one overriding characteristic, it is probably wrong. Advice, as to specific actions or

decisions should never be taken from any source unless there is full knowledge of the specific situation. Just like your treatment plans, your financial plans should at least be based on the consensus of trained, experienced, and well thought of professionals and integrated with the client's goals.

If you are really ready to think more deeply about financial planning, consider using the templates presented in this chapter to get your basic value and financial information in front of yourself. When you are comfortable with your information, it could be time to schedule interviews with some trained financial planners to assist you to grow further in your financial planning experiences.

REFERENCES

Kiyosaki RT, Lechter SL. Rich Dad, Poor Dad: What The Rich Teach Their Kids About Money That the Poor and Middle Class Do Not! New York, NY: Warner Books. 2000.

Vohwinkle J. Choosing a financial planner. Available at http://financialplan.about.com. Accessed 6/03/08.

ADDITIONAL RESOURCES

Free online financial planning tools are available at: http://www.About.com; http://www.fidelity.com; http://www.finance.cch.com; http://www.finplan.com.

Books:

Berson SA. Modern rules of personal finance for professionals. Chicago, IL: American Bar Association. 2008.

Gwartney JD, et al. Common sense economics: What everyone should know about wealth and prosperity. New York, NY: St. Martin's. 2005.

Nissbaum M, et al. Ernst and Young's personal financial planning guide. New York, NY: John Wiley. 2004.

Opdyke JD. The wall street journal complete finance guidebook. New York, NY: Three Rivers Press. 2006.

Author Index

Subject Index

Note: Page numbers followed by an f denote figures; those followed by a t denote tables.